Decontamination and Device Processing in Healthcare

Decontamination and Device Processing in Healthcare

Second Edition

Gerald McDonnell
Vice President of Microbiological Quality and Sterility Assurance at Johnson & Johnson

Georgia Alevizopoulou
Senior Clinical & Education Manager at STERIS Corporation

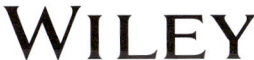

This edition first published 2025
© 2025 John Wiley & Sons Ltd

Edition History
[1e in 2012 by Wiley Blackwell]

All rights reserved, including rights for text and data mining and training of artificial technologies or similar technologies. No part of this publication may be reproduced, stored in a retrieval system, or transmitted, in any form or by any means, electronic, mechanical, photocopying, recording or otherwise, except as permitted by law. Advice on how to obtain permission to reuse material from this title is available at http://www.wiley.com/go/permissions.

The right of Gerald McDonnell and Georgia Alevizopoulou to be identified as the authors of this work has been asserted in accordance with law.

Registered Offices
John Wiley & Sons, Inc., 111 River Street, Hoboken, NJ 07030, USA
John Wiley & Sons Ltd, New Era House, 8 Oldlands Way, Bognor Regis, West Sussex, PO22 9NQ, UK

For details of our global editorial offices, customer services, and more information about Wiley products visit us at www.wiley.com.

Wiley also publishes its books in a variety of electronic formats and by print-on-demand. Some content that appears in standard print versions of this book may not be available in other formats.

Trademarks: Wiley and the Wiley logo are trademarks or registered trademarks of John Wiley & Sons, Inc. and/or its affiliates in the United States and other countries and may not be used without written permission. All other trademarks are the property of their respective owners. John Wiley & Sons, Inc. is not associated with any product or vendor mentioned in this book.

Limit of Liability/Disclaimer of Warranty
While the publisher and authors have used their best efforts in preparing this work, they make no representations or warranties with respect to the accuracy or completeness of the contents of this work and specifically disclaim all warranties, including without limitation any implied warranties of merchantability or fitness for a particular purpose. No warranty may be created or extended by sales representatives, written sales materials or promotional statements for this work. This work is sold with the understanding that the publisher is not engaged in rendering professional services. The advice and strategies contained herein may not be suitable for your situation. You should consult with a specialist where appropriate. The fact that an organization, website, or product is referred to in this work as a citation and/or potential source of further information does not mean that the publisher and authors endorse the information or services the organization, website, or product may provide or recommendations it may make. Further, readers should be aware that websites listed in this work may have changed or disappeared between when this work was written and when it is read. Neither the publisher nor authors shall be liable for any loss of profit or any other commercial damages, including but not limited to special, incidental, consequential, or other damages.

Library of Congress Cataloging-in-Publication Data
Names: McDonnell, Gerald, author. | Alevizopoulou, Georgia, author.
Title: Decontamination and device processing in healthcare / Gerald
  McDonnell, Georgia Alevizopoulou.
Other titles: Practical guide to decontamination in healthcare
Description: Second edition. | Hoboken, NJ : John Wiley & Sons Ltd., 2025.
  | Preceded by: A practical guide to decontamination in healthcare /
  Gerald McDonnell, Denise Sheard. 2012. | Includes bibliographical
  references and index.
Identifiers: LCCN 2024046213 (print) | LCCN 2024046214 (ebook) | ISBN
  9781394206162 (paperback) | ISBN 9781394206179 (adobe pdf) | ISBN
  9781394206186 (epub)
Subjects: MESH: Cross Infection–prevention & control | Infection
  Control–methods | Equipment Contamination–prevention & control |
  Decontamination–methods | Safety Management
Classification: LCC RA761 (print) | LCC RA761 (ebook) | NLM WX 167 | DDC
  614.4/8–dc23/eng/20241204
LC record available at https://lccn.loc.gov/2024046213
LC ebook record available at https://lccn.loc.gov/2024046214

Cover Design: Wiley
Cover Image: © Gerald McDonnell

Set in 9.25/11.5pt MinionPro by Straive, Pondicherry, India

Printed in Singapore
M125777_241224

Contents

Foreword to the second edition, vi

Foreword to the first edition, vii

Glossary of terms, viii

Acknowledgments, xv

1 Introduction, 1

2 Basic anatomy, physiology, and biochemistry, 18

3 Medical and surgical procedures and facilities, 50

4 Instrumentation, 67

5 Microbiology and infection prevention/control, 102

6 Chemistry and physics, 130

7 Point-of-use treatment and transport, 156

8 Cleaning, 169

9 Disinfection, 218

10 Inspection, assembly, and packaging, 257

11 Sterilization, 289

12 Storage and distribution, 355

13 Safety, 366

14 Management and quality, 389

15 Special interest topics, 432

Index, 455

Foreword to the second edition

Much has changed in the areas of decontamination and device processing since the publication of the first edition, *A Practical Guide to Decontamination in Healthcare*. First, there has been a better appreciation of the impact of device processing – including best practices in cleaning, disinfection, and sterilization – on patient safety. Reports about lapses in device decontamination and processing have been published, including instances of microbial contamination of devices used in surgical, medical, and endoscopic procedures that, in some instances, led to patient infections. Of note were multiple reports of device-associated transmission of antibiotic-resistant strains of bacteria (such as carbapenem-resistant Gram-negative bacteria and methicillin-resistant Gram-positive bacteria). In addition, other impacts on patient safety were reported due to undetected device damage and device-associated toxicity from lapses in best practices (e.g. inadequate device inspection, lack of attention to device manufacturer's instructions for use, and inappropriate use of chemicals and antimicrobial processes during device processing). Therefore, similar to the central tenets of infection prevention and control and public health, we must continue to evolve the basic principles and practices for safe medical device use.

Given these reports about device-related contamination and associated risks, it is no surprise that there has been a concerted effort to improve and even innovate the way we can comply with best practices. Examples include the harmonization of requirements internationally; the focus on dedicated education, training, and career advancement for device processing professionals who often dedicate their careers to this area; the development and introduction of new technologies to ensure reliable processes in equipment and device processing; and the emphasis on collaboration between device manufacturers, testing labs, regulatory agencies, and device users. Standard nomenclature is also important. For example, the word "decontamination" can encompass the removal of contaminants (including microorganisms and other materials such as blood) to specified levels, but the more recent universal term "processing" is now internationally accepted as referring to all activities to prepare a new or used healthcare product for its intended use. Both terms are now reflected in the title of the book. Other recent standard requirements include the harmonization of requirements for instructions for use (with particular emphasis on device processing in standards such as ISO 17664 Parts 1 and 2), cleaning endpoints, and disinfection. Ensuring that staff in processing areas are educated, trained, and competent will ensure that they can benefit from a strong career pathway and that they will be considered essential healthcare employees who are valued throughout for their vital contributions to patient care and infection prevention.

International best practices have been subsequently published or updated, including those from the World Health Organization (WHO) and the World Federation for Hospital Sterilisation Sciences (WFHSS), as well as those from the United States such as from the Association for the Advancement of Medical Instrumentation (AAMI). Further, professional organizations, such as the Healthcare Sterile Processing Association (HSPA), lend valuable support, education, certification, and other resources for device processing professionals worldwide. Finally, the surgical, medical, and device processing profession is experiencing technological and procedural innovations, such as robotic surgery and innovative equipment and automation tools, as well as a heightened emphasis on the environmental and safety impacts of products and processes. Many of these related requirements and best practices have now been incorporated in this second edition.

With these valuable updates, *Decontamination and Device Processing in Healthcare*, 2nd edition, will continue to serve as an essential reference for students interested in learning and understanding the basics of decontamination, processing, and infection prevention.

Damien Berg, BA, BS, CRCST, AAMIF
Vice President of Strategic Initiatives
HSPA (Healthcare Sterile Processing Association)
USA, 2024

Foreword to the first edition

Having spent a lifetime's career in healthcare and in particular developing a great interest in the decontamination of medical devices and other patient associated equipment, I am greatly honoured and privileged to be invited to write this foreword.

This text book is intended for worldwide use as a reliable reference book for those interested in the science, technology and practice of decontaminating devices. As such, the book provides great detail, translated into easy reading and understanding.

In the opening chapter we see the scene set through a look at past notable events relating to decontamination practices. A basic introduction is then given to the associated areas of anatomy and physiology, microbiology, chemistry and the various types of medical/surgical devices the reader is likely to be confronted with in practice. This is followed by a detailed description of each step in the decontamination process, including cleaning, disinfection, inspection, sterilization and storage, with a final consideration being given to the key aspects of safety and management.

Bear in mind that although the principles of decontamination remain the same internationally, their interpretation is necessarily different according to where you are practising. This is brought about by varying cultures, national economics, and availability of resources, both human and material, and the perception of safe health-care in differing situations. Within this book, therefore, you will find a variety of solutions to similar problems aimed at giving the most appropriate advice to suit local circumstances.

The book provides a comprehensive approach and guide to all aspects of device decontamination and is essential reading for all involved in the reprocessing of re-usable devices either in healthcare or similar situations.

Gillian A. Sills Consultant and Director of Education
IDSc (Institute for Decontamination Sciences)
UK, 2012

Glossary of terms

Many general terms are used throughout the book, such as "cleaning," "disinfection," "sterilization," "decontamination," and so on. These are specifically defined here. They can have very specific meanings and are often misused in the literature, including in regulations. Definitions can vary from country to country or depending on their use in certain applications. Some definitions continue to evolve, but wherever possible internationally accepted definitions are used here. Further definitions related to specific discussions in the book, for example in the chapters on anatomy, physiology, and biochemistry (Chapter 2), microbiology and infection control/prevention (Chapter 5), and chemistry (Chapter 6) are provided in the respective chapters.

Aeration Removal of volatile chemical residuals to a predetermined level.

Anatomy The study of the structure of living things.

Anion Negatively charged atom or molecule, with examples being Cl⁻ (the chloride ion) and OH⁻ (the hydroxide ion).

Antibiotic Drug that kills or inhibits the growth of bacteria and some fungi by interfering with their normal functions. They are used to prevent ("prophylactic") or treat bacterial and some fungal infections.

Anti-infective Drug that can kill or inhibit the growth of infectious agents. These drugs are usually specific in the way they work; they are typically classified as antibacterials, antifungals, antivirals, and antiprotozoal agents.

Antimicrobial Ability to inactivate or suppress the growth of microorganisms. This can include a process (e.g. application of heat) or a product (e.g. drugs or disinfectants). Antimicrobials include drugs that are particularly used therapeutically within patients to control infections. These are called anti-infectives and include antibiotics, antifungals, and antiviral agents. These are generally specific in their activity, being active against a very limited range of microorganisms. For example, antibiotics only work against some kinds of bacteria (and sometimes some fungi) and most antiviral agents only target certain classes of viruses. These are not discussed in any further detail in this book. The antimicrobial chemicals that are used in disinfection and sterilization applications are called "biocides" or "microbiocides."

Antisepsis Inactivation or inhibition of microorganisms in or on living tissues, such as the skin, mucous membranes, or wounds. An antiseptic is a product used for this purpose. Hand hygiene is an example of antisepsis, including the use of hand washes (soap-based products, water-based applications) and hand rubs (alcohol-based products, waterless applications).

Antiseptic Chemical, product, or process used for antisepsis. In some countries antiseptics are labeled as disinfectants or antiseptic disinfectants. They are often further classified based on their particular use, to include hand washes, hand rubs, hygienic hand disinfectants, pre-operative preparations ("pre-op preps"), and surgical scrubs (or "surgical hand disinfectants").

Archaea A group of unicellular, prokaryotic microorganisms that are distinct from bacteria. In general these microorganisms are not described as being pathogenic to humans, plants, or animals, but are found to survive in extreme environmental conditions (such as hot springs).

Asepsis Prevention from contamination with microorganisms.

Aseptic technique Activities designed to limit the risk of the introduction of microbial contamination.

Assurance of sterility Qualitative concept comprising all activities that provide confidence that a product is sterile. This implies an end-to-end concept that considers all processes that are required in the development, manufacture, and delivery of a sterile labeled product for its intended use.

Bacteria Also known as *eubacteria*. A class of microorganisms that are prokaryotic (no defined nucleus) and unicellular (one-celled, in comparison to multi-cellular organisms). Examples include *Bacillus*, *Staphylococcus*, and *Pseudomonas*.

Bactericidal Ability to inactivate bacteria. This term applies to any agent or product that can kill vegetative bacteria, but may not include bacterial spores (see *sporicide*).

Bioburden Population of viable (or detectable) microorganisms on or in a product or other material. Note: the bioburden from patient-derived materials such as bodily fluids (or "soil") may include non-viable (abiotic) substances such as proteins and lipids.

Biochemistry The study of the chemical processes in living organisms and the structure and function of cells and their components.

Biocide Chemical or physical agent that can inactivate living organisms. Chemical biocides include chlorine, iodine, alcohols, and hydrogen peroxide. Physical biocides include heat and radiation. "Microbiocides" or "microbicides" are those biocides that are effective against microorganisms. Subcategories of microbicides include bactericides and viricides.

Biofilm Community of microorganisms (either single or multiple types). They often develop on or in association with types of surfaces or interfaces.

Biological indicator (BI) Test system containing viable microorganisms providing a defined resistance to a specified sterilization or disinfection process.

Carbohydrate An essential structural component of cells/microorganisms and a source of food/energy. They include sugars (such as sucrose, glucose) and starch. Also known as "saccharides."

Cation Positively charged atom or molecule, with examples including Na^+ (the sodium ion) and Ag^+ (the silver ion).

Cell From the Latin for "small room," a cell is the basic structural and functional component of living organisms. Humans, for example, are multi-cellular organisms consisting of many billions of cells and cell types (such as muscle cells and skin cells), while bacteria are single celled. They can be further sub-classified into two groups based on their basic, microscopic structure: prokaryotic cells (prokaryotes) and eukaryotic cells (eukaryotes). Prokaryotes are considered smaller and often simpler in structure, while eukaryotes are larger and more compartmentalized.

Chelating agent A compound that attaches to a component (e.g. metal ion) and forms a stable complex. It therefore removes metal ions from water or another solution.

Chemical indicator (CI) Test system that reveals change in one or more pre-defined process variables based on a chemical or physical change resulting from exposure to a process (e.g. a color change).

Chemistry The study of chemicals and chemical reactions.

-cidal A suffix (the ending of a word) that means the ability to kill a group of microorganisms. As an example, sporicidal designates the ability to kill bacterial spores. Other terms include bactericidal (kills bacteria), fungicidal (kills fungi), and viricidal (kills viruses). In certain countries these terms are defined by the demonstration of being able to pass certain standardized tests (e.g. a known level of kill in a defined test against certain types of microorganisms). Compare *–cidal* to *–static*.

Clean Visually free of soil and quantified as being below specified levels of analytes. Soil can be any unwanted contaminant(s), including patient materials and process residues. Analytes can include any chemical substance that is the subject of chemical analysis, such as detergents or human tissue components (e.g. proteins, hemoglobin). In many applications a visually clean endpoint might be acceptable and might not require the quantification of specified analytes, but in other cases more defined chemical (or analyte) analysis is required.

Cleaner A formulation designed for cleaning purposes. Also referred to as a "detergent," because it contains chemicals known as detergents (or surfactants).

Cleaning Removal of soil to the extent necessary for further processing (e.g. disinfection, sterilization) or for intended use. "Soil" most often consists of various forms of contaminants, as we typically observe in device processing.

Cleaning chemistry A formulation (or mixture of chemicals) designed for cleaning purposes. Cleaning chemistries are often referred to as "detergents," but detergents are usually only one part of these mixtures that can include biocides, enzymes, buffers, chelating agents, and other components.

Conductivity Measure of the concentration of ions and therefore various metals and molecules in solution (such as water).

Contaminant Material (e.g. chemical, biochemical, or microbiological) not intended to be part of a product or process. Examples of contaminants include soils, protein, dirt, detergents, product residuals, particulates, and microorganisms.

Contamination Presence of material (e.g. chemical, biochemical, or microbiological) not intended to be part of a product or process. The presence of dirt or "soil" can include various materials, chemistries, and bioburden microorganisms. Depending on the situation, contamination may be visible (e.g. a blood spill) or invisible (e.g. the presence of microorganisms). Contamination of a device (e.g. an endoscope) following patient use is generally referred to as being "soiled."

Critical water Water that is extensively treated to ensure that microorganisms and inorganic/organic materials are removed to meet a defined specification.

Cyst (or oocyst) In microbiology, a dormant form of a microorganism, particularly made by protozoa.

Decontamination Removal of contaminants to specified levels. A decontamination process can include a cleaning (physical removal) and/or an antimicrobial (e.g. disinfection) process, depending on the defined level previously specified as being appropriate for a specified purpose, and is often a combination of these processes. Decontamination is intended to render a surface or item safe for handling, use, or disposal. In many cases decontamination is at least a two- or even three-step process, to include cleaning and disinfection and/or sterilization; however, cleaning alone or a multi-step process of cleaning, disinfection, and sterilization may also be required for decontamination, depending on the final use of the surface/item. In this book and in the literature, the terms "decontamination" and "processing" or "reprocessing" are often used interchangeably.

Detergent A compound, or a mixture of compounds, intended to assist cleaning. Detergents are a sub-class of surface-active agents ("surfactants"). Also commonly referred to as cleaners or cleaning chemistries, but detergents are only one part of these mixtures.

Device Any instrument, apparatus, appliance, material, or other article that is intended to be used for the purpose of diagnosis, prevention, monitoring, treatment, or alleviation of disease or other medical/surgical use. A reusable device is designed to be used many times on different patients, being provided with detailed instructions on how it can be safely reprocessed between each patient. A single-use device (SUD) has been designed by a manufacturer to be used on a single patient only and then discarded. The terms "device" and "instrument" are used interchangeably throughout the book.

Diagnosis A variety of observations and/or tests that can be performed in order to identify ("diagnose") the cause of a particular disease or medical problem, and provide the supporting evidence of such as the cause.

Disinfectant Chemical and/or physical agent used for disinfection. Other terms can be used internationally to refer to disinfectant types such as "germicide," "fumigant," "high-, intermediate-, or low-level disinfectant" and "sterilant" (see *disinfection*).

Disinfection Process to inactivate viable microorganisms to a level previously specified as being appropriate for a defined purpose. Other terms, such as pasteurization, sanitization, and antisepsis, are forms of disinfection. Methods include the use of chemicals, combinations of chemicals, and/or non-chemical disinfectant modalities such as using heat. Different "levels" of disinfection have been defined for specific applications, such as high-, intermediate-, and low-level disinfection. The exact meaning and usage of these terms may vary from country to country. A low-level disinfectant is expected to inactivate vegetative bacteria (except mycobacteria), enveloped (lipid) viruses, and fungi, but not necessarily fungal or bacterial spores. An intermediate-level disinfectant is expected to inactivate all vegetative bacteria, including tubercle bacilli, lipid and some non-lipid viruses, and fungal spores, but not bacterial spores. A high-level disinfectant is expected to inactivate all forms of microbial life except for large numbers of bacterial spores, when used in sufficient concentration and under suitable exposure conditions.

Drug A medicine that has a physiological effect when ingested or otherwise introduced into the body.

D value Time or dose required under stated conditions to achieve inactivation of 90% of a population of the test microorganisms.

Endospores Types of spores that are produced within a cell, such as bacterial spores.

Endotoxin Components of certain types of microorganisms that are released only on the death and disintegration of their cells. The most common are high molecular weight complexes that contain lipopolysaccharide (LPS), protein, and phospholipid originating from the outer membrane of Gram-negative bacteria. Although these are naturally occurring, even in the body (e.g. from bacteria in the intestine), higher levels of endotoxins can cause fever (pyrogenic) when injected into the body.

Environmental control Application of engineering and/or procedural systems to maintain conditions in a defined space within specified limits. An example is the use of cleanrooms and air filtration systems to reduce contamination in a room/environment.

Enzyme A protein molecule that speeds up a chemical reaction but is not changed during the process. They are widely used in formulation with chemicals for cleaning applications (e.g. enzymatic cleaners) because of their ability to break down (or "digest") various types of molecules found in soils (such as proteins, lipids, and carbohydrates). Enzymes are classified based on mechanism of action, to include proteases (enzymes that break down proteins) and lipases (enzymes that break down lipids).

Epidemiology A branch of science dealing with the transmission and control of disease; an "epidemiologist" is a specialist in this area.

Eukaryotic Defines a type of cell that is much larger than that of bacteria and contains a well-defined nucleus and other organelles; examples of eukaryotic cells include those of fungi, protozoa, plants, and humans (see the section on human cells).

Exotoxin Toxin produced from a microorganism while it is fully functional (e.g. the tetanus toxin from *Clostridium tetani*).

Formulation A combination of ingredients, including active and inert ingredients, into a product for its intended use. Examples include liquid chemical cleaning and disinfection formulations. Although products used for antisepsis, disinfection, and cleaning have common names such as "enzymatics," "alkalines," "peracetic acid," and "glutaraldehyde," these only refer to the active ingredients and their individual activities can vary dramatically. The benefit of a formulation is to optimize the activity of these ingredients while minimizing any negative effects (such as poor water quality, surface damage, and loss of activity over time).

Fumigation Delivery of a disinfectant to an area by aerial dispersion, usually in the form of a gas, vapor, or aerosol.

Fungi A group of cell wall–containing eukaryotic microorganisms, which can be further sub-divided into molds (or filamentous fungi, as they can form long filaments or lines of cells) and yeast (unicellular, single-celled forms).

Germ and germicide A germ is a general term referring to any microorganism, but is often used to refer to bacteria in particular (e.g. in the United States). Therefore, germicidal refers to a product or process that kills microorganisms, but sometimes only refers to bactericidal activity (as in US Environmental Protection Agency disinfectant registrations). As "germ" is a general term for a microorganism; its use in decontamination is discouraged as it can be misleading.

Guideline Document used to communicate recommended procedures, processes, or usage of particular practices.

Hardness Concentration of calcium and magnesium ions in water, expressed as parts per million (ppm) or milligrams per liter (mg/L) of calcium carbonate ($CaCO_3$) equivalents.

Helminths A large group of multicellular eukaryotic microorganisms that include worms (such as tapeworms and roundworms) and flukes. Examples include *Ascaris* and *Taenia*.

Hydrophilic (polar) Refers to "water-loving," being a substance that attracts and can absorb water; compare to lipophilic, meaning "lipid-loving."

Hydrophobic (non-polar) A substance that repels and does not absorb water ("water-hating"); compare to lipophobic, meaning "lipid-hating."

Hygiene Conditions and practices that help to maintain health and prevent the spread of diseases, particularly those caused by pathogenic microorganisms.

Inactivation Loss of the ability of microorganisms to grow and/or multiply.

Indicator For microbiological quality, a test system that indicates by measuring, recording, or detecting. Microbiological quality indicators can include parametric (e.g. mechanical or electrical sensors), chemical, or microbiological test systems. Examples include biological indicators, chemical indicators, and temperature probes.

Infection Invasion and multiplication of microorganisms in humans or another host. The presence of microorganisms does not necessarily imply an infection risk. Infection will depend on factors such as the strain (or type) of microorganism, the infectious dose, the susceptibility of the host, etc.

Infection prevention/control Discipline concerned with preventing the spread of microorganisms and infection; it is therefore part of the branch of the science known as epidemiology. Often used interchangeably, "prevention" is more correctly used to describe practices to prevent infection, while "control" may also include practices to control the infection after it has taken place (e.g. isolation precautions, antibiotic or other drug-based therapy, etc.). Prevention strategies including antisepsis, disinfection, and vaccination; control strategies may include the use of anti-infectives (drugs) to treat or even prevent infections, investigating outbreaks, and managing outbreaks of infection. Experts in this area may be known as infection control practitioners, infection preventionists, or epidemiologists.

Inorganic Non-carbon-based molecules. Inorganic chemistry is the study of non-carbon-based molecules such as table salt (NaCl) or water (H_2O). The exception to this rule is a group of chemicals like the carbonates (such as calcium carbonate, $CaCO_3$, and sodium carbonate, Na_2CO_3) that are known as "inorganic carbon."

ISO International Standards Organization.

Label An identification indication on a product or other article. This can include the manufacturer, its address, product/item identification (e.g. serial or part number), instructions for use, etc. A product label can include what is physically written on the product (the attached label), but also any other accessory information such as additional instructions for use, the safety data sheets (SDSs), and technical literature.

Lipid An essential structural component of cells/microorganisms and a source of food/energy. They are generally described as being insoluble in water (hydrophobic) and include fats, oils, and cholesterol.

Load Defined product, equipment, or materials to be processed together within an operating, sterilization, or decontamination cycle.

Matter Any living or non-living thing that takes up space.

Medicine The science of and ability to heal. "Medical" refers to the study and practice of medicine.

Microbiology The study of microorganisms.

Microorganism Entity of microscopic size, including bacteria, fungi, protozoa, and viruses.

Minimum effective concentration (MEC) Lowest concentration of a chemical or product that achieves a claimed activity.

Minimum recommended concentration (MRC) Lowest concentration of a chemical or product specified for use in a process.

MSDS See *safety data sheets (SDS)*.

Nucleic acid A class of macromolecules that make up the genetic material of cells and viruses. There are two main classes, DNA (deoxyribonucleic acid) and RNA (ribonucleic acid).

Nosocomial Acquired or occurring in a hospital or healthcare facility. A nosocomial infection is an infection acquired in a healthcare facility.

Oocyst See *cyst*.

Operating cycle Complete set of stages of a process that is carried out in a specified sequence. An example is a steam sterilization cycle.

Organic Carbon-based. Organic chemistry is the study of carbon-based molecules, which are a diverse group including proteins, lipids, and plastics (e.g. polyurethane and polypropylene). The exception to this rule is a group of chemicals, like the carbonates (such as calcium carbonate, $CaCO_3$, and sodium carbonate, Na_2CO_3), that are known as "inorganic carbon." Strictly speaking, "organic" refers to chemicals with carbon (C) and hydrogen (H).

Packaging system Combination of a sterile barrier system and protective packaging.

Parasite   A microorganism that can live in or on a host (animal, plant, or other organism) without benefiting or killing the host, but may cause damage/sickness.

Pasteurization   Heat-based disinfection process used to reduce levels of pathogenic and spoilage microorganisms to a level previously specified as being appropriate for a defined purpose.

Pathogen   Disease-causing microorganism.

pH   A measure of the activity of hydrogen ions (H^+) in a solution and, therefore, its acidity or alkalinity. The pH value is a number without units, between 0 and 14, that indicates whether a solution is acidic (<7), neutral (~7, generally 6–8) or basic/alkaline (>7).

Physiology   The study of how living structures function.

PPE   Personal protective equipment.

Preservation   Control of the multiplication of microorganisms or prevention of microbial contamination.

Pressure   The effect that occurs when a force is applied on a surface or the force applied per unit area. For example, atmospheric pressure is the pressure exerted by the earth's atmosphere and at sea level is known to be ~101.3 kPa (= 14.7 lb in^{-2}, 1 bar, 760 mmHg, or 760 Torr).

Prion   Transmissible agent that is composed entirely of protein material and that does not appear to have a unique, associated nucleic acid.

Process   A designed sequence of operations or events, possibly taking up time, space, expertise, or other resources, which produces some outcome.

Process challenge device (PCD)   Item providing a defined resistance to a cleaning, disinfection, or sterilization process and used to assess the performance of a process.

Processing   Activity to prepare a new or used healthcare product for its intended use. Processing (or reprocessing) is used to describe steps such as cleaning, disinfection, and/or sterilization as well as other steps (e.g. inspection, maintenance) for the preparation of a new or used medical device for patient use. Processing steps are commonly conducted prior to patient use and in accordance with the manufacturer's instructions for use.

Product family   Group or sub-group of products characterized by similar attributes determined to be equivalent for evaluation and processing purposes.

Prokaryote   A type of cell that is considered less organized in structure than eukaryotic cells; bacteria are the most common examples of prokaryotic cells.

Protein   An essential structural and operational component of cells/microorganisms and a source of food/energy. They are made up of nitrogen-containing molecules known as amino acids, and examples of protein include enzymes, collagen, and keratin.

Protozoa   A diverse group of cell-wall-free, unicellular, eukaryotic microorganisms. Examples include *Cryptosporidium* and *Plasmodium*.

Pyrogen   Substance that causes fever reactions at sufficient amounts. A fever is an increase in temperature, and in a human is defined as any body temperature above the normal of 98.6°F (37°C). Many microorganisms produce pyrogens (known as toxins), which can be an important cause of disease or other patient complications. Examples include bacterial endotoxins and some types of exotoxins.

Qualification   Activities undertaken to demonstrate that utilities, equipment, or methods are suitable for their intended use and perform properly. With decontamination equipment, this can include installation (IQ), operational (OQ), and performance qualification (PQ). Installation qualification refers to evidence that equipment has been provided and installed in accordance with its specification; OQ indicates that the installed equipment operates within pre-determined limits when used in accordance with its operational procedures; and PQ refers to evidence that the equipment consistently performs in accordance with pre-determined criteria and meets its specification.

Qualitative   The quality of something, usually referring to the various types of chemicals present in a sample.

Quality   A measure of meeting an expectation or a standard. In device decontamination, this will be to provide a device that is safe for patient use and to meet the requirements of those needing to use the device (medical/surgical staff). Quality control (QC) is a procedure or set of procedures to ensure that a manufactured product or performed service adheres to a defined set of criteria or meets the requirements of a customer. Quality assurance (QA) is similar, being a procedure or set of procedures intended to ensure that a product or service under development (before work is complete, as opposed to afterwards) meets specified requirements. QC and QA are often expressed together as quality assurance and control (QA/QC). A quality management system (QMS) describes the organizational structure, procedures, processes, and resources needed to implement quality management in any facility.

Quantitative   The amount of something (from "quantity"), for example the various amounts of a type of chemical in a given sample.

Regulation   A rule or order issued by a country, community, or administrative agency, generally under authority granted by statute, that enforces or amplifies laws enacted by the legislature and has the force of law.

Reprocessing   See *processing*.

Resistance   The ability (natural or acquired) of a microorganism to survive treatment with an anti-infective or biocide.

Resistivity   The ability of water (or any liquid) to resist the flow of electricity; a measure of the resistance of water and the inverse of conductivity (being the ability to transmit electricity).

Reusable (medical) device   Device designated or intended by the manufacturer as suitable for processing and reuse.

Safety The condition of being protected from danger, harm, or injury.

Safety data sheet (SDS) Document provided with a chemical product by the manufacturer/supplier that describes any chemicals that are present, and pertinent safety information, including safe handling and emergency procedures. Sometimes called material safety data sheets (MSDS).

SAL See *sterility assurance level*.

Sanitization Removal, reduction, or inactivation of microorganisms. The preferred term is "disinfection."

Self-contained biological indicator (SCBI) Biological indicator presented such that the primary package intended for incubation contains the incubation medium required for incubation and recovery of the test microorganism.

Soil Natural or artificial contamination on a device or surface following its use or simulated use. Contamination on a surface following a patient procedure (also see *contamination* and *bioburden*).

Spore A stage in the reproductive cycle of certain types of bacteria and fungi, where the cell becomes condensed in a thick coat. It is a dormant, reproductive structure of a microorganism that is adapted for dispersal and surviving for extended periods of time in unfavorable conditions. They form part of the life cycles of various types of fungi and bacteria. Bacterial spores are also known as endospores. Sporulated microorganisms can survive much longer in the environment and are also more resistant to inactivation by antimicrobial agents. Many spores are known to be highly resistant to disinfection and even sterilization methods.

Sporicide Agent that inactivates microbial spores.

Standard Document that specifies the minimum acceptable characteristics of a product or material, issued by an organization that develops such documents. Note: publication of standards can include international and/or local standards. Standard organizations include ISO (International Standards Organization).

–static A suffix (the ending of a word) that refers to the ability to inhibit the growth of a group of microorganisms, but not to kill. Examples include bacteriostatic (inhibits vegetative bacteria), fungistatic (inhibits the growth of fungi), and sporistatic (inhibits the growth of spores, generally bacterial and fungal spores).

Sterilant (or sterilizing agent) Chemical or physical (e.g. heat) agent that can be used for sterilization, but is only effective for sterilization when provided as part of a defined process.

Sterile Free from viable microorganisms.

Sterile barrier system Package that minimizes the risk of ingress of microorganisms and allows aseptic presentation of the sterile product at the point of use.

Sterility State of being sterile, based on the probability of the presence of viable microorganisms.

Sterility assurance level (SAL) The probability of a single viable microorganism occurring on a product after sterilization. This is generally expressed as 10^{-n}. For example, it is common in healthcare applications to use an SAL of 10^{-6}, implying a probability of <1 in a million chance that an item may be contaminated when a starting population of 10^6 (or one million) of the test microorganism is present on the test surface.

Sterilization Validated process used to render an item free from viable microorganisms. This will include a wide range of microorganisms (bacteria, viruses, fungi, etc.), including bacterial spores that are considered some of the more resistant forms to inactivation.

Sterilization cycle Predetermined sequence of stages performed in a sterilizer to achieve a product free of viable microorganisms.

Surfactant Surface active agent. An agent that can emulsify oils/fats and holds dirt in suspension. They are widely used in cleaning chemistries. Detergents are a sub-class of surfactants.

Surgery A specialty in medicine that investigates or treats disease or injury by an operative procedure. Surgical procedures (or "operations") involve entering the body or body cavities by incision (breaking through the skin or other area of the body).

Thermolabile Readily damaged by heat.

Total dissolved solids (TDS) Sum of all ions in a solution, often approximated by means of electrical conductivity or resistivity measurements.

Total organic carbon (TOC) Measure of organic (or carbon-based) substances that are present in a solution or on a surface. Strictly speaking, this excludes "inorganic carbon" such as carbonates. In water analysis it is usually residual carbon material from natural microbial, plant, and animal decomposition.

Toxicity Quality of being toxic or poisonous.

Toxin Foreign substance that is capable of inflicting damage on a host cell. Most toxins are generated by microorganisms. They are poisonous ("toxic") substances. Toxins produced by many types of pathogens are the primary cause of the signs and symptoms of infection, such as an increase in temperature and tissue damage. They can be further sub-classified based on how they are produced by a microorganism (endotoxins or exotoxins) or by what type of microorganism they are produced by (e.g. mycotoxins are produced by certain types of fungi). Many toxins, such as endotoxins, are also "pyrogens," referring to their ability to cause a dramatic rise in body temperature.

Utility water Water as it comes from a potable source. The quality or purity of utility water can vary significantly depending on the region or areas, and seasonally. It may be sufficient for certain device processing applications, but often requires further treatment to achieve a desired and consistent specification.

Validation Confirmation process through the provision of objective evidence that the requirements for a specific intended use or application have been fulfilled. This is a documented procedure for obtaining, recording, and interpreting the results required to establish that a process will consistently yield a product complying with pre-determined specifications.

Vegetative   In microbiology, refers to an actively growing and multiplying form of a microorganism. The opposite of a vegetative form would be a dormant form of a microorganism (e.g. bacterial and fungal spores or protozoan cysts).

Verification   Provision of objective evidence that specified requirements have been met. This will include a documented procedure for obtaining, recording, and interpreting results to confirm that pre-determined specifications have been met.

Viable   Indicates that something is alive and capable of reproducing.

Virucide   Agent that inactivates viruses to make them non-infective.

Virus   A class of microorganisms that cannot replicate without a living, susceptible host cell (human, plant, or bacterial). They are therefore called "obligate parasites." They have no cell structure typical of other microorganisms (see *eukaryote* and *prokaryote*).

Washer-disinfector   A machine that cleans and disinfects medical devices and other articles used in the context of medical, dental, pharmaceutical, and veterinary practice.

Worst case   Condition or set of conditions within the specified operating range that pose the greatest risk(s) of process or product failure.

z value   Change in temperature of a thermal sterilization or disinfection process that produces a tenfold change in D value.

Acknowledgments

The authors would like to thank sincerely all those who critically reviewed various sections and chapters of the book. Their feedback was invaluable. They include:

Richard Bancroft, UK
Damien Berg, USA
Andrew Ellis, Australia
Paula Freeman, Ireland
Dhouha Hamdani, Qatar
Sulisti Holmes, UK
Xana Jardine, South Africa
Nancy Kaiser, USA
John Kimsey, USA
Sue Klacik, USA
Stephen Kovach, USA

Sofia Kravvariti, Greece
Terra Kremer, USA
Nicole Lapanaitis, Australia
Heike Martiny, Germany
Terry McAuley, Australia
Geraldine McNulty, UAE
Ian Moone, UK
Val O'Brien, UK
Richard Schule, USA
René Vis, Netherlands

1 Introduction

What is device processing?

> As to diseases, make a habit of two things – to help, or at least to do no harm.
> *Of the Epidemics*, Hippocrates (~400 BC)

Health is an important subject to all. It affects us as individuals, our families, and the communities in which we live. Our health is improved by promoting well-being and preventing disease or other negative health impacts. A disease may be defined as any effect that impairs/harms the body's normal function and therefore can have an impact on our health (mild, moderate, or even severe). Diseases can be infectious or non-infectious (such as cancer, effects of drug abuse, stress, effects of toxic chemicals, etc.). Infectious diseases are a leading cause of sickness and death worldwide. They are caused by living organisms that cannot be seen by the naked eye, known as "microorganisms," such as viruses and bacteria. It is estimated that infectious diseases that affect our breathing, digestive, and immune systems are responsible for ~17% of human deaths worldwide (the next highest cause of death is coronary heart disease at ~12%). These rates are averaged across the whole world, but are even higher in lower-income regions. Examples of advances in health efforts in the last 200 years in particular to reduce these risks in the general public include improving drinking water quality (chemical and microbiological), immunization practices (vaccination), and safe handling/disposal of waste. Many of these efforts influence our daily lives, but the risk of infectious disease significantly increases when we are sick or when our bodies are otherwise compromised (e.g. when undergoing a surgical procedure, or if we have an existing sickness). For these reasons, healthcare institutions (such as hospitals and clinics) have many procedures and practices in place to control the spread of infectious disease within these facilities, and to protect patients, staff, and the general public. The prevention of harm is an important philosophy in medical practice and is the basis of the Hippocratic oath traditionally taken by medical staff stating "first, to do no harm" or in Latin *primum non nocere* (in Greek ὠφελέειν ἢ μὴ βλάπτειν), often attributed first to the Greek physician Hippocrates. Such procedures are collectively referred to as "safe" or "infection control/prevention" practices that prevent the spread of disease or other negative effects to or between patients (or to/from staff or visitors within these facilities). These practices include:

- Immunization.
- Isolation of patients with specific diseases.
- Hand hygiene.
- Decontamination of equipment and various surfaces.

As "contamination" refers to something being "dirty" or "soiled," "decontamination" is the means to render it safe for handling, use, or disposal. Dirt or soil may include things like dust, patient materials (such as blood, feces, various tissues from surgical procedures, etc.), and associated microorganisms that can cause disease. In this book, the terms "decontamination," "reprocessing," and "processing" are used interchangeably. In healthcare facilities a variety of physical and/or chemical products or processes are used for decontamination. These include:

- Cleaning, the removal of soil to make something "clean."
- Disinfection, the antimicrobial reduction of microorganisms; other widely used terms that refer to disinfection can include antisepsis, pasteurization, sanitization, and fumigation.
- Sterilization, the complete eradication of all microorganisms.

These are all methods of decontamination and are explained further in this book. Examples of specific decontamination practices include:

- Hand and skin hygiene, including routine hand disinfection and preparation of the skin for a surgical procedure.
- Taking surgical or medical instruments that have been used on one patient and decontaminating them in preparation for use on another.
- Cleaning and disinfection of linens or other materials (including patient bed sheets, sterile towels and cotton fabrics).

Decontamination and Device Processing in Healthcare, Second Edition. Gerald McDonnell and Georgia Alevizopoulou.
© 2025 John Wiley & Sons Ltd. Published 2025 by John Wiley & Sons Ltd.

- Disinfection of water for drinking or sterilization of water and other liquids (such as saline or glucose) for injection or infusion into the body.
- Cleaning and disinfecting environmental surfaces such as table-tops, contact surfaces, floors, and bedrails.
- Sterilization of contaminated waste materials for safe disposal (including incineration or burning).

In some cases decontamination is a one-step process, for example sterilization of contaminated waste materials, but it is most often a two-step process to include cleaning (the physical removal of soil) and disinfection or sterilization (as the antimicrobial processes to inactivate the various types of microorganisms that we cannot see). For reusable medical and surgical instruments this will normally include at least cleaning and disinfection, but will often include sterilization, this being the highest level of safety. Decontamination is therefore an integral part of infection prevention and should not be underestimated.

A brief history of decontamination

It is clear from many ancient documents that decontamination practices have been considered to have health benefits. This was before a true understanding of the existence of microorganisms such as bacteria and viruses. Examples include:
- In approximately 1400–1200 BC (estimated to be at the time of Moses), a sanitary code was outlined in the Leviticus, Numbers, and Deuteronomy chapters of the Bible. It was noted even at this time, when dealing with disease, that hands should be washed under running water and that there was a value in boiling water to make it safe for drinking or other purposes.
- The Ebers Papyrus, a medical document from about 1500 BC, describes a method of combining animal and vegetable oils with alkaline salts to form a soap-like material used for treating skin diseases, as well as for washing hands.
- The world's oldest known medical text outlines the procedures for wound management practiced by the Sumerians (~2000 BC). The wound was cleansed with beer (which contained alcohol) and then bandaged with a cloth soaked in wine and turpentine. The practice of using alcoholic beverages and turpentine would remain the treatment of choice until the modern era.
- Similar examples of wound, water, or air treatments have been described by the ancient Greek and Roman cultures. Aristotle (384–322 BC), a Greek philosopher, also described boiling to treat water. Homer (~850 BC), in his epic poem the *Odyssey*, described the use of sulfur as an area disinfectant.
- Ancient methods of preserving foods from rotting during storage (which we now know is caused by microorganisms) included drying, heating, and use of sugar or vinegar.

From these ancient times to the 19th century, infection was a major cause of death and suffering (mortality and morbidity) in humans. It would take many thousands of years for the microbiological origin and reasons behind the transmissibility of infection to be discovered. A recurring theme in history was the belief that epidemic diseases were spread by something in the air. Hippocrates (460–370 BC) was an ancient Greek doctor and is often referred to as the father of medicine, and as the source of the Hippocratic oath discussed earlier. He put this belief into practice when attempting to drive the plague (now know to be a bacterial disease) out of Athens by lighting fires of aromatic wood in the streets. This belief that diseases were spread by something in the air continued throughout history.

Many ancient physicians well understood that when the skin was broken in any way (by a wound or during attempts at surgery) the risks of bad things happening was significantly increased. It was unknown at the time that wound infections were caused by various types of microorganisms, particularly bacteria, with dramatic consequences, including destruction of limbs and death. Infections in such cases of skin damage were the major contributor to death and suffering, which is why surgical procedures were attempted only as a last resort. Through the ages operations were performed with little regard for a "clean" environment. Surgeons' hands, rarely washed, were placed directly into the patient's wounds. Frequently, onlookers were encouraged to "take a feel" for educational purposes. Surgical instruments used in such procedures were crudely wiped, placed back into their velvet carriers, and reused, some having been sharpened on the sole of the surgeon's boot. The floors of the surgical wards were covered with whatever came from the patient, which could include feces, urine, blood, and pus, and hygiene practices in other areas of such facilities (if indeed dedicated facilities were used) were also unknown at the time. Not surprisingly, surgical site infection was the major contributor to morbidity and mortality rates, occurring after practically all operations and taking the lives of almost half of all surgical patients.

Hippocrates was one of the first recorded as holding an opinion on the cause of such problems, stating that the formation of pus (suppuration) was not a natural part of the healing process and should be avoided. His recommendations for managing wounds included cleansing with wine, applying a bandage, and then pouring wine on the bandage. Another Greek physician, Claudius Galen (~AD 130–200), recommended soap for both medicinal and cleansing purposes. He, however, disagreed with Hippocrates' view that the formation of pus was not a normal occurrence; he believed that pus was essential for wound healing. It is often considered that this was originally an Arabic idea. Unfortunately, the generation of pus in a wound (suppuration) was actively encouraged by surgeons in traumatic and painful procedures. This disagreement would continue to be debated for centuries.

One thousand years later, the Italian Theodoric Borgognoni (1205–1298) challenged Galen's view of suppuration. He dedicated his career to finding the ideal conditions for wound healing and became one of the most famous surgeons during the Middle Ages. He argued that a wound should be maintained clean and closed (sutured) to control infection (and preserve life). Because his views were contrary to the established teachings, he was denounced by his colleagues and even by the local church. Indeed, the surgeon would often welcome the signs of suppuration, depending on how it looked. Wounds were classified into two categories: those with suppuration and those without. Wounds with "laudable pus" (a creamy yellow ooze) tended to run a chronic course, taking months to heal, but the patients were generally free of other negative signs and did not die. Wounds with a thin, watery discharge were often associated with a fatal outcome, with the patient dying of sepsis within days. It is not therefore surprising that even the most conscientious surgeons preferred and even encouraged the formation of pus. Galen's doctrine of suppuration would remain the rule for wound management until the late 19th century.

In addition to wound infection, general standards of public hygiene and their impacts on public health were not widely appreciated. In Europe, following the fall of the Roman Empire in AD 467 many simple hygiene practices were neglected. Examples included a decline in bathing habits, lack of personal cleanliness, and unsanitary living conditions (lack of waste disposal, etc.). It is well appreciated that such conditions contributed heavily to the great plagues of the Middle Ages, and especially to the Black Death (caused by a type of bacteria) of the 14th century. At the same time, it was understood that contact with sick individuals could rapidly spread a disease, as highlighted by the fear associated with bacterial diseases such as leprosy and the Black Death; in fact, infected bodies have been used over the ages as effective weapons in battles and sieges. Equally, infected bodies and materials were often dealt with by burning (incineration).

Hieronymus Fracastorius (1478–1553) suggested that the cause of infectious disease was from invisible living "seeds" (*seminaria contagionum*). He even at this period described three modes of disease spread: direct contact with infected persons, indirect contact with surfaces (fomites), and airborne transmission. Ambroise Paré (1510–1590), considered one of the fathers of modern surgery, believed that infection was introduced from the environment. In 1625 Francis Bacon described some methods to prevent or control wound infections, such as by the use of salt or excluding air contact. In the 1670s Antonie van Leeuwenhoek is often considered one of the first microbiologists to observe individual, live microorganisms by using a simple microscope he designed. He called these animalcules or "little animals." He also described the first direct evidence of disinfection in observing the death of animalcules treated with pepper (in water) or vinegar (a type of acid). Similar disinfection studies were described shortly after by Edmund King and John Pringle. It could be argued that this was the start of the modern era of understanding infectious diseases and their control, but even then the "microbial theory" remained debated for the next few centuries.

In the meantime, the benefits of disinfection practices continued to be better understood. Ancient disinfection methods had been previously recognized, such as the benefits of storing water and other liquids in copper or silver vessels (as a preservative method from the release of copper or silver into the water), burning with fire (as a method of incineration), and boiling water. In the modern era further advances were made such as:
- In 1680 Denis Papin developed the first recognizable steam-generating machine.
- In 1774 Carl Wilhelm Scheele discovered chlorine and its antimicrobial effects.
- In the 1830s William Henry published studies on the "disinfection power of increased temperatures."
- In the mid-1800s copper sulfate, zinc chloride, and sodium permanganate, acids, alkalis, sulfurs, and alcohols were recognized as disinfectants.

In the late 1840s Dr. Ignaz Semmelweis, while working in the maternity wards of a Vienna hospital, observed that the mortality rate in a delivery room staffed by medical students was up to three times higher than in a second delivery room staffed by midwives. Expectant mothers were terrified of the room staffed by the medical students. Semmelweis observed that the students were coming straight from their lessons in the autopsy room to the delivery room. He believed that they were carrying infectious agents from the lab to their patients. When he implemented a hand-washing protocol at the hospital the mortality rate dropped to less than 1%. Today he is recognized as the father of hand hygiene, one of the most important measures to be taken by healthcare practitioners to reduce cross-contamination. Due to the lack of indoor plumbing at the time, it was difficult to get water to wash hands, making this an unpopular idea. In order to make the water comfortably warm, it would have to be heated over a fire. Besides, contact with water was associated with diseases such as malaria and typhoid fever. Unknown to Semmelweis, similar results had been described a few years previously by the American scientist Oliver Wendell Holmes. Both suggestions fell on deaf ears. Semmelweis, for his efforts, was committed to an asylum and died of a blood infection.

Despite the earlier work by others such as van Leeuwenhoek, the prevailing theory at the time was known as "spontaneous generation." This is often originally attributed to the Greek philosopher Aristotle (384–322 BC) and simply regards the origins of life as being from inanimate matter or non-living substances. Many famous names in the modern history of infection control, such as Pouchet, Nightingale, and Virchow, contributed to this debate.

Louis Pasteur was born in 1822 in France and in 1857 he proposed the "germ theory of disease," which is regarded as one of the most important discoveries in infection prevention history. The theory proposed that most infectious diseases are caused by germs; he also specifically described the existence of bacteria. In the 1860s Pasteur commenced his antispontaneous generation experiments and demonstrated that "microorganisms are present in air but not created by air," thereby disproving the concept of spontaneous generation. This was vigorously debated for many years after, with many leading scientists refusing to accept this idea, but the modern era of microbiology had begun. Pasteur proved that protection from air, by sealing or providing a tortuous path, prevented contamination; if a growth liquid (food or media) was exposed to air it resulted in contamination by microorganisms. With the development of the germ theory by Pasteur and its subsequent application to surgical practices, surgeons were able to operate with a substantially reduced risk of infection. Pasteur was also able to show that bacteria could be killed by various processes. "Pasteurization" is a heat-based process to control microorganisms that still bears his name and he also designed some simple steam cabinet sterilizers (with Charles Chamberland in 1880).

During the 1700s–1800s, various scientists described the phenomenon that by injecting healthy people with fluids (such as blood) from patients suffering from certain diseases, particularly with milder or similar types of disease, they could be protected from that disease. This became known as vaccination and was previously described by the Chinese, Indians, and Turks. Wortley Montagu and Jenner used such methods to prevent smallpox, a prevalent infectious disease at the time and now eradicated. Pasteur also developed vaccination methods (e.g. against rabies). Vaccination is now an important part of public health, including the prevention of common diseases such as measles, mumps, seasonal flu, and more recently COVID-19. Polio, a virus that can cause a serious disease, has all but been eradicated due to immunization.

Pasteur's work accelerated other investigations in microbiology and infection control/prevention. As an example, Agostino Bassi (1773–1856) described the use of a variety of disinfectants in the control of different diseases such as cholera (a bacterial disease); these included alcohol, acids, and chlorine. Joseph Lister (1827–1912), a professor of surgery in Glasgow, Scotland, quickly noticed the connection between Pasteur's work and the suppuration of wounds. He concluded that microbes in the air were most likely causing the infection and had to be destroyed before they entered the wound. Lister began to clean wounds and dress them using a solution of carbolic acid (phenol). Little did he know that at the same time other European surgeons were already practicing similar methods with other chemicals. In 1867 he published a paper on antisepsis, stating that "all the local inflammatory mischief and general febrile disturbance which follow severe injuries are due to the irritating and poisoning influence of decomposing blood or sloughs." Lister started applying phenol to compound fracture wounds; the wounds often healed without infection. The application of germ theory to wound healing changed the practice of surgery. Lister also campaigned for heat or chemical sterilization (and for surgeons to use something other than sawdust swept up from the floors of the mills for surgical dressings).

During the Franco-Prussian war (1870–1871) antiseptic practices were shown to have an impact on saving soldiers' lives. German surgeons were beginning to practice antiseptic surgery, using sterilized instruments and materials. In 1876, Lister presented his ideas at the International Medical Congress in Philadelphia. William W. Keen (1837–1932) attended the presentation and became one of the first American surgeons to implement Lister's ideas. During the American Civil War (1861–1865), Keen was one of the first physicians in the world to adopt aseptic surgical technique. Infectious disease was the cause of 90% of the deaths on both sides rather than direct death from military trauma. While bayoneting killed fewer outright, minor scratches from other injuries often festered into mortal wounds. Keen recommended and practiced the following surgical set-up in hospitals at the time:

- All carpets and unnecessary furniture were removed from the patient's room.
- Walls and ceilings were carefully cleaned the day before the operation, and the woodwork, floors, and remaining furniture were scrubbed with carbolic solution. This solution was also sprayed in the room on the morning preceding but not during the operation.
- The day before the operation, the patient was shaved, scrubbed with soap and water and ether, and covered with wet corrosive sublimate dressing until operated on, and then ether and mercuric chloride washings were repeated.
- The surgical instruments were boiled in water for two hours, and sponges for use during the procedures were treated with carbolic acid before use.
- The surgeon's hands were cleaned and disinfected with soap, water, and alcohol.

It is interesting to note that many of these practices are still in use today (such as washing or the use of alcohol on the hands), while others are not (such as the use of mercury). As the knowledge on the use of various chemicals improved, it was realized that while many of these practices could kill or prevent the growth of microorganisms, many could also do harm to human health (or were "toxic" in either the short or long term).

As scientific knowledge expanded during the late 19th century so did the advancement of infection prevention. Another important milestone was when Robert Koch (1843–1910), a German physician and competitor of Pasteur, was able to demonstrate the cause-and-effect relationship between a specific bacterium (*Bacillus anthracis*) and the disease anthrax. He used a sequence of experimental steps to directly relate a specific microbe to a specific disease; these steps of disease association, isolation, inoculation, and re-isolation became known as Koch's postulates. These still form the basis of defining an infectious agent today. In 1882 Koch also discovered the causative agent of tuberculosis, the bacterium *Mycobacterium tuberculosis*. Tuberculosis was estimated as the cause of one in seven deaths in the mid-19th century; interestingly, in the 21st century tuberculosis is once again a major problem due to the development of drug (antibiotic)-resistant forms of the bacterium. Koch also published a book in 1881 (*Über Desinfection* or *On Disinfection*) that described various types of disinfectants and the differences in their abilities to kill various types of microorganisms (with *Mycobacterium tuberculosis* and *Bacillus anthracis* being particularly difficult to inactivate, the latter due to its ability to form heat/chemical-resistant spores). Other advances before the end of the 19th century included:

- In 1883, Gustav Neuber introduced the use of sterile gowns and caps during surgery.
- In 1890, William Stewart Halsted introduced surgical gloves after he commissioned the Goodyear rubber company to fashion gloves for his nurse to protect her hands from the mercuric chloride solutions used to disinfect the instruments. Rubber gloves were routinely used after 1890.
- In 1891, Ernst von Bergmann introduced routine heat sterilization of instruments, which proved superior to chemical methods used at the time.
- In 1897, Johannes von Mikulicz-Radecki introduced the use of surgical masks.

During the early part of the 20th century a variety of other chemicals began to be used for infection prevention purposes, including hydrogen peroxide, various types of phenols, dyes, and quaternary ammonium compounds. During the 1920s Sir Alexander Fleming (1881–1955), working in London, made the accidental discovery of penicillin, one of the first and most widely used antibiotics. Antibiotics are drugs used to treat or prevent bacterial infections. It was not until the Second World War (in the 1940s) that penicillin was widely introduced as an extract from the fungus (another type of microorganism) known as *Penicillium*. This led to a revolution in the development and manufacturing of various types of antibiotics (such as tetracycline and methicillin). It seemed that bacterial infections might be something of the past, but quickly it was shown that bacteria could develop resistance to antibiotics and in the present day there are fewer antibiotics available to treat a greater variety of antibiotic-resistant bacteria (such as methicillin-resistant *Staphylococcus aureus*, MRSA, and multi-drug-resistant *Mycobacterium tuberculosis*, MDR-TB).

Despite this, antibiotics became and remain widely used for treating bacterial infections and also for preventing them (known as prophylaxis, such as when given prior to surgery). With increasing rates of antibiotic-resistant bacteria today, there is a refocus on efforts to prevent infection by isolating and eliminating any variable that could pose a risk, including decontamination practices.

Up until the 1940s, medical/surgical supplies were mainly decontaminated (or "reprocessed") and maintained in the surgery or patient care area in which they were to be used. Under this system there was duplication of both time and equipment at various locations within larger healthcare facilities, and it was difficult to maintain consistently high standards. As the number and variety of surgical procedures grew and the types of medical/surgical devices, equipment, and supplies increased, it became apparent that centralized processing areas were needed for efficiency, economy, and patient safety. The work of scientists such as W.B. Underwood and J.J. Perkins was instrumental in encouraging healthcare facilities to establish separate and distinct areas/departments with specialized expertise and direct responsibility for providing clean and sterile medical/surgical supplies and equipment to patient care areas. These areas are referred to by a variety of names, such as decontamination service (DS), central sterile services department (CSSD), sterile services department (SSD), sterile processing center (SPC), and theater sterile services unit (TSSU), to mention but a few. It was also in the 1940s that various organizations (such as the British Medical Research Council) advocated that in order to reduce surgical sepsis and other associated infections in healthcare facilities, "fulltime special officers" should be appointed to supervise the control of infection. These officers became experts in infection control and prevention practices within facilities, such as infection prevention and control nurses and doctors. Further recommendations included the establishment of an infection control committee with multidisciplinary representatives, including doctors, nurses, and administrators. It is now normal practice worldwide to employ infection prevention and control specialists and to have established infection control committees with a mandate to monitor and prevent hospital- or healthcare-acquired infections (HAIs).

Advances in various sterilization methods, including those based on steam, dry heat, and even low-temperature chemical methods, such as those based on ethylene oxide, became standard practices in the preparation of surgical devices. Focus was also placed on the variety of devices and instruments that were being developed and used on patients, both medically and surgically. Examples included flexible endoscopes that allowed internal structures of the body to be examined by entering through natural openings (such as through the mouth). During the 1950s a classification system was proposed by Dr. E. Spaulding that suggested devices could be considered as critical (entering the "sterile" areas of the body, including blood contact), semi-critical (contacting non-intact skin or mucous membranes), and non-critical (intact skin contact). While sterilization was recommended for critical devices, various levels of disinfection (ranging from low to high level) could be safely used for the other device classification. New types of high-level disinfectants (sometimes even referred to as "sterilants"), such as those based on glutaraldehyde, became widely used as effective and more rapid alternatives to heat and chemical sterilization methods. Medical/surgical devices continue to show new innovations, including replacement parts of the body (e.g. hips and knees), as well as allowing for robotic surgery. In parallel, newer and even safer disinfectants and sterilization processes have been developed to meet the processing demands for traditional and advanced instrumentation. Safety requirements can include consideration of risks to the patient, those applying the technology (e.g. facility staff), devices or surfaces being treated, and the environment. But it is also important to note that disinfectants and sterilants kill different forms of life and can, when not controlled correctly, have negative impacts on human health.

Our knowledge of the various different types of microorganisms that cause infections has continued to develop. Examples include the ever-increasing types of bacteria, fungi, and protozoa that are implicated as causing various diseases. At the end of the 19th century, a further group of infectious agents were first described that appeared to be much more basic in nature than previously considered: viruses. It was not until the 1930s, with the invention of powerful electron microscopes, that their nature was truly understood. Viruses are now well known as the causative agents in many diseases such as measles (the measles virus), acquired immune deficiency syndrome (AIDs)/human immunodeficiency virus (HIV), flu (influenza), hepatitis (e.g. hepatitis A and B viruses), and some forms of cancer (e.g. papillomavirus). During the 1970–1980s further groups known as "prions" were identified as causative agents in diseases such as "mad cow disease" in animals and humans. Indeed, the range of microorganisms that are implicated in disease continues to expand.

In the modern era, with increasing microbial resistance to drugs (not only in bacteria but in other microorganisms) and greater risks of infections (e.g. with the use of more invasive surgical procedures, types of drugs, etc.), there is a much greater emphasis than ever before on the prevention of infection. Decontamination and process practices play a central role in infection prevention strategies and ensuring patient safety.

Goals of decontamination and the Spaulding classification

Decontamination is the removal of contaminants to specified levels, and decontamination practices are designed to render devices, instruments, and materials safe for handling, use, and/or disposal. It has already been highlighted that the primary goal is to reduce or even completely remove microbial contamination, but in fact it is more than that. Overall, it is to ensure safety: safety for the patient, staff, the devices, and even the environment. The endpoints of decontamination should include:

- To reduce or completely remove microbial contamination to a level that is safe for use by medical staff and with/in a patient.
- To ensure that no toxic substances remain on the surface that could cause other negative patient reactions. This can include patient soil (even in some cases at low concentrations), water or decontamination chemistry (e.g. cleaning and disinfection chemicals) residues, and even parts of microorganisms that have been killed (e.g. toxins).
- To ensure that the decontamination process does not damage the device or surface and that the process is therefore "compatible" with the device. Negative effects can include visual and undetected damage that may lead to device failure or breakage over time and during use. Even cosmetic changes in the device can sometimes impact its practical use (e.g. loss of color-coding marks or labeling).
- A final concern is the impact of decontamination on the environment. On the positive side, decontamination reduces the risks to the general public from exposure to contamination. But equally it requires the use of energy (e.g. generation of steam or use of an automated washing disinfection process), large quantities of water, and many different types of chemicals/materials. The negative effects of chemicals and materials need to be minimized, particularly in the use and disposal of chemicals that have a minimum impact on the environment. There are other issues that may need to be considered, such as costs, but these are secondary to the primary aim of patient and staff safety.

Given the range of potential decontamination opportunities in healthcare facilities, various methods are considered acceptable under different situations to ensure safety. First, inanimate objects are treated separately to animate (or living) ones. Consider, for example, the various types of physical and chemical antimicrobial methods that can be used on medical and surgical devices; these will include various heat and/or chemical methods, but many of these could not be safely used on the skin. Disinfection of skin (or antisepsis) can include the washing of hands and the preparation of the skin for an injection or surgical incision. Only a limited number of antimicrobial methods may be used, due to the sensitive nature of the skin. Therefore, the decontamination of the skin (and mucous membranes) is considered separate to various hard surfaces such as tables, benches, and surgical devices. Second, different classification systems can be used that define the level of decontamination that is applicable depending on the use of the surface, device, or instrument. The most widely used classification for medical/surgical devices is known as the Spaulding classification (as introduced briefly in the previous section). During the 1950s, Dr. Earl Spaulding defined the minimum levels of disinfection/sterilization to be employed according to the infection risk associated with a device/surface when used with a patient. The emphasis was on microbiological and infection risk. But it was clearly stated that the first step was to ensure that the contact surfaces were visually clean; this was to safeguard the effectiveness of any antimicrobial process/product, as the presence of soil or dirt can interfere with its activity. The required use of the device then dictates the recommended antimicrobial process:

- Non-critical devices or surfaces are considered to have the lowest risk to patients, being any surface that only contacts intact skin. Examples could include table tops, bedrails, and chairs, as well as some medical devices such as stethoscopes and blood pressure monitoring cuffs. For such non-critical devices, cleaning alone may be sufficient (to physically remove microorganisms and visual signs of soiling). In other cases, disinfection (to a low level) may be recommended, including the effectiveness against certain types of viruses (especially enveloped viruses such as influenza and HIV), most bacteria, and some fungi. Cleaning and disinfection may sometimes be performed in a one-step process, but are often achieved using a two-step process of cleaning followed by disinfection. Remember, disinfection only reduces the level of microorganisms present and is not expected to completely remove all microorganisms.
- Semi-critical devices pose a higher risk as they may come into contact with mucous membranes or non-intact (broken) skin. These devices may include a variety of endoscopes, probes, or even reusable thermometers. In these cases, meticulous cleaning and disinfection are recommended, but at a higher level of disinfection to ensure the inactivation of a wider range of microorganisms. This would include certain types of microbes that are considered more difficult to kill, such as non-enveloped viruses (e.g. polio- or noroviruses), fungi, and mycobacteria. As before, cleaning is a necessary first step, followed by disinfection.
- Critical devices pose the highest risk as they enter or have contact with a normally "sterile" (or microorganism-free) area of the body, such as the blood or tissue. Cleaning followed by sterilization is recommended for these devices. Sterilization is a process used to render a surface or product free from viable microorganisms, including bacterial spores. Sterilization therefore includes disinfection, but provides a greater level of safety.

Note that in this system a device can change its classification depending on how it is used with a patient. For example, the same device may be critical when used for a surgical procedure or semi-critical if used for a non-invasive diagnostic purpose. Although other classification systems may be used (e.g. class 1, 2a, 2b, and 3), the Spaulding classification is a practical and widely used system worldwide. Examples of other systems include the classification of antiseptics as being used with water (e.g. with soap-based hand washes) or without water ("waterless," such as alcohol hand rubs) or for use for routine hand hygiene, higher-risk applications (such as in preparation for surgery by surgeons, using surgical scrubs, or on patients using a pre-operative skin preparation antiseptic), and even therapeutic applications (such as treatment of skin acne or fungal infections).

These exact requirements ensure the safety and effectiveness of cleaning, disinfection (including antisepsis), and sterilization products/processes, which vary from country to country and region to region. Different guidelines, standards and regulations can be consulted or are even required to be followed to ensure such products/processes are effective. These will include compliance with international standards (see the section "Where to start"), demonstrating effectiveness using standardized test methods (for antimicrobial efficacy and toxicity), routine or periodic tests, and compliance with local registration requirements. As these can vary considerably, those purchasing or using decontamination products should take care to ensure that they do provide the required level of effectiveness and safety.

The decontamination process

A summary of the various processing steps for patient-used devices, instruments, and materials is given as a guide in Figure 1.1. The central cycle is typical for all devices, where non-critical or semi-critical devices can include disinfection steps, and semi-critical or critical devices can include sterilization (often but not always utilizing packaging to allow for sterile presentation immediately prior to use).

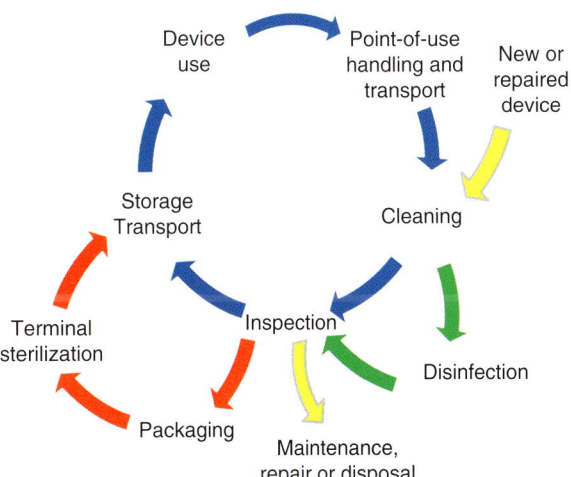

Figure 1.1 Processing cycle.

Healthcare devices can be classified in a variety of ways, such as their purpose of use, materials of construction, and the risk of contamination/infection transmission to a patient (as defined by the Spaulding classification, in the previous section). Another classification is when the device is labeled for single use (on a single patient) or reuse (may be used with many patients). A single-use device can be defined as a device that has been provided by a manufacturer to be used on a single patient. These are usually discarded following use on that patient, although in some cases they may be used a number of times with the same patient. They can include implantable devices (devices that are inserted and maintained within the body that can be for a short time or in many cases for years). They can be provided immediately ready for use (e.g. already clean and sterile) or require processing prior to use.

A reusable device has been designed to be used on a patient, decontaminated (or processed), and then used again. Depending on the manufacturer's instructions, the number of reuse cycles can be defined and this can include a maximum number of times (e.g. 2, 5, or 10) or where the device is no longer needed, damaged, unsafe to use, or otherwise needs to be replaced. The emphasis is therefore placed on ensuring that the device is safely handled, decontaminated, and fit for purpose between patients. The decontamination cycle describes this process used in healthcare facilities. Devices can enter the cycle either as new from the manufacturer or as already used for their intended use. The various steps in the process are briefly discussed here and in more detail in the subsequent chapters of this book. They include:

- Point-of-use (post-procedure) handling and transport (Chapter 7). Medical or surgical procedures using devices and materials can be performed in various locations within a healthcare facility. Post-procedure it is important that these are handled correctly, to include not being damaged or lost and not posing any safety risks to staff, visitors, and subsequent patients. This can include sorting (e.g. disposable from non-disposable items following surgical use) and then safely containing and transporting them to an area designated for decontamination. There may be specific pre-cleaning or safe handling instructions to be performed at this point. These steps are typically recommended to be done within the same area where they are used ("point of use"), but may be conducted in a separate, adjacent room/area or at another location.
- Cleaning (Chapter 8) is the removal of contamination (or "soil") from an item to the extent necessary for its further processing and its intended subsequent use. This can include the removal of patient materials (blood, tissues, etc.), microorganisms, and even different chemicals used during a procedure (e.g. cements, gels, etc.). Cleaning may be the only decontamination step required (e.g. for some non-critical devices/surfaces), but is always a required step before any further decontamination steps in the cycle (such as disinfection and/or sterilization). This is because soil can interfere with the effectiveness of these processes and can cause other patient risks. In some cases, such as with non-critical devices/surfaces, cleaning can be combined with disinfection.
- Disinfection (Chapter 9) is the antimicrobial reduction of microorganisms from a surface to a level determined to be appropriate for its intended further handling or use. Microorganisms can be very different in their structures, with some easier to kill than others. They also are different in their abilities to be able to cause problems to human health (e.g. their ability to cause disease). This will be considered in further detail. Different levels of antimicrobial activity (disinfection or sterilization) may be required, depending on the risk associated with the device/surface. In some cases only disinfection is used to render the device safe for use. In others disinfection is an interim step, being applied first (to reduce the risk of handling devices) and followed by packaging and sterilization. Sterilization may also be applied to the device without disinfection. If this is conducted without sterile packaging, the device is only safe for immediate use with or on a patient, as it can become recontaminated on storage or further handling. Many devices can leave the decontamination cycle at the disinfection stage for patient use (following some inspection to ensure they are safe for use and, where appropriate, interim storage).
- Inspection and, where appropriate, packaging (Chapter 10). Prior to direct patient use or further decontamination, devices or materials are checked for cleanliness, functionality, dryness, and so on. Devices may be identified at this point for repair or even disposal (although this may occur at any stage during the decontamination cycle, right up to the point of patient use). They may then be safely transported to a site of patient use or for further assembly/packaging in preparation for sterilization. Specifically, sterile packaging is designed to protect a single device or set of assembled devices during sterilization, storage, and transport, for future use with or on a patient. At this stage, surgical devices can often be assembled in dedicated trays designed for specific types of surgical procedures (Chapter 3). Note that there may be other practices where devices are covered or stored in various ways prior to use on a patient to prevent cross-contamination, but care should be taken to ensure that such practices are safe and effective.
- Sterilization (Chapter 11) is a process used to render a surface or product free from viable organisms, including those that are particularly hard to kill such as bacterial spores. Following sterilization, devices may be transported for direct patient use or, when correctly packaged, stored until required for the patient procedure.
- Storage and distribution (Chapter 12). The correct storage (if applicable) and distribution of reusable devices to the next point of use are essential to complete the decontamination cycle.

In addition to these steps in the decontamination cycle, the acquisition of devices and other materials used during the decontamination process is discussed, as well as the safe handling of wastes. Consideration is also given in specific chapters to basic principles that are important to decontamination practices, such as:

- Human anatomy and physiology (Chapter 2).
- Different types of medical and surgical procedures (Chapter 3).
- The variety of medical and surgical devices used (Chapter 4).
- Principles of microbiology and infection prevention/control (Chapter 5).
- Basic understanding of chemistry and physics (Chapter 6).
- Safety considerations (Chapter 13).
- Management and quality principles (Chapter 14).

The design of a decontamination area

Decontamination (or processing) areas may be at or adjacent to the patient procedure area (e.g. a TSSU or decontamination room/area), at a remote location within the hospital (e.g. a CSSD or decontamination service departments), or at a completely different facility (e.g. a regional or contract sterilization facility). Despite the location, the primary purpose of the area, department, or facility is to ensure the safe processing of devices. It should be dedicated and appropriate for that purpose. The area should be designed to:

- Allow for the safe processing of devices and/or materials, should they require cleaning alone; cleaning and disinfection; or cleaning, disinfection, and sterilization, as examples. Safety considerations should include patient as well as staff and visitor risks.
- Ensure it can meet the workload demands to maintain a supply of reusable devices. This will include costs (budget), available space, equipment, and staffing requirements.
- Reduce the risk of accidental mixing of "dirty," "clean," or disinfected/sterilized devices or cross-contamination. This will include workflow design.

An important factor in managing an effective decontamination service is good area design and workflow. Workflow must allow for the logical flow of devices from being dirty to clean to disinfected/sterile. Such workflow systems are designed to prevent the accidental mixing of dirty and clean (or decontaminated) devices/materials. Such areas may be part of a room, a dedicated room, or a whole, purposely built decontamination department or facility. Examples of area layouts that highlight such workflows are shown in Figure 1.2.

Maintaining good workflow implies proper functioning and coordination between distinct decontamination areas. These include:

- "Dirty" area: here devices/materials are received, disassembled, and decontaminated. For non-critical equipment this can include cleaning and disinfection. For washing the area can include a manual cleaning area alone, but consideration should also be given to include automated washers or washer-disinfectors. For manual cleaning of semi-critical or critical devices, a double (two) or even triple (three) sink arrangement is optimal, one or two for cleaning and one for rinsing. Automated washers or washer-disinfectors are often preferred in these areas and can be provided as single- or double-door designs. Double-door designs allow for the physical separation of the dirty and clean areas of the decontamination area, where dirty devices enter on one side and exit on the opposite side, most commonly into a separate room.
- "Clean" area: cleaned, and most often disinfected, devices/materials are inspected in this area and reassembled or prepared for use. For semi-critical or critical devices this area is also used for packaging and subsequent sterilization (when applicable). There may be provisions made for specific transfer methods (e.g. transfer hatches) between physically separated department designs (for example for the return of devices that have been inspected and found not to be clean; Figure 1.2).
- Sterilization area (if applicable), where devices/materials are subjected to a sterilization process.
- Processed goods storage and distribution: this may be at the same area or in a separate, designated area of the facility (e.g. with other sterile stores).

Serious consideration should always be given to the correct layout of a decontamination area/facility. Too often the layout of decontamination areas is found to be inadequate.

The area should be designated for device decontamination purposes only (e.g. not mixed with recreation or food or drink preparation areas) and of ample size for the required procedures/workload. These can include single or multiple room/area designs (Figure 1.2). In single room set-ups, correct layout, standard procedures, and staff training are essential to prevent cross-contamination. These risks are particularly minimized in larger, physically separated area designs (Figure 1.3). It is important to remember that in addition to the receiving, decontamination, and storage/dispatch of reusable devices/materials, provision should also be made for the handling of supplies or raw materials for the decontamination process. This will include chemicals, packaging materials (single use or reusable), labels, indicators, and so on. Equally, the area can have many items (contaminated or non-contaminated) that will be designated for waste disposal and will need to be considered. Areas will also be required to allow for staff to prepare themselves to enter/exit the different areas (e.g. gowning, washing hands, etc.). Finally, any equipment within the area (and their associated utilities such as electricity, water/steam supply, drainage, etc.) will require periodic maintenance and testing; therefore access to such equipment should be considered and present minimum disruption to the decontamination

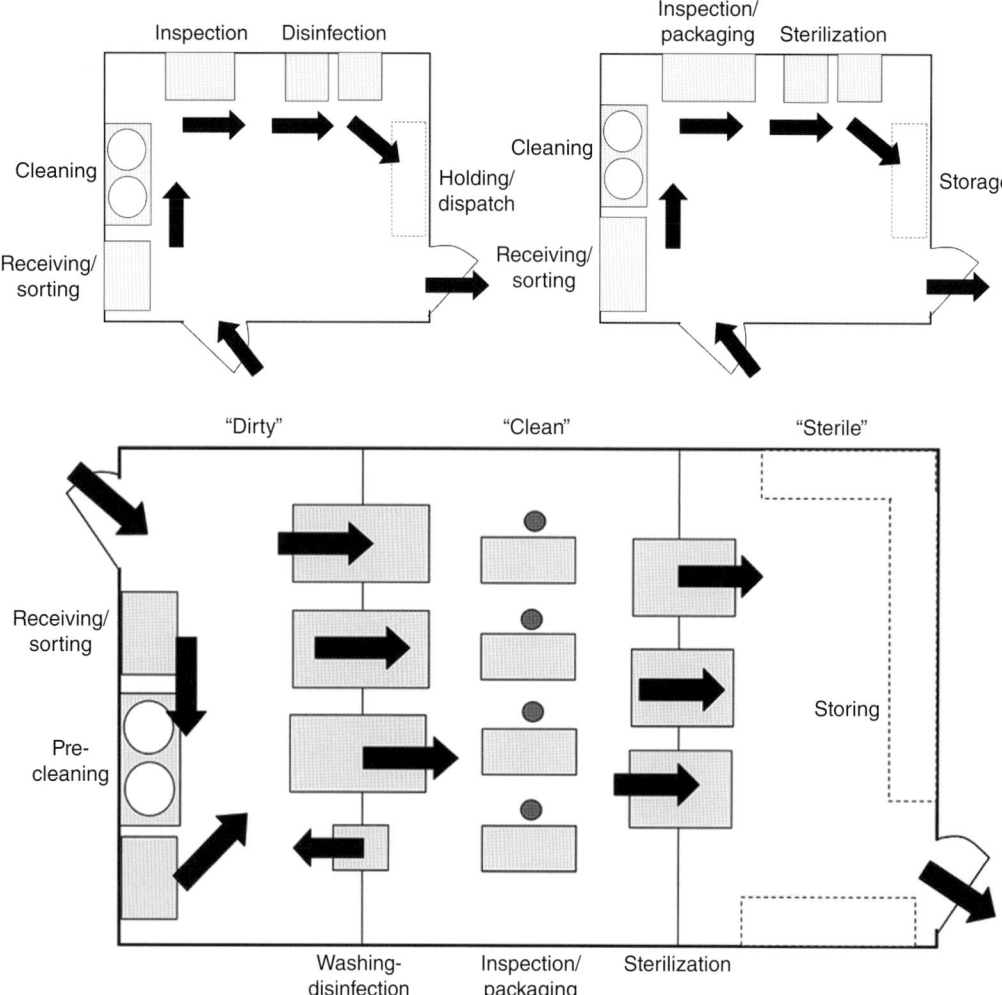

Figure 1.2 Examples of decontamination area/facility workflow plans. On the upper panel are examples of single rooms for cleaning–disinfection (left) and cleaning–sterilization (right). In the disinfection example, devices are received in one area, passed through the process, and held in a separate area waiting for release for the new patient procedure. The sterilization example is identical, but in this case the devices/sets are packaged, sterilized, and adequately stored ready for patient use. The lower panel shows a typical physically separated area design, designated areas for receiving/pre-cleaning, cleaning disinfection, inspection–packaging, sterilization, and storage. Physical separation in this case is enabled by using two-door designs of washer-disinfector machines and sterilizers (which open on one end for loading and on the other for unloading); note that an additional pass-through hatch is shown between the clean and dirty areas, to allow for devices that have not been adequately cleaned to pass back to the dirty area for additional cleaning.

needs of the facility. It goes without saying that these utilities should be of the correct capacity and quality to meet the decontamination needs of the facility.

There are many other environmental concerns to be considered in the design of a decontamination area. These include the following:

• Access to the area should be limited and controlled. This should prevent any unauthorized person from entering the area without permission.

• Comfort of staff: temperature and humidity control (air conditioning), in particular in areas where heat-associated equipment (such as steam sterilizers and thermal washer-disinfectors are used) is used. Consideration should also be given to ensure there is adequate lighting (particularly for inspection areas) and noise control.

• Ventilation: the cleaning area, in particular for manual cleaning, can pose a safety risk to staff and visitors (from microorganisms, patient tissues, and various chemicals used

Figure 1.3 The layout of a modern decontamination facility, designed to have physical separation between dirty, clean, and sterile storage/dispatch areas.

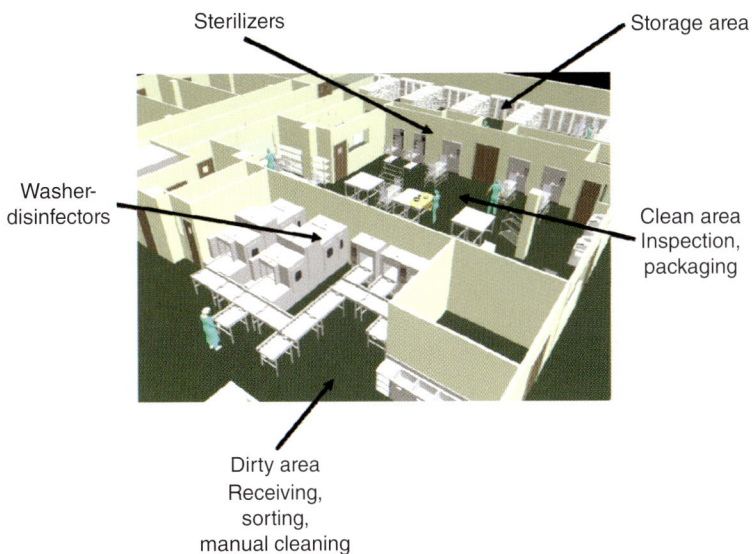

in the cleaning process). These areas should be adequately ventilated, typically providing ~10–20 air changes/hour. It is also recommended that these areas should have dedicated air handling systems and be maintained at ambient pressure or even at a slight negative pressure (e.g. −5 to −10 Pa) that acts to keep contamination within the area. Equally, the clean or sterile packaging area should also be similarly ventilated (~10–20 air changes/hour), reducing any risks of airborne contamination, and under a slightly positive pressure (e.g. +10 Pa) to keep contamination out.

- The area should be designed to allow for periodic cleaning or, particularly in dirty areas, handling of accidental spillages.
- Sterile or otherwise decontaminated items should be stored in a suitable area designed to reduce any potential for cross-contamination such as from the air, water, damage, etc. Sterile packaged items may be compromised by exposure to extremes of temperature and humidity.
- Staff/visitors should have access to hand washing facilities, separate to those used for cleaning devices, before entering or leaving the areas.
- For larger facilities/departments, provisions may need to be made for management offices, general staff areas (for resting or eating and drinking) and storage that are separated from the decontamination area.

An effective management system should be in place to control the entire decontamination system, from patient use to the next patient use. This may require a coordinated effort from all staff involved, particularly in larger facilities: that will include operating room, transport, decontamination, and inventory control staff as examples. For the decontamination process, written procedures should be in place and staff trained on these procedures to ensure that the various decontamination steps are conducted correctly. Once established procedures are in place, deviations to them should not be tolerated. If deviations are demanded by medical/surgical staff due to patient needs, it is recommended that written authorization is obtained from management that accepts any associated patient risk. In many, if not most, countries these areas of healthcare facilities are considered regulated and therefore it is mandatory that specific controls and procedures are in place.

For effective decontamination, other considerations will include:

- Adequate water supply: this will include cold and hot tap (potable) water, and may also include the provision of a higher water quality for rinsing and other purposes (e.g. for generation of steam). Water, and the various types of chemicals and other materials that can be present in it, can play an important role in the safe decontamination of devices and patient safety.
- Sufficient draining or liquid waste disposal, with consideration of any local or regional requirements regarding disposal of chemicals or other materials into drains.
- Automated decontamination processes (for cleaning, disinfection, and sterilization) are preferred over manual methods. Any equipment provided should be installed correctly and periodically verified to be fit for purpose; for example, any equipment that requires temperature control should be routinely checked to ensure it is working at the expected, set temperatures, and only authorized staff should be able to change cycle parameters. Equipment will require periodic maintenance and testing.
- Staff and visitor safety is important: safety equipment (personal protective equipment, PPE), such as safety glass/face shields and proper gloves (e.g. heavy duty for cleaning), should be provided and used. Specific safety equipment will depend

on the various procedures or equipment being used within the area.
- International, regional, and local guidelines and standards regarding decontamination should be considered.

A correctly designed decontamination area is the first step to ensuring patient safety, but is closely followed by the second, staff training. Designated and qualified staff should be trained on the correct procedures (including equipment used) for decontamination within the area and have sufficient allocated time to ensure a quality process. It is important that training should be conducted when any changes in these procedures are made, such as the introduction of new equipment, chemicals, devices, and so on. Periodic retraining should also be considered to ensure that standards are maintained.

Where to start

This book provides a practical guide to decontamination principles and practices from an international perspective. As introduced in the previous section, this includes many background concepts to the subject, such as an introduction to anatomy, chemistry, and microbiology, as well as detailed consideration of the various steps of the decontamination process. This book should be used in conjunction with available international, regional, and local regulations, standards, and guidelines. These will include local requirements for decontamination practices, including quality control, the design of decontamination facilities, minimal steps for device/materials processing, waste disposal, use of chemicals, selection of equipment and their use, and so on.

Regulations are rules or orders issued by a region, country, community, or administrative agency, under legal authority, and have the force of law. Depending on the region or country you live in, there may be various laws or directives concerning the safe provision or use of medical/surgical equipment, as well as various products and processes used for decontamination. Examples, at the time of writing, include:
- European Union (EU). The CE mark (CE) stands for Conformité Européenne or "European conformity," which when attached to a device (or device labeling) is a manufacturer's claim that it meets all the requirements of applicable European legislation. This can vary depending on the type of product, with examples including:
  ○ The EU Medical Device Regulation (EU 2017/745, which replaced Directive 93/42/EEC on medical devices and Directive 90/385/EEC on implantable medical devices). This regulation covers the essential requirements for any medical device, defined as any instrument or other article (used alone or in combination) intended to be used for human beings for the purpose of diagnosis, prevention, monitoring, treatment, or alleviation of disease, etc. Medical devices are further sub-classified based on their use and risk to patients. Examples of their use include duration of use (transient or <60 minutes, short term at 60 minutes to 30 days, and long term at >30 days) or being non-invasive, invasive, or implantable. Risk to patient classifications are rated from classes 1 to 3, with class 1 being lower risk and class 3 being higher risk. Similar (but often different) classifications are used in many other parts of the world. For the EU, class 1 devices are low risk, and either do not touch a patient or if they do only touch intact skin (similar to non-critical devices described earlier under the Spaulding classification system). Examples include beds, wheelchairs, and many types of reusable surgical instruments. Class II devices are separated into two subtypes and include many devices that contact injured skin or mucous membranes or invasive devices. Class IIa are considered low–medium risk, such as hearing aids and many types of surgically invasive devices intended for short-term use, and class IIb are medium–high risk, such as many surgical devices used to administer a medicinal product using a delivery system, or implantable devices. Class III are the highest risk and include many types of implantable devices such as those in direct contact with the heart, joint or spinal disc replacements, or many devices controlling or monitoring implantable devices. It is important to note that the classification of devices under the regulation is the responsibility of the manufacturer in collaboration with the local regulatory bodies, and the information given here is only a guide. Equipment and products used in the processing of devices (disinfectants, sterilizers, etc.) are also considered "medical devices" under this regulation (typically classes IIa and IIb). The manufacturer, with reference to the "essential" requirements of the regulation as well as other standards (international and/or European) that are specific to the type of device/equipment, ensures compliance and should provide a certificate (or "declaration") of conformance. In most cases this is reviewed and approved by an independent organization known as a Notified Body. Note that separate regulations may be in place for specific types of medical devices, such as *in vitro* diagnostic medical devices under EU regulation 2017/746.
  ○ Machinery Directive (2006/42/EC), defining essential health and safety requirements for machinery. "Machinery" is any assembly using moving parts and therefore would apply to equipment like washers and sterilizers. Compliance is similar to that described for the Medical Devices Directive.
  ○ Biocidal Products Directive (98/8/EC). "Biocides" are defined active substances/preparations supplied to destroy, deter, render harmless, prevent the action of, or otherwise exert a controlling effect on any harmful organism. Interestingly, this includes the use of chemical disinfectants/sterilants

on general surfaces, but excludes their specific use on medical devices (since when used as such they are required to meet the requirements of the Medical Devices Directive). In addition to these essential requirements, a series of specific test methods have been under development in Europe that should be used to confirm any disinfectant efficacy claims (e.g. kills bacteria or viruses). These methods are discussed in further detail in Chapter 9.

○ REACH (Registration, Evaluation, Authorisation and Restriction of Chemicals); Regulation (EC) 1907/2006. This regulation concerns the production and use of any chemical, with an emphasis on human and environmental health. This would include a wide range of chemicals used, for example, in cleaning chemistries or chemical disinfectants. Other directives/regulations apply to specific types of chemicals such as biocides (98/8/EC, as discussed earlier) and detergents (regulation (EC) 648/2004).

These directives are applicable for all EU countries and compliance allows for the devices to be legally sold in all countries; however, in some cases additional requirements can be put in place in individual countries.

- United States of America:
  ○ The US Food and Drug Administration's (FDA) Center for Devices and Radiological Health (CDRH) is responsible for regulating those who manufacture, repackage, relabel, and/or import medical devices sold in the United States. Medical devices are classified based on their risk, to include class 1, 2, and 3 (from low to high risk). These include surgical devices and decontamination processes such as washer-disinfectors, sterilizers, and device disinfection chemistries. Class 2 (such as sterilizers and device disinfectants) and class 3 devices, specifically, require a formal approval by the FDA known as a Premarket Notification 510(k) or Premarket Approval (PMA). In either case, the safety and efficacy of a product/process are reviewed and formally approved prior to selling in the United States. The FDA also provides guidance documents to manufacturers regarding device/process-specific requirements, such as for sterilizers or high-level disinfectants/sterilants, and device processing validation requirements and instructions.
  ○ The Environmental Protection Agency (EPA) regulates the use of general/environmental surface disinfectants under the Federal Insecticide, Fungicide, and Rodenticide Act (FIFRA). Note that any disinfectants used on medical devices are registered for use in the United States by the FDA, while those for environmental surface disinfection should be registered by the EPA. It refers to biocides or antimicrobial chemistries as "antimicrobial pesticides." The EPA requires that special tests (such as those described by AOAC International) are used to ensure disinfectant efficacy, as well as for any human and ecological risks from exposure. The EPA also provides guidance documents on various aspects of disinfectant use and registration, such as testing for specific antimicrobial claims and dental issues.

- Australia:
  ○ The Therapeutic Goods Administration (TGA), a division of the Department of Health and Aged Care, is the regulatory authority for therapeutic goods, including medical devices and their processing methods. Medical devices are registered under the Therapeutic Goods Act 1989 and the Therapeutic Goods (Medical Devices) Regulations 2002. All products are required to be listed in the Australian Register of Therapeutic Goods (ARTG), unless specifically exempt, before they can be supplied in Australia. The Office of Devices Authorisation (ODA) is responsible for initial registration of medical devices, while the Office of Product Review (OPR) is responsible for any post-registration issues. Devices are also classified based on risk, ranging from low (class I) to high (class III or active implantable devices separately). Device disinfectants, for example, are considered class IIb devices. Liquid chemical disinfectants are considered under the Therapeutic Goods (Standard for Disinfectants and Sanitary Products) Order 2019, known as TGO 104. But this excludes antiseptics (disinfectants used on the skin), sterilants, and disinfectants specifically used for water treatment. The TGA also provides various guidance documents such as infection control guidelines for the prevention of transmission of infectious diseases and reducing public health risks associated with reusable medical devices.

- Canada:
  ○ Medical devices regulations are under the authority of the Food and Drugs Act. Health Canada (under the Medical Devices Directorate) monitors and evaluates all medical devices to assess their safety, effectiveness, and quality before they are authorized for sale in Canada. Medical devices are classified based on risk, ranging from class 1 to class 4. For example, equipment/products used for disinfecting or sterilizing a medical device are classified as class 2. Health Canada also provides guidelines such as for processing instructions for use and reporting problems with medical devices.

As can be seen from this brief but not exhaustive review, specific country/region requirements can be complicated and are regularly updated or changed. These laws/directives generally control the legal marketing and use of medical/surgical devices, as well as requirements for decontamination, within those specific areas. It is the responsibility of the healthcare facility to understand these requirements and ensure that they are correctly applied. Many of these regulations are general in their content, but they can also be associated with more detailed requirements included in various standards and guidelines. Examples of different standard/guideline organizations are shown in Table 1.1.

Standards are documents that specify the minimum acceptable characteristics of a product or material, issued by a

Table 1.1 Examples of various standard and guideline publishing organizations internationally. This list is by no means exhaustive.

Title	Notes
International Organization for Standardization (ISO)	A non-governmental, international body based in Geneva, Switzerland Develops draft standards through technical committees (e.g. ISO/TC 198 *Sterilization of healthcare products*) that are then approved by a majority of country (national) member bodies[1] ISO collaborates closely with the International Electrotechnical Commission (IEC) on all matters of electrotechnical standardization and with CEN on harmonized international standards[2]
Comité européen de normalisation/European Committee for Standardization (CEN)	A not-for-profit European organization based in Brussels, Belgium Develops draft standards through technical committees (e.g. CEN/TC 204 *Sterilization of medical devices* and CEN/TC 216 *Disinfectants and antiseptics*) that are then approved by European country (national) member bodies[3] CEN collaborates closely with CENELEC (Comité européen de normalisation en électronique et en électrotechnique/European Committee for Electrotechnical Standardization) on matters of electrotechnical standardization and with ISO on the development of harmonized international standards[2]
British Standards Institution (BSI)	National standards body in the United Kingdom BSI also uses the "Kitemark" to indicate that a product has been independently tested to conform with a relevant British Standard
Deutsches Institut für Normung (DIN)	National standards body in Germany
Association française de normalisation (AFNOR)	National standards body in France
American National Standards Institute (ANSI)	National standard and guideline bodies in the United States
Association for the Advancement of Medical Instrumentation (AAMI)	AAMI develops standards and recommended practices, with many being approved by ANSI as American National Standards. For example, a TIR (Technical Information Report) provides guidance on a particular aspect (e.g. use of disinfectants/sterilants in various applications or the design, testing, and labeling of reusable devices)
ASTM International (previously known as the American Society for Testing and Materials)	Standards body based in the United States, focused on the development of test method (e.g. chemical and microbiological) standards
AOAC International (previously known as the Association of Analytical Communities)	Standards body based in the United States, focused on the development of test method (chemical and microbiological) standards
Standardization Administration of China (SAC)	Standards body in China Mandatory standards are prefixed with "GB," while recommended standards can be prefixed with "GB/T"
Standards Australia and/or New Zealand	Standards bodies in Australia and New Zealand Joint Australian (AS) and New Zealand (NZS) Standards and Guidelines are often developed (known as AS/NZS). An example is AS/NZS 4187 (2014) on processing of reusable devices in health service organizations (replaced in Australia by a new AS5369 standard on processing for health- and non-health-related facilities)

[1] Examples of national standard bodies include BSI (UK), AFNOR (France), DIN (Germany), and AAMI (United States), see the table.
[2] The Vienna Agreement (1991) is an agreement on technical cooperation between ISO and CEN in the development of standards. As an example, ISO/TC 198 *Sterilization of healthcare products* and CEN/TC 204 *Sterilization of medical devices* cooperate to develop harmonized standards in the processing or sterilization of devices. An example of a harmonized standard is EN ISO 14937 *Sterilization of healthcare products – general requirements for characterization of a sterilizing agent and the development, validation and routine control of a sterilization process for medical devices*. Despite these efforts, sometimes the standard is not adopted in all countries or modifications of the standard are made/published by the national standards body.
[3] CEN members are the national standards bodies of different European countries. Members should comply with the CEN/CENELEC regulations that stipulate that a European Standard should be given the status of a national standard without any alteration.

standards organization (e.g. International Organization for Standardization, ISO, and Comité européen de normalisation (CEN), the European Commission for Standardization). Most countries will have some legal requirements, directly or indirectly, regarding decontamination of reusable devices/materials; these are typically included in different standards or guidance within a given country/region. International standards (such as those developed by ISO) are continually under development for different aspects of decontamination procedures and practices. A summary of some of these standards is provided in Table 1.2. Other regional (e.g. CEN within Europe) and local standards and best practice guideline documents are also important to consider, and are mandated in certain countries (Chapter 14). Guidelines are documents used to communicate regional recommended procedures, processes, or usage of particular practices; they are often considered best practice at the time of their writing and can be frequently updated. During the course of this book, different standards and guidelines are referenced for each phase of the decontamination cycle.

Particularly important standards that should be considered in decontamination are the ISO 17664 series on information to be provided by the medical device manufacturer for the processing of medical devices, be they critical, semi-critical, or non-critical (Table 1.2). Although it is the responsibility of the healthcare facility to safely decontaminate reusable items, it is the responsibility of the suppliers of these items to provide detailed instructions on how they should be safely processed. These instructions should be validated as effective by the manufacturer. These standards have been recently updated to apply to the wider range of medical device types, as well as to provide greater and more consistent processing instructions. Instructions provided should include:

- The device manufacturer and its contact information.
- Device(s) by model number, and device description or generic type.
- Any appropriate warnings or limitations, such as care on handling (e.g. sharp edges) or restrictions on processing conditions (e.g. "cannot be immersed in water" or "electrical hazard").
- Service life of a device, based on a specific number of processing cycles or some other type of end-of-life indication.
- Instructions on handling the device at its point of use and for transport to a decontamination area. Examples include inspections, pre-cleaning, care in handling, etc.
- Instructions on preparation for decontamination, including disassembly. The use of specific tools and procedures may need to be described, depending on the device design.
- Cleaning instructions. These will include recommendations for the types or restrictions (e.g. due to damage risks) of cleaning chemistries, conditions, equipment, and procedures to be used. Preference is given to providing at least one automated cleaning method (which may include some manual steps), but full manual cleaning methods are to be specified if automated cleaning is not possible and/or desired to meet specific needs. Methods used for inspection of cleanliness, in particular for areas of the device known to be difficult to clean, will also be important.
- Disinfection (if applicable). As for cleaning, automated disinfection (typically using moist heat methods) is preferred, but manual procedures can be described where automated processes cannot be employed. Methods should include applicable thermal and/or chemical disinfection methods, equipment required, and requirements for rinsing (in particular with chemical disinfection to ensure the device is safe for patient use or further processing). As for other parts of the decontamination process, the quality of water used will also be an important consideration.
- Drying (if applicable). Instructions for the drying of the device should be provided. This may or may not include the consideration for using chemicals that aid in the drying process (e.g. alcohols or rinse aids).
- Maintenance, inspection, and testing. This will include instructions for periodic testing, lubrication, inspections, reassembly, etc. to ensure that the device can be safely used on the next patient. Inspection is a particularly important variable here and can sometimes require diligent and specific requirements (such as inspection of moving parts, internal lumens, etc.).
- Packaging (if applicable), in preparation for storage and/or terminal sterilization.
- Sterilization (if applicable). At least one method of sterilization should be provided, but the instructions may also include restrictions on what should or should not be applied, such as should not be immersed, should not be subjected to low pressure levels, or should not exceed certain temperatures.
- Storage. Any recommendations for the time or conditions of storage prior to use, if required.
- Transportation. When applicable, instructions may be required to reduce the risk of device damage or compromising cleaning, disinfection, or sterilization during transport to the place of use.

Processing instructions are essential in order to ensure patient safety. They require close cooperation between medical/surgical device manufacturers, processing staff, those using the devices with patients, and the suppliers of cleaning, disinfection, and sterilization products/processes. Although it is often impractical for manufacturers to provide detailed instructions to meet individual requirements for each country (due to historical requirements in these countries or specific and changing guidelines), it is important that they consider local decontamination standards and guidelines. In the absence of adequate instructions, it may not be possible to ensure patient safety and the healthcare facility may decide not to use such devices/materials.

In conclusion, this book has been written for a wide interdisciplinary, international audience, and while it discusses the

Table 1.2 Examples of international standards that consider various decontamination aspects. These may or may not apply to a given region or country and the associated dates can change over time depending on periodic updates to the standard requirements.

Standard Number[1]	Title	Description
ISO 13485 (2016)	*Medical devices – quality management systems – requirements for regulatory purposes*	The requirements for the development, implementation, and monitoring of a quality management system for the manufacturer of medical devices. Generally for device manufacturers, but can also apply to healthcare facilities decontaminating devices
ISO 17664-1 (2021)	ISO 17664-1:2021 *Processing of health care products — Information to be provided by the medical device manufacturer for the processing of medical devices. Part 1: Critical and semi-critical medical devices*	Instructions to be provided by the device manufacturer to ensure safe processing of critical or semi-critical medical devices
ISO 17664-2 (2021)	ISO 17664-2:2021 *Processing of health care products — Information to be provided by the medical device manufacturer for the processing of medical devices. Part 2: Non-critical medical devices*	Instructions to be provided by the device manufacturer to ensure safe processing of non-critical medical devices not intended to be sterilized
ISO 15883 series	*Washer-disinfectors. General requirements, definitions and tests*	Design, performance, and testing of washer-disinfectors, including cleaning and disinfection requirements. Provided in a series. Part 1 describes the requirements for all washer-disinfectors, Part 5 specifies updated performance requirements and test method criteria for demonstrating cleaning efficacy, and other parts provide more details on specific types of machines (e.g. surgical instruments and flexible endoscopes)
ISO 9398 series	*Specifications for industrial laundry machines*	Series of standards on laundry machines, including definitions, testing of capacity, and consumption characteristics
ISO 14937 (2009)	*Sterilization of healthcare products – general requirements for characterization of a sterilizing agent and the development, validation and routine control of a sterilization process for medical devices*	Development, validation, and routine control of any sterilization process used for healthcare devices and other materials
ISO 17665-1 (2006)	*Sterilization of healthcare products – moist heat. Part 1: requirements for the development, validation and routine control of a sterilization process for medical devices*	Development, validation, and routine control of moist heat (steam) sterilization processes for devices
ISO 20857 (2010)	*Sterilization of healthcare products – dry heat – requirements for the development, validation and routine control of a sterilization process for medical devices*	Development, validation, and routine control of a dry heat sterilization process for devices
ISO 11135 (2014)	*Sterilization of health-care products — Ethylene oxide — Requirements for the development, validation and routine control of a sterilization process for medical devices*	Development, validation, and routine control of an ethylene oxide sterilization process for medical devices

[1] International standards, as published by ISO, are designated by a specific number but also the date of issue (as they are periodically updated). When (and if) the standard is accepted regionally or within a specific country it may be designated, for example, BS EN ISO xxxx (designates a harmonized standard for the United Kingdom, European Union, and international) or AMMI ISO xxxx (designates a US-AAMI version of an international standard); note that in such cases modifications specific to that region or country may be included before publication in these areas. All attempts are made internationally to harmonize such standards, but at the time of writing this is not always possible.

basic principles of decontamination and related guidelines, it should not be used as a replacement for local legislative or guidance documents issued in particular countries or regions. However, regardless of your location, the same basic principles should be applied to decontamination practices throughout the world, using a combination of processes that include as a basic minimum adequate cleaning, inspection, and disinfection and/or sterilization in order to render a reusable item safe for further use on patients and for handling by staff. Decontamination and processing of reusable devices and materials is essential in minimizing the risk of transmission of infectious agents and other patient risks.

2 Basic anatomy, physiology, and biochemistry

Anatomy is the study of the structures of living things and physiology is the study of how these structures function. This chapter gives a brief introduction into human anatomy and physiology, and in particular aims to give a basic understanding of the many terms that are used during surgical or interventional procedures. Similar language is used for the anatomy and physiology of animals, which may be a helpful introduction to some readers. Microbiology and microorganisms are specifically discussed in Chapter 5.

Let us consider the structure of the human body, from what we can see down to the very basis of life itself (see Table 2.1). The human body is a complex, organized structure of various systems. There are 11 systems to consider and each one has a unique function. As an example, the digestive system consists of various parts that allow us to eat and drink, breaking down food into various components, allowing nutrients to be absorbed into the body, and ridding the body of any remaining wastes. Each system can be subdivided into individual organs. In the digestive system organs include the mouth, stomach, and intestines (small and large). It is important to note that many organs have shared functions; examples include the mouth being used for breathing (as part of the respiratory system) and for eating/drinking (the digestive system).

Each individual organ is made up of various tissues that work together to perform a specific function. There are only four basic types of tissues in the adult body: epithelial, nervous, muscular, and connective:

- Epithelial tissues provide coverings or linings to organs, in addition to forming various types of glands that can produce substances (or secretions). Examples of epithelial tissues include the epithelium (or outermost) layer of the skin (where specific glands excrete sweat) and, in the case of the stomach, the inner mucous membrane (containing mucus-producing glands) and outer serous membrane. Other examples are glandular tissues, which produce hormone chemicals that secrete into the bloodstream and function to direct other cells in the body to act or respond.
- Nervous tissue allows for communication within the body directly.

Table 2.1 The various human body structures and examples.

Structures	Examples
Systems	Nervous, respiratory, digestive, and cardiovascular systems
Organs	Stomach, heart, kidney, liver, brain
Tissues	Epithelial, muscular, nervous, connective tissues
Cells	Nerve, muscle, skin, blood cells
Molecules	Water (H_2O), proteins, carbohydrates, lipids, nucleic acids
Atoms	Carbon (C), hydrogen (H), oxygen (O), nitrogen (N)

- Muscular tissue allows for movement (i.e. in the beating of the heart). There are three types of muscular tissue: cardiac, smooth, and skeletal. Cardiac and smooth muscle are controlled by involuntary commands, whereas skeletal muscle can move by way of voluntary commands.
- Connective tissue provides support and connections (i.e. bones, blood).

It should be noted that the four basic tissue types can be further sub-divided into specific kinds based on their structures and functions, such as the many kinds of muscle and connective tissues.

When the structural and functional integrity of tissues is compromised, the result can lead to disease of the organ that is composed of these tissues. Pathology is the study and diagnosis of disease through examination of the whole body, including the various organs, tissues, and cells. To explore further the structure of the various types of tissues, microscopic examination is now required. Specifically, histology is the science that studies the microscopic structure of organs and tissues. Each type of tissue is made up of specialized cells that are similar in function and structure. A single cell is the basic unit structure and function of life. Human cells are found to be in different shapes and sizes, depending on their function and structure, and are organized together to give the various types of tissues. Despite these differences, cells are all essentially of the same basic design (Figure 2.1).

Decontamination and Device Processing in Healthcare, Second Edition. Gerald McDonnell and Georgia Alevizopoulou.
© 2025 John Wiley & Sons Ltd. Published 2025 by John Wiley & Sons Ltd.

Figure 2.1 Human cell structure. Examples are given (top) of the various different shapes of cells that can be observed, but they practically all have the same essential structure (shown below).

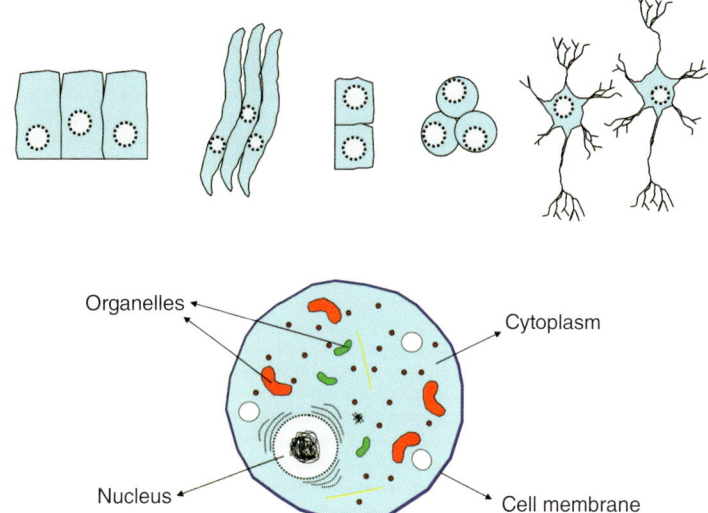

As we begin to look into the structure of these cells, we now consider the science of biochemistry. This is the study of the chemical processes in living organisms, focusing on the structure and function of cells and their components. Human cells consist of an outer cell membrane, enclosing a liquid-like cytoplasm (Figure 2.1). The cytoplasm holds various different structures (known as "organelles") that provide the various functions to the cell. Organelles are composed of macromolecules such as proteins, lipids, and carbohydrates, with each type of cell having a unique mix of organelles based on the primary function of the cell. Key organelles include mitochondria (which make energy in the cell), microfilaments (allowing for movement and support), lysosomes (which contain enzymes for food digestion and destruction for invading microorganisms), and the nucleus. The nucleus is particularly prominent and is separated from the rest of the cell by a further membrane. This is the heart of the cell, containing the genetic material DNA (deoxyribonucleic acid). In human cells the DNA is organized into specialized structures called chromosomes, of which most cells in the body contain 46 (23 pairs, one of each pair inherited from the mother and the other from the father). These are important structures, as the DNA is like a blueprint for the cell and is made up of individual genes. It is the expression (whether they are turned off or on) of these genes that allows the cell to produce all the necessary molecules (biomolecules) that are required for cell structure and function (described in the following section). It is therefore the same gene expression that allows the cell to survive or die, divide, communicate with other cells, and change structure or function, and essentially dictates during the development of the human body whether that cell becomes any of the various types of cells that make up the tissues and organs. It is quite a remarkable structure.

All cells are made up of four basic structures, referred to as biomolecules: proteins, lipids, carbohydrates, and nucleic acids. Their structures can vary from simple to very complex, but they combine together to perform all the functions and provide all the structures of the cell. Each chromosome, for example, that was described as being present in the nucleus of the cell contains one long thread of DNA (a nucleic acid), which is wrapped around various types of proteins. The cell membrane is made up of a double layer of lipid-based molecules (one to the outside and one to the inside), but includes various types of proteins integrated into the lipid structure, such as "glycoproteins" (proteins that have attached carbohydrates). Examples of each type of biomolecule are given in Table 2.2. If we look at one of the structures of these biomolecules (for example, starch), we find that it is made up of a basic unit of structure (glucose) that is itself constructed from various different types of chemical elements (Figure 2.2).

Chemistry is the study of chemicals and chemical reactions. Chemical elements are the essential building blocks of chemistry, including all living and non-living things. Examples include oxygen (also known by its chemical symbol O), nitrogen (N), calcium (Ca), silver (Ag), and gold (Au). Elements can exist on their own (e.g. gold, silver) or combine together to form molecules (e.g. H_2O, the chemical symbol for water, made up of two hydrogens and one oxygen). A molecule is therefore made up of two or more elements. There are over 100 types of elements that have been identified, but only six are actually used in the different types of biomolecules that make up the various cells, tissues, organs, and systems of the body: carbon, hydrogen, nitrogen, oxygen, sulfur, and phosphorus.

Table 2.2 Examples of the four biomolecules that make up cellular structure and function.

Biomolecule	Examples	Basic unit
Nucleic acids (polynucleotides)	DNA, RNA	Nucleotides
Proteins (peptides, polypeptides)	Enzymes, keratin, albumin	Amino acids
Carbohydrates (saccharides)	"Sugars," starch, cellulose, polysaccharides	Monosaccharides
Lipids	Fat, oil, glycolipids, sterols	Structurally diverse but many based on fatty acids

DNA, deoxyribonucleic acid; RNA, ribonucleic acid.

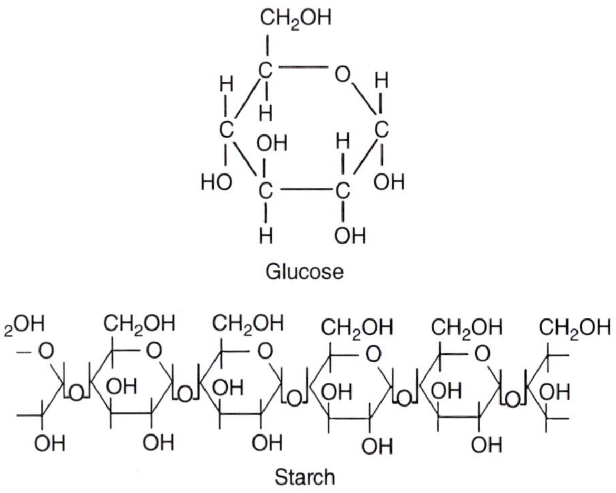

Figure 2.2 The chemical structure of glucose and starch, types of sugars or carbohydrates. Glucose is made up of atoms from three types of chemical elements: carbon (C), hydrogen (H), and oxygen (O). The chemical way of describing glucose is $C_6H_{12}O_6$, with the numbers of each type of element identified. Note that starch is essentially a polymer of glucose, consisting of long lines of glucose bound together.

As shown in Figure 2.2, glucose and starch (which are types of carbohydrates) are made up of only three elements (hydrogen, oxygen, and carbon). One unit (or molecule) of glucose is actually composed of 6 carbon (C), 12 hydrogen (H), and 6 oxygen (O) atoms and can be written in chemical terms as $C_6H_{12}O_6$. Starch is a polymer of glucose, being a rather large molecule consisting of repeated units of glucose linked together. In another example, DNA is a polymer of nucleotides. In the structure of DNA there are only four types of nucleotides (as defined by their bases: adenine, thymine, cytosine, and guanine); it is remarkable to think that all the genes in human DNA are made up of only these four types and it is their sequence that dictates all the structure and functions that make us human and all different.

Anatomy terminology

In surgical or diagnostic practice there are a number of key definitions that will help you understand the terminology that is frequently used. The human body can be examined in an upright position, with the palms of the hands turned out (Figure 2.3). This is referred to as the anatomical position. In this position, the body can be considered as having five major sections: the head, neck, trunk/back, upper limb, and lower limb. The front of the body is considered as the "anterior" and the back as the "posterior." A summary of the different regions of the body, with both their common and anatomical names, is given in Figure 2.3. Many of these terms may already be familiar to you. These regions can be further sub-divided. For example, the trunk (or torso) can be sub-divided into various regions from the top of the chest to just above the pubic area, such as the epigastric (just below the nipples), umbilical (the area of the belly button), and hypogastric (upper pubic) regions.

Another position of the human body under examination when the body is face up on a surgical table is referred to as being in a "supine" position, the most commonly perceived position for surgical procedures and in contrast to being face down (in the "prone" position). In fact, the surgical procedure may take place in a variety of positions, depending on many factors such as the type of surgery, the surgeon, and available surgical equipment.

Next let us consider some of the most common terms that are used to describe the position of one part of the body in relation to another part, which are also referred to as "directional" terms. For the purpose of this description, the same anatomical position is considered with a single line drawn through the center of the body from the top to the bottom, referred to as the "midline." The most widely used directional terms are summarized in Figure 2.4. These terms can be used to refer to various organs and structures both on the outside of (external) and inside (internal) the body.

Before we describe the various anatomical systems, there are a number of defined body spaces, known as "cavities," that should be mentioned. A cavity may be defined as a space within the body that contains, supports, protects, and separates the various internal organs. In the human body a cavity can be either open or closed from the external environment. For example, open cavities consist of the oral, nasal, and alimentary (or digestive) cavities. There are two major closed cavities within the body, the ventral and the dorsal, which can be further sub-divided as follows (Figure 2.5). The dorsal cavity is made up of the cranial (containing the brain) and vertebral (containing the spinal cord) areas. The ventral cavity, the largest

Basic anatomy, physiology, and biochemistry 21

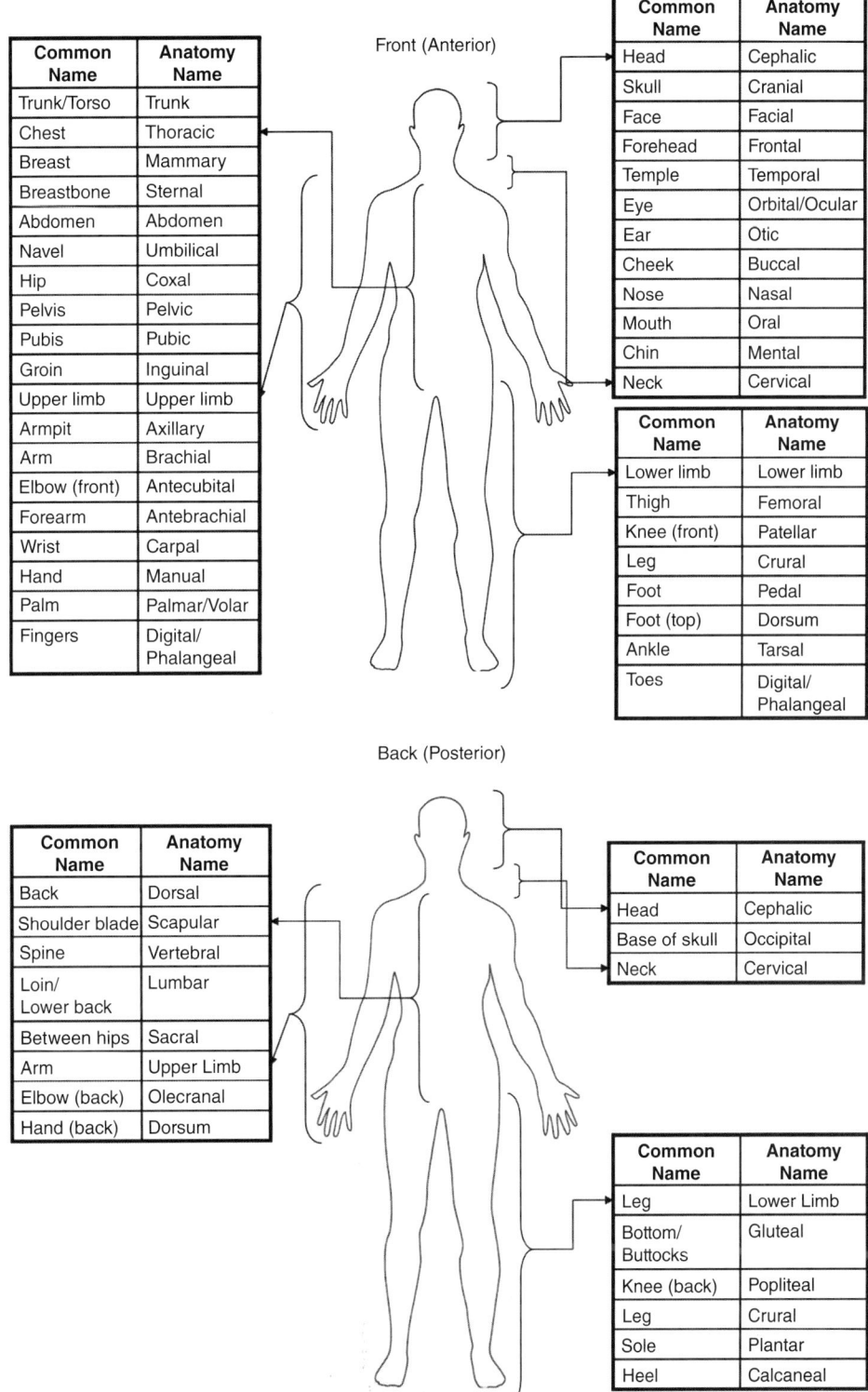

Figure 2.3 Common and anatomical names for various parts of the human body.

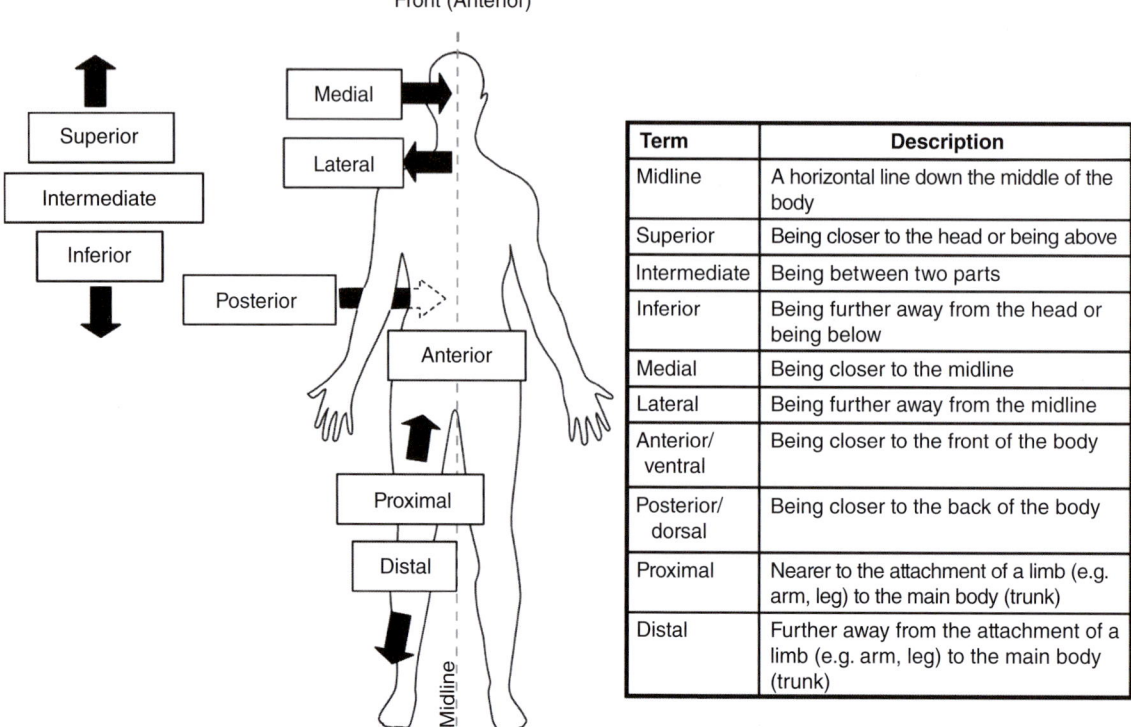

Figure 2.4 The most common directional anatomical terms used in anatomy.

body cavity, is divided into two parts, the thoracic and the abdominal pelvic area, which are separated by the diaphragm. The thoracic cavity contains the lungs (referred to as the "pleural cavity") and the other organs in the area (such as the heart, esophagus, and trachea within the mediastinal cavity); the heart may be considered to be a separate area in its own right known as the "pericardial cavity." The abdominal-pelvic cavity is sub-divided into two sections: the abdominal (including the stomach, liver, pancreas, and most of the intestines) and the pelvic (including the bladder and reproductive organs).

The anatomical systems of the human body

All in all, the human body is a complex organization of systems. There are 11 major systems of the human body and these are summarized in Table 2.3. A very brief description in alphabetical order of each system, their functions, and the major organs are described in the following sections.

Cardiovascular

The cardiovascular system consists of the heart, various blood vessels, and the blood itself that circulates around the body (Figure 2.6). Blood is a type of connective tissue consisting of two parts: the plasma (a watery-type liquid) and various types of cells/cell fragments (often called the "formed elements"). Plasma is similar to the "interstitial" fluid that surrounds the various cells in the body and to the lymph that circulates through the lymphatic system (see the section on the lymphatic system). The blood moves around the body through the various types of blood vessels and is pumped by the heart.

Structure

Blood consists of two major components: the plasma and the cell/cell fragment component. The plasma is a pale, yellow liquid that consists of ~92% water, the remainder being various types of plasma proteins and other components (such as nutrients, waste products, and dissolved gases). The cell/cell fragment part consists of red blood cells (RBCs), white blood cells (WBCs), and platelets. They are all produced in a process known as hemopoesis, primarily from the red bone marrow of the skeletal system (see the section on the skeletal system). The platelets are not cells but cell fragments, produced from specialized cells known as megakaryocytes; they are primarily involved

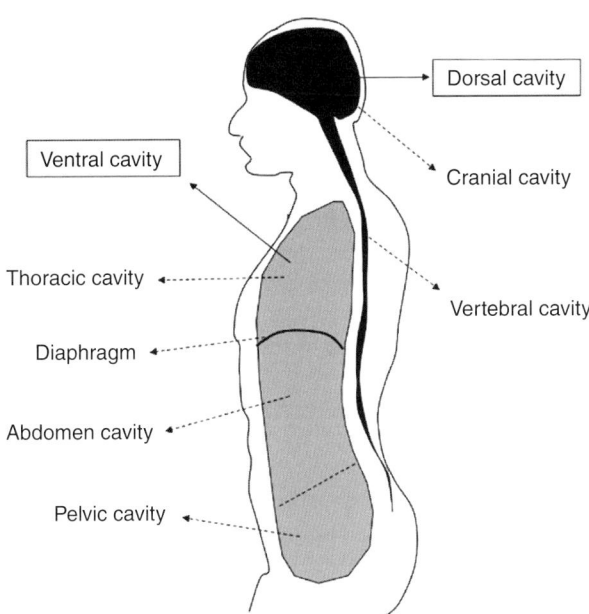

Figure 2.5 Major and minor human body cavities. Note that the abdominal and pelvic cavities are not physically separated and are continuous. This cavity is also referred to as abdominopelvic (a dotted line shows the approximate area of separation). The diaphragm physically separates the ventral cavity into the thoracic and abdominopelvic cavities.

in the generation of blood clots to prevent the loss of blood from the cardiovascular system (e.g. due to blood vessel rupture or skin cuts). RBCs and WBCs are living cells. RBCs (also known as erythrocytes) give blood its characteristic red color due to the presence of a unique protein (or pigment) called hemoglobin. Hemoglobin plays an important role in the transport of oxygen through the blood (and in a certain part carbon dioxide). WBCs (also known as leukocytes) consist of many different types of cells such as neutrophils, eosinophils, lymphocytes, and monocytes; they are all involved in the body's immune system, protecting the body from the invasion of various types of microorganisms (e.g. bacteria and viruses).

The blood is carried through the body via a series of blood vessels (the vascular system). They are referred to as arteries, arterioles, capillaries, venules, and veins. Blood vessels are similar but vary in their individual structures. For example, arteries have thicker muscle layers in their structure than most veins. The arteries are larger vessels that take blood from the heart to the various organs and parts of the body. Arteries subdivide into arterioles and then into capillaries that supply the various cells of the body. Conversely, venules and then the larger veins take blood back to the heart. The blood vessels have various names depending on the areas of the body they provide blood to. Examples include:

- Coronary: to and from the heart muscle tissue.
- Pulmonary: to and from the lungs.

Others have specific names, such as the aorta (the largest artery in the body providing blood to the body) and the vena cava (superior and inferior veins being two of the main veins from the upper and lower parts of the body, respectively).

The heart lies slightly to the left side of the thoracic cavity, just above the diaphragm in an area known as the mediastinum (Figure 2.7). It does vary in size depending on the individual, but is approximately the size of a clenched fist in the same person. From the outside in, the heart consists of an external membrane (the pericardium) and a three-layered wall (consisting of an epicardium, myocardium, and endocardium layer, from the outside in). The myocardium contains the muscle cells of the heart that are responsible for its pumping action. The endocardium is the innermost layer that lines the cavities of the heart and forms part of the heart valves. The heart is divided into four inner chambers (Figure 2.7) that make up two distinct pumping systems (a "right" and a "left" system). Each pumping system consists of an upper chamber (called an atrium) and a lower chamber (the ventricle; Figure 2.7). In each system the blood enters the atrium from the supplying veins, passes into the lower ventricles, and is pumped out into the various arteries. The right system is called the pulmonary system, which takes blood being returned from the body and pumps it to the lungs to take up oxygen. The left system receives the oxygenated blood returning from the lungs and pumps it to the rest of the body through the aorta. In both cases, the blood flowing through the heart is controlled by the muscles and four major valves (two in each system) to ensure a one-way flow of blood.

Functions

The cardiovascular system has three major functions: transportation, protection, and regulation:

- Transportation: blood carries various substances to and from the various cells of the body. Nutrients absorbed from the digestive system (see the section on the digestive system) and oxygen from the lungs (see the section on respiration) are transferred to cells through the interstitial fluid surrounding them. Similarly, various wastes (including carbon dioxide) are taken up by the blood and transferred to different organs for elimination from the body (such as the skin, lungs, digestive system, and kidneys).
- Protection from disease/damage: blood (in particular the platelets) can form clots that stop the loss of blood from the cardiovascular system (e.g. due to a cut on the skin) and allow for a platform from which the body can repair the damage.

Table 2.3 A summary of the anatomical systems of the human body.

System	Common names	Organ and component examples	Function
Cardiovascular	Circulatory system, blood	Heart, veins, arteries	Circulation of blood around the body Carries oxygen, nutrients, and wastes to and from cells Regulates temperature and water levels Defends against disease and repairs damaged tissues
Digestive	Eating, drinking, waste disposal	Mouth, stomach, intestines, rectum	Food intake, digestion, nutrient adsorption, and waste elimination

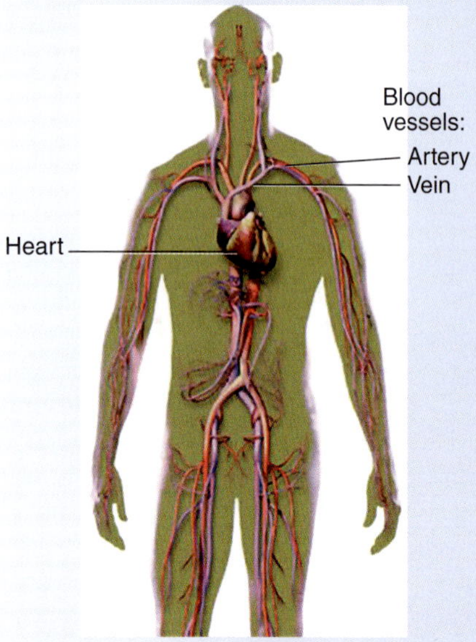

Figure 2.6 The cardiovascular system.

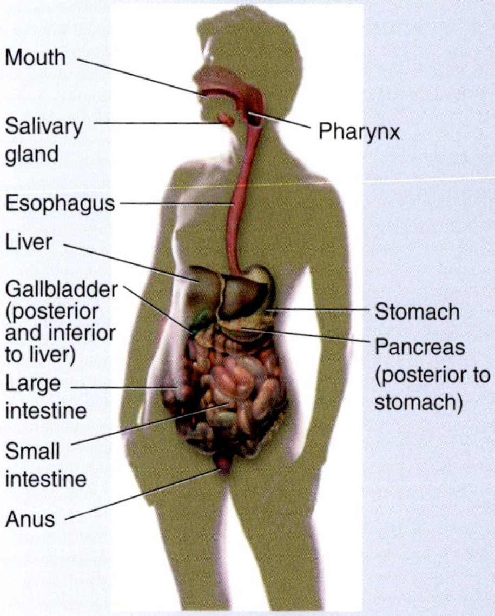

Figure 2.8 The digestive system.

Basic anatomy, physiology, and biochemistry 25

Table 2.3 (cont'd).

System	Common names	Organ and component examples	Function
Endocrine (see Figure 2.9)	Hormones	Adrenal glands, pituitary glands, ovaries, testes, thyroid	Controls various functions in the body by releasing special chemicals known as hormones (e.g. insulin, estrogen, and testosterone)
Integumentary	Skin	Skin, hair, nails	Senses (touch, taste, pain, etc.), protection, temperature regulation

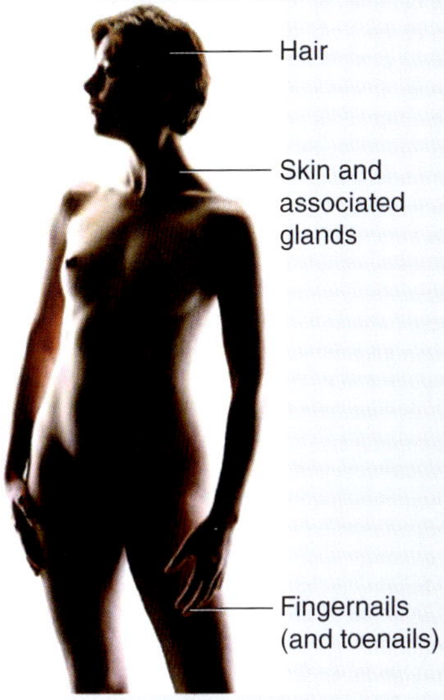

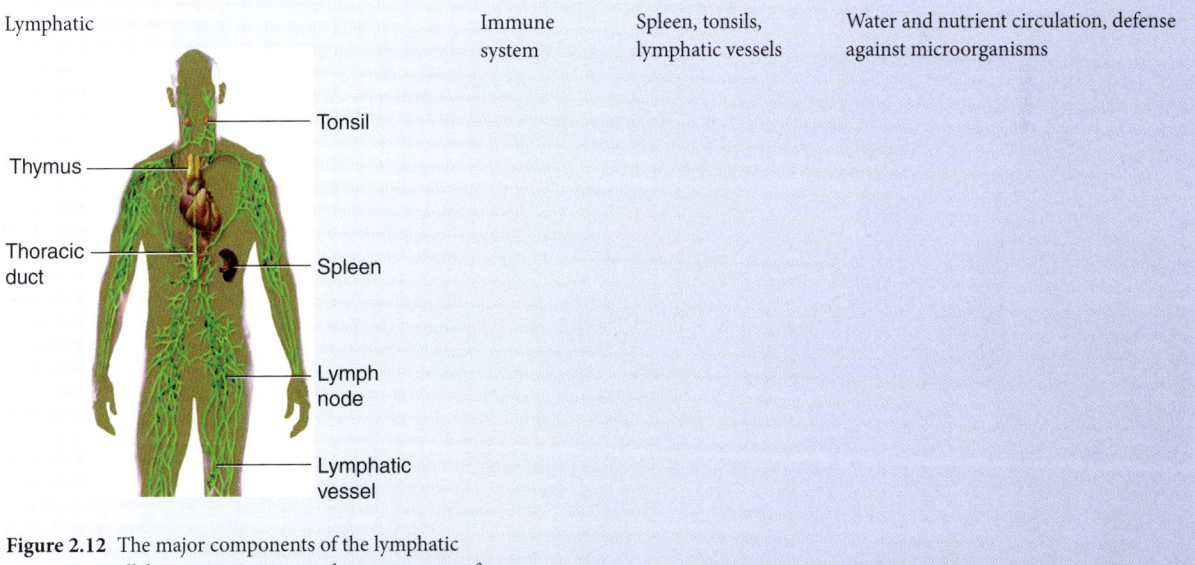

Figure 2.10 The integumentary (or "skin") system.

Lymphatic	Immune system	Spleen, tonsils, lymphatic vessels	Water and nutrient circulation, defense against microorganisms

Figure 2.12 The major components of the lymphatic system, a parallel transport system to the venous part of the circulatory (blood) system.

(continued)

Table 2.3 (cont'd).

System	Common names	Organ and component examples	Function
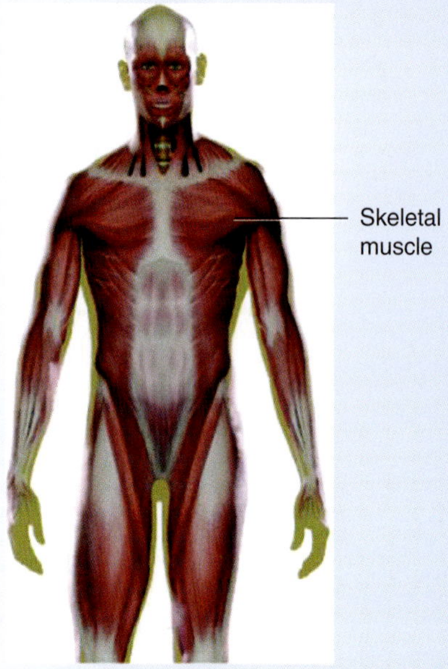 Muscular	Muscle, movement	Biceps, triceps, hamstrings	Movement, heat generation

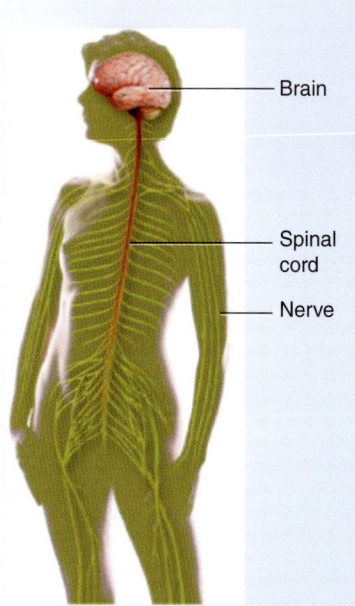

Figure 2.13 The muscular system.

System	Common names	Organ and component examples	Function
Nervous	Nerves, brain	Brain, spinal cord, optic nerve	Regulates the body's activities

Figure 2.14 The nervous system.

Table 2.3 (*cont'd*).

System	Common names	Organ and component examples	Function
Reproductive	Sex	Testes, ovaries, uterus	Reproduction

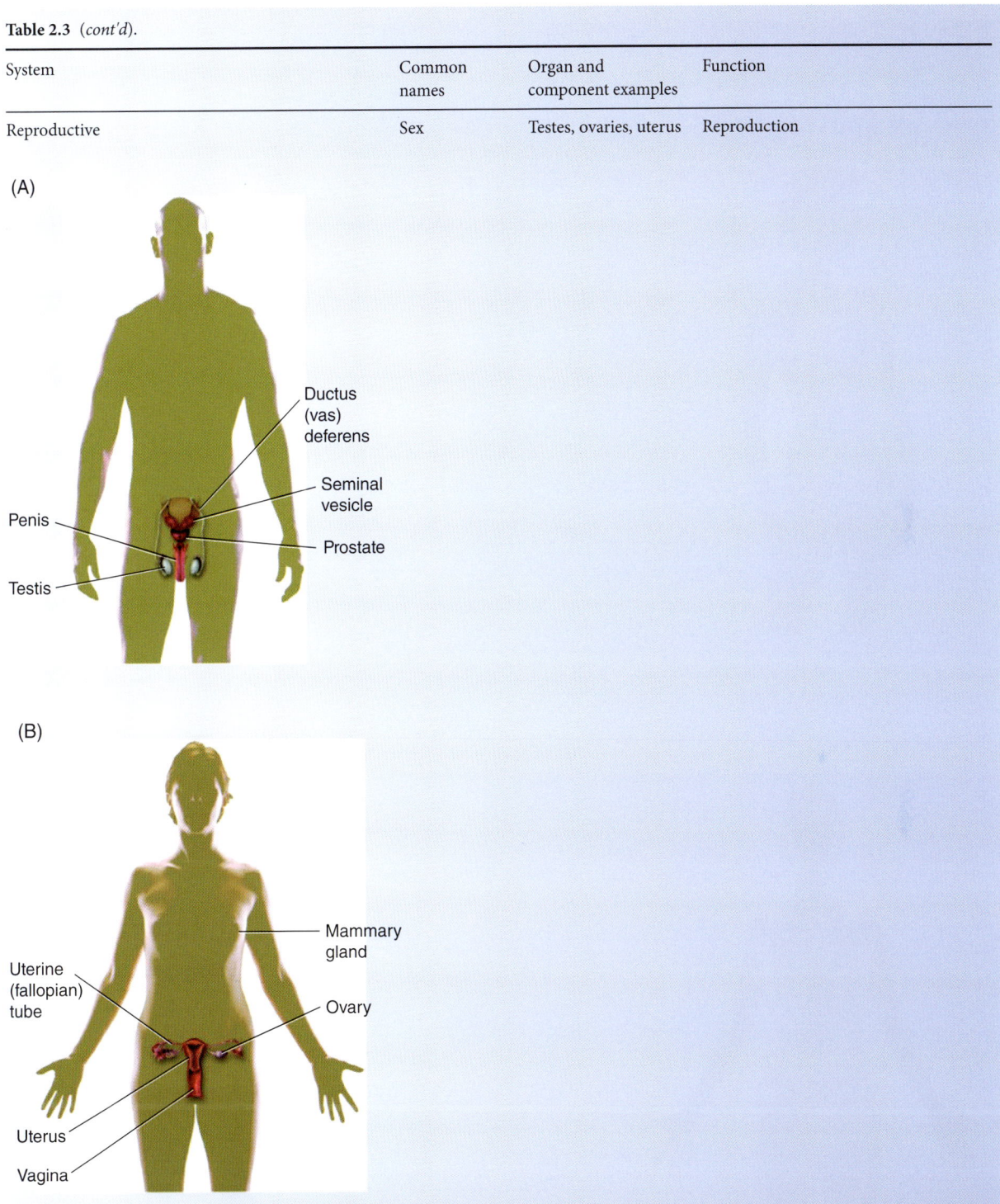

Figure 2.16 The reproductive system, showing the major components of (A) the male and (B) the female systems.

(*continued*)

Table 2.3 (cont'd).

System	Common names	Organ and component examples	Function
Respiratory 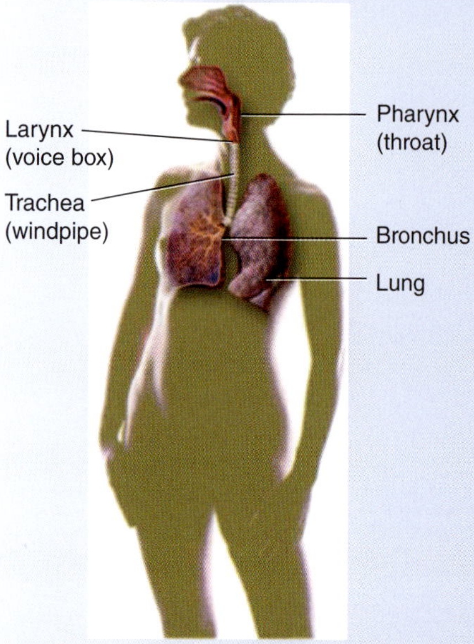	Breathing	Lungs, larynx, bronchus	Bringing in oxygen and removing wastes such as carbon dioxide Speaking
Skeletal (including dental)	Bones, teeth, skeleton	Skull, femur, pelvis, molars	Body support and protection

Figure 2.17 The respiratory system, consisting of the upper and lower tracts/systems.

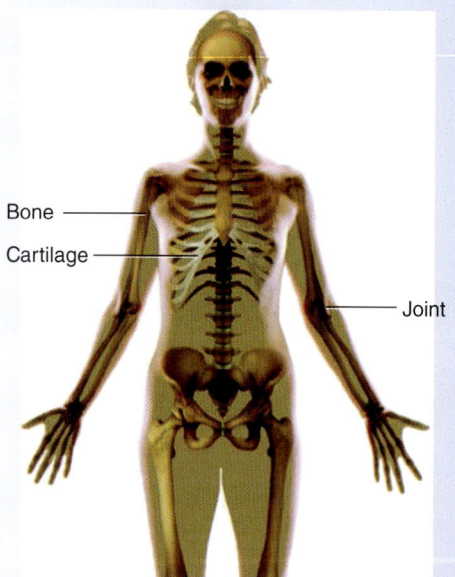

Figure 2.18 The skeletal system.

System	Common names	Organ and component examples	Function
Urinary	Urine, excretion	Kidneys, bladder	Urine generation and excretion, maintaining mineral balance

Table 2.3 (cont'd).

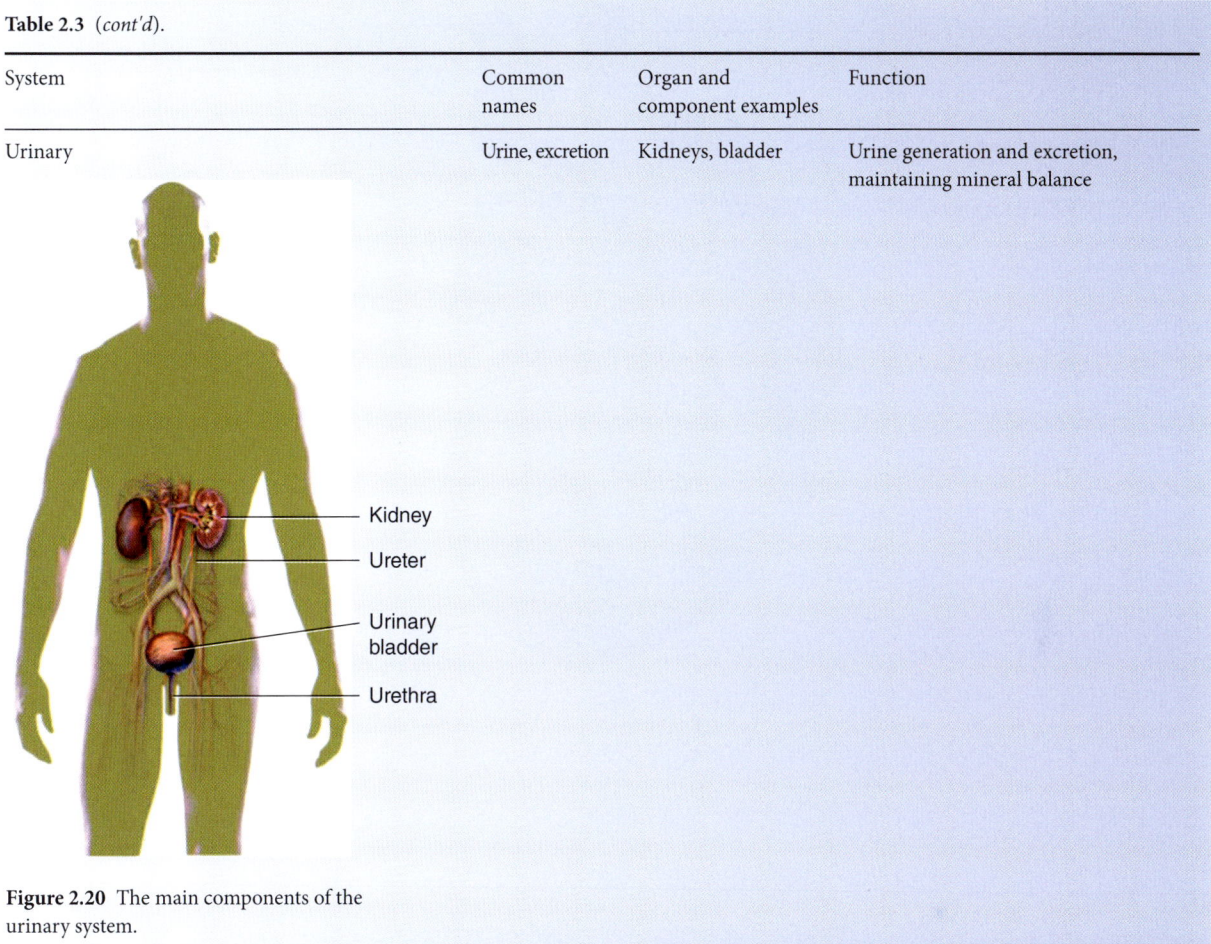

Figure 2.20 The main components of the urinary system.

The blood also contains various types of cells (WBCs) and proteins (such as antibodies) that are actively involved in the body's immune system to protect it against the invasion of various microorganisms and associated diseases.
- Regulation: the blood system is involved in regulating the different body fluids, temperature, and pH balance (how acidic or alkaline the blood is; see Chapter 6) to ensure proper functioning of the various organs and body parts.

Additional comments

Hematology is the study of blood, the tissues that form blood, and the various types of blood diseases and disorders. Different blood types are defined in hematology. For example, the ABO-type system of defined blood type is based on the presence of different types of proteins (in this case referred to as antigens) that are present on the surface of RBCs; individuals with only type A or B antigens are called types A or B, respectively; those with both A and B are called type AB; and those with neither are called type O. Similar antigens are used to define an individual as being type Rhesus$^+$ or Rhesus$^-$ (being the presence or absence of another type of antigen). These are important where the blood is being taken from one person and placed into another in a process known as transfusion, to ensure that the recipient does not have an adverse reaction to the transfused blood.

Other commonly used terms in the study of blood are "septicemia" (commonly known as blood poisoning), describing where microorganisms (particularly bacteria and their associated toxins) have entered the blood during an infection (Chapter 5), and "hemorrhage," describing the loss of a large amount of blood from the system either internally (inside the body) or externally (outside the body).

Cardiology is the study of the heart and associated diseases. An important example is coronary artery disease or disease of the arteries supplying the heart muscles. This is a leading cause of death in humans due to the development of restrictions in these blood vessels, which can in its most severe case lead to heart attacks. These conditions can be

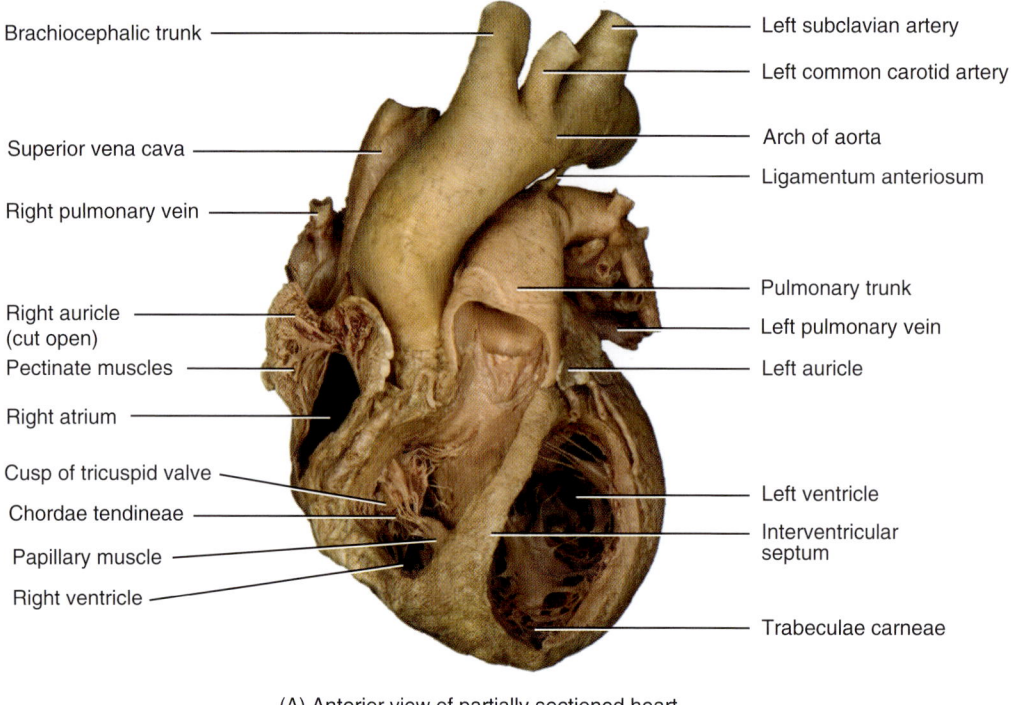

(A) Anterior view of partially sectioned heart

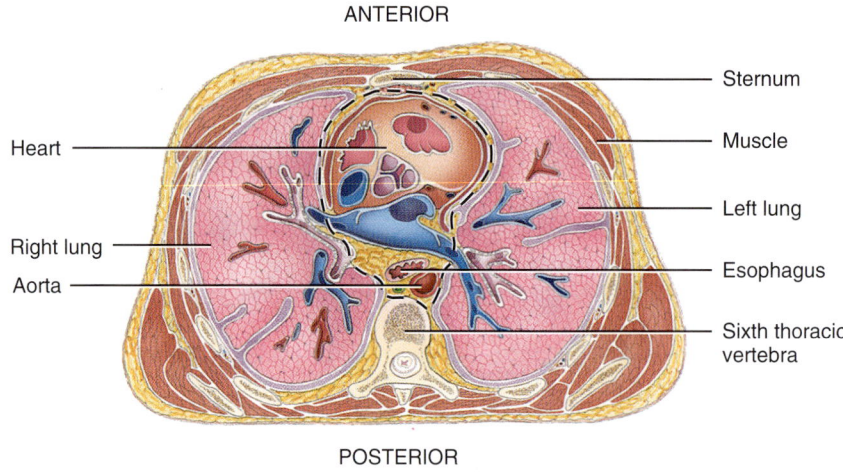

(B) Inferior view of transverse section of thoracic cavity showing the heart in the mediastinum

Figure 2.7 (A, B) The position and structure of the heart. Source: Reproduced with permission from Tortora et al. (2011) / John Wiley & Sons.

treated surgically in a procedure known as coronary artery by-pass grafting (CABG or by-pass surgery), where a blood vessel from another part of the body is taken out and attached to the affected artery to by-pass the blockage. Alternatively, this can be treated non-surgically by percutaneous transluminal coronary angioplasty (PTCA or balloon angioplasty), where a special type of device (known as a balloon catheter) is entered into the affected area, inflated to squash the blockage, and then withdrawn. Medical device technologies based on catheter designs (e.g. cardiac catheterization or coronary angiogram) for the treatment or diagnosis of coronary diseases (or using the bloodstream for access to various parts of the body) continue to develop in complexity.

Digestive

The digestive system is responsible for the breakdown ("digestion") and absorption of the various foods and nutrients required for the structure and function of the body. The system consists of two parts: the gastrointestinal (GI) tract (or alimentary canal) and its associated organs (such as the liver and pancreas; Figure 2.8). The alimentary canal part is a continuous tube or tract that starts at the mouth, goes through the esophagus, stomach, small and large intestines, and rectum, and exits at the anus. It is extremely long (~6.5 m in length in a typical adult), but is folded in a way to fit into a smaller area. The basic structure in humans is described further in this section, but it is essentially similar in other mammals, although distinct in other ways (e.g. some mammals have a multi-chambered stomach, as opposed to a single-chambered human stomach).

Structure

The GI tract, being one long continuous tubular structure, is made up of the same basic structure along its length, although there are distinct differences that reflect the various functions of the different areas of the tract (e.g. the stomach is primarily for mixing and initial digestion, in contrast to the optimal structure in the small intestine for absorption of the various nutrients). The structure consists of four layers, from the outside in to the body: the outer serosa layer, the muscularis externa (containing various types and thicknesses of muscle tissue depending on the particular part of the GI tract), the submucosa (which is rich in blood vessels and nerves), and finally the inner mucosa layer (including the innermost lining of epithelial cells that secrete fluids such as mucus and are also responsible for the absorption of nutrients to be taken up by the blood system). The GI tract consists of various organs; starting at the entry point these are the mouth, pharynx, esophagus, stomach, small intestine, large intestine, rectum, and anus. The first part of the tract is referred to as the upper GI, extending from the mouth to the stomach, with the lower GI referring to the intestines and rectum/anus.

In addition, the accessory organs to the digestive system include the salivary glands, the liver, the pancreas, and the gall bladder. These are briefly described in the following section.

The entry of the digestive system is the mouth (the oral or "buccal" cavity), which includes three types of accessory organs, namely the salivary glands, the tongue, and the teeth (for further discussion on the teeth, refer to the skeletal section). This area provides initial mechanical digestion of food (by mastication or chewing), as well as providing taste (or "gestation") due to the location of special sensory organs mainly on the surface of the tongue (known as taste buds). The accessory salivary organs (three types known as the parotid, submandibular, and sublingual glands) produce a watery-type secretion (known as saliva) in the mouth, which aids in lubrication and chemical digestion. Saliva consists mainly of water (~99%), but contains various types of enzymes (amylase and lipase) and salts. Enzymes are protein molecules that speed up a chemical reaction (but are not themselves changed in doing so); their primary role in digestion is the breakdown of various types of food molecules. In this case amylase breaks down starch (a type of carbohydrate) and lipase breaks down fats (types of lipids) into smaller parts to allow their absorption further down the GI tract. More discussion of enzymes and their use in cleaning chemistry applications is given in Chapter 6.

The food next moves into an area after the mouth known as the pharynx (or the throat), which acts in swallowing and passing food/liquids into the esophagus. The esophagus is a tube that runs from the pharynx to the stomach. Swallowing, or deglutition, is controlled by voluntary muscle contraction in the upper esophagus to force food into the lower esophagus, where a process known as peristalsis ensures that the food is pushed along to the stomach. Both the pharynx and the esophagus produce mucus, which aids in this process by lubrication. The stomach is an enlarged, J-shaped organ that acts as a mixing and digesting area before the intestine. As part of the digestive process it produces gastric juice (produced by gastric glands) and provides a more acidic environment for digestion. Gastric juice contains a low concentration of hydrochloric acid (HCl) and enzymes, such as pepsin (a protease) and gastric lipase, which work optimally under acidic conditions; it is the combination of enzymatic and acidic processes that digests the various foods.

The stomach also controls the rate of entry of food into the first part of the small intestine called the duodenum. Further digestion in this area is dependent on various other organs associated with the GI tract: the liver, gall bladder, and pancreas, all adjacent to the duodenum. The liver is the largest organ in the body and is divided into lobes. Its structure is primarily made up of specialized cells known as hepatocytes; these cells perform many key roles in body metabolism including, as part of the digestive process, secretion of a substance known as bile (which is involved in the digestion and absorption of lipids). Other important functions include controlling carbohydrate (glucose) levels in the blood, controlling lipid and protein metabolism, detoxification of various substances harmful to the body, and nutrient storage (including carbohydrate, vitamins, and minerals). Bile is stored in the gall bladder, located just outside the liver (Figure 2.8). The pancreas is also located adjacent to the duodenum and has two key functions: the majority of the cells that make up the pancreas are involved in the digestion process and produce pancreatic juice (its so-called exocrine function) and a smaller proportion of cells (known as the "islets of Langerhans") specifically produce hormones as part of the endocrine system (see the section on the endocrine system) and are therefore referred to as the endocrine function; the hormones include glucagon and insulin, both involved in the maintenance of glucose levels in the blood. Pancreatic juice contains multiple enzymes involved in the digestion of carbohydrates (e.g. amylase and trypsin), a lipase and others, in combination with water and salts.

The small intestine is made up of three regions (from the stomach to the large intestine): the duodenum, the jejunum, and the longer part known as the ileum. It is in the small intestine that digestion continues and particularly absorption of nutrients into the body takes place, primarily due to its length and increased surface area resulting from the presence of many folds and finger-like projections known as villi on its internal surface. Specific types of cells produce mucus (known as goblet cells) and absorb nutrients ("absorptive cells"). Digestion is performed over time by a combination of the presence of bile, pancreatic juice, and the production of intestinal juice. Intestinal juice is at a slightly neutral pH (pH 7.6) and is made up of primarily water, mucus, and further enzymes (including those breaking down protein and carbohydrate). In all, about 90% of nutrients and water is absorbed in the small intestine. The remaining material next moves into the larger intestine, which is sub-divided into four regions known as the cecum, colon, rectum, and the anal canal. It is in this area that any final absorption takes place, but particularly water, various vitamins, and minerals, with any remaining material considered as feces and passed out of the body. The inner wall of the large intestine also contains specific absorptive and goblet (mucus-secreting, but in this case not enzyme-secreting) cells, but does not have the same convoluted structure as the small intestine. Large amounts of bacteria are also present in the large intestine, which can play an important role in the digestive and adsorption processes.

Functions

The major role of the digestive system is the acquisition of nutrients for the body, which can be sub-divided into four functions:
- Ingestion, including the eating of food and drinking of liquids. This is performed in the mouth in combination with various accessory organs such as the tongue and teeth, to provide mixing.
- Digestion, which is performed both mechanically (e.g. in the mouth with the aid of teeth and in the stomach) and chemically. Chemical digestion includes the use of both acid and alkaline pH conditions, as well as the various enzymes produced during passage through the GI tract. During this process the various proteins, carbohydrates, and lipids are broken down into smaller, absorbable molecules that are taken up by the body.
- Absorption, or the uptake of nutrients into the body (the blood system; see the section on the cardiovascular system) is performed by specialized epithelial cells lining the inner surfaces of the system, and particularly in the small and large intestines.
- Defecation or waste removal, with the ridding of feces from the system.

In addition to their digestive functions the pancreas and liver, as accessory organs of the system, have other key roles. The pancreas is a major part of the body endocrine system (see the section on the endocrine system) and the liver is involved in toxic substance detoxification, nutrient metabolism, and storage.

Additional comments

Gastroenterology is the study of the structure, function, and diseases of the stomach and intestines, while proctology specifically relates to the lower part of the GI tract (the rectum and anus).

Flexible endoscopes are instruments (or devices) that are used for minimal invasive diagnostic and surgical procedures (Chapters 4 and 15). Although they were initially designed for diagnostic purposes, for the direct visualization of various internal parts of the body and in particular the digestive system, they are being increasingly used for surgical procedures penetrating the internal surface of the various parts of the system. There are many types of endoscopes designed for use in different areas of the GI tract. These include:
- Colonoscopes: for "lower endoscopy" viewing, particularly the large intestine, by entering the anus.
- Gastroscopes: for "upper endoscopy" viewing of the stomach by insertion through the mouth.
- Duodenoscopes: for observing the duodenum and associated ducts (e.g. to the liver, gall bladder, and pancreas) by insertion through the mouth and through the stomach.

Endocrine

The endocrine and nervous systems (see the section on the nervous system) work together to control the various functions of the body. In the nervous system this is controlled by a connecting system of specialized cells (called neurons) that rapidly communicate with each other and various organs. In the endocrine system this is due to the production of specialized chemical substances, known as hormones. The system is made up of a diverse number of organs known as the endocrine glands and parts of other organs that contain endocrine tissue (Figure 2.9).

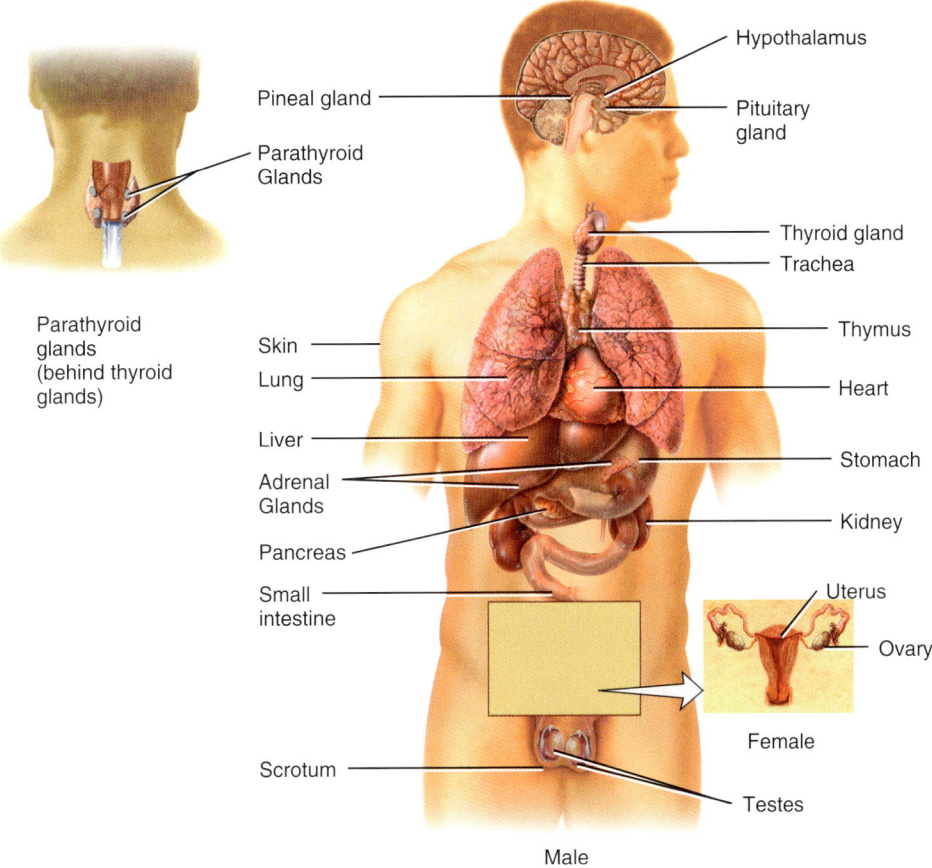

Figure 2.9 The endocrine system. The location of the major endocrine glands is shown, in addition to various other parts of the body that contain endocrine tissue. Source: Reproduced with permission from Tortora et al. (2011) / John Wiley & Sons

Structure

Endocrine tissue, either as part of a whole organ (specifically known as a "gland") or as part of another organ with other functions, is composed of specialized cells that produce the various different types of hormones. Glands are defined as specialized groups of cells within the body that secrete various substances and are sub-divided in anatomy into two types: endocrine and exocrine glands. The endocrine glands secrete hormones into the body (being taken up into the blood, which then transfers them to the various cells of the body) and exocrine glands secrete substances into specialized ducts for transfer to and even outside the body, for example the sweat glands in the skin (see the section on the integumentary system) and the various digestive glands (see the section on the digestive system). A summary of the major endocrine glands, the hormones they produce, and their specific effects is given in Table 2.4. Many glands are primarily involved with hormone production (such as the adrenal and thyroid glands, which are known as the primary endocrine glands), while other organs are involved in many other functions for other systems. In addition to the organs listed in Table 2.4, these secondary organs include:

- The kidneys (urinary section), which produce many hormones such as erythropoietin that controls RBC production.
- The heart (cardiovascular section), which produces a hormone known as atrial natriuretic peptide (ANP) that is involved in controlling blood pressure.
- Various parts of the GI tract (see the digestive section), which produce hormones that regulate digestion, such as gastrin, produced in the stomach and stimulates the local production of acid, and secretin, produced in the duodenum and stimulates secretion from the pancreas (see the section on the endocrine system), the kidneys (see the section on the urinary system), and the testes/ovaries (see the section on the reproductive system).

Hormones are released at very low concentrations but have powerful effects on the cells they contact. However, not all cells are capable of reacting with the various hormones when

Table 2.4 A summary of the major primary endocrine glands and secondary organs that contain endocrine tissue, with examples of the associated hormones they produce and their functions.

Endocrine gland/organ	Hormones produced	Function(s)
Major glands		
Hypothalamus	Hypothalamic releasing and inhibitory hormones	Controls the release of various hormones from the pituitary gland
Pituitary gland	Major hormone-producing gland of the body, including: • Human growth hormone (somatotropin) • Thyroid-stimulating hormone (thyrotropin) prolactin • "Gonadotropins" • Antidiuretic hormone (vasopressin)	Produces many hormones that control the functions of other endocrine glands: • Stimulates production of a range of hormones that regulate growth and metabolism • Control of the thyroid gland • Milk production from the mammary glands • A number of hormones involved in controlling the ovaries/testes • Controls water loss from the body
Pineal gland	Melatonin	Involved in regulating the body's "biological clock" or rhythms Other hormones and functions are proposed but are not fully defined
Thyroid gland	Thyroid hormones (thyroxine, triiodothyronine)	Multiple functions including growth and cell metabolism
Parathyroid gland	Parathyroid hormone (parathormone)	Bone breakdown ("reabsorption"; see section on the skeletal system)
Thymus	Thymosin Thymic factor	Controls the production of cells involved in immunity (e.g. T-cells, see section on the lymphatic system)
Adrenal glands	Produce a variety of hormones including aldosterone, cortisol, epinephrine ("adrenaline")	Water/salt blood level control Stress response (affecting glucose metabolism) Stress response ("flight or fight")
Secondary organs (examples)		
Pancreas	Variety of hormones, but particularly glucagon and insulin	Blood sugar (glucose) level control Glucagon raises and insulin decreases levels in the blood
Ovaries (in females)	Female sex hormones (e.g. estrogens and progesterone)	Regulate the female productive cycle and female body characteristics
Testes (in males)	Male sex hormones (e.g. testosterone)	Regulate the production of sperm and male body characteristics

they are released, which will depend on the types of cells and the specific hormone. Hormones are often classified into three types based on structures:
• Amino acid-derived, specifically from the amino acids tyrosine and tryptophan (e.g. thyroxine, adrenalin).
• Peptide or protein based (e.g. insulin).
• Lipid based (e.g. testosterone).

Functions
The endocrine system and the nervous system (see the section on the nervous system) are the informational and signaling systems of the body, essentially controlling the various body functions. The major roles of the endocrine system are:
• Controlling body growth and metabolism.
• Controlling the expression of male or female characteristics and reproduction (the process of generating offspring).
• Control of body rhythms and stress responses.
• Regulation of body fluids, metabolism, various secretions, and some immune (protection) functions.

The specific functions of some of the major hormones produced from the endocrine system that have been described in some detail are given in Table 2.4.

Additional comments
Endocrinology is the study of the endocrine system, including associated diseases. Hormone balance is important to the various functions of the body, so much so that even slight imbalances can have significant physiological and emotional effects. For example, the various forms of diabetes are due to the inability of the body (specifically the pancreas) to produce or to use insulin effectively. Insulin is involved in stimulating (and therefore controlling) the

lowering of glucose levels in the blood. Diabetes remains a major cause of death in humans. Other examples of endocrine-based diseases include polycystic ovary syndrome, hypothyroidism, osteoporosis, and Addison's disease.

Growth factors are substances (or chemicals) that stimulate cell production, growth, differentiation (into the various types of cells), and even cell death. They include various types of hormones and cytokines. Cytokines are in many ways similar to hormones; they are protein-based substances, with examples including the interleukins. They all essentially allow communication between cells/organs. In addition to their natural functions in the body, various growth factors are also used artificially in the treatment of certain blood and cancer diseases.

Integumentary

The integumentary system includes the skin and its associated structures. The name takes its origin from the Latin meaning "to cover the body" (Figure 2.10).

The skin is actually the largest system in the body. It includes the skin itself, but also the various external structures attached to the skin that we can see, such as hair and nails, and those within the skin structure that we do not see, such as sweat glands and sensory receptors. Dermatology is the study of the structure and treatment of the integumentary system and its associated diseases.

Structure

If we section ("cut through") and examine the structure of the skin microscopically we find that it consists of three layers: the outer epidermis, the inner dermis, and the lower hypodermis (or subcutaneous) layer (Figure 2.11). The epidermis is a thin, external layer of cells (a type of epithelial tissue; see the introductory section); it is a tough structure, composed of high concentrations of a certain type of protein called keratin that protects the more sensitive internal layers from damage. It is also this area that gives the skin color due to the production of a specific pigment known as melanin. The epidermis is continually growing from the inside out, accumulating more keratin as it grows, to eventually become released from the surface as skin flakes or in obvious excessive conditions such as "peeling" following sunburn or with dandruff. Beneath the epidermis is the dermis layer, which is primarily composed of different types of tissues (connective tissues containing proteins such as collagen and elastin). The dermis gives the skin flexibility, but also strength. It is within this layer that we see many of the associated structures of the integumentary system, like the various glands, receptors, and the basis for hair attachment, but in addition this layer includes blood vessels and nerves that provide nutrients/remove wastes (blood vessels) and allow for various sensing reactions (nerves). Glands include those that

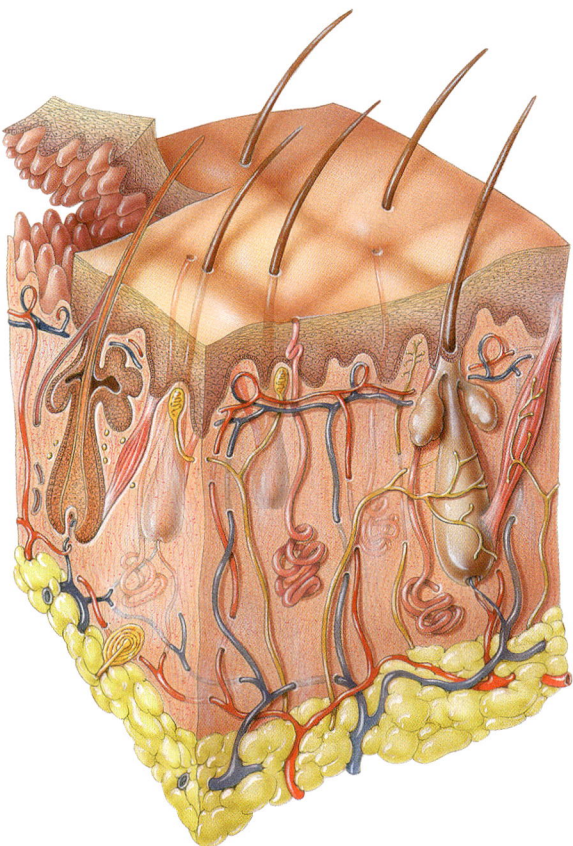

Figure 2.11 The structure of the skin, with associated components. Source: Reproduced with permission from Tortora et al. (2011) / John Wiley & Sons.

produce sweat ("sudoriferous") and oil ("sebaceous") glands. Finally, the subcutaneous (or "below the skin") layer is the innermost and is strictly not considered part of the true skin structure. This area also includes larger blood vessels and nerves supplying the dermis, but in particular is where fat (technically included in a further type of tissue known as "adipose tissue") is stored.

The main accessory structures of the skin are the hair, nails, and glands. The hair is based in the dermis and grows out through the outer layers. The outer portion of the hair that we see is made up of dead cells containing keratin and other proteins. Nails are the same, but are more packed or dense to give them a harder, clear structure; the lower part of the nail is actively growing (alive), but then becomes inactive and dead as the structure grows out of the tips of fingers/toes. The final structures are glands; these are defined as groups of specialized cells or even organs (as in the case of the pancreas; see the section on the digestive system) that produce various types of substances. These include hormones (referred to as the endocrine glands and discussed in the section on the endocrine system) and the exocrine glands, which secrete salt, enzymes, water, and other liquids. Examples of exocrine glands in the skin are the sebaceous and sudoriferous (sweat) glands. The sebaceous glands are generally associated with the base of hairs in the dermis (Figure 2.11) and secrete an oily liquid known as sebum (a mixture of proteins, lipids, and salts); acne in teenagers, although a complicated condition, is often associated with overproduction of sebum, although sebum has an important role in the various functions of skin (such as preventing drying). The sweat glands of various types (e.g. eccrine and apocrine) are also found in the dermis, but extend up to and at the surface of the epidermis (as in the case of the sweat pores on the skin surface). They produce mainly a mixture of water and salts, but may also include various types of proteins, lipids, and other chemicals; it is interesting to note that in their excreted form they have little to no odor, but their presence on the skin can also allow for the growth of various types of bacteria/fungi that naturally live on or in the skin (see later discussion) and it is these that give rise to the various smells associated with sweat. The sweat glands aid in regulating body temperature, protection from microorganisms (such as bacteria), and disposal of wastes. A further example of a modified sweat gland is the mammary gland (or breast); this actually gives the name to "mammals" or a group of animals that have these types of glands and produce milk as food for their young.

Overall, the skin is a remarkable, active, and resilient structure.

Functions

The skin has many functions, many of which are not obvious. The most important and well-described of these are as follows:
- Outer covering for and protection of the internal organs of the body. The skin essentially keeps us together. In addition to the obvious protection mechanism to prevent physical damage, including active repair of this damage as observed during wound healing, it also provides chemical inhibition to various types of microorganisms (such as bacteria and viruses) that may otherwise infect, damage, and even penetrate the skin. A further mechanism is the production of melanin, which in addition to giving the color to the skin also offers some limited protection against damaging ultraviolet rays from the sun.
- Detection of various environmental conditions and sensory functions, such as cold, heat, chemical or microbial irritation (e.g. itching), and pain, which in itself is a protective mechanism for the body to prevent more serious damage.
- Temperature control, by sweat production and heat insulation (afforded by adipose tissue in the subcutaneous layer).
- Waste disposal, via sweat for example, which can include ammonia and urea as breakdown products within the body.
- Adsorption (the accumulation or taking up) of some substances that can occur at the skin surface, including some vitamins (A and D) and gases (oxygen, but to a limited extent). Medicine has often made use of this fact by the application of drug-impregnated patches to the skin.
- Vitamin D synthesis – vitamin D is essential to human life and the skin is involved in its production.
- Blood reservoir – up to 10% of the total blood in the body can be contained within blood vessels in the skin (particularly the dermis), which allows the body to control the need for blood (oxygen) at various times and control the body temperature.

Additional comments

As the outermost external structure of the body, the skin not only contains the various types of human cells, but actually co-exists with an even greater number of other microorganisms (Chapter 5). The actual numbers and types of microorganisms will depend on many factors, such as lifestyle and wet/dry areas of the skin. In general, the microbial flora or ecosystem of the skin is considered as "resident" and "transient." The resident types are found on the skin of most people and are considered permanently present, including a variety of bacteria (e.g. *Staphylococcus* such as *S. epidermidis*, *Micrococcus*, *Propionibacterium*, and *Corynebacterium* species) and fungi (*Candida* and the dermatophytes such as *Microsporum*). Transient microorganisms are any that are temporarily picked up by the skin and can include viruses (e.g. noroviruses), a variety of fungi, and bacteria such as *S. aureus* (including MRSA strains), *Clostridium difficile* (in vegetative and spore forms), and *Escherichia coli*.

Hand washing and skin cleaning therefore play essential roles in preventing the transmissions of microorganisms from a patient or contaminated surface (such as a medical or dental instrument) to another person (including yourself). This topic is further considered as an important strategy for infection prevention and control (Chapter 5).

Lymphatic

In parallel to the circulatory (or blood) system, which transfers various nutrients, chemicals, and gases around the body (see the section on the cardiovascular system), there is another transport system known as the lymphatic system. This system is closely linked to the structure and functions of the circulatory system. It consists of various lymphatic tissues/organs, a series of lymph vessels, and a watery substance that flows through the system known as lymph.

Structure

The lymphatic system is composed of the lymph, lymph vessels (conducting system for the lymph), and various lymphatic tissues and organs (Figure 2.12).

The lymph is essentially the same as the interstitial fluid that surrounds the various cells of the body. As a clear fluid, it is mostly composed of water (~92%) and various types of proteins, lipids/fats, minerals, hormones, and WBCs (see the section on the structure of the cardiovascular system). The WBCs are involved in protecting the body against the attack of various microorganisms, as part of the immune system (discussed later in this section). The blood system provides various components to this fluid, which exchanges nutrients (in) and wastes (out) of the various cells of the body. Part of this fluid exchanges back into the blood veins and through the circulatory system; the other part drains into the lymph system, where it is then referred to as lymph. The lymph is filtered into a network of lymph capillaries that come together to form larger lymph vessels. Lymph capillaries and vessels are similar in this sense to the structure of the veins (see the section on the cardiovascular system). The vessels further drain into larger lymph trunks and finally into two major ducts (the thoracic and right lymphatic ducts), which are located just below the neck and feed directly into specific veins in this area.

The lymphatic system tissues and organs are distributed around the body, being associated with the lymph vessels. Lymphoid tissue itself consists of connective tissues, with associated types of WBCs (in particular the lymphocytes). These consist of two major types:
- Primary tissues/organs, being the thymus and bone marrow. It is in these that the lymphocytes (known as T- and B-lymphocytes) are made.
- Secondary tissues/organs, including the lymph nodes and lymphatic follicles present in various organs such as the tonsils, skin, and spleen.

The lymph nodes vary in size and are present along the various lymph vessels through which the lymph passes on its return to the blood system. This allows for a close interaction with the various types of immune cells present, and they act as natural filters for the body to remove unwanted agents. The spleen is the largest organ consisting of lymphoid tissue in the body; in addition to its role in the lymphoid system, it is responsible for the removal of aged RBCs from the blood. Overall, there is a close connection between the circulatory and lymphatic systems of the body.

Functions

The lymphatic system has essentially three major functions in the body:
- Provides defense against the various microorganisms or other foreign substances found in the body, playing a vital role in the immune system.
- Links to the functions of the digestive system; various lipids and lipid-soluble materials (such as vitamins A, D, E, and K) are taken up by the lymph and transported to the blood through the lymphatic system.
- Controls the levels of fluids around the various cells of the body, by draining into the lymphatic circulatory system and transferring lymph back to the blood system.

Additional comments

Immunity (or the body's resistance) is the ability of the body to protect itself against disease or damage. The human immune system consists of two main parts:
- Innate, non-specific immunity: this consists of the various organs, tissues, cells, and substances that we are born with and that defend the body from microorganisms in a non-specific manner. It can be further sub-divided into the front line of defense (such as the skin and mucous membranes, which provide a physical barrier to attack from these agents) and the second line of defense. The second line includes types of cells known as phagocytes, the body's inflammation and fever reactions, and the production of various antimicrobial chemicals (such as cytokines, further discussed in the section on the endocrine system under additional comments). The innate system also interacts and actually activates adaptive immunity.
- Adaptive, specific immunity: this is composed of various types of cells (known as T- and B-lymphocytes) that recognize and attack the presence of various microorganisms when they encounter them in a specific way. Therefore, this type of immunity is constantly developed through life, based on what we are exposed to. In addition to the specific reactions to the invading microorganism, this type of immunity provides a memory to the immune system, acting quickly against the microorganism if it is experienced in the future.

The adaptive response is the basis of immunization (or vaccination), where the body is exposed to a part of or an injured microorganism, allowing for the development of the response in the absence of disease. Examples include the BCG (Bacillus Calmette–Guérin) vaccine against tuberculosis (a disease caused by bacteria known as *Mycobacterium tuberculosis*), COVID-19 vaccines against severe acute respiratory syndrome coronavirus 2 (SARS-CoV-2), the virus that caused initial coronavirus disease in 2019, and the MMR vaccine (a combined vaccination against three viral diseases: measles, mumps, and rubella).

When immunity is lowered (in patients this is described as being "immunocompromised"), the body can become very susceptible to infection from the various types of disease-causing microorganisms (which are known as pathogens; see Chapter 5). A common example is observed during the progression of the disease known as AIDS (acquired immune deficiency syndrome). This is caused by a virus known as HIV (human immunodeficiency disease), which actively attacks the human immune system. The virus specifically attacks certain types of T-lymphocytes, which over time are no longer available as part of the adaptive immune response. This leads to the patient becoming immunocompromised and open to infection by a variety of bacteria, viruses, and fungi. It is the combination of infections with these microorganisms that eventually leads to death in these patients.

Muscular

The muscular system (Figure 2.13), consisting of the various sizes and shapes of muscles, makes up about 45% of the body mass and is distributed around the body. It is the action of these various muscles that provides movement, internally and externally, in coordination with various other systems such as the nervous, circulatory, and skeletal systems.

Structure

Muscle cells (also known as myocytes or muscle fibers) are arranged into bundles ("fascicles") that are combined to give individual muscles. In the body there are three principal types of muscle tissue: skeletal, cardiac, and smooth tissues. This classification is based on their structures, locations, and functions. Skeletal muscles are primarily associated with the bones, being attached through specific connective tissues known as tendons (also see the section on the skeletal system); they are often referred to as "voluntary" muscles as they work when we decide to use them (e.g. for lifting and walking). Muscle tissues allow for movement by contracting and relaxing, primarily under control of the nervous system, and expending energy. Cardiac tissues, as the name would suggest, are found in the walls of the heart; their control is considered "involuntary" in that we do not decide if they work or not and they play an important role in the pumping of blood (by the heart) around the circulatory system. Smooth muscles are also considered involuntary and are located within the structures of various other systems, such as blood vessels, the stomach and intestines, the skin, uterus, and eyes.

Functions

The primary functions of the muscular system are:
- Allowing for movement, including walking and lifting, as well as providing support and posture.
- The action of various tissues that allow for the passage of various substances through the body, including the intestines, airways, and blood/lymph vessels.
- Heat generation: the heat generated by movement is used by the body to regulate the body temperature, which is necessary for normal metabolism.

Additional comments

Myology is the study of muscles. All muscles of the body have specific names, such as the orbicularis oris (surrounding the mouth), rectus abdominus (in the belly), deltoid (shoulder), and soleus (lower leg).

Muscle cells consume a lot of energy during movement, which is generated by the production and expenditure of a chemical known as ATP (adenosine triphosphate); ATP is also used by other cell systems such as in bacteria. Note that ATP detection methods are sometimes used to evaluate bacterial contamination and/or the presence of residual, patient soil on instrument surfaces (Chapter 8).

Some common medical problems associated with muscles include strains and tendonitis. A strain (also known as a tear or pulled muscle) is due to the muscle becoming torn or broken, generally due to some kind of physical exertion (e.g. in sports). Tendonitis may be caused by similar exertion, injury, or disease, leading to inflammation of the tendons.

Nervous

The nervous system, together with the endocrine system (see the section on the endocrine system), is responsible for communication and control in the body. The nervous system senses various stimuli (both outside and within the body) and can cause a reaction to what it senses, as well as providing control of walking, talking, exercising, and so on, and higher-order effects such as memory. Its major components are the brain, spinal cord, and various nerves around the body (Figure 2.14).

Structure

Nervous tissue is made up of two unique types of cells: nerve cells (known as neurons) and glia cells ("neuroglia" or "glia"). Neurons are specialized cells that conduct signals (nerve impulses) along the nervous system; they can respond to various types of stimuli (e.g. heat sensors in the skin), cause an effect to happen (e.g. movement away from a source of heat), and even lead to the development of memory (e.g. hot may not be good). The glia cells support, maintain, and protect the neurons.

The nervous system can be considered in two ways: functionally and anatomically. Functionally, the system can be considered in three parts: sensory (those parts that detect various stimuli, both external to and within the body), motor (those that cause an effect, such as stimulating a muscle to move in connection with the skeletal system), and integrative (connecting between the sensory and motor functions, including the storing of information). Anatomically the nervous system can be sub-divided into two parts: the central nervous system (CNS), consisting of the brain (in the skull) and the spinal cord (which runs from the brain through the vertebral column of the back), and the peripheral nervous system (PNS), consisting of all the nerves extending from the spinal cord and through the rest of the body. The peripheral system includes various nerves (consisting of neurons, glia, connective tissue, and blood vessels), ganglia (groups of neurons), and sensory receptors (e.g. in the skin, responding to various stimuli).

Think of the brain as a central computer that controls the body by sending and receiving messages between the brain and various parts of the body through the spinal cord and a network of peripheral nerves. When the brain receives a message it sends a reply instructing the body in how to act. For example, if you touch a hot surface the nerves in the skin automatically send a message to the brain that registers as pain and sends a message back telling the muscles in the hand to pull away.

The brain is one of the larger and more complex organs of the body. Different areas have been identified as dealing with different functions, such as speech, hearing, smell, sight, movement, salivation, and so on. Some of these centers are concerned with the information coming into the brain (sensory areas) and others are concerned with sending messages from the brain and making things happen (motor centers). The brain can be further sub-divided into three main sections (Figure 2.15):

- The forebrain (or "cerebrum") is the main part of the brain and itself is sub-divided into various sections known as lobes (e.g. the frontal lobe). In addition, various parts of the forebrain have been mapped to the control of various body functions, such as vision to the back of the cerebrum and speech/hearing more centrally.
- The midbrain is located underneath the middle of the forebrain, and is considered the master coordinator for all the messages going in and out of the brain.
- The hindbrain sits underneath the back end of the forebrain and consists of the cerebellum, pons, and medulla. The cerebellum is responsible for balance, movement, and coordination. The pons and the medulla, along with the midbrain, are often referred to as the "brainstem." The brainstem takes in, sends out, and coordinates all of the brain's messages. It also controls many of the body's automatic functions, like breathing, heart rate, blood pressure, swallowing, digestion, and blinking. If an individual has an injury to the brainstem they generally cannot survive without significant medical assistance.

The spinal cord extends from the hindbrain and through the vertebrae of the back (approximately to the lumbar area of the back); different nerves extend from the cord at various intervals along its length into particular parts of the body.

The CNS (brain and spinal cord) is surrounded by three layers of protective membrane known as the meninges.

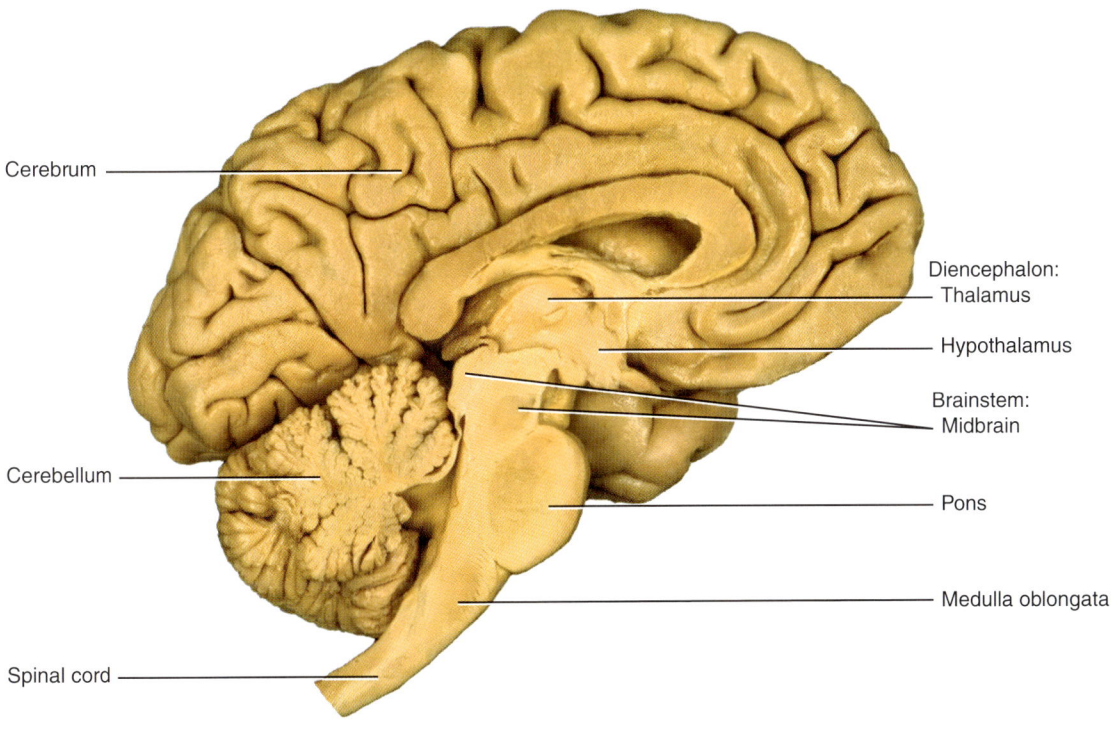

Sagittal section, medial view

Figure 2.15 The basic structure of the brain, with main sections indicated. Courtesy of Mark Nielsen, The University of Utah, Salt Lake City, UT, USA.

These layers are called, from the outside in, the dura mater, arachnoid, and pia mater. Between the inner two layers of the meninges is a water-like substance known as cerebrospinal fluid (CSF); this is a colorless fluid that is composed mostly of water, as well as various chemicals and nutrients. It is the combination of bones (the skull or vertebrae), the meninges, and the CSF that protects the CNS from movement and damage.

Functions

The nervous system is overall responsible for communication and control in the body, by reacting to various stimuli and causing reactions around the body. These include:
- Sensing, such as the five senses (sight, taste, touch, hearing, and smell). This includes both external and internal environment sensing, as well as other functions such as movement and balance.
- Motor effects, causing movement or other responses to occur around the body (e.g. movement of muscles and release of hormones).
- Control and coordination of the various functions of the organs and systems of the body, including collaboration with the endocrine system and its associated hormones.
- Memory and intelligence.

Additional comments

Neurology is the study of the nervous system (including its functions and associated diseases) and therefore a neurologist is a specialist in this area. Encephalopathy is any disorder of the brain.

Neurons are unique cells in the body as they do not have the ability to divide or reproduce; therefore they survive for the whole of our lives unless they are lost due to injury or disease. Therefore, loss or degeneration of neurons can lead to severe disease in patients, such as Parkinson's disease, Alzheimer's disease, and Creutzfeldt-Jakob disease. Damage to the brain or spinal cord can lead to a variety of effects, including coma (a state of unconsciousness), encephalitis (inflammation of the brain, for example due to a virus infection), meningitis (inflammation of the meninges due to infection), dementia (loss of intelligence ability, often associated with the progression of age), and paralysis (loss of function/control of one or many limbs).

Reproductive

Reproduction is the process of generating offspring. In humans and animals this is achieved by "sexual" reproduction, where the goal is the union of specialized cells (known as "gametes") in a process known as fertilization. The introductory section explained that most cells of the body contain the nucleic acid DNA in organized structures known as chromosomes; there are 46 chromosomes (23 pairs) in each cell, with the exception of the gametes that only contain one set (only 23 chromosomes). The male gametes are called sperm (or spermatozoa) and are produced in the testes (or testicles) and the female gametes are called oocysts and are produced from the ovaries. The testes and ovaries are organs known as "gonads." During fertilization (in the female), the gametes join together to form a new cell known as a zygote that contains 46 chromosomes (half from the mother and half from the father) and develops by cell division into an embryo. Over time, referred to as gestation or pregnancy, the embryo develops into a fetus, which when fully developed is born (during parturition or labor) as an infant.

The human reproductive system in males and females consists of the gonads (which not only produce the gametes but also the sex hormones as part of the endocrine system; see the section on the endocrine system), a system of ducts (to store and/or transfer the gametes), accessory glands, and supportive structures (such as the penis in males and the vagina in females).

Structure

The male reproductive system (Figure 2.16(A)) consists of the testes (or testicles, held in the scrotum), various ducts (such as the epididymis that is attached to each testicle, storing the sperm, and vas (or ductus) deferens that transports the sperm from the epididymis to the urethra and out of the penis during ejaculation), accessory glands (such as the seminal vesicle and prostate gland), and supportive structures (in this case the penis and scrotum). The sperm are developed in the testes and the different associated glands add various substances to this (for transportation and protection purposes) to produce semen for ejaculation from the male system into the female system. The testes also contain specific cells that produce the male sex hormone testosterone as part of the endocrine system (see the section on the endocrine system).

The female reproductive system (Figure 2.16(B)) consists of the ovaries (on either side of the uterus), the uterine (or Fallopian) tubes (which transfer the oocysts released from the ovaries into the uterus), the uterus (where fertilization usually occurs, as well as the development of the fetus), the vagina (for receiving the penis during sexual intercourse and for passage of the fetus out of the system during birth), and also the mammary glands (or "breasts," for the production of milk and feeding of the newborn). The ovaries produce, develop, and release the female gametes (oocysts) during a process known as ovulation during the female reproductive cycle. The cycle ends in menstruation ("period") or in fertilization and fetus development. Similar to the testes, the ovaries also produce various female sex hormones, such as progesterone and the estrogens, as part of the endocrine system (see the section on the endocrine system).

Functions

The primary function of the reproductive system is to produce offspring and the survival of the species. For this purpose the specific functions include:

- Generation of gametes (sperm in the testes and oocysts in the ovaries).
- Sexual intercourse.
- Fertilization and development of the fetus (in the female, specifically in the uterus).
- Nourishment during development of the fetus, delivery, and initial feeding (with milk) of the newborn infant.
- Production of the various sex hormones that determine the principal male or female traits (see the section on the endocrine system).

Additional comments

Gynecology is the branch of medicine that specializes in the study of the health, associated diseases, and disorders of the female reproductive system. Similarly, andrology is the branch of medicine associated with the male system. Both branches are closely related to urology, or the study of the urinary tract or "urogenital" system (see the section on the urinary system). In medical literature, a female is often designated by the symbol ♀ and a male by the symbol ♂.

Respiratory

Cellular respiration is the process used in human cells to produce energy (in the form of a molecule called ATP) from the various nutrients acquired through the digestive system (see the section on the digestive system). In addition to nutrients, cells also require oxygen (O_2) for respiration and the respiratory system provides a mechanism of acquiring oxygen for the body by breathing in air (which contains ~21% oxygen). In addition, the system expels a further gas (carbon dioxide, CO_2) that is a by-product of respiration; at high levels this can be toxic to human cells, and therefore it is continually removed and expelled from the body. The respiratory system works closely with the cardiovascular (blood) system (see the section on the cardiovascular system) to take in O_2 (inspiration) and expel CO_2 (expiration). The system consists of various airways that passage air into the system and the lungs that allow gas (O_2 and CO_2) exchange. As examples of accessory functions, the respiratory system allows for speech and the sense of smell.

Structure

The respiratory system (Figure 2.17) is generally divided into two parts: the upper tract and the lower tract. The upper tract consists of the nose/mouth and pharynx (in the head/neck region) and the lower tract includes the larynx (voice box), trachea (windpipe), bronchi, and lungs (in the neck/thoracic cavity region).

The upper respiratory system channels air into the lower system and is mostly shared with the digestive system (mouth and pharynx; see the section on the digestive system). The nose and mouth provide the entry/exit points for air. The nose structure is part of the skull (being bone), but also a more flexible tissue known as cartilage (at the outer part of the nose; see the section on the skeletal system). Internally it contains the nasal cavities that extend back and deep into the head, below the brain and above the oral cavity (mouth); the nasal and oral cavities join at the back of the throat. The nasal passages are covered by mucous membranes that secrete mucus and also contain specialized sensing cells that are responsible for "olfaction" (the sense of smell). The area extending from the back of the nasal passages and the mouth, down toward the lower tract, is known as the pharynx (or throat). Muscles in the pharynx play a role in digestion (swallowing) and contain the tonsils (part of the lymphatic system; see the section on the lymphatic system). For device and surgical reference, the pharynx is subdivided into three sections, from the back of the nose down: the nasopharynx, oropharynx, and laryngopharynx. The pharynx channels air through the system and at the base of the laryngopharynx is the point at which the respiratory and digestive systems separate, at the larynx (voice box). The larynx connects to the trachea (windpipe); it contains cartilage in its structure that gives it strength but also contains the inner vocal cords (made of mucous membrane folds). Vibrations of the cords on the passage of air across them give sound. The trachea also has an internal mucous membrane layer and a rigid, external cartilage ring structure. The trachea separates into two bronchi just as they enter into either lung. The lungs are found in the thoracic cavity, in the rib cage, and on either side of the sternum (see Figure 2.18 and the section on the skeletal system). Each lung is maintained in a separate sub-cavity and is protected by a pleural membrane. The lung itself is divided up into different lobes and contains the various extensions of the bronchi and other supportive tissues (such as connective tissues, blood vessels, and lymph vessels). As the bronchi enter the lungs they further sub-divide to give a continuous airway deep in the lung structure; bronchi sub-divide into smaller-diameter bronchi and even smaller bronchioles, similar to the roots of a tree and changing structure (e.g. losing cartilage) as they get smaller in size. At the ends of each bronchiole are alveolar ducts and various grape-like sub-divisions called alveoli. The alveoli are lined with specialized types of cells that allow for the diffusion (or passage) of gases in and out of the various capillary blood vessels of the lungs.

Functions

The primary functions of the respiratory system include:
- Intake of oxygen and removal of carbon dioxide as part of cellular respiration (the generation of energy in the body).

- Regulation of water and heat content in the body, along with other systems, as both are also expelled during expiration (breathing out).
- Regulation of the acidity/alkalinity (pH) levels in the blood, due to gas and water exchange.
- Providing the ability to speak/make sounds and smell, through associated organs and receptors.

Additional comments

The medical specialty dedicated to the lungs and associated parts of the respiratory system is known as pulmonary medicine (or pulmonology); therefore, the term "pulmonary" is linked in some way to this system. Specifically, the ENT ("ear, nose, and throat") specialty is known as oto-rhino-laryngology.

Anesthesia is defined as the ability to block or take away the sensation of pain. It is important during surgical and other procedures. Anesthetics can include processes and, more commonly, various types of drugs. Local or regional anesthesia has an effect at a certain region or even smaller area of the body; in these cases the drugs work outside the brain and are applied directly to the region/area in preparation for surgery/a procedure. In contrast, in the case of "general" anesthesia the drugs work on the brain and can cause the patient to partially or fully lose consciousness ("sleep") and not be awoken even when in pain. A variety of drugs are used for anesthesia. General anesthesia is usually administered to a patient intravenously (through a vein) or more commonly by inhalation (breathing) through the lungs. In the latter case the drugs are mixed with a carrier gas and are absorbed into the body through the respiratory system. This can be a complex process in preparing, administering, monitoring, and reviving the patient; those specializing in anesthesiology are called anesthesiologists or anesthetists.

Asthma, where a patient is diagnosed with repeated difficulty in breathing, is due to reoccurring inflammation of the lungs and associated airways (particularly the bronchi, which become narrower and restrict the passage of air); the condition can range from mild to severe, even leading to respiratory failure and death. Its exact cause is often unclear, but it is known to be affected by the genetics of the patients and his/her environment. Other diseases/conditions of the respiratory tract include:
- Laryngitis: inflammation of the inner membranes of the larynx, often associated with a loss of voice and commonly due to microbial infections.
- Bronchitis: inflammation of the bronchi (mucous membranes), often associated with viral infections such as influenza (common cold) but also some bacteria.
- Pneumonia: inflammation of the lungs, also commonly due to a wide range of microorganisms including bacteria (such as *Streptococcus pneumoniae* and *Mycobacterium tuberculosis*), viruses, and fungi.

Upper respiratory tract (ENT) endoscopy and bronchoscopy are types of procedures using special types of devices known as endoscopes (see Chapters 4 and 15) for direct visualization of the upper and lower respiratory tracts, respectively.

Similar to the various types of flexible endoscopes described for use in the GI tract, various types of rigid and flexible endoscopes are designed for use in the respiratory tract, including ENT scopes and bronchoscopes (Chapters 4 and 15).

Skeletal (including dental)

The human skeletal (or bone) system consists of 206 bones that are organized in a structure known as the skeleton (Figure 2.18). It is the skeleton structure that gives the body its characteristic shape and support. In the study of anatomy, the skeleton is sub-divided into two parts: axial and appendicular. The axial skeleton consists of the central part of the structure, including the cranium (skull), vertebral column (running down the back), sternum (the long flat bone in the center of the chest), hyoid bone (in the neck), and the associated ribs (in the chest). The appendicular skeleton consists of the pectoral (or shoulder) girdle, consisting of two clavicles (collar bones) and two scapula (shoulder blades) bones, the pelvic (or hip) girdle, consisting of two coxal or hip bones, and their associated limbs (the arms and legs, respectively, also known as the upper and lower limbs).

In addition to the skeleton, the dental system is considered briefly in this section. It is made up of the teeth (or "dentes") in the mouth and contains specific organs associated with both the skeletal and the digestive system (see the section on the digestive system).

Structure

Due to their strength and structure, it is a common misconception that bones are dead; bones are actually active, continuously regenerating structures consisting of unique types of cells and tissues. Bone (or osseous) tissue is made of four types of bone cells: osteogenic cells, osteoblasts, osteocytes, and osteoclasts. Osteogenic cells are actively dividing cells in the inner bone structure, which subsequently stop dividing and develop into osteoblasts and then osteocytes. The osteoblasts produce an external matrix that surrounds the cells, which gives bone its unique, hardened structure. This matrix consists of 25% water, 25% collagen (a type of protein), and 50% salt crystals. The crystals are made up primarily of hydroxyapatite (a combination of two salts: calcium phosphate [$Ca_3(PO_4)_2$] and calcium hydroxide [$Ca(OH)_2$]) mixed with other salts (e.g. calcium carbonate) and ions (e.g. fluoride). It is the combination of collagen and salt crystal production and deposition that gives bone strength, in a process known as calcification. As the osteoblasts become entrapped in the calcification process, they develop into osteocytes; osteocytes are not dormant but are actively involved in maintaining bone structure in the exchange of nutrients and waste materials with blood supply. As bone is generated, it is also continuously broken down by the final type of bone cells, the osteoclasts. These specialized cells are found in the inner bone structure and break down the bone tissue by the production of acids and enzymes (this process is referred to as reabsorption).

There are two main types of bone tissue, compact (or "dense") and spongy (or "cancellous") bone, which differ in overall structure; in general, compact bone tissue is found on the surface of bones and spongy tissue in the interior. Finally, as an active structure, the various bones are supplied by nerves (the nervous system), muscles, and a blood supply (as part of the cardiovascular system). A brief summary of the major parts and bones of the skeletal system is given in Table 2.5.

A joint (or "articulation") is where two bones meet, and is designed to allow for movement between bones and for mechanical support. There are many types of joints that vary in structure, including fibrous, cartilaginous, and synovial

Table 2.5 The various types of bones in the skeletal system.

Skeletal structure	Common name	Description
Axial cranium	Skull, head	The skull is composed of various cranial and facial bones The cranial bones surround and protect the brain The facial bones give the face structure and support, while also supporting the dental system (teeth) and, along with the cranial bones, other organs such as the eyes, nose, and ears Examples of facial bones include the mandible or lower jaw bone that is the only movable bone in the skull, carrying the lower teeth, and the maxillae, supporting the upper teeth
Vertebral column	Spine or backbone	Consists of 33 bones known as vertebrae arranged in a column They protect the spinal cord and give upright support They are further sub-divided into the cervical (neck), thoracic (chest or upper back), lumbar (loin or lower back), and sacral (consisting of four fused bones) vertebrae and the coccyx (four fused bones)
Sternum ribs	Breastbone ribs	Large flat bone in the center of the chest 24 bones arranged in 12 pairs They all are attached to the vertebrae and some are also attached to the sternum The ribs and sternum provide protection to the main organs in the chest, such as the heart and lungs
Appendicular pectoral girdle	Shoulder	Consists of two clavicles (collar bones, along the front) and two scapulae (shoulder blades, to the back) Can be considered part of, and are attached to, the upper limbs
Upper limbs	Arms	Consist of 30 bones and divided into three areas (from the girdle end down): the humerus (upper arm), the ulna and radius (forearm), and the hands The hands are divided into 8 carpal bones (carpus or wrist), 5 metacarpals (the palm of the hand), and 14 phalanges (making up the fingers and thumb; each bone is a *phalanx*)
Pelvic girdle	Hips	Two hip bones (coxal or pelvic bones) They are joined together at the front (anterior) of the body and interact with the vertebral column (the sacrum) Can be considered part of, and are attached to, the lower limbs There is a distinct difference between the structures of male and female pelves
Lower limbs	Legs	Consist of 30 bones, similar to the upper limbs, and divided into four areas (from the girdle end down): the femur (upper leg), the patella (kneecap), the tibia and fibula (lower leg), and the feet The feet are divided into 7 tarsal bones (tarsus or ankle), 5 metatarsals (in the center of the foot), and 14 phalanges (making up the toes)

joints. In all of these cases, muscles are attached to bones by specialized structures known as tendons (or sinews). Ligaments join bones together and fascias connect muscles to each other. All of these are similar in structure, composed of collagen fibers.

Special consideration should also be given to the dental system or teeth. They are associated (in the mouth) with the mandible (lower jaw) and maxillae (upper jaw) bones of the cranium (Table 2.5). Humans have 20 deciduous (or primary) and 32 permanent (or secondary) sets of teeth. The first set develop early in life, consisting of (from the back of the mouth forward and on each side of the mouth) two molars, one canine, and two incisor teeth in each jaw. These are lost typically between the ages of 6 and 12 and replaced by the permanent teeth, consisting of (from the back of the mouth forward and on each side of the mouth) three molars, two premolars, one canine, and two incisor teeth in each jaw (Figure 2.19); the innermost molars (known as the third molars or "wisdom" teeth) are often not formed or displayed in the mouth.

A single tooth consists of three sections: the outer and visible crown, the neck (at the gum line), and the root (Figure 2.19). From the outside in, a tooth has an external covering of white enamel composed of hydroxyapatite (composed of calcium phosphate and calcium carbonate, and stronger than even bone structures). Within the enamel is the dentin layer, also an extremely strong structure consisting of calcified connective tissue (produced by cells known as odontoblasts) and a central space known as the pulp cavity, consisting of connective tissue, nerves, blood, and lymph vessels. Teeth are embedded and supported in the mouth by the periodontium. This consists of four parts: the cementum (part of the tooth, surrounding the dentin in the root of the tooth; Figure 2.19), periodontal ligaments, alveolar bone, and gingiva (or "gum"). The ligaments attach the tooth (specifically the cementum) to the alveolar bone, which is covered externally by the gingiva (consisting of mucosal tissue).

Functions
There are five main functions of the skeletal system:
- Providing support to the body and its structures, such as various types of attached tissues and associated organs.
- Protection for various essential organs, including the lungs, brain, and heart.
- Allowing for movement, with the interaction of the muscular system.
- Blood cell production: some bones contain a specific type of tissue known as red bone marrow (or myeloid tissue). These include the hip bone, ribs, femur, and humerus. This tissue produces various types of blood cells, such as RBCs, WBCs, and platelets (see the section on the cardiovascular system). These cells are produced in the marrow and broken down in the liver.
- Storage: the bone provides storage of various types of essential minerals (such as calcium and phosphate) and lipids (triglycerides). The triglycerides are stored in "yellow bone marrow," which is primarily made up of adipose (or "fat") tissue. Triglycerides are an important source of energy and yellow marrow is most commonly found in the inner parts of bones such as the femur, tibia, and humerus. The dental system is used for biting and grinding food, as part of the digestive system (see the section on the digestive system).

Additional comments
Cartilage is a similar structure to bone, but is more flexible in structure. It is a type of connective tissue made up of specific cells known as chondrocytes, which also produce an extracellular matrix including protein (collagen or elastin) fibers and a gel-like substance (chondroitin sulfate). Cartilage is primarily found at the end (or joints) of bones as well as in specific structures such as the nose, ears, and bronchial tubes (see the section on the respiratory system).

"Osteo-" is a prefix associated with bone. Examples include the various types of bone cells (e.g. osteoblasts) and associated diseases. Osteoarthritis is a joint-based disease, where the cartilage around the bone ends in joints degenerates (or breaks down) over time due to wear and tear. Similarly, rheumatoid arthritis (RA) is also associated with degeneration of cartilage, but in this case due to the body's reaction against itself. In these cases the body's immune system (see the section on the lymphatic system) reacts against the joint structure, leading to damage and breakdown. A further commonly used suffix is "arthro-," which is in reference to a joint; examples include arthroplasty (a surgical procedure relating to the reconstruction or replacement of a joint) and arthroscopy (the surgical examination and repair of the interior of a joint by minimally invasive surgery (MIS) using a specific type of endoscope known as an arthroscope).

Rheumatism refers to any naturally (not due to infection or injury) occurring pain associated with the skeletal system (including the bones, tendons, ligaments, and associated muscles).

A "fracture" is a break in any bone. Examples include open, closed, simple, multi-fragmentary, and stress fractures. An open (or compound) fracture is where the bone breaks and penetrates through the skin so that it can be seen; a closed fracture is therefore where the bone does not break through the skin. A simple fracture is when the bone breaks along one line, while multi-fragmentary (or *comminuted*) fractures are more serious in that the bone is broken at multiple sites. A stress fracture is composed of smaller or minor fractures in the bone but not necessarily showing any obvious break in the bone.

Dentistry is the science of diagnosing, preventing, and treating diseases of the teeth, gums, and related structures of the

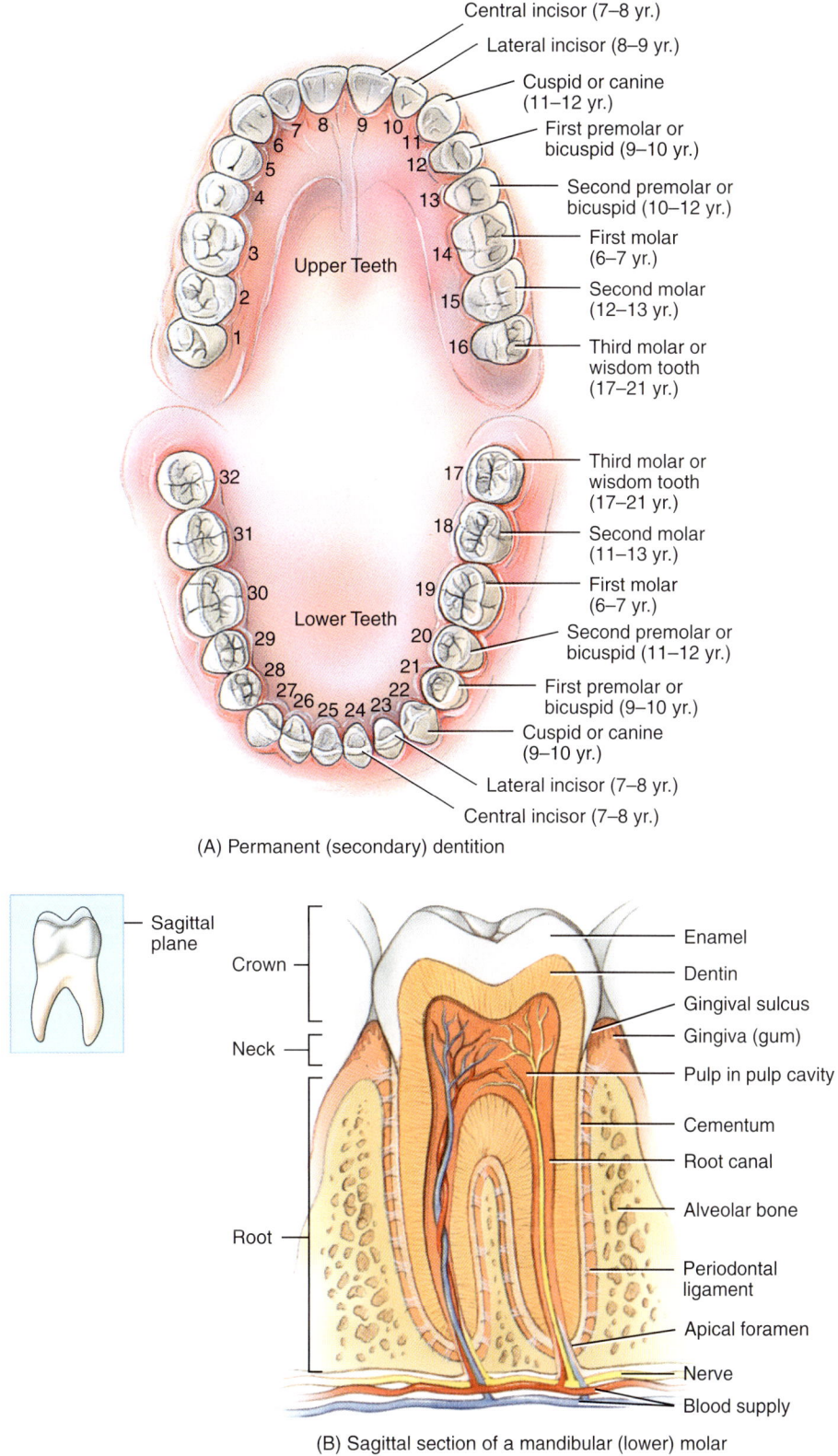

Figure 2.19 The dental system. (A) The permanent teeth of an adult human (third molars shown) and (B) the structure of a tooth. Source: Reproduced with permission from Tortora et al. (2011) / John Wiley & Sons.

mouth. Specifically, endodontics is concerned with the more inner structures of the teeth (the pulp, root, and alveolar bone) and periodontics relates to those tissues around the teeth (such as the gums). Orthodontics is concerned with the prevention and correction of teeth alignment within the mouth.

Urinary

The urinary (or excretory) system works closely with the cardiovascular system (see the section on the cardiovascular system) for waste disposal and maintenance. It consists of the kidneys (two) and a series of transport tubes and storage vessels. The kidneys are constantly filtering the blood to remove various wastes (such as urea and ammonia that can be toxic at high concentrations in the body), but also in reabsorbing back into the blood various components (such as water and salts) necessary for fluid/electrolyte balance; the end result is a concentrated liquid waste known as urine. The urine is initially stored in the body and then discharged from the body during urination.

Structure

The urinary system includes the kidneys, ureters, bladder, and urethra (Figure 2.20).

The kidneys are the main organs of the system and are responsible for most of its primary functions. Internally they are divided into two distinct areas: the external cortex and the internal medulla. Blood enters the kidneys and is transferred via the blood vessels to specialized structures known as nephrons, which start in the cortex and extend into the medulla. At the cortex level, the blood vessels make contact with the entry to the nephrons and, under pressure, cause various components of the blood to filter into nephrons. The resulting fluid (which is notably some 100 times the volume of the final urine) then passes through the rest of the nephron structure, where various components are reabsorbed back into the surrounding blood supply (such as water and minerals) and further exchange of wastes from the blood vessels to the nephrons can occur. The resulting urine is collected by various tubules in the medulla region that combine to exit the kidney structure into a ureter tube that extends from each kidney to collect in the bladder for storage. The bladder acts as a hollow reservoir. When the bladder fills, this creates a pressure that triggers the requirement and eventually necessary release of urine through the urethra and out of the body. The release of urine from the body is referred to as urination or micturition.

Functions

The urinary system functions include:
- The removal of various wastes and foreign chemicals (such as drugs and/or their by-products) from the blood and release from the body.
- Regulation of blood composition and volume. In addition to the removal of water, salts, and wastes, essential chemicals (such as water, sodium, and calcium) can be reabsorbed, pH levels are regulated (by uptake of ions), and blood pressure can be controlled.
- The kidneys produce some hormones as part of the endocrine system (see the section on the endocrine system), including erythropoietin that is involved in the control of RBC production.

Additional comments

Urology is the branch of medicine that deals with the urinary system, while nephrology particularly relates to the study of the kidneys. The term "renal" also pertains to the kidneys. There is a physically close relationship between the urinary and reproductive systems (see the section on the reproductive system), which are often medically referred to together as the genito-urinary (or urogenital) system.

Urinalysis is analysis of the urine for the purpose of medical diagnosis or monitoring. A urine sample is taken from a patient and can be subjected to various chemical and (if required) microbiological analyses as an indication of health or disorder. Urine is normally ~95% water, with the remaining 5% containing various chemicals such as urea, uric acid, ammonia, and minerals/salts (such as sodium and potassium). In various conditions the composition of urine can change dramatically and can indicate different internal disorders, diseases, diets, and so on. Urine, for example, is generally free of bacteria and the presence of certain types of bacteria can be indicative of a urinary tract infection (called a UTI). Chemically, the presence of blood (and therefore bleeding) may indicate damage to the various tissues/components of the system.

The system can be very robust, but when it is not working effectively it can be life threatening. Dialysis is a medical intervention that can act as an alternative, artificial system and is used in patients with damaged or diseased kidneys. "Hemodialysis" uses a machine to take blood from a patient, remove the wastes in the machine, and then return it to the patient. "Peritoneal" dialysis is performed within the patient, where a sterile fluid is added into the abdominal cavity and the surrounding peritoneal membrane that encloses the cavity acts as a substitute membrane for the exchange process with the blood; the fluid is maintained for a given time and then removed/discarded.

Like with many other natural orifices of the body, endoscopes can be used for the direct visualization, investigation, and treatment of various parts of the urinary system. Procedures include cystoscopy (investigating the bladder by entry through the urethra) and ureteroscopy (entry through the urethra and bladder to access the ureters).

Additional structures

There are two additional structures of the body that are briefly introduced and described in this section. These are the eyes and the ears, both of which work closely with the nervous system for the full scope of their functions.

Eyes

The eyes (Figure 2.21) are responsible for the sense of sight (the detection of light). They are ball shaped and associated with the skull (see the section on the skeletal system). From the outside we can see some of the internal structures at the front of the eye, including the sclera (the white surface that surrounds most of the eye), the iris (which is colored), and the central pupil (the central black circle). The front of the eye contains various structures such as the cornea, pupil, iris, and lens; they are all involved in allowing light to enter and be focused into the eye. Most of the eye's innermost wall is a specialized surface known as the retina. The retina contains the photoreceptors that respond to the presence of light; there are two types of receptors known as the rods (which react to dimmer light, showing blacks, whites, and grays) and the cones (which react to show various other

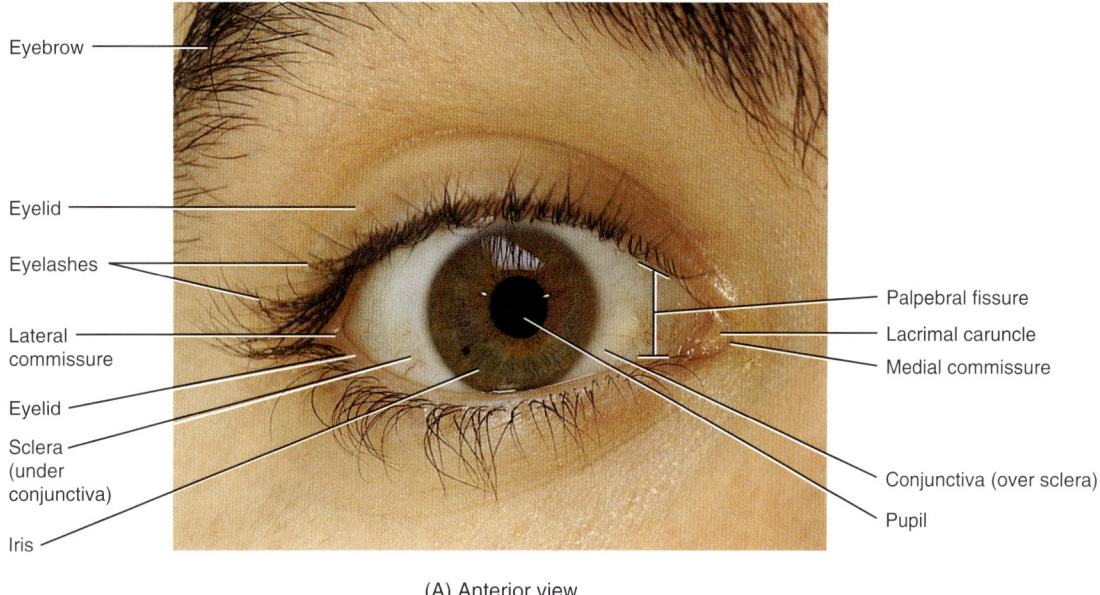

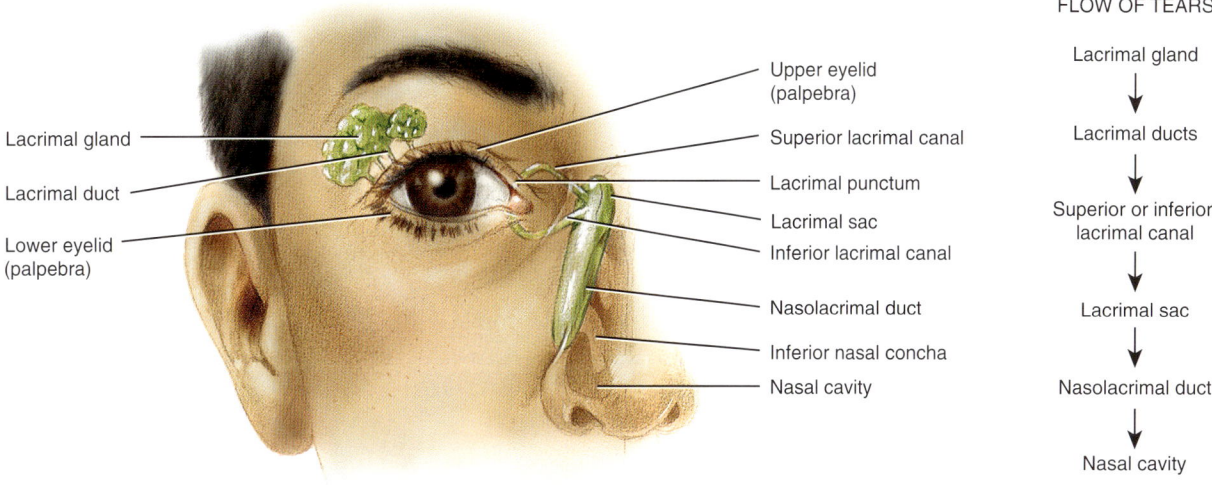

Figure 2.21 (A, B) The external and internal structures of the eye. Source: Reproduced with permission from Tortora et al. (2011) / John Wiley & Sons.

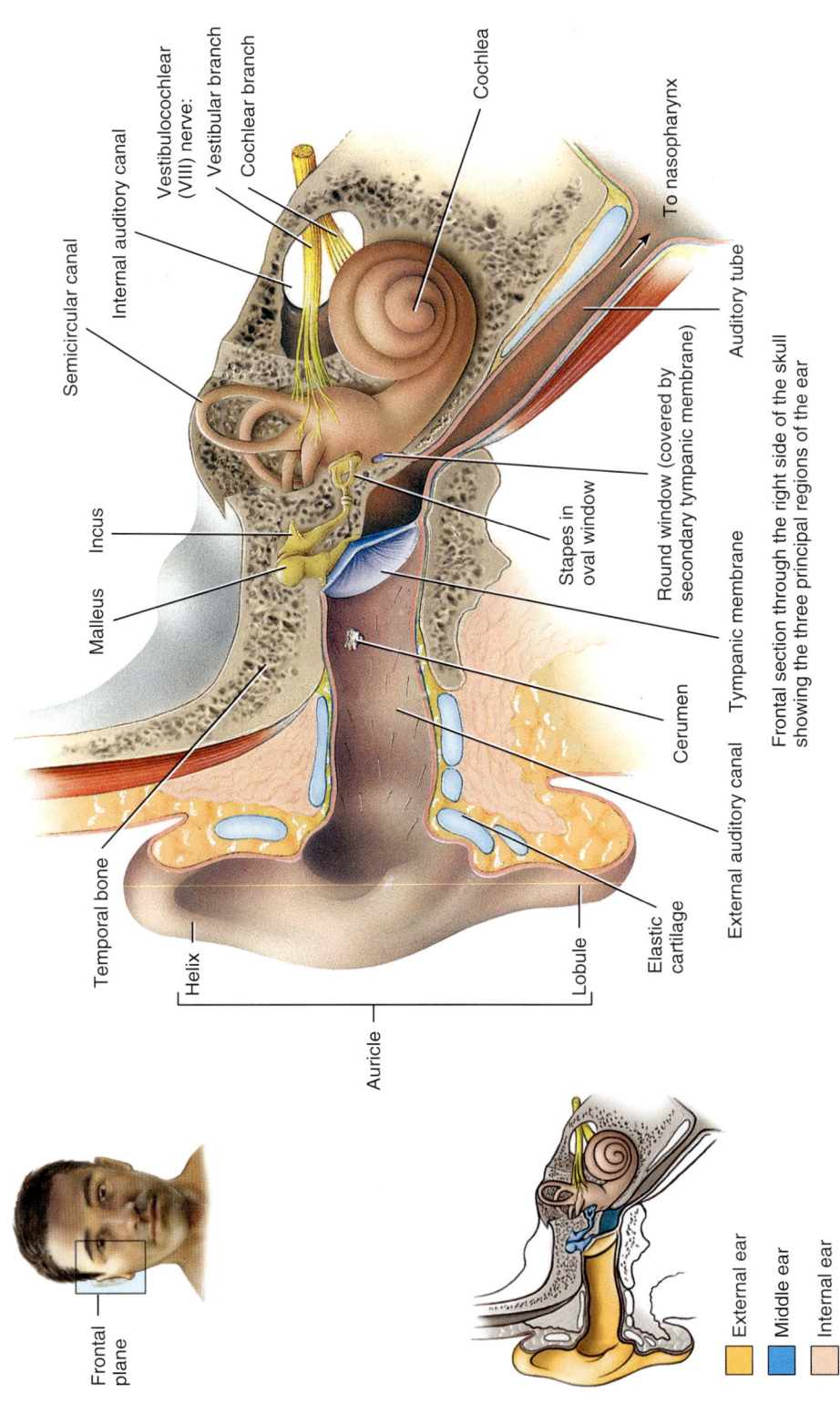

Figure 2.22 The external and internal structures of the ear. Source: Reproduced with permission from Tortora et al. (2011) / John Wiley & Sons.

colors). These receptors convert light to nerve pulses along nerve fibers that collect at the back of the eye to form the optic nerve. The eyeball is filled with a jelly-like substance known as vitreous humor that helps maintain the eyeball shape and protects the retina.

Ophthalmology (or optometry) is a medical specialty dealing with the eye and associated structures. The terms "ocular" and "optic" pertain to the eye and/or to light (e.g. fiber-optic or ocular diseases).

Ears

The ears (Figure 2.22) are responsible for the sense of sound (detection of vibrations). They are located on either side of the head and project into the skull. The ear structure consists of three areas: the outer, middle, and inner ear. The main, external part of the ear is called an "auricle" and functions in funneling sound waves into the ear. The auricle leads to the entry into the ear, along the auditory canal and to the eardrum (known as the tympanic membrane); the outer ear consists of the region from the auricle to the eardrum. The middle ear, on the other side of the eardrum, is a small cavity containing some of the smallest bones in the body known as the ossicles: malleus (hammer), incus (anvil), and stapes (stirrup). In that order the joint formed by these three ossicles provides a link from the eardrum to the oval window, a membrane that separates the middle and inner ear. The middle ear is also linked, by the auditory (or Eustachian) tube, to the upper pharynx (see the sections on the digestive and respiratory systems). The inner ear (or "labyrinth") consists of a series of fluid-filled channels, such as the semicircular canals and the cochlea. Sound is detected by directing sound waves into the outer ear, leading to vibrations on the eardrum; these vibrations are amplified through the bones of the middle ear and the interaction of the stapes along the oval window causes pressure changes in the inner ear structures. These pressure changes are converted into nerve pulses along a network of nerves in the inner ear that combine and leave the ear structure as the vestibulocochlear nerve. Although the ear detects sound, it is the transmission and interpretation of the signals that are transmitted to the brain that also form differentiation of language, music, and so on. In addition to hearing, the ear plays an important role in maintaining body balance.

Otology is the study of the ear and accessory structures, including various diseases and disorders. The ear, nose, and throat are all connected through the pharynx (see the sections on the digestive and respiratory systems) and are often considered under the same medical specialty (ENT) and by ENT specialists.

3 Medical and surgical procedures and facilities

The word "medical" refers to the study and practice of medicine, which is the science of and ability to heal. Generally it refers to the course of action concerned with the diagnosis, management, and especially non-surgical treatment of diseases, either of one particular organ system or of the body as a whole. Examples of medical interventions include observation (visually inspecting the patient's skin color, weight, teeth, temperature, blood pressure, and pulse rate) and specific therapeutic treatment (prescribing drugs, dialysis, chemotherapy, wound therapy, etc.). An important medical term that is worth defining is "diagnostic," which refers to a variety of observations and/or tests that can be performed in order to identify (diagnose the cause of) a particular disease or medical problem and to provide the supporting evidence such as the cause. Examples of diagnostic procedures include various types of endoscopy, cardiac stress tests, blood tests, X-rays, and so on. The term "surgical" refers to a specialty in medicine that investigates or treats disease or injury by an operative procedure. Surgical procedures (or "operations," "surgery") involve entering the body or body cavities by natural orifices or incision (breaking through the skin or other area of the body). Surgical specialties focus on the various operative and instrumental techniques to treat disease/injury, generally classified according to the organ, organ system, or tissue involved (Chapter 2). It should be pointed out that surgical procedures can be performed to treat disease or injury and may also be performed to improve function, to enhance body appearance (such as in cosmetic surgery), and even for religious reasons (such as circumcisions and tattoos). A variety of instruments and devices can be used with, on, or in patients during the procedures. When these are reused from patient to patient, device processing plays an essential role in reducing any health risks.

Medicine can be further sub-divided into three areas of care – primary, secondary, and tertiary:
- Primary care is care provided by health professionals who have first contact with a patient seeking treatment. This contact most often occurs in a doctor's office, outpatient clinic, nursing home, school, etc.
- Secondary care is provided to patients who are generally referred to hospitals, specialists, and specialized clinics by primary care providers, for either diagnosis or further specialist treatment.
- Tertiary care is specialized, highly technical care that includes diagnosis and treatment of disease and disability. Various types of diagnostic, surgical, and medical procedures can be performed in any of the areas mentioned depending on the nature of the procedure, risks of patient complications, and available facilities. Minor procedures can be considered routine and are performed in a physician's office, dental office, or opticians, whereas more complicated procedures require a full medical team and are usually restricted to dedicated hospital or clinic settings. These facilities can range from a procedure room to a specially designed area equipped with modern imaging, lighting, equipment, and self-contained air-handling systems (Figure 3.1).

Despite the design of these facilities, and regardless of the economic status of different geographic regions of the world, the same essential policies and procedures can be enforced to ensure the safe processing of reusable instrumentation and devices used for these procedures. The various different types of instruments are described further in Chapter 4. As outlined in Chapter 1, in the section on goals of decontamination and the Spaulding classification, a variety of medical and surgical instrumentation is used across the world; a standard system is recommended for the processing of instrumentation and devices based on the risk to an individual or patient. This system, known as the Spaulding classification, is based on the use of the instrument or device on a patient, and recommends a higher standard of processing (e.g. disinfection or sterilization) as the risks of the introduction of microbial contamination to that patient are considered greater. For example, if an instrument is introduced into or comes in contact with a patient's blood supply or sterile space, it carries a higher risk to that patient than a procedure that would only touch the intact skin. This classification system is not always as simple to apply as it appears, given the design of a facility or area in which a

---

Decontamination and Device Processing in Healthcare, Second Edition. Gerald McDonnell and Georgia Alevizopoulou.
© 2025 John Wiley & Sons Ltd. Published 2025 by John Wiley & Sons Ltd.

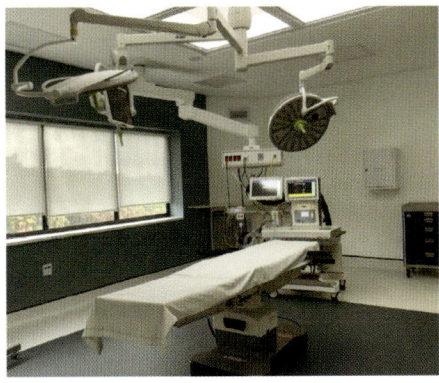 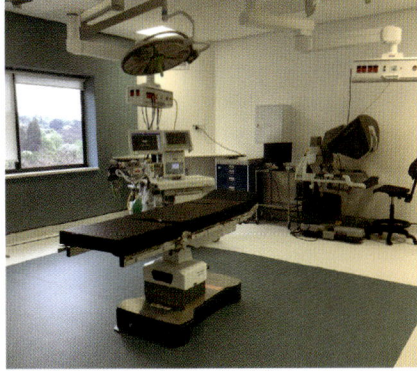 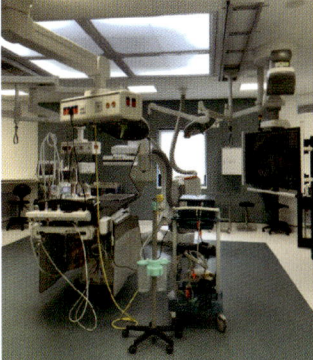
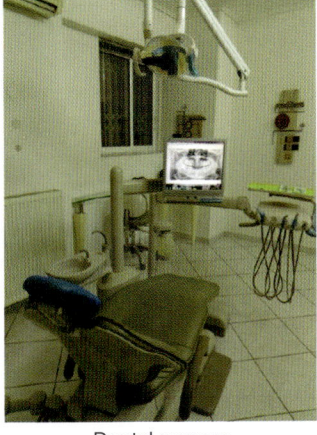 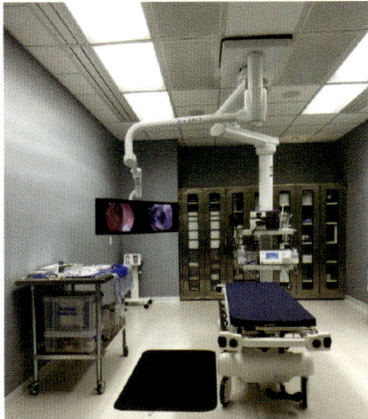 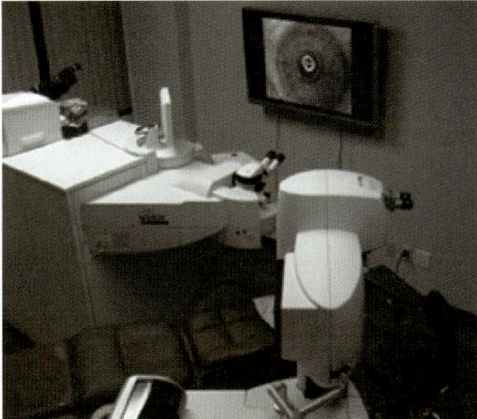

Operating room (OR)   OR with robotic surgeon console   Hybrid OR

Dental surgery   Endoscopy suite   LASIK eye surgery

Figure 3.1 Examples of the various types of facilities in which medical and surgical techniques are in use worldwide. Although the design and investment in such facilities can range dramatically depending on the patient procedure and country-specific economic situation, the essential practices of device processing should remain the same.

medical or surgical procedure is being conducted. It is expected that the highest levels of processing standards should be applied to the higher-risk surgical instruments and devices that enter essentially sterile areas of the body, such as those used in neurosurgery (into the brain or spinal cord), orthopedic surgery (e.g. knee and hip implants), and cardiothoracic (e.g. heart) surgery. Most, if not all, of these types of procedures should be conducted with sterile instruments and devices and in dedicated operating rooms (ORs). However, procedures that may also be considered as requiring sterile instrumentation and techniques are often performed in other facilities such as dental practices, cosmetic surgery clinics, and tattoo parlors, where the person's blood system may be entered. Although the design of such facilities may be dramatically different, the processing standards should remain the same as the risk to the individual is just as high.

Historical methods of surgical intervention often were associated with exposing internal body organs and tissues to the air for long periods of time, therefore exposing the patient to a greater risk of infection. Newer methods and techniques of medical and surgical interventions (e.g. using various types of endoscopic instrumentation for minimally invasive surgery, MIS) are less invasive than historical methods, shortening the surgery time and reducing trauma to the patient. The complex equipment used today for these procedures can present a challenge, as it is often more difficult to perform safe and effective device processing and can therefore result in an increased risk of infection or other patient complication.

An infection is a type of disease caused by microorganisms (Chapter 5). Surgical site infections (SSIs) are defined as infections that occur in or around surgical sites (usually incisions), typically when microorganisms are introduced at the time of surgery (e.g. when a contaminated device is introduced into a patient). SSIs can be, but are not always, acquired during an operation, either from the OR environment, medical equipment, or staff ("exogenous") or from microorganisms on the patient's skin ("endogenous"). The risk of infection is also dependent on the patient's general health, length of the procedure, wound classification, and so on. Other predisposing factors include the surgical technique used, the presence of foreign bodies, such as implants, drains, or pre-operative shaving (if used), and the experience and skill of the surgical team. A clean OR environment with sterile (or correctly decontaminated) equipment, with restricted access and appropriately attired staff, can go a long way to reducing the risks of SSIs.

Procedures and techniques

When a cure is unlikely naturally over time or through medication alone, various medical, diagnostic, and surgical procedures can be performed to identify causes and alleviate disease and suffering. A variety of devices and instrumentation can be used to perform these procedures. The terms "instrument" and "device" are used interchangeably throughout this book as generally meaning any inanimate object that is used for medical, diagnostic, or surgical procedures. In some countries terms such as "medical device" are used specifically from a legal point of view. This topic is discussed further in Chapter 4.

Medical and surgical procedures can be categorized according to their urgency, body system involved, department they are conducted in (e.g. dedicated ORs for specialized procedures such as orthopedics, cardiac, or neurosurgery, since different equipment is used), type of procedure, degree of invasiveness, and any special instrumentation that may be used (e.g. an endoscopic suite or catheterization laboratory). Based on the diagnosis and need for surgical intervention, patient admission is generally classified according to the organ, organ system, or tissue involved (Chapter 2). Dentistry, while being a separate discipline from medicine, is also considered part of the medical field. There may also be various options on how the procedure will be performed, for example:
• Elective procedures – these may not be essential but may improve the quality of life. The patient can choose if and when to have the procedure.
• Required procedures – these need to be done to prevent future complications, but do not necessarily have to be done immediately.
• Emergency procedures – often a matter of life or death and are required due to an urgent medical or traumatic event.

Medical procedures are generally performed in hospitals, doctor's offices, clinics, dental offices, and so on, and are supported by a multidisciplinary group of professionals, often referred to as the medical team, consisting of experts in various disciplines of medicine who collaborate to better serve their patient's needs.

The medical team

The healthcare medical team consists of physicians, surgeons, registered nurses and nurse practitioners, clinical pharmacists, dieticians, physical therapists, social workers, microbiologists, occupational therapists, and others. Depending on the medical discipline, a multidisciplinary team cares for the patient throughout his/her stay. In many cases a smaller team or even an individual may be responsible for immediate care, such as in the case of emergency treatment or local surgery and dental procedures.

Types of medical disciplines

Examples of the most common types of medical disciplines are given in Table 3.1.

Medical equipment

Medical equipment is designed to aid in the diagnosis, monitoring, or treatment of medical conditions. It includes a variety of devices and it is not within the scope of this book to describe all of these in detail.

Two of the most obvious examples of simple and widely used medical devices are:
• A stethoscope used to listen to breathing, lung, and heart sounds
• A Baumanometer/blood pressure machine used to check a patient's blood pressure (BP)

More complicated examples include:
• Therapeutic equipment, used to assist with patient treatment, including infusion pumps and dialysis equipment.
• Life support equipment, used to maintain a patient's basic bodily functions (breathing, kidney function), such as medical ventilators, anesthetic machines, heart–lung machines, extracorporeal membrane oxygenation (ECMO), and dialysis machines.
• Diagnostic equipment, such as electrocardiography (ECG), a non-invasive transthoracic recording of the electrical activity of the heart captured and externally recorded by skin electrodes and direct imaging devices. The range of diagnostic

Table 3.1 Types and descriptions of medical disciplines.

Discipline	Explanation
Alternative medicine	Acupuncture, chiropractic, homeopathy, naturopathy, osteopathy
Cardiology	Disease of the cardiovascular system dealing with congenital heart defects, coronary artery disease, heart failure, valvular heart disease, and cardiac emergencies
Critical care medicine	Deals with life support and management of critically ill patients, often in an intensive care unit (ICU)
Dermatology	Skin and its appendages (hair, nails, sweat glands, etc.)
Emergency medicine	The primary management of medical emergencies, often in hospital emergency departments or at point of injury
Endocrinology	The endocrine system (i.e. endocrine glands and hormones; see Chapter 2) and its diseases, including diabetes and thyroid diseases
Gastroenterology	The alimentary tract and associated organs (see Chapter 2)
Geriatrics	Care of elderly patients
Hematology	Deals with the blood, the blood-forming organs, and blood diseases
Hepatology	Liver and biliary tract, usually a part of gastroenterology
Immunology	Deals with the immune system
Infectious disease	Diseases caused by biological agents
Medical genetics	Diagnosis and management of hereditary disorders
Nephrology	Diseases involving the kidneys
Neurology	Diseases involving the central, peripheral, and autonomic nervous systems (see Chapter 2)
Neurophysiology	Physiology or function of the central and peripheral nervous systems
Nuclear medicine	The study of various systems of the body, for diagnostic and therapeutic reasons, using radioisotopes or radioactive methods. An example is using a PET (positron emission tomography) scanner and radioactivity sources such as Technetium99m
Obstetrics/gynecology	Deals with childbirth, reproductive, and fertility medicine, the female reproductive system, and associated organs (see Chapter 2)
Oncology	Cancer and other malignant diseases (due to uncontrolled growth of tissues)
Ophthalmology	Diseases of the visual pathways, including the eyes, brain, etc.
Pediatrics	The medical care of infants, children, and adolescents (newborn to 16–21 years, depending on the country)
Palliative care	Pain and symptom relief and emotional support in patients with long-term or terminal illnesses
Pathology	The study and diagnosis of disease, including studying tissues, organs, and the whole body (e.g. an autopsy) and by other laboratory analysis (e.g. analyzing blood and urine samples)
Psychiatry	The diagnosis, treatment, and prevention of cognitive, perceptual, emotional, and behavioral disorders
Pulmonology/respirology	The lungs and respiratory system (see Chapter 2)
Radiology	Imaging of the human body, e.g. by X-rays, computed tomography, ultrasonography, and nuclear magnetic resonance tomography
Rheumatology	Autoimmune and inflammatory diseases of the joints and other organ systems (e.g. arthritis and other rheumatic diseases)
Urology	The urinary tract system of males and females, and the male reproductive system (see Chapter 2)

imaging equipment that is available, giving the ability to look into the body without the need for surgery, exemplifies some of the greatest advances in medicine in recent years. Traditionally X-rays were used for this purpose, in particular to view damaged (broken or fractured) bone. But technological advances now include:

- Magnetic resonance imaging (MRI), an imaging technique used in radiology to visualize detailed internal structures.

The imaging makes it possible to differentiate between healthy and unhealthy/abnormal tissue, and it is especially useful in imaging brain, muscles, and heart, and in cancer diagnosis.
  ○ Computed tomography (CT), a medical imaging X-ray procedure that uses ionizing electromagnetic radiation (tomography) for processing the X-rays.
  ○ Positron emission tomography (PET), a nuclear medicine imaging technique that produces a three-dimensional image or picture of functional processes in the body.
  ○ Cardiac catheterization, a procedure used for both diagnostic and interventional purposes to determine and/or treat various heart conditions. It involves passing a thin catheter into a chamber or vessel of the heart.

As a note, a catheter is a flexible or rigid tube that is inserted into the body for the purpose of introducing or withdrawing a fluid, creating an opening (e.g. for another device), or to keep any passageway open; examples include cardiac (in the heart), intravenous (into a vein), and urine (into the bladder to collect urine, e.g. Foley) catheters. In cardiac surgery a thin flexible catheter is inserted into the chambers of the heart and associated blood vessels, either via the femoral artery in the groin or the radial artery in the wrist. The catheter is inserted using a long guidewire and moved toward the heart. Once the catheter is in position the guidewire is removed. The cardiologist can view the progress of the catheter on a video screen and may insert a further device or contrast medium (a type of dye) through the catheter to treat a specific condition or provide further visualization. This procedure is usually performed using a local anesthetic that is injected into the skin at the point of entry (wrist/groin) to numb the insertion area.

A summary of some examples of common medical and diagnostic procedures performed in hospitals and clinics is given in Table 3.2.

Surgical procedures

Surgical procedures are generally performed by a surgical team in a dedicated OR (surgical theater/suite). The basic surgical team consists of experts in operative procedure, pain management, and overall or specific patient care. The surgical team is responsible for patient care during the peri-operative period. This period includes the pre-, intra-, and post-operative management of the patient from preparation for the surgical procedure to surgery itself and through to discharge:
• Pre-operative care is the preparation and management of a patient prior to surgery. It can include both physical and psychological preparation.
• Intra-operative care is the management of the patient during the operative procedure while in the OR. The intra-operative period begins when the patient is transferred onto the table in the OR and ends when the patient is transferred to the recovery area. During this period the patient may be anesthetized, prepped, and draped, and the operation is performed.
• Post-operative care is the management of the patient after the procedure until discharge.

The basic makeup of any surgical team will depend on the type of surgery to be performed (discipline), the precise procedures (complexity, etc.), and the location and the type of anesthesia (the induced loss of pain) that will be used. The team may include surgeons, anesthesiologists, nursing and technical staff who are trained in general surgery or in a particular surgical specialty. Complicated specialized surgeries require larger teams. Minimally invasive procedures require specialized expertise as well as dedicated instruments and equipment.

Surgical team members

Surgical team members can include a few or many qualified persons, depending on the complexity of the surgical procedure. These generally include the surgeon, an anesthesiologist, and various nursing staff.

The surgeon generally leads the surgical team and is responsible for performing the surgery in an effective and safe manner. Surgeons are qualified doctors who have undergone further intensive training in surgical procedures. The anesthesiologist is responsible for ensuring the safety of the patient and reducing the stress of the operation, including pain relief. Anesthesiologists are qualified physicians with advanced training in anesthesia, which can be defined as the induced or controlled loss of sensing pain. Anesthesia may or may not be associated with falling asleep (loss of consciousness); examples include local and general anesthesia, referring to methods used to render part of the body free from pain (but remaining conscious) and putting the patient "to sleep" (unconscious and loss of pain), respectively. Anesthesiologists are therefore directly or indirectly involved in all three stages of surgery (pre-operative, operative, and post-operative) due to their focus on pain management and patient safety before, during, and after surgery. An anesthetist is often a registered professional nurse who is trained to administer anesthetics and supports the anesthesiologists.

Nursing staff are an important part of the surgical team. They are involved in care, assistance, and pain management throughout the peri-operative period. Specific nursing staff will include the scrub and circulating nurse. The scrub nurse is a qualified nurse who assists the surgeon during an operation by passing instruments, sutures, and so on. A circulating nurse is an integral part of the peri-operative team who manages the flow of patients and materials in the surgical suite, ensuring a safe and comfortable environment. The circulating nurse is a non-sterile member of the team.

Table 3.2 Common medical procedures.

Procedure	Explanation
Acupuncture	A commonly used alternative medicine procedure to theoretically rebalance patterns of energy flow ("Qi") through the body that are essential for health. Any disruption of Qi is believed to be responsible for disease. The most common procedure involves penetration of the skin by thin, solid, metallic needles for manual/electrical stimulation of acupuncture points.
Amniocentesis	A non-surgical procedure where a sample of fluid is removed from the amniotic sac (fluid-filled structure inside the pregnant uterus within which the baby lives) for analysis. Fluid is removed by placing a long needle, often guided using ultrasound imaging, through the abdominal wall into the amniotic sac.
Apheresis	A medical procedure that involves removing whole blood from a donor or patient and separating or selectively removing individual components so that one particular component can be removed. The procedure involves passing the blood from the person through a machine and then back into the patient. For example, plasmapheresis is the removal of blood plasma (a colorless watery fluid of the blood in which the various blood cells are carried; Chapter 2).
Atherectomy	The removal of plaque, usually from the coronary vessels.
Biopsy	The removal of a sample of tissue from the body for diagnostic/examination purposes. A biopsy may be performed in an operating room, clinic, or doctor's office by surgery or needle aspiration. Examples include a breast or liver biopsy.
Blood transfusion	Blood previously taken from a patient or from another person (donor) is administered directly into a patient via an intravenous catheter.
Bone marrow aspiration	A medical procedure used to withdraw bone marrow, the blood-forming portion of certain bones (Chapter 2). A special needle is inserted into the hip bone or sternum (chest bone) to withdraw a sample.
Chemotherapy	The use of toxic chemicals (drugs) for treating disease. Antibiotic chemotherapy is used to treat bacterial infection (Chapter 5). Cancer chemotherapy uses low concentrations of highly toxic drugs that may reduce or destroy fast-growing and abnormal human tissue (such as in the cause of "tumor" or cancer development). In the treatment of cancer, chemotherapy can cure (no signs of the disease) or control (reducing the size of a tumor) the disease. Chemotherapy may be administered intravenously (through a vein), orally (by mouth), by injection, topically (applied to the skin), intra-arterially (directly into the artery that is feeding the cancer), or intra-peritoneal (directly into the peritoneal cavity; Chapter 2). Allowing multiple administration of the drug is often assisted by using a catheter that is surgically placed, or a port placed under the skin and connected to a large vein.
Collagen injections	Cosmetic injections used to give the skin a plumper, smoother appearance.
Computerized axial tomography (CAT) scan	A CAT scan produces a computer-generated image of the structures within the body, to assist in diagnosing tumors, fractures, bony growth, and infections in the organs and tissues. Data from multiple X-ray images is converted into pictures on a computer screen.
Coronary angiogram	Using a cardiac catheter, this procedure shows up the structure of the coronary arteries to detect any narrowing or damage. A doctor inserts a small catheter (diameter of 23 mm) through the skin into an artery (in the groin or the arm), which is guided, with the assistance of a fluoroscope (a special X-ray viewing instrument), to the coronary arteries. A small amount of radiographic contrast (an iodine solution), which is easily visualized with X-ray images, is injected into each coronary artery. The X-ray images that are produced are referred to as an angiogram.
Dialysis	The movement of fluids and chemicals across a semipermeable (selective) membrane. Medically, dialysis is used to correct fluid and electrolyte imbalances and remove waste products. It replaces kidney function (urinary system; Chapter 2) by artificially filtering and cleansing the blood of excess fluid, minerals, and wastes. There are two main types of dialysis: hemodialysis and peritoneal dialysis. During hemodialysis the blood is removed from the patient and circulated through a dialysis machine, where the dialysis takes place and then the blood is returned to the patient. Peritoneal dialysis uses the patient's own body tissues (peritoneal cavity) to act as a filter. A "dialysis catheter" is inserted through the abdominal wall into the abdominal cavity. Dialysis fluid ("dialysate") is infused into the abdominal cavity, allowed to exchange (dialyze) in the body, and then removed.
Electrocardiogram (EKG)	Usually the first and most simple test used to diagnose any coronary artery disease (CAD). It is a non-invasive test used to measure underlying heart conditions by measuring the electrical activity of the heart via positioning leads around the heart and on the arms and legs in standard locations. Information about the electrical activity of the heart is recorded on a screen.

(continued)

Table 3.2 (cont'd).

Procedure	Explanation
Endotracheal intubation	A medical procedure to assist breathing, where a tube is inserted through the mouth into the trachea (the large airway from the mouth to the lungs). The endotracheal tube artificially opens a passage through the upper airway allowing air to pass freely to and from the lungs. It can be connected to a mechanical ventilator to provide artificial respiration. The tube is inserted through a device known as a laryngoscope, which allows the practitioner to see the upper portion of the trachea, just below the vocal cords.
Lumbar puncture (LP)	A sampling procedure used to diagnose or even treat diseases associated with the cerebrospinal fluid (CSF; Chapter 2). In some cases the CSF is removed to decrease spinal fluid pressure in the patient.
Magnetic resonance imaging (MRI) scan	A radiology technique using magnetism, radio waves, and a computer to produce images of internal body structures. The MRI scanner looks like a long tube (into which the body is placed) that is surrounded by a giant circular magnet. The magnet creates a strong magnetic field that is used to produce a very faint signal from the various parts of the body. These are detected by the scanner and processed by a computer to give an image. MRI can be used to detect small structural differences throughout the body.
Pacemaker insertion	A pacemaker is a small device that controls the heart (cardiac) rhythm using electrical impulses. A battery-operated pacemaker is placed in the chest or abdomen through a small incision.
Pap smear	A medical sampling procedure in which a sample of cells is removed from a woman's cervix (the bottom end of the uterus) and sent for microscopy in order to detect pre-malignant (before-cancer) or malignant (cancer) changes.
Percutaneous transluminal coronary angioplasty (PTCA) or percutaneous coronary intervention (PCI)	An angioplasty is a non-surgical procedure that involves the insertion of a small balloon catheter into an artery in the groin (femoral) or arm (brachial), which is advanced past the narrowing in the coronary artery. The balloon is then inflated to enlarge the narrowing in the artery. As part of this procedure, a stent (a stainless steel wire-mesh design) can be inserted into the coronary artery to assist in keeping it open; during a PCI the balloon (angioplasty) is removed and the stent remains in the artery to keep it open. If successful PCI can relieve chest pain and improve the prognosis of individuals with unstable angina, minimizing the risk of a heart attack without having the patient undergo open heart coronary artery by-pass grafting (CABG) surgery.
Restoration of dental caries	Caries is any kind of progressive bone, including teeth, that decays or is damaged over time. Dental caries is therefore tooth decay caused by bacteria in the mouth. During a routine procedure a dentist uses a drill, air abrasion instrument, or laser to remove the decayed areas of the tooth. Once the decay has been removed, the tooth is prepared by cleaning the cavity of bacteria and debris, and then restored using a "filling." If the tooth has extensive decay or if there is a risk of infection or injury to the tooth's pulp, this may require a more serious surgical intervention by extraction (removal of the tooth) and endodontic therapy (known as a "root canal"). A root canal involves the removal of the outer and lower tooth, which can be reconstructed with a replacement, artificial tooth (including the outer "crown").
Ultrasonography (sonography) and echocardiography	Ultrasonography (an "ultrasound") is a radiological technique using high-frequency sound waves to produce images of the structures within the body. Echocardiography uses ultrasound to visualize the heart. There are several types. During transthoracic procedures a transducer that transmits high-frequency sound waves (ultrasound) is placed on the chest; these sound waves bounce off the heart structures, producing images and sounds that can detect heart damage and disease. In transesophageal echocardiogram (TEE) the transducer is inserted through the esophagus for the same purpose but placed closer to the heart, allowing for a clearer picture. A further example is a stress echocardiogram, which is performed prior to and just after exercise in order to measure the motion of the heart's walls and pumping action when stressed.

Surgical techniques

There are many different surgical techniques that may be used depending on the type of surgery to be performed, available equipment, the surgeon or patient's preference, and the patient's anatomy or physiological condition at the time. A summary of the major different types is given in Table 3.3. Despite continuing improvements of surgical techniques, there is still considerable variation in the literature as to the optimal management technique.

Surgical disciplines and common procedures

There are a number of different surgical specialties or disciplines generally classified depending on the area of the body on which the procedures may be performed, for example the brain, stomach, liver, intestines, appendix, breasts, heart, and so on.

Table 3.3 Various types of surgical techniques.

Technique	Explanation
Cosmetic surgery	Performed to improve the appearance of an otherwise normal surface structure of the body.
Laser surgery	Involves the use of a laser, allowing the surgeon to precisely cut tissue instead of using a physical knife (scalpel) or similar surgical instruments. An example is LASIK (laser-assisted in situ keratomileusis) surgery, a special type of laser-assisted eye surgery for correcting eyesight.
Microsurgery	Involves the use of an operating microscope positioned above a small incision allowing the surgeon to visualize small structures.
Minimally invasive surgery (MIS)	A surgical technique that involves minimal or a limited number of incisions (holes) on the skin to insert specially designed instruments into a body cavity or structure ("keyhole procedure"). Natural orifices, such as the alimentary canal and the bellybutton (navel, "umbilicus"), are also used. The surgeon can see into and directly operate in the body through the use of associated devices. MIS is associated with a lower rate of post-operative patient implications compared with a conventional approach for the same operation, including reducing the associated tissue trauma, pain, and bleeding, lowering risks of infection, promoting rapid healing, and cosmetically leaving smaller scars.
Open surgery	Procedures that require a large incision to access the relevant area of skin and tissues to allow the surgeon direct access to the internal structures or organs involved, e.g. the removal or repair of an internal organ such as a gall bladder.
Reconstructive surgery	Involves reconstruction of an injured, mutilated, or deformed part of the body (including the teeth in dental surgery).
Robotic-assisted surgery (RAS)	Makes use of a surgical robot that controls the surgical instrumentation, by indirect or voice activation, under the direction of the surgeon.
Tattooing	A tattoo is a marking made by inserting indelible ink into the dermis layer of the skin.
Transplant surgery	Replacement of an organ or body part by removing the diseased organ and replacing it with a donated healthy organ.

Depending on the capabilities and specialties of any facility and the associated staff, a number of common procedures may be performed. The most common surgical specialties include:

- General surgery – general surgeons operate on almost any part of the body. They confirm the diagnoses provided by primary care or emergency physicians, then perform the necessary procedures to correct or alleviate the problem. If a specialized procedure is involved, they will often refer the patient to a relevant specialist.
- Cardiothoracic surgery – this is a common surgical specialty and often with very high demands. The cardiothoracic surgical team treats pathological conditions within the chest, including the heart and its valves, the lung, esophagus, and chest wall and blood vessels.
- Neurosurgery – neurosurgical teams specialize in surgery of the nervous system, including the brain, spine, and peripheral nervous system, and their supporting structures.
- Oral and maxillofacial surgery – maxillary facial surgical teams deal with surgical problems of the head and neck; that is, the ears, sinuses, mouth, pharynx, jaw, and other structures of the head and neck.
- Reconstructive and plastic surgery – surgery on abnormal structures of the body due to injury, birth defects, infection, tumors, or disease. These teams also perform cosmetic surgery to improve a patient's appearance.
- Transplantation – these teams specialize in specific organ transplant techniques, such as heart and heart–lung transplants, liver transplants and kidney/pancreas transplants. These highly intricate surgeries require very advanced training and technological support.
- Urology and renal transplantation – these teams deal with the kidneys, kidney stones, bladder, urethra, and ureters and coordinate with transplant team members.
- Gastrointestinal surgery – the team specializes in problems of the digestive tract (stomach, bowels, liver, and gall bladder).
- Vascular surgery – diagnosis and treatment of arterial and venous disorders such as aneurysms, lower-extremity revascularization, and other problems.
- Pediatric surgery – specially trained to perform procedures on infants and children. These teams work closely with specially trained anesthesiologists, and are experts in childhood diseases of the head, neck, chest, and abdomen, with training in birth defects and injuries.
- A range of other types of surgical procedures are listed in Table 3.4.

Table 3.4 Examples of specific surgical procedures.

Procedure	Explanation
Adeno-tonsillectomy	Removal of the adenoids and/or tonsils, generally due to chronic infection.
Amputation	Cutting off a body part, usually a limb or digit. Replantation involves reattaching a severed body part.
Appendectomy	Surgical removal of the appendix, a small appendage that branches off the large intestine.
Arthroplasty	The surgical reconstruction or replacement of a joint.
Cesarean section	Surgical delivery of a baby through an incision in the mother's abdomen and uterus.
Cholecystectomy	Surgical removal of the gall bladder because it is infected, cancerous, or has an accumulation of gallstones.
Coronary artery by-pass	Grafting (surgically taking a portion of living tissue from one part of an individual to another part, or from one individual to another) of veins or arteries, taken from the leg or chest, from the aorta to the coronary artery, in order to by-pass vessels that are blocked.
Hemorrhoidectomy	Removal of hemorrhoids in the lower rectum or anus.
Hysterectomy	Surgical removal of a woman's uterus (womb). This may be performed either through an abdominal incision or intravaginally, and may or may not include the removal of fallopian tubes and ovaries.
Inguinal hernia repair	Inguinal hernias are usually found in men and are protrusions of part of the intestine into the muscles of the groin. These can be surgically repaired.
Mastectomy	Removal of all or part of the breast, usually performed to treat breast cancer.
Partial colectomy	Removal of part of the large intestine (colon) to treat cancer or ulcerative colitis.
Prostatectomy	Removal of all or part of the prostate gland in males, which surrounds the neck of the bladder. A prostatectomy may be performed for an enlarged or cancerous prostate. It can be done as a minimally invasive procedure using a rigid cystoscope or as an open procedure.
Restoration of dental caries	Dental caries is progressive tooth decay and can be minor or serious. Serious cases may require surgical intervention by extraction (removal of the tooth) and endodontic therapy (known as a "root canal"). A root canal involves the removal of the outer and lower tooth, which can be reconstructed with a replacement, artificial tooth (including the outer "crown").
Skin grafting	Detaching healthy skin from one part of the body to repair areas of lost or damaged skin in another part of the body. Usually performed when the wound is too large to be repaired by stitching or natural healing.
Surgical endoscopy	The use of specific types of devices (endoscopes) and accessories through tiny incisions, called portals, to allow the surgeon to visualize and operate within a patient. A form of minimally invasive surgery used for a variety of procedures including appendectomies, gallbladder surgery, oophorectomy, repair of shoulder and knee ligaments, etc.
Tattooing	A tattoo is a puncture wound made by penetrating the skin with a needle and injecting ink into the area, usually creating some sort of design. What makes tattoos so long-lasting is that the ink is not injected into the dermis, which is the second, deeper layer of skin. A tattoo machine is a handheld electric instrument that uses a reusable or disposable handle and disposable needle system. On one end is a sterilized needle, which is attached to tubes that contain ink. A foot switch is used to turn the machine on and off, which moves the needle in and out while driving the ink into the skin. Medical tattooing is used to conceal a condition or the effects of a treatment, for example after breast reconstruction or simply marking the precise position where radiotherapy is applied.
Tracheotomy (tracheostomy)	A tracheotomy is a surgically created opening in the trachea (the breathing tube). It is kept open with a hollow tube called a tracheostomy tube. This is performed to by-pass an obstructed upper airway that prevents oxygen from reaching the lungs, to clean and remove secretions from the airway, or to deliver oxygen directly to the lungs. Commonly performed in an intensive care unit, emergency room, or operating theater during emergency situations or on very ill patients.
Wound debridement	Surgical removal of foreign material and/or dead, damaged, or infected tissue from a wound or burn in order to facilitate effective healing.

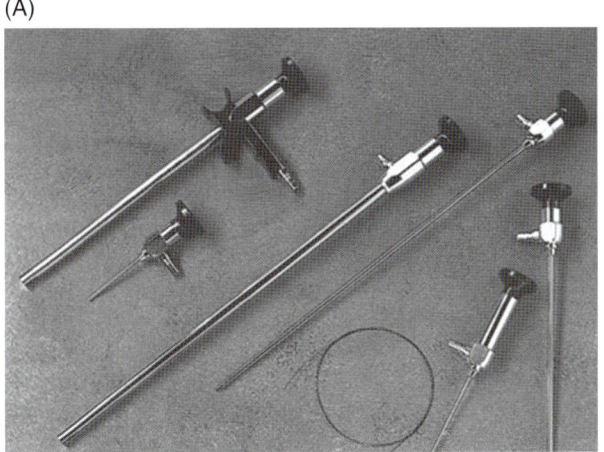 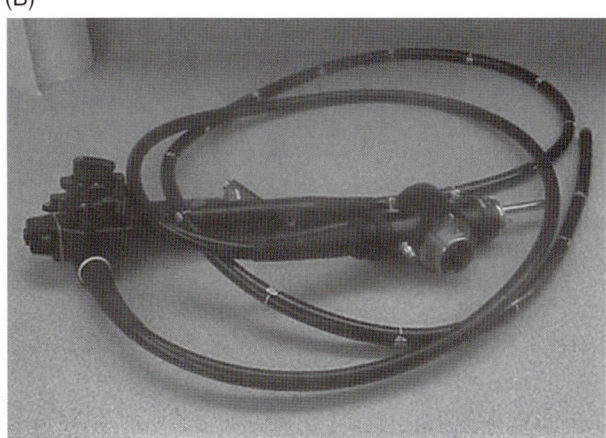

Figure 3.2 Examples of (A) rigid and (B) flexible endoscopes used for endoscopic procedures.

Endoscopy and endoscopic procedures

Endoscopy means looking inside. The word is derived from the Greek *endon*, meaning "within," and *scopeo*, meaning "examine." Endoscopy therefore refers to any procedure to look inside the body, for medical, diagnostic, and surgical purposes, using a device known as an endoscope. Endoscopes are advanced, sophisticated medical instruments that serve both a diagnostic and a therapeutic role. They vary greatly in terms of design, construction, materials, intended use, and so on (Figure 3.2). Endoscopes are most usually inserted into the body through existing orifices, such as the mouth and rectum, but in certain cases small incisions may be made so that otherwise inaccessible body areas may be examined. The design, morphology, and types of the various endoscopes are discussed in more detail in Chapter 4.

Endoscopy is one of the fastest-growing areas of medical and surgical practice used for patient care. It has evolved and matured so rapidly during the past few decades that it has transformed the practice of medicine and the approach to traditional, well-established medical procedures. Merely from a classification standpoint, endoscopy is grouped under what are referred to as minimally invasive procedures. By definition, that is any procedure, surgical or diagnostic, that is used to assess the interior surfaces of an organ causing minimal damage of biological tissues at the point of entrance of the instrument(s). One way in which endoscopic procedures can be defined is based on the area of the body on which they are performed (Table 3.5).

Endoscopic procedures comprise a significant percentage of healthcare across the world. They are increasingly popular among both patients and medical staff due to the clinical benefits they are associated with. By eliminating the large incisions, typical of open surgery, pain and recovery times are significantly reduced; less trauma is associated with limited discomfort and little or no scarring. Physicians and surgeons champion endoscopy for its efficacy, allowing greater flexibility and patient management. Coupled with the tremendous growth in the adoption of various cancer screening programs, the volume of the endoscopic procedures is estimated to rise even further. Advances continue to progress with both diagnostics and the ability to perform more and more therapeutic procedures, such as those involved with robotic-assisted surgery (RAS) and with more surgical procedures being performed through natural body offices, such as natural orifice transluminal endoscopic surgery (NOTES).

The operating/procedure room

Medical procedures, due to their nature and range, can be conducted in a variety of settings, ranging from at home to the general practice doctor's office, clinics, dedicated hospitals rooms, or ambulatory (outpatient) surgical centers (ASCs). Some of these procedures require specialized instruments (such as MRI scanners and dialysis machines) and are therefore limited to where the equipment is available; but with technological advances in both medical and diagnostic equipment, even complex instrumentation is becoming more widely available, miniaturized, and mobile. Surgical and critical medical procedures pose an increased risk of infection and other complications to the patient; for this reason, these procedures are usually conducted in specifically designed and dedicated areas. These include various designs of operating and dedicated procedure rooms. An operating room, also called surgical theater or suite, is usually a purpose-built,

Table 3.5 Examples of various types of endoscopic procedures.

Procedure	Explanation
Arthroscopy	An arthroscope is inserted into a joint to examine or treat the interior of the joint.
Bronchoscopy	A procedure performed to inspect the respiratory system including the lungs, larynx (voice box), vocal cord, trachea, and bronchi. Lung tissue can be biopsied and lung contents can be sampled using a variety of methods (such as by aspiration or washing) through the bronchoscope. Bronchoscopes are commonly flexible in design but may also be rigid.
Colonoscopy	Visualization of the colon by inserting a flexible device (colonoscope) through the anus and into the colon. Typically used for diagnosis (e.g. causes of bleeding and colon cancer screening), but also for some surgical techniques. Samples of the colon can be removed for further analysis using specific accessories such a biopsy forceps.
Cystoscopy	Examination of the urinary tract. A cystoscope is inserted through the urethra to examine the urethra and bladder cavity.
Endoscopic retrograde cholangiopancreatography (ERCP)	Using a duodenoscope inserted through the mouth and through the upper digestive system, particularly for investigations and procedures in the duodenum (between the stomach and small intestine), including the bile duct (connecting the liver/gall bladder to the duodenum).
Gastroscopy	A flexible gastroscope is inserted through the mouth into the upper digestive system to visually inspect the lining of the esophagus, stomach, and upper duodenum. It is also possible to perform minor procedures (polpectomy) and take tissue samples via a gastroscope.
Hysteroscopy	Examination of the vagina and uterus. Introduction of a hysteroscope through the vagina.
Laparoscopy	A laparoscope is inserted through a small incision and used to visualize and aid a surgical procedure in the abdominal cavity using other devices (as an example of minimally invasive surgery). The procedure is performed with other instruments inserted through additional incisions in the abdominal wall, to include inspection (for diagnostic purposes) and surgical removal (e.g. ovaries and fallopian tubes in women).
Laryngoscopy	A laryngoscope is inserted through the mouth into the oropharynx to inspect the larynx and to assist with intubation.
Sigmoidoscopy	A sigmoidoscope is introduced into the anus to examine the rectum and the lower part of the large intestine (known as the sigmoid colon).

enclosed area with ample space to accommodate the patient, surgical staff, and equipment. Historically, the term "operating theater" referred to a non-sterile, tiered theater or amphitheater in which medical students and others could watch surgeons perform surgery.

The area is primarily designed to accommodate any defined surgical procedures and reduce contamination risks, but also other patient/staff considerations (such as patient dignity, access to equipment/supplies, etc.). It should be easy to maintain and clean, with limited and controlled access. Most modern ORs are designed with specialized air-handling systems that maintain temperature/humidity, keep the area under a positive pressure (slightly pressurized, to keep out contamination), filter the incoming air (to remove microorganisms and other particles), and control the flow of air in the room to reduce any cross-contamination risks. In addition, the OR may also have a backup electricity supply to ensure an uninterrupted power supply in case of a blackout/power outage. Furniture, fittings, and equipment should be limited to the minimum required for the types of surgery that are conducted in the area. Standard equipment consists of the operating table (also known as surgical table), the anesthetic delivery unit, surgical lights, booms (also known as equipment booms or equipment management systems, EMSs), cardiac monitor, various surgical displays, diathermy machine, suction, oxygen, and various other gases. In addition, there are movable tables to set instruments on that can be pulled in or pushed back as needed and mobile or stationary cabinets for storage of medicine or accessories. Regardless of the facility or use, each piece of equipment serves its own vital purpose in the OR. Typical designs and equipment for ORs are further discussed in the next section.

Operating room setup

Each OR should have an adjacent preparation (or "scrub") room or have access to a scrub area common to a few rooms. This area is designed to allow staff to prepare to enter the aseptic ("sterile") OR area, namely to apply hand washing and gowning up (wearing dedicated gowns, clothing, and footwear), but is also used for storage of supplies used during surgery (including fluids, blankets, surgical supplies, etc.) as well as pre-warming (in a warming cabinet). The scrub area is most commonly adjacent to (outside) the OR and is equipped with a sizable sink and antiseptics (surgical "scrubbing"; Chapter 9, section on antiseptics; Figure 3.3).

Once in the OR, some of the typical equipment found in the area is shown in Figure 3.4. The OR should be set up such that the patient, surgeon, scrub nurse, and other assisting staff are comfortable, close enough to handle instruments, and have good visualization of each other, any surgical equipment, and video monitors.

Central to any OR is the surgical table that is used for a patient to lay on during a surgical procedure. The table may be adjusted depending on the procedure and can range in complexity from a simple table to a fully adjustable surgical table that can be raised, lowered, and tilted in any direction to meet the need of the surgeon and the surgical procedure. General operating tables are designed to perform a wide range of procedures, while others are designed for specific procedures, for example orthopedic tables.

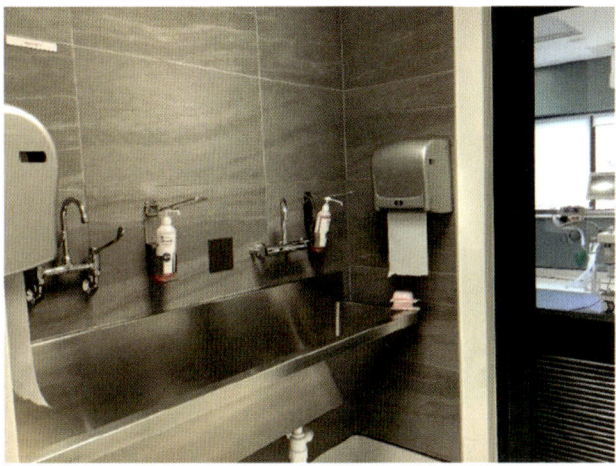
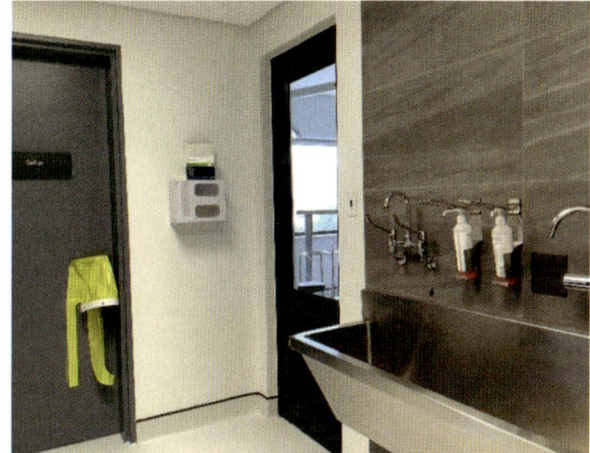

Figure 3.3 A typical scrub area, showing sinks and available antiseptics for hand washing prior to entering the operating room.

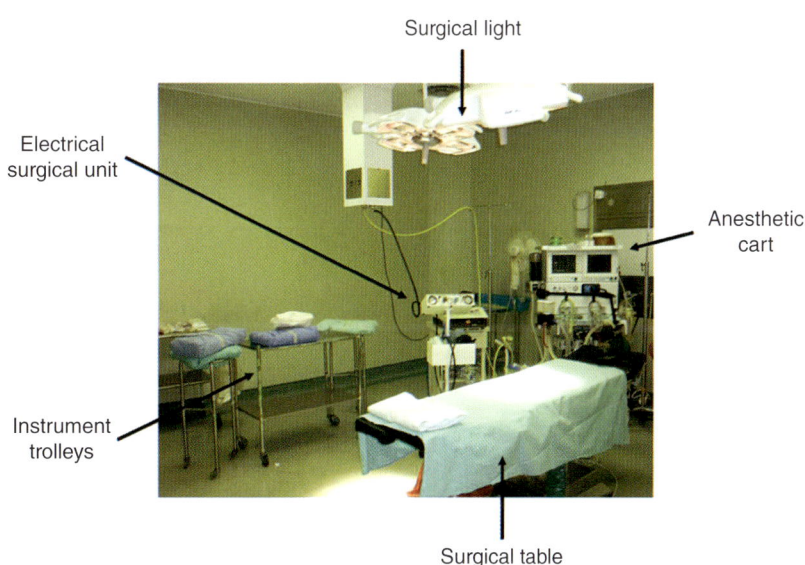

Figure 3.4 A typical operating room design with room equipment highlighted.

Directly overhead is an adjustable surgical light that provides the artificial light required for direct illumination of the surgical site. The source of the light is from one or more lamps, often called bulbs or tubes. LED lights or halogen lights are two common types of surgical lights. Adequate light intensity, minimal shadowing and heat production, appropriate field size and depth of field, natural coloring, and light fixture maneuverability are critical for a successful operation. In many cases, dedicated sterile light handle covers are used to allow the surgeon to adjust the light position aseptically during surgery.

Modern designs of surgical lights and tables may be voice controlled, to allow easy, non-touch access to control features of this equipment.

Many of the more modern ORs will include surgical booms that are used to centralize all surgical support equipment and utility services in the OR. They are essential to hide any electrical cords to reduce tripping hazards, house multiple electric and gas outlets for electrical power needs and medical gases, and can also provide access to a smoke evacuation system, intravenous support, and other organizational tools. Surgical booms are typically adjustable and can be positioned in a variety of locations, mounted on the ceiling or around the room.

As most surgical procedures are performed under anesthesia, an anesthetic delivery unit and cart are usually placed at the head of the operating table. This allows the anesthesiologist to work in an area that minimally affects the surgical staff but with direct access to monitor the patient's health during surgery.

Depending on the complexity of the procedure being performed, a number of movable stainless steel instrument trolleys or "back tables" and "Mayo" stands (device/instrument stands) are available. These are used to lay out and position instruments before, during, and after surgical use by the scrub nurse and/or other support staff. Other movable equipment may include waste disposal carts/trolleys with disposable bags.

An electrosurgical unit that is used to control bleeding is usually available and is placed on the side of the table. This uses an electric current to cut, coagulate, and desiccate (dry) tissues, particularly to reduce blood loss during surgery.

As discussed in the introduction to this chapter, most modern ORs are designed with specialized air-handling systems. These are not just designed to maintain the area as a comfortable environment (for temperature and humidity), but also to reduce the risks of microbial contamination from the air in the room. ORs are usually under positive air pressure relative to the surrounding corridors/areas, forcing air out of the room and minimizing any "dirty" air flowing into the room. The internal air is constantly being replaced, for instance ~20–25 changes per hour of high-efficiency particulate air (HEPA). This is generated by passing the air through HEPA filters mounted on the incoming air in the ceiling; these filters are designed to remove most bacteria and fungi (typically larger than ~0.2 μm in diameter). The air currents provide a downward stream of air through the room (especially around the patient) and are taken out at floor level (Figure 3.5).

As minimally invasive procedures become the new standard and various technology including computer-assisted, robotic, endovascular, and imaging equipment is adopted by the surgical team to improve operation outcomes and overall efficiency, the OR design and setup are reconfigured. Hybrid, digital, and integrated multipurpose OR setups are considered in addition to conventional ones. Hybrid OR requirements are usually based around imaging, like CT, MRI, C-arm, or other types of imaging brought into surgery. A digital OR is a setup in which software sources, images, and video data are all connected to and displayed on a single device. OR integration (ORi) is the connection of image and video in the OR to improve workflow, procedure guidance, and peer collaboration. An example of an integrated OR is shown in Figure 3.6. In general, these newer setups all share the common goal of improving safety to positively impact patient outcomes and simplify workflows for the surgeon and surgical team.

Other current trends in the OR are associated with a greater design emphasis on patient privacy before, during, and after the operation, as well as increasing OR size and storage space, while maintaining flexible, modular designs.

Principles of aseptic (or "sterile") technique

Any medical or surgical procedure should be performed using an aseptic technique, particularly within a designated OR. Aseptic technique refers to practices and procedures to prevent microbial contamination and to maintain an essentially "sterile" or "clean" area. This is an important concept in that it helps minimize any risks of contamination and therefore the development of infection following a medical or, particularly, a surgical procedure. Aseptic technique is practiced in many ways in pre-, intra-, and post-operative procedures, including pre-surgical scrubbing, gowning, and wearing sterile gloves, the design of air-handling systems within the OR, use of sterilized surgical devices, and so on. The setup of an OR for a procedure follows the same aseptic technique practices. An aseptic (or "sterile") field is established in the OR and is separated from the unsterile area, such as contaminated areas and equipment. Only sterile instruments are used when performing surgical procedures and these must all be reprocessed once they have been used or become contaminated (i.e. handled in an unsterile manner, or allowed to touch an unsterile surface).

Important aspects of aseptic technique are the divisions of working areas around and within ORs. These are traditionally divided into three working areas:
- Unrestricted:
  - General area outside the OR complex.

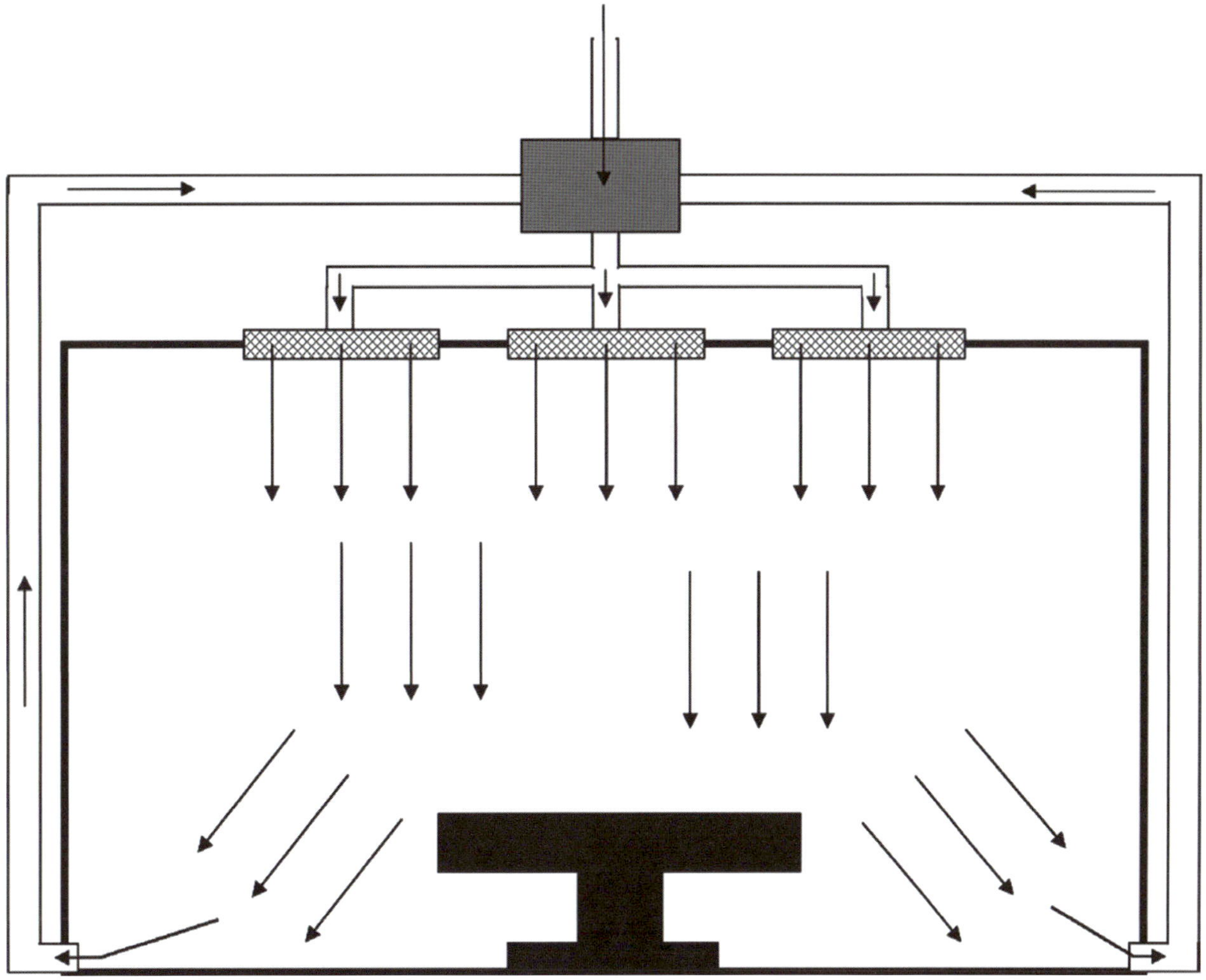

Figure 3.5 An air-handling system, showing the flow of air (as arrows) through the room in a downward motion from entry at the top of the room (gray box at the top), through a dedicated air-handling system, through high-efficiency particulate air (HEPA) filters (three shown) on entry into the room, and air returning to the system at the bottom of the room. The air is constantly being passed through the filters that remove bacteria/fungi, providing a clean flow of air over the patient area (representation of a surgical table shown in the center, in black). The principle of controlling the pressure and quality of air can be applied to any controlled environment (often referred to as "clean") procedure room or area, such as in laboratories, pharmacies, intensive care units, and processing areas.

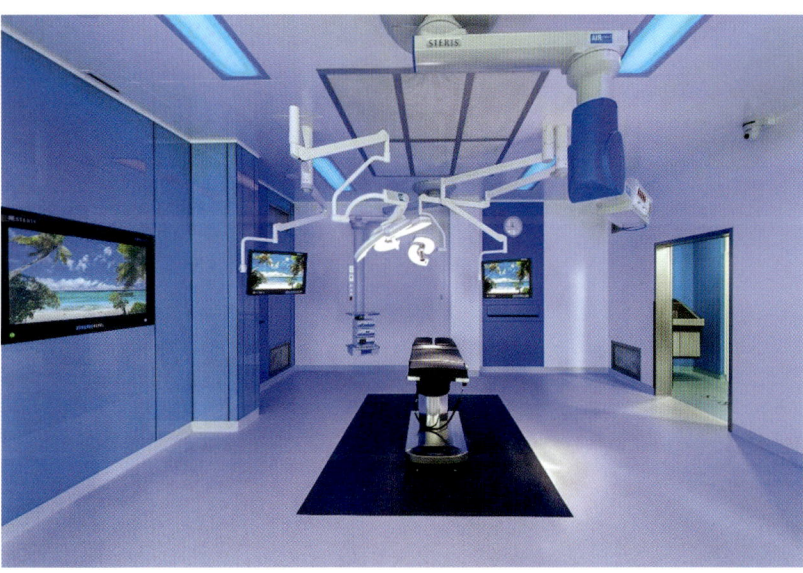

Figure 3.6 An operating room (OR) integration system is designed to simplify and streamline the OR by consolidating data, access to video, and controls for all of these devices at a central command station, allowing the surgical staff to perform many of their tasks efficiently without needing to move around the OR area.

64 Decontamination and Device Processing in Healthcare

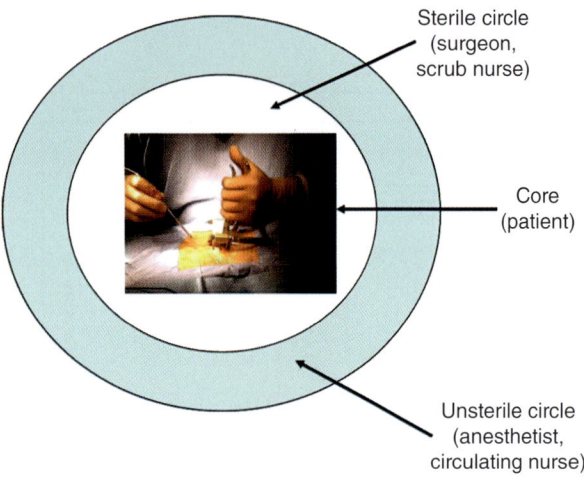

Figure 3.7 The three areas of a restrictive procedure room.

- The actual restricted procedure room is further sub-divided into three areas (Figure 3.7):
  ○ The core or center is the patient on whom the procedure is being performed.
  ○ The "sterile" circle is the area directly around the patient where the person/people (surgeon, scrub nurse, etc.) are operating using sterile instruments.
  ○ The unsterile area is where associated support staff (i.e. anesthesiologist, circulating nurse, etc.) are performing their duties within the procedure room.

Pre-operative procedures

Pre-operative care is the preparation and management of a patient prior to surgery. It can include both the physical and psychological preparation of the patient, including reviewing medical history, checking for any allergies, skin disinfection, physical/medical examination, and so on. In parallel, the surgical staff are preparing to receive and operate on a patient in the OR.

When "setting up" for a procedure, before the full surgical team are present, a scrub nurse will begin to open the sterile items following specific aseptic guidelines. Any devices within packages or containers will be checked to ascertain that they have been sterilized (e.g. for a reusable device that the sterilization chemical indicators have changed color on correct exposure to a sterilization process), that they have not been tampered with, and that the packaging is intact. If the scrub nurse is satisfied that the sterile barrier has not been compromised, before opening the package it must be positioned on a clean, dry, usually covered, flat surface at the level of the sterile field (Figure 3.8).

  ○ Street clothing is worn.
  ○ Patient receiving area, changing rooms, office.
- Semi-restricted:
  ○ Midway between an unrestricted and a restricted area.
  ○ Restricted to authorized personnel only.
  ○ Theater attire must be worn.
  ○ OR complex passages/corridors, reprocessing area (if present).
- Restricted:
  ○ Where procedures are performed.
  ○ Authorized personnel only.
  ○ Scrub area, procedure room, sterile supplies stores.

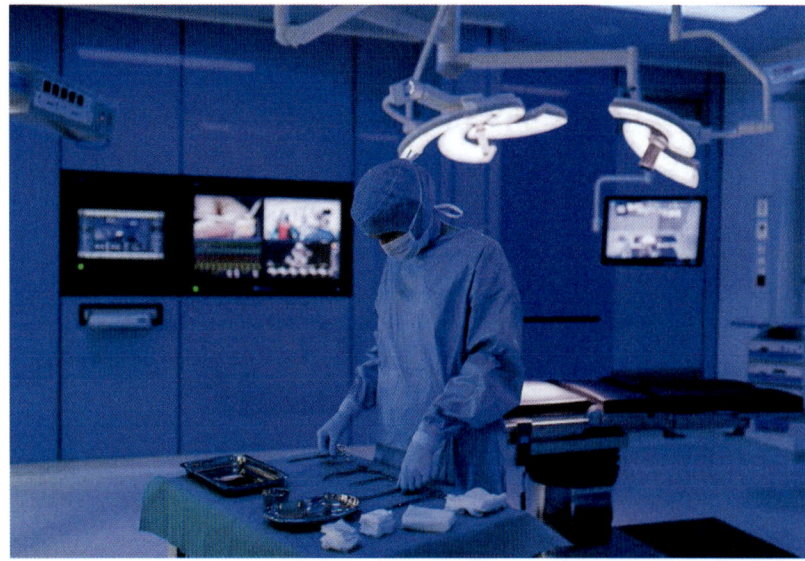

Figure 3.8 Setting up for a surgical procedure within the operating room.

The external seal is then broken and the top layer of wrapped packs is unfolded (note: sterile packages are usually double-wrapped; see Chapter 10 on sterile barrier systems and materials). If using a rigid container, the container is placed on a solid, clean surface and checked to see that it is sealed and dry and that any filters are correctly in place; the lid is then removed according to the manufacturer's recommendations, making sure there is no contact between the lid and the inner rim or any part inside the container.

Following surgical hand washing, the remaining sterile layer(s) can be unwrapped, depending on whether a sequential or simultaneous wrapping technique is used; the inner trays are removed from the container, taking care not to touch the sides of the containers. The scrub nurse will then check any in-pack sterilization indicators and that all instruments are present for the procedure.

All staff entering the operating area should at least wear surgical scrubs and surgical masks that cover all hair, including sideburns, and the neckline as well as covering the nose and mouth. Jewelry, nail polish, and artificial nails should not be worn. Sterile surgical gowns should be worn over surgical scrubs by all staff working within the sterile circle and participating directly in the procedure.

Surgical hand scrubbing should be performed by all staff prior to entering the sterile area and participating in the procedure. As an additional precaution, staff working in the sterile circle should wear at least one pair of sterile surgical gloves, with double gloving being recommended for procedures with a high risk of puncture, such as orthopedics. Gloves should be changed immediately after any accidental puncture during a procedure.

Intra-operative procedures

The patient is the "core" or center of the sterile area. This will also include any OR staff directly involved in the procedure wearing sterile surgical attire, the operating table, other accessory equipment, and any furniture that is covered with sterile drapes, such as trolleys and stands.

After the skin preparation is complete, the patient will be fully covered with sterile drapes or other such materials; no part is uncovered except the operating field and areas needed for the administration and maintenance of anesthesia and fluids.

It is generally recommended that anyone working in the sterile circle must adhere to sterile or aseptic techniques using only sterile items, such as instrument sets, drapes, sponges, and so on. Strictly speaking, gowned and gloved personnel directly involved with procedures are only considered sterile on their front and from the chest down to the level of the patient. Sterile personnel must always keep their hands within sight, in front of the body, and below shoulder height. Sterile personnel should always face the sterile area. Generally, the scrub nurse, surgeon, and surgeon's assistant work within this area. In addition, only the tops of the sterile draped table, instrument trolley, and Mayo stand are considered sterile. All items used within the sterile area should be sterile. Once a sterile drape has been placed in this area it should not be moved, as this may compromise the sterile field. Sterile personnel may only touch sterile items or areas and may not leave the sterile area. Items are brought to the sterile area by "non-sterile" personnel, such as the circulating nurse. Sterile items should be opened and presented so that the scrub nurse can safely take the item, avoiding any contact with the wrap or peel pack, or the item can be opened and carefully placed onto the sterile field. Peel packs, for example, are opened by separating the seal halfway open and folding the top down halfway, before presenting the contents. While assisting "sterile" personnel, unsterile personnel remain in the unsterile area and avoid crossing into or between sterile areas. The anesthesiologist/anesthetist deals with the patient's airway and generally does not come into contact with the sterile operative area or sterile area.

Surgical items should not be dropped onto the sterile field as they may fall off the sterile field or could cause other items to be displaced, contaminating the sterile field. A device may be inadvertently dropped on the floor during a procedure; in such situations the level of potential contamination may be low but is still considered significant. It is best that the device is replaced with alternative, sterilized devices. As an alternative, an immediate-use steam sterilization process (previously known as "flash" sterilization) can be employed (Chapter 11). These are generally steam sterilization processes, specifically developed for rapid treatment to reduce any surface contamination risks; sterilization cycles in these cases are developed for non-wrapped devices, where the device is placed directly into the sterilizer, exposed, and quickly removed to proceed with the surgical process. This is usually performed in a sterilizer located in an area adjacent to, or even within, the OR. Immediate use sterilization should not be considered as a replacement for normal decontamination processes (in particular for wrapped devices), as it is generally not designed for such applications.

On completion of the actual procedure, but typically before the surgical opening is closed ("sutured"), the scrub nurse should check that all instruments, sponges, or any other items used during the surgery are present. If everything is accounted for, any healthcare contaminated waste and heavily soiled items will be segregated at the point of use (Chapter 7).

Post-operative procedures

Similar to pre-operative procedures, a series of procedures are performed post surgery to ensure the well-being of the patient. Soiled sponges and any biological contaminants are directly discarded as per hospital policy on handling healthcare contaminated waste. Particular attention should be paid to the correct handling of disposable sharp devices, such as scalpel blades. Sharps are usually disposed of into specific sharps containers. This can include any single-use tips, such as an electrosurgical tip that has been removed from its handle. All disposable scalpel blades are safely removed from their handles using a hemostat or needle holder and discarded.

Soiled instruments should be placed into containers for transport to a processing area outside the OR. Practices at this stage can vary from hospital to hospital, but it is generally good practice that devices are not allowed to dry during transport and storage, prior to processing; this is discussed in further detail in Chapter 8 as an important part of the decontamination cycle. Any linens should also be separated. These can include single-use, disposal materials that are directly disposed of as healthcare waste, or linens that are collected and reprocessed as hospital laundry (Chapter 15, the section on surgical and medical laundry). A hospital policy should be in place to describe the containerization and transport of contaminated equipment/linens to any applicable processing area(s).

All horizontal surfaces and surgical furniture, such as tables and trolleys, are recommended to be cleaned/surface disinfected between procedures. At the end of a theater "list" (a series of procedures in a row) the entire surgical area is typically also cleaned and disinfected (Chapter 9, in the section on antiseptics). In some cases ORs are closed to further procedures for longer periods of time while the area is being disinfected. Care should be taken to review any manufacturer's instructions provided with surface/environmental disinfectants; in general, cleaning should be performed first, but can be combined with disinfection depending on the product claims and instructions. Chemicals (cleaner and disinfectant) should never be mixed (unless specified) and, if required, should always be prepared according to manufacturer's instructions.

4 Instrumentation

Humankind has learned to heal from the birth of civilization. Hippocrates (born in 460 BC), considered by many to be the father of medicine, is believed to have said, "What cannot be cured with medicaments is cured by the knife; what the knife cannot cure is cured with the searing iron; and whatever this cannot cure must be considered incurable." Today, medicine offers us numerable treatment medications, diagnostic and therapeutic interventions, as well as a plethora of instruments and devices that assist healthcare professionals to cure the sick.

There is evidence that surgical instruments and devices have been used for thousands of years (Figure 4.1). Archeologists have discovered primitive knives that would have been used for surgical procedures as early as 5000 BC. One of the oldest surgical procedures is trepanation, a surgical intervention in which a hole is drilled or scraped into the human skull. Rough trephines, instruments used to cut out a round piece of the skull, have been discovered and associated with Neolithic (2500 BC) sites in many places. It is believed that trepanation was used by shamans to release evil spirits and to alleviate headaches and head trauma-associated infections from war-inflicted wounds. Surgeons and physicians in India have used sophisticated surgical instruments since ancient times. Sushruta (circa 500 BC) was probably the most important surgeon in ancient history, often known as the "father of surgery." In his text *Sushruta Samhita* he described over 120 surgical instruments and 300 surgical procedures, and classified human surgery into eight categories. Surgeons and physicians in Greece and the Roman Empire developed many instruments made from bronze, iron, and silver, such as scalpels, lancets, curettes, catheters, tweezers, specula, trephines, forceps, probes, dilators, tubes, surgical knives, and so on.

The first instruments were certainly made by men who made armor and cutlery, but some were also made by other metal workers such as silversmiths. Instrument making only became a modern profession in the 18th century. The invention of more advanced surgical instruments was directly linked to the discovery of anesthesia and modern sterile techniques. These developments allowed the penetration of the body cavities, namely the skull, the thorax, and the abdomen. Due to the increased severity of war-inflicted wounds by shot, shrapnel, and cannon, amputation sets were more widely described and used.

During the 19th century and the first decades of the 20th century an explosion of new instruments occurred, with hundreds of new surgical procedures being developed. New materials, such as stainless steel, chrome, titanium, and vanadium, were available for the manufacturing of these instruments. The invention of stainless steel in 1913, by English metallurgist Harry Brearley, brought about perhaps the greatest change to the manufacture of surgical instruments. While working on a project to improve rifle barrels, Brearley accidentally discovered that adding chromium to low-carbon steel gives it stain resistance. Precision instruments were developed for neurosurgery, microsurgery, ophthalmology, and other applications in the second half of the 20th century. Energy-based power tools were also developed, such as diathermy, ultrasound, and surgical tools for endoscopic surgery. Advances were made from the 1950s with the introduction of rigid and flexible endoscopes that could be used for direct observation within the body for diagnostic, therapeutic, and surgical procedures. Endoscopes paved the way in the development of minimally invasive surgery (MIS, Chapter 3), which has experienced a surge in popularity over the past few decades and led to the conversion of several surgical tools into minimally invasive equivalents; finally, in the 21st century we see continuous advances in 3D enhanced imaging, navigation- and image-guided systems, as well as the wide spread of robotic-assisted surgery (RAS), all of which have revolutionized the way surgery is performed. In the near future, artificial intelligence (AI) will be added to RAS, giving robots the ability to learn and even make decisions. New and ever-changing surgical techniques and advances in the medical field create a continual need for new technology that brings along the development of a variety of new instruments. Today there are more than 5000 surgical instrument types available in different shapes and sizes, made from various materials, that perform at least one essential function.

Decontamination and Device Processing in Healthcare, Second Edition. Gerald McDonnell and Georgia Alevizopoulou.
© 2025 John Wiley & Sons Ltd. Published 2025 by John Wiley & Sons Ltd.

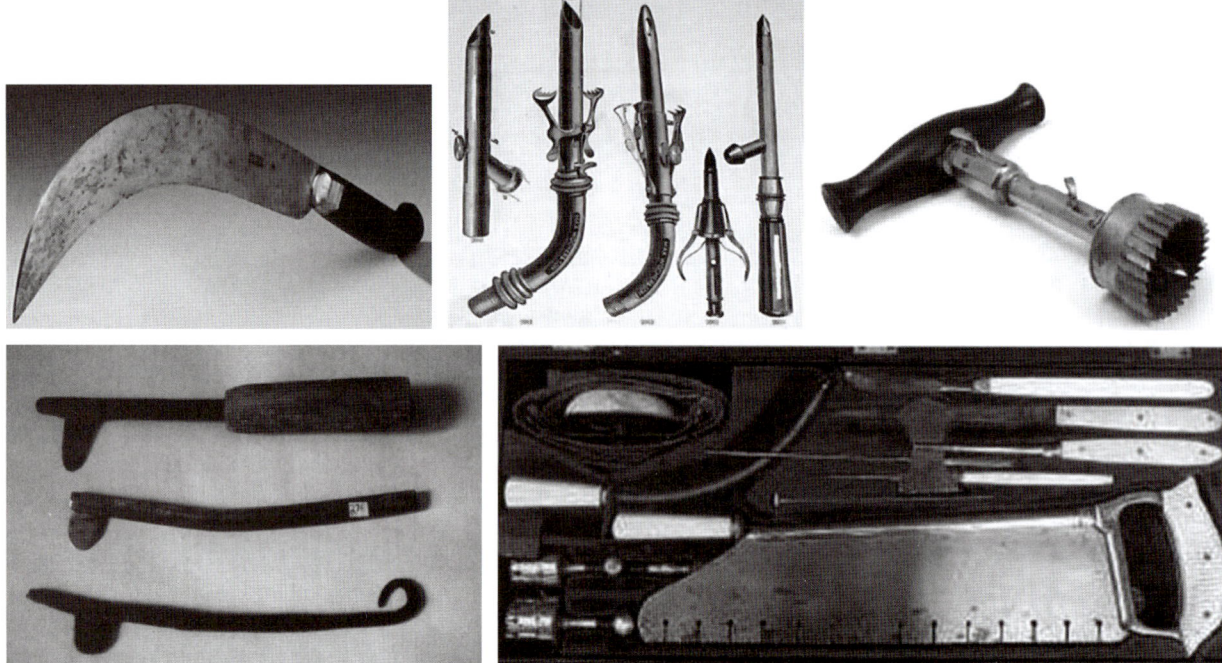

Figure 4.1 Examples of older surgical device designs.

Instruments represent a significant investment in any healthcare facility and a good understanding of what they are, how they are made, and how they are used, handled, and maintained is important. In this chapter the various types of surgical instruments are discussed.

Single-use, limited-use, and reusable medical devices

Instruments can be classified in a variety of ways, such as for what purpose they are used, their construction materials, and the risk of contamination/infection transmission to a patient.

A common classification that is used internationally is based on how the device is used and the risks associated with it:
- Class 1: considered low risk and includes most types of non-invasive devices, meaning that they do not penetrate through or into the body. Examples are surgical lights, surgical tables, examination gloves, packaging materials, and stethoscopes.
- Class 2: considered medium risk, which can include various types of the most invasive devices (or even products that are used with such devices) that penetrate into or through the body. (Note: in some countries this is even sub-divided further into sub-classes such as Classes 2a and 2b.)
- Class 3: considered the highest risk, which can include various types of implantable devices (those that can remain in the body long term or even permanently).

This is a general example, as the exact classification of a device can be different, depending on various rules or regulations in individual countries or regions, and such a classification may change over time.

Another important division to consider in this section is whether the device is designed for multiple use (reusable), limited use (semi-reusable), or single use (disposable).

A reusable device is a device that has been designed to be used many times on multiple patients. In such a case, attention is required to ensure that the device is safely handled and processed between patients. Collaboration between the user of the device and the manufacturer is essential. It is the responsibility of the device manufacturer to provide clear, detailed instructions on how safe handling and processing need to be carried out, while users must ensure that these instructions are followed correctly and consistently, in order to mitigate the risk of patient infection and/or other complications. Useful documents to reference are the ISO 17664 international standard series on *Processing of health care products – Information to be provided by the medical device manufacturer for the processing of medical devices*. These standards apply to critical/semi-critical (Part 1) and non-critical (Part 2) medical devices and include information for processing prior to use or reuse of the medical device.

Many types of reusable medical devices have an indefinite lifetime, which means they do not have a defined number of uses (or reuses). In these cases the end of the device's life is based on inspection of any damage, whether it is no longer operational, or other end-of-life indications (e.g. loss of labeling or color). These should be defined by the manufacturer in the instructions for use (IFU), which include maintenance and inspection requirements (see Chapter 10). Good examples include testing the sharpness of scissors used for the surgical cutting of tissues, testing of power tools for sufficient power or working mechanisms, and inspection of endoscopic devices to ensure the lenses (used to view various parts of the body) are clear and not broken. In some cases the device may have a limited number of use times defined, but require more detailed inspection or maintenance before being used further. Attention to this detail in the manufacturer's IFUs is essential.

A semi-reusable medical device may be considered a device that is intended only for a defined, specified number of uses. These can include devices labeled as only reused for a set number of processing cycles (e.g. 2, 10, or 20 times). Examples include certain types of robotic instruments that are designed for and labeled as having a limited shelf life. The device is processed in line with the manufacturer's guidance. The number of times an instrument is processed should not be exceeded. The count is documented and records of reuse are maintained. Such records are typically also included with inspection requirements to ensure that the devices are fit for purpose and have not been unexpectedly damaged due to surgical/medical use or during handling/processing.

A single-use device (SUD) can be simply defined as a device that has been designed and provided by a manufacturer to be used on a single patient and then disposed of. Under this definition the device may be used multiple times on the same patient, although this depends on the design of the device and the instructions given by the manufacturer on how it should be safely used. The internationally recognized symbol that designates an SUD is shown in Figure 4.2. It is important to note that many SUDs are provided non-sterile and are required to be cleaned and sterilized prior to patient use (see later in this chapter, and Chapter 15, the section on loan devices, sets, and implants). Some are designed to be processed multiple times (or even indefinitely), but once used on or with a patient are not allowed to be processed further. Examples include implantable screw sets that are designed for use in trauma or orthopedic surgical procedures. The screw sets can be provided non-sterile, are processed prior to surgical use, and some of the implants are used for the surgical procedure, but all are not used during that procedure. If the remaining screws have not been soiled, damaged, or used, they can be labeled for processing in preparation for the new surgery.

Other types of SUDs have not been designed or labeled by the manufacturer to be processed. They can be labeled as single use and not to be resterilized (Figure 4.2). However, in many parts of the world healthcare facilities and manufacturers will decide to process such devices and allow them to be used on other patients. In some countries reuse of SUDs is considered illegal, while in others it is accepted under specific conditions. Although often debated, users can justify the processing of such devices based on economic and environmental benefits. But processing of a SUD may alter its characteristics so that it may no longer comply with the original manufacturer's specifications and thus its performance may be compromised. The reuse of SUDs can affect their safety, performance, and effectiveness, exposing patients and staff to unnecessary risk. Any decisions regarding the processing of SUDs should not be taken lightly and should be considered at the highest level of any healthcare facility, in collaboration with infection prevention/control and written approval by management. This subject is considered in further detail in Chapter 15.

Materials used in the manufacture of instruments

Over the years surgical instruments have been made from many different types of materials including metals, plastics, and synthetics. Stainless steel has been the metal of choice for making surgical instruments for decades, but other metals, such as titanium, copper, aluminum, chromium, and even silver and gold, are also widely used. In addition, various types of plastics, polymers, and synthetic materials are used, especially with single- or limited-use instruments, while new materials are also regularly introduced. Instruments that are made of a mixture of different material types are also available. The selection of the appropriate material is not a simple task; a few physical properties are considered in advance that satisfy the design, use, and regulatory requirements in making a surgical instrument. Some of these are biocompatibility, ductility and malleability, durability (managing wear and tear), flexibility,

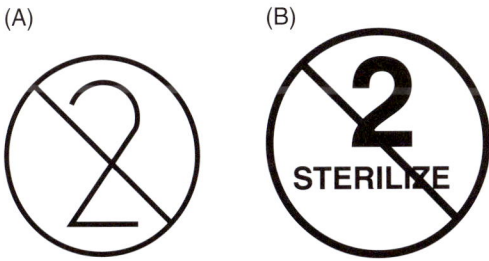

Figure 4.2 The internationally recognized symbols for (A) do not reuse the device and (B) do not resterilize.

ability to withstand high temperatures and chemicals, resistance to corrosion, magnetic behavior, low glare effect, functionality, and ergonomics (being lightweight), although other characteristics are sometimes considered.

The most commonly used material still today to produce a surgical instrument is stainless steel, also known as corrosion-resistant steel (CRES), inox steel, or just inox (from the French word *inoxydable*, meaning stainless). Steel is an alloy, a further chemical term used to describe a compound of different metals (mixed together by heating at high temperatures). The various types of stainless steel alloys are made up of a combination of basic elements (Chapter 6). These include iron, carbon, and chromium, but also other metals such as silicon, nickel, nitrogen, molybdenum, titanium, aluminum, niobium, copper, nitrogen, sulfur, phosphorus, selenium, and manganese. Properties of the final stainless steel alloy are tailored by varying the amounts of these elements. Other examples of alloys, which may also be used to manufacture instruments, include bronze (a mixture of copper and tin) and brass (an alloy of copper and zinc).

High-grade, low-rusting stainless steel has been widely used because it is strong, hard, resistant to heat, and resistant to corrosion. Note that it is stain*less* steel, not stain-*proof* steel. Corrosion is damage to any metal due to the effects of chemicals (including oxygen, in a process known as oxidation that forms oxides such as ferric oxide, Fe_2O_3, more commonly known as rust). Despite this, even with the use of high grades of stainless steel, over time/use and especially when not correctly cared for, instruments will corrode or be otherwise damaged, causing a variety of problems, including perforation (pitting), loss of strength, degradation of appearance, breakage, and accumulation of chemical (scale or rust) deposits that can lead to adverse patient outcomes.

There are over 80 types of stainless steel manufactured, but only about 20 of them are widely used for making surgical instruments. These fall into two main categories: martensitic (the 400 series) and austenitic (the 300 series). The difference is due to the ratio of chromium, nickel, and iron in the stainless steel alloy and the choice is determined according to the desired physical properties. Some types of steel can be "hardened" (made more hard wearing), others cannot, depending primarily on the carbon content. The 400 series is hard steel that contains a greater carbon content and no nickel (with very few exceptions). It is mainly used when strength and cutting edges are required, such as with ophthalmic instruments and the various scissors, osteotomes, and hemostats. The 300 series contains iron, carbon (e.g. 0.15%), chromium (16%) and nickel/manganese. This is the most common forms of stainless steel and is often referred to as "surgical" stainless steel. Examples of instruments using 300 series stainless steel include retractors, suction devices, and cannulas. Surgical stainless steel grades are usually considered easier to clean, disinfect, and sterilize, as well as being stronger and corrosion resistant. Examples include 304 (contains iron with <0.08% carbon, 17–20% chromium, 8–11% nickel, <2% manganese, <1% silicon, <0.045% phosphorous, and <0.03% sulfur) and 316 L (essentially the same but with a lower <0.03% carbon level, denoted by the L, and 2–3% molybdenum). The higher percentage of chromium gives the metal its scratch and corrosion resistance. The chromium also combines with oxygen in the atmosphere to form a thin, invisible layer of chrome-containing oxide (a chemical molecule, see Chapter 6), called a "passive" film or layer. If the metal is cut or scratched and the passive layer is disrupted, this can allow the formation of rust (ferric oxide) or the regeneration of the chrome-containing oxide that recovers the exposed surface and protects it from further oxidative corrosion of the iron. The nickel provides a smooth and polished finish.

Other widely used metals and molecules include titanium, tungsten carbide, copper, aluminum, chromium, molybdenum, and a certain amount of silver and gold. Titanium is widely used in the manufacture of implants used to repair fractures, for example plates and screws. It has proven high biocompatibility, which means that body tissue will adhere to it but not react adversely, and has non-magnetic and anti-glare properties. Titanium is also used in the manufacture of microsurgical instruments, where its light weight is an important factor in avoiding surgeon fatigue. Tungsten carbide is an alloy of tungsten and carbon. It is an extremely hard metal, harder than steel, and is renowned for its exceptional durability. It is typically used in the manufacture of needle holders, scissors, pin cutters, pliers, and wire tighteners, to name a few devices. It is usually soldered or welded to the jaws or working ends of instruments, because it increases sharpness and gripping ability.

Some lightweight instrument parts and cases are manufactured from aluminum, which has often been treated with an electrochemical process called anodization (therefore referred to as "anodized" aluminum). This process forms an oxide layer on the surface of the aluminum that offers good corrosion resistance. The oxide layer can also be colored with pigments/dyes. Aluminum is often used for manufacturing orthopedic devices, as it is lighter than stainless steel. Finally, precious metals, such as gold, platinum, and silver, are highly malleable and ductile, which allows them to be shaped into intricate forms without breaking or becoming brittle, thus they are often used to make prosthetics, tubes, and probes.

Besides metals, a range of plastics are used in the manufacture of medical and surgical devices, especially in the last few decades. They are strong and lightweight, but they are mainly preferred because they are more easily processed than metals, opening up additional design options using complex shapes and with integrated parts. Plastics are complex chemical (organic, carbon-containing) molecules called polymers. Each polymer consists of several thousand repeating units (monomers).

Plastics are usually classified by the chemical structure of these polymer chains. Some are naturally occurring, but most modern plastics used for devices are artificially manufactured (synthetic). Examples of plastics include nylon, polystyrene, polypropylene, polycarbonate, polyvinyl chloride (PVC), and polyethylene. Many plastics have the prefix "poly," which means "many." This is followed by the name for the monomer from which the plastic is derived, so the name is source based. Most of these are specially formulated to withstand high temperatures, such as polytetrafluoroethylene (PTFE, also known as "Teflon"), polyethylene terephthalate (PET), and ultra-high molecular weight polyethylene (UHMWPE), while others will not, including polyurethane and low-density polyethylene (LDPE). This is an important consideration in the processing cycle, as some devices can be heat disinfected or sterilized while others will be restricted to only low-temperature chemical treatment methods (Chapters 9 and 11).

Finally, in the last decade there have been advances in biotechnology in the manufacturing of 3D-printed devices, instruments, and equipment. 3D printing, also known as additive manufacturing (AM), is a process that allows the creation of solid objects directly from raw materials and a digital file by an additive process. Various 3D-printed items are already used for patient and healthcare professional education, training, pre-surgical, and surgical use, and as personalized implants. Customized implantable devices are already widely available, with further advancements expected in the development of customized instruments. In environments where surgical equipment is not readily available, such as when operating surgical hospitals in war zones, spacecraft, or areas where natural disasters occur, the potential advantages of functional 3D-printed surgical instruments are enormous. Durable metals, such as stainless steel and titanium, as well as medical-grade polymers are already used to print surgical guides, prototypes, and prosthetics. Evaluation is still ongoing to find appropriate materials that can be printed without additional finishing (e.g. removal or burrs) and processing for surgical use. Essentially, 3D printing is an alternative manufacturing process in which we can expect to see further developments and applications in the future, but the requirements of processing are similar (at this time) to other reusable devices.

It is not unusual to see a variety of materials being used for the manufacture of medical and surgical devices, depending on their required purposes. This can be very complicated considering the range of materials (metals, alloys, plastics, glass, adhesives, electrical components, etc.) that can be used, their various grades or methods of generating these grades, and different surface finishes. Such flexibility in the choice of materials gives the widest range of options for device design to meet the needs of surgeons, physicians, and patients. Given the range of materials that can be used, it is important to consider all instructions provided by the manufacturer of these devices (see the section on single-use, limited-use, and reusable medical devices) to ensure that the various materials are not damaged (or have limited damage) over time and reuse.

Device manufacturers and suppliers

Quality standards

In the simplest terms, the manufacturer is responsible for making a device to a defined quality standard. Defining quality can be difficult depending on your perspectives and expectations, but a reasonable definition is the provision of a product or service to a defined, consistent standard. It is not always the case that the same company designs, manufactures, and provides/sells a device to a healthcare institution. If there is a single company or a range of companies involved in the process, they all have responsibilities to provide the device in a safe and effective manner for its intended use. In general, this will apply not only to those involved in designing and making the product, but also those directly involved in selling or providing it in a given geographic region (e.g. in the European Union or a specific country like India). It is also important to note that by definition in some regions of the world a processing department may be considered a "manufacturer" because it takes a device and renders it fit for use in or on another patient; therefore, many of the quality requirements on those who make the device may also be applicable to those processing the device for patient use.

An important quality requirement for any manufacturer is having a quality management system (QMS), where there is a documented organizational structure with the relevant procedures, processes, and resources needed to implement quality within the organization. International standards are available that define these requirements. For example, ISO 9001 *Quality management systems – requirements* defines these requirements for any type of organization, while ISO 13485 *Medical devices – quality management systems – requirements for regulatory purposes* is more specific about those requirements for medical devices. ISO 13485 provides guidance on developing, implementing, and maintain a quality system, with the emphasis on having this correctly documented, supported by management, and correctly resourced. This standard has become the minimum quality requirement for medical device manufacturers worldwide. Compliance with this standard should be initially and periodically verified by an approved ("accredited") third-party organization such BSI Group or TÜV; the relevant ISO standard is assessed and, if satisfactory, a certificate confirming that the organization complies with the requirements of the standard is issued. An important aspect to such a quality system is to reduce the risk of something going wrong. Risk analysis with any product, process, or service is therefore a further aspect of quality management. Guidance on risk management is provided in further medical device-related standards such as ISO 14971 *Medical devices – application of risk management to medical devices*. This standard provides guidance on all aspects of risk management; determining the safety of a medical device throughout its life cycle is considered by the manufacturer. Further discussion on quality management and associated standards for processing departments is given in Chapter 14, in the section on quality management.

Manufacturing process

The making of surgical instruments is considered a highly developed craft that has respected many traditions over centuries of practice. While new manufacturing techniques are developed as medical practices evolve, the true craft changes very little. Every instrument starts out as an idea, followed by a series of steps to design the device and ensure that it is fit for purpose. A variety of processes can then be used. It is outside the scope of this book to describe all of these processes, but some detail is given here regarding typical manufacturing processes for metal surgical devices.

The first step involves the common metal device manufacturing processes known as "hot forging," "cold forging," or laser cutting. These are all used to make the basic device design, known as a "blank." During hot forging, pre-cut pieces of stainless steel or other metal bars are heated to very high temperatures and shaped/forged under the weight of a giant drop forge weighing many tons. The quality of the forgings is critical, as errors or poor quality cannot be corrected later in the process. Cold-forged blanks are made out of sheet metals or bars. Instead of being shaped under heat, they are shaped/forged using the force of hammers. Laser cutters are used to cut out or mill the desired shape of device, particularly for precision instruments.

Once the instrument manufacturer has verified the quality of the blanks to be used, the next step in the process is milling and/or turning. In the case of surgical forceps, this process is used to create the basic shape of the box lock, jaws, and ratchets of the device (see the section on basic, everyday instruments).

Once all the parts are made, the instrument may need to be assembled. On a two-part instrument there is generally male and female parts, which are assembled depending on the type of hinge used. A typical forceps has a box lock, which is created by widening the female part under heat and inserting the male part; the hinge can then be secured with a pin or screw. At this point the shape of the metal is still quite rough and it will need to be filed and ground into its final shape.

Now that the instrument is in its final shape it will generally need to be further tempered or hardened. This is necessary to make the instrument hard enough to withstand the rigors of use. The stainless steel is heated to a very high temperature and then cooled until it has reached the required hardness; this is a crucial part of the manufacturing. If the steel is too soft, it will wear out or bend prematurely; if the steel is too hard, it will be brittle and break too easily. The correct hardness is usually defined and tested as part of quality control, for example being measured in units called Rockwell Hardness (HRC). A typical hardness range for a needle holder without tungsten carbide inserts is HRC 40–48. For scissors, the hardness range may be HRC 50–58.

When the correct hardness has been attained, the manufacturer will typically need to further fine tune the shape and mechanism of the instrument. All unwanted sharp edges, burrs, and so on are removed. Scissors and other cutting instruments are sharpened and adjusted. It is at this point that an instrument is transformed from a piece of stainless steel into the precision instrument a surgeon will rely on. Once this is completed, the instrument is polished in order to create a homogeneous surface, which determines the final appearance or finish of the instrument. There are three types of instrument finishes: mirror finish, which is shiny (reflects light); dull or satin (does not reflect light); and ebonized or black. Most instruments have a dull silk matte or satin finish, which is a gray-colored surface that reduces glare in the operating room, an important property that limits eye fatigue and prevents distraction during procedures. Ebony finish is a black coating that is often used in laser surgery to prevent beam reflection. It also allows for better color contrast because it does not reflect the color of tissues. Finally, the instruments may be electro-polished. This process chemically removes foreign substances and makes the surface even more corrosion resistant, creating a thin protective layer known as the passive or passivation layer. If properly cared for during use, these passive layers can actually protect the device over time, ensuring the longevity of the instrument. The manufacturing process then continues with rigorous inspection and testing. New instruments feel stiff and are more magnetic. As they age, they soften and the magnetism gradually wears off. The next and final part of the process is instrument marking.

Instrument marking

Instruments can be marked with a variety of symbols, labels, or unique identification codes (UICs). These are usually limited and minimal (especially on any part of the device that would enter a patient), but can include manufacturer's name, logo, device model, and/or serial number. Any instrument markings should preferably only be done at the time of manufacture by the manufacturer. They may be visible (e.g. color coating and model number) or invisible (e.g. a code inserted into the device and detected using a specific sensor). UICs are numerical or alpha-numerical codes that are defined through a coding system for the identification of a specific device on the market. They have become widely used (and often mandatory) in and on medical devices, either as provided in the device

Figure 4.3 Examples of labeling systems used with medical devices/instruments. Similar systems are used to label instrument sets (a set of instruments for a particular procedure).

design (by the manufacturer) or with/on a device at the site of use (by healthcare staff or a third party). Examples of these labeling systems include those that are visible and read directly by the eye, bar codes, two-dimensional data matrix, and radio-frequency identification devices (RFIDs). Examples are shown in Figure 4.3. International efforts have harmonized the coding systems used with medical devices; an example is the GS1 identification standards that are used for tracking and identifying products worldwide.

Although it is not recommended by manufacturers, instruments are often directly labeled post manufacture. This can include the use of engraving, laser etching, indelible (water-insoluble) markers, adhesive tapes, and so on. Such procedures may provide problems: unapproved engraving can damage the surface of the device (in the case of stainless steel leading to removal of the passivation layer and corrosion), while other labels/tapes may present problems to staff and patients during surgical or medical use. Labels and tapes should never be placed on areas of the instrument that are directly handled by staff or used directly in/on a patient; they can pose an infection risk and can become dislodged/introduced into a patient during a procedure. Etching, laser marking, or other similar marking methods should also be done in collaboration with the device manufacturer to limit any safety risks.

Today, individual device marking/labeling systems have become widespread, but a variety of systems are used internationally. Similarly, various labeling systems used to identify surgical and medical instrument sets are widely used for tracking and traceability purposes (there are further details in Chapter 14).

Surgical instrument types and descriptions

Instruments range from basic forceps to delicate microsurgical instruments to air/battery-powered drills and complex endoscopic equipment. They have a variety of different angles, curves, lengths, tip lengths, sizes, and serrations, which are necessary to accommodate the different types of procedures and anatomical structures as well as the medical staff's preferences.

Surgical instruments are designed to be minimal in design, cause as little damage as possible, and are generally named either according to the action they perform (e.g. scalpel), the name of the inventor (e.g. Mayo forceps), or the kind of surgery they are used for (e.g. osteotome). They can be classified in a variety of ways, including type of surgery, handheld or robotic, powered or non-powered, and so on. In this section some of the most commonly encountered surgical instruments are described, based on their surgical use.

Basic, everyday instruments

Scalpels or a pair of scissors (Figure 4.4) is the instrument of choice to cut or separate skin, fat, fascia, muscles, and so on. Dissecting forceps (Figure 4.5) hold, clamp, or pull tissue, or are used to stop bleeding. A handheld or self-retaining retractor (Figure 4.6) holds an incision, wound, or cavity open while a surgeon works or holds tissues or organs out of the way during surgery. Dilators keep open (or wider) a natural opening or

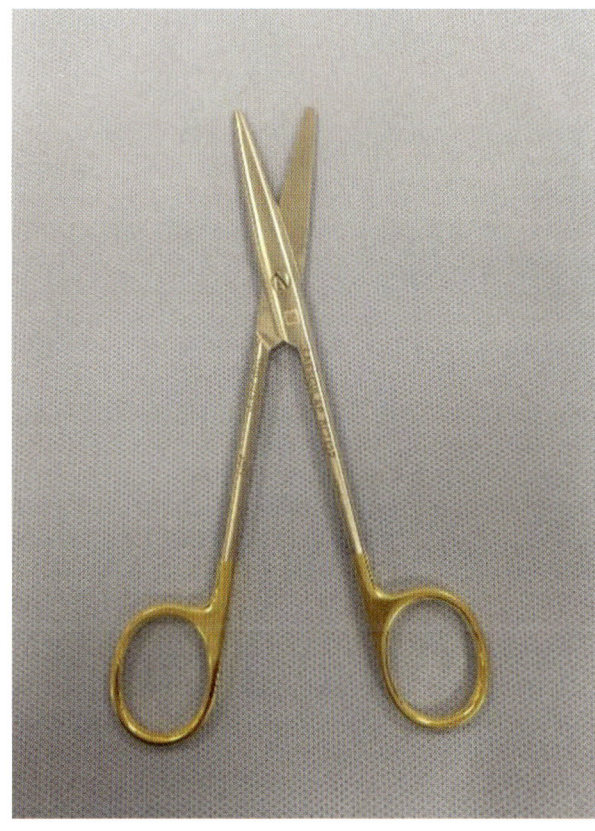

Figure 4.4 A pair of surgical scissors.

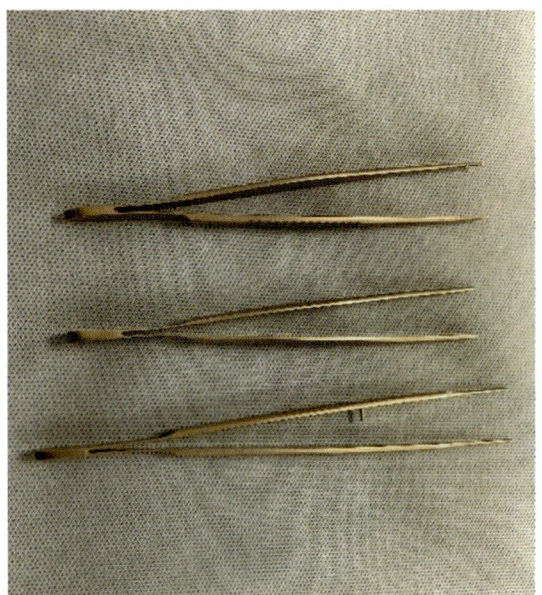

Figure 4.5 Examples of dissecting forceps.

(A)

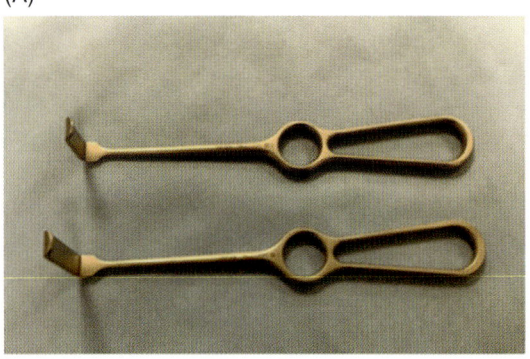

(B)

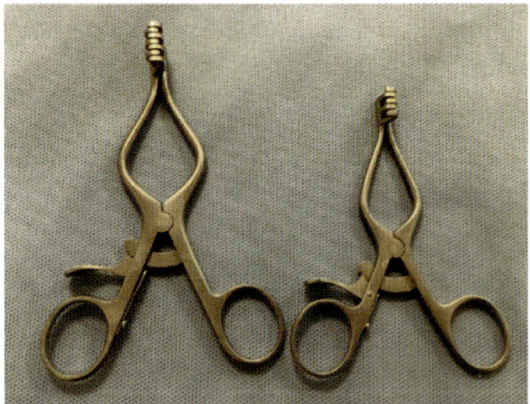

Figure 4.6 Examples of retractors, showing (A) handheld and (B) self-retaining designs.

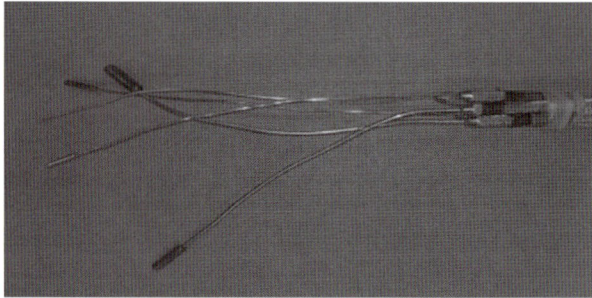

Figure 4.7 Examples of dilators.

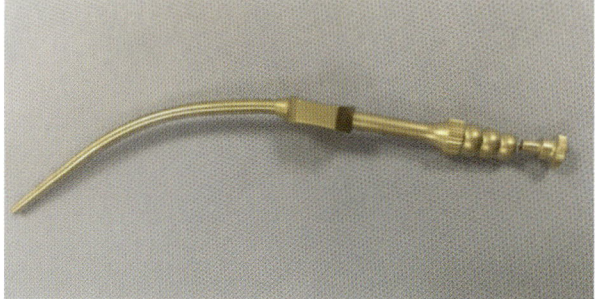

Figure 4.8 A suction nozzle.

orifice ("dilated") to inspect various body cavities (Figure 4.7). A suction nozzle (Figure 4.8), attached to a suction source within the operating room, suctions fluids (such as blood) from cavities during procedures. A needle holder (Figure 4.9) holds a suturing needle for closing wounds ("anastomosis") and for other procedures. Some instruments have serrations or "teeth" at their ends to strengthen their grip on body tissues, or elsewhere along the device to aid the surgeon in holding it (Figure 4.10). These may be coarse or fine, run lengthways or crossways, run the length or only part of the blade, be curved or straight, long or short. A ratchet allows surgeons to control their grasp or vary the tension they are applying through the instrument. Ratchets vary in size and strength, with some having a self-retaining clasp at the handle for ease of use.

A common term in many of these instruments is the "joint." This is the junction of the instrument that allows the working (patient) end to be opened and closed (Figure 4.11). There are various types of joints:
- Hinge joint: the shaft of the device is stable and only the end of the device ("jaw") moves, either one or both jaws.
- Box joint: a box joint is fused in the factory and cannot be taken apart for repairs. A joint pin is electrically fused during manufacturing through the outer elements of the hinge before the hardening step; this strengthens the joint and therefore the instrument. Even if the pin fractures during use, the fused

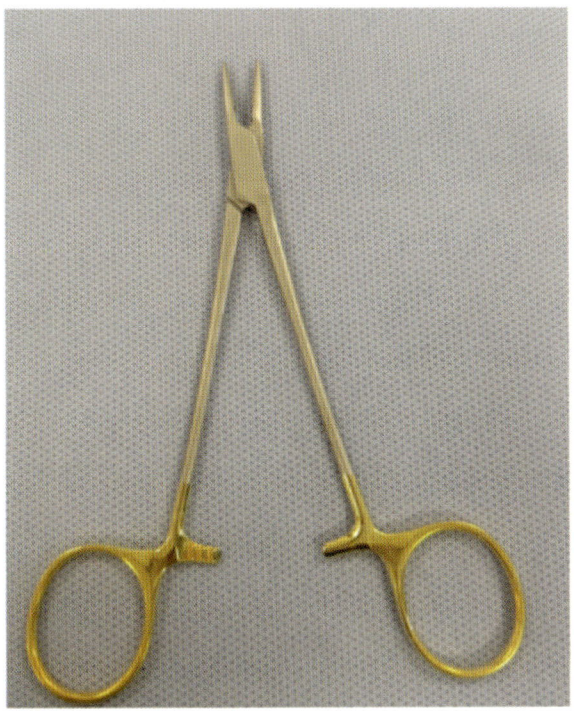

Figure 4.9 A needle holder. A gold handle on scissors, forceps, or needle holders means they have tungsten carbide inserts on the working surfaces (Note the clamping mechanism or ratchet; see the section on instruments used for clamping and occluding.)

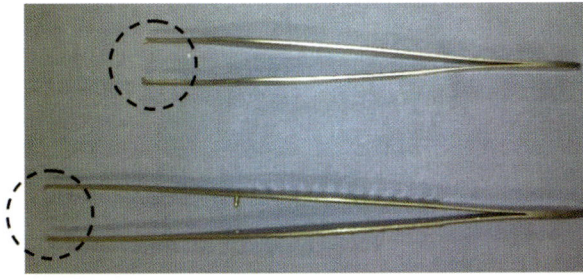

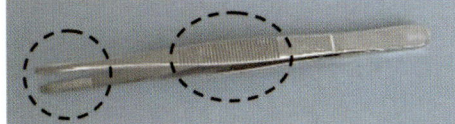

Figure 4.10 Examples of serrated instruments.

box hinge prevents broken-off parts of the pin from falling out of the instrument and into the patient.
- Screw joint: a screw joint is used on instruments that can be sharpened as it allows the instrument to be completely disassembled to ensure effective sharpening, for example scissors, bone nibblers, bone cutters, etc.

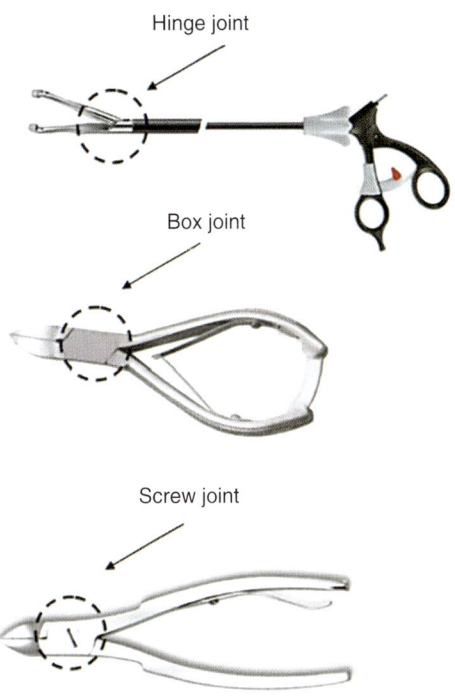

Figure 4.11 Various types of joints on instruments.

Instrument classification

Surgical instruments can be classified in a variety of ways. In this chapter the most frequently used instruments are considered based on their surgical use:
- Cutting and dissecting:
  ○ Scalpels
  ○ Knives
  ○ Scissors
  ○ Bone cutting
  ○ Other sharp dissectors
  ○ Blunt dissectors
- Grasping and holding:
  ○ Delicate forceps
  ○ Adson/Gillies forceps
  ○ Bayonet forceps
  ○ Strong-toothed forceps
  ○ DeBakey forceps
  ○ Diathermy forceps
  ○ Lane tissue forceps
  ○ Babcock forceps
  ○ Vulsellum forceps
  ○ Bone holders
- Clamping and occluding:
  ○ Hemostatic forceps
  ○ Crushing clamps
  ○ Vascular clamps

- Exposing and retracting:
  - Handheld retractors
  - Malleable retractors
  - Hooks
  - Self-retainers
- Suturing or stapling:
  - Needle holders
  - Clip appliers
- Suction irrigation/aspiration
- Dilation
- Measuring
- Powered tools
- Viewing:
  - Rigid and flexible endoscopes
- Microsurgery
- Unique dental instruments
- Unique robotic surgery
- Other miscellaneous instruments (e.g. mallets, thermometers, blood pressure cuffs)

This discussion is not exhaustive of the range of devices in surgical use.

Instruments for cutting and dissecting

A scalpel is a very sharp blade used for surgery (Figure 4.12). Scalpel blades are loaded or mounted onto BP handles, named after Charles Russell Bard and Morgan Parker, founders of the Bard-Parker Company. The blades are available in various shapes and sizes, and the blades used will depend on where and how the surgeon needs to cut. For example, a general surgeon will make a skin incision into the abdomen using a 21 or a 20 blade. A plastic surgeon will make an incision on the face using a 15 blade. Different shapes and sizes of scalpels fit onto different sizes of BP handles. BP handles are also available in various shapes, lengths, and sizes (Figure 4.12). Size 3, 4, and 7 BP handles are commonly used. For example, a 15 and an 11 blade will fit onto a size 7 BP handle.

Scissors are probably one of the most common cutting tools, both for tissues and also for various other accessories during a procedure (e.g. sutures, bandages, etc.). The various parts of a pair of surgical scissors are shown in Figure 4.13.

A variety of scissor types are used surgically (Figure 4.14). There are two types of Mayo scissors: curved and straight. Curved scissors are used for dissecting tough tissues and tend to be used by orthopedic surgeons and gynecologists. Mayo straight scissors are used mostly to cut sutures and dressings. McIndoe and Metzenbaum scissors are used for fine dissection and tend to be used by general and vascular surgeons. Littler scissors are fine dissecting scissors used by plastic surgeons and hand surgeons. Potts angled scissors are used to make incisions into vessels, and are therefore commonly used by vascular and general surgeons. Potts scissors are available in various angles.

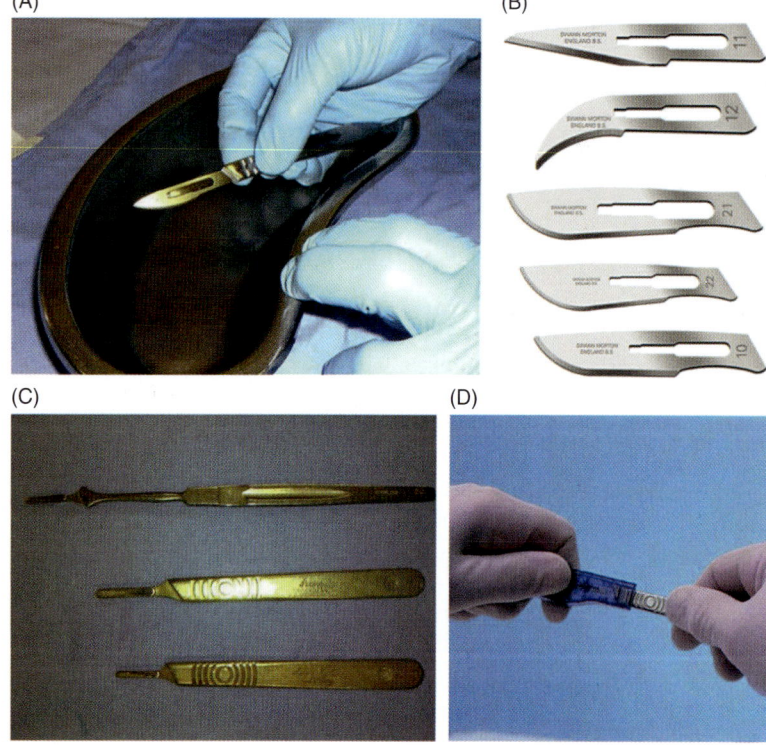

Figure 4.12 (A) A scalpel blade and associated BP handle. Also shown are examples of (B) various different types of scalpel blades; (C) BP handles (3, 4, 7); and (D) a disposable scalpel blade remover.

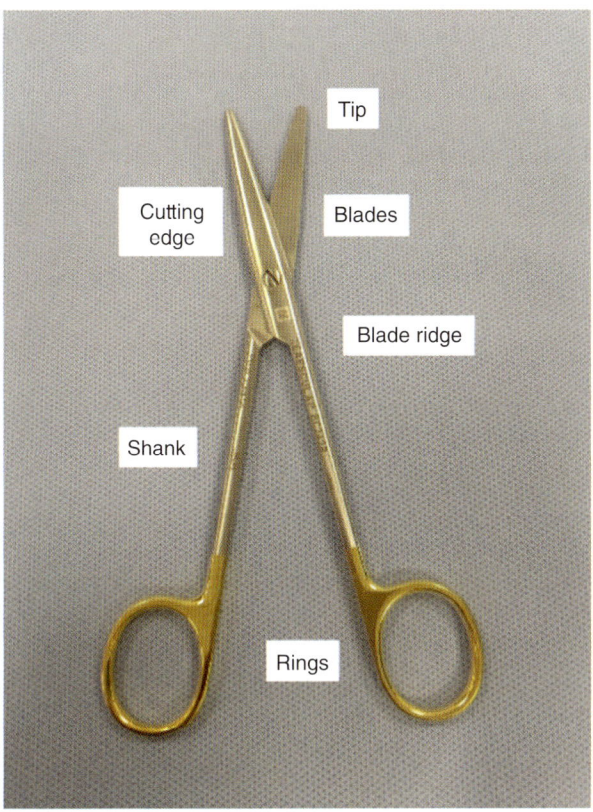

Figure 4.13 The various parts of a pair of scissors. Note the gold handle on the scissors, which means they have tungsten carbide inserts on the working surfaces.

There are many types of instruments that are able to cut through bone and cartilage (bone cutters). They are commonly used by neurosurgeons, orthopedic surgeons, and plastic surgeons. An example is bone rongeurs, which are also known as bone "nibblers" (Figure 4.15). The term "rongeur" is derived from a French word meaning "to nibble." Nibblers can be single or double action (depending on the hinge mechanism). The double-action movement of a bone nibbler reduces the amount of hand strength needed to close the jaws. Other, simpler instruments with no moving parts are also used on bone, including periosteal elevators, chisels, osteotomes, gouges, mallets, and curettes (Figure 4.16). Periosteal (e.g. Freer) elevators are used for scrapping and elevating the periosteum (a tough membrane material that covers bone) away from the surface of the bone. Normally this procedure is performed prior to the surgeon either cutting or drilling the bone. Osteotomes are designed to cut bone, chisels to shave and shape bone in one plane or level, and gouges are used to shave bone into a curved surface. Osteotomes are used for splitting bone and they have a gradual bevel (or slant) on both sides (Figure 4.16). Chisels have a bevel on one side that provides a controlled direction of cut by using the bevel. Chisels are used for chipping pieces of bones away. These instruments may be curved or straight and are available in a variety of widths. Handles may be flat, square, hexagonal, or round.

Other types of sharp dissectors include various types of biopsy forceps, punches, curettes, and snares (Figure 4.17). A snare is a loop of wire that is put around a pedicle of tissue to dissect it, as in the case of a tonsil snare. The snare is looped around the tonsil and pulled tight; the wire cuts through the tissue as it pulls back into the instrument to extract the tissue. A curette removes tissue by scraping it away. As examples, uterine curettes can have a sharp or a blunter tip and are available in different sizes depending on the volume of tissue that is required to be scraped out of the uterus; a Volkmann bone curette (also known as a Volkmann spoon) is used in many different types of surgery (Figure 4.18). Blunt dissection (tissue separation, without cutting) is also desired during some surgical procedures and can be done using a scalpel handle, the blunt side of a scissor blade, or a "swab on a stick," for example a swab loaded on to a Kocher forceps (see the next section).

Instruments used for grasping and holding

Tissue is grasped and held in place for the surgeon to work on using a variety of forceps, such as when inspecting, cutting (e.g. in the case of a biopsy forceps), or even suturing (stitching). The specific type of forceps surgeons will select will depend on the type of tissue or surgical material they need to grasp or hold (Figure 4.19). Delicate or fine forceps are used on delicate tissues such as during eye surgery or certain types of plastic surgery. Forceps are often named after their inventors, with examples being Adson, Gillies, and Kocher forceps (Figure 4.20). Adson forceps are often used by surgeons when suturing the skin (closing a wound using stitches/sutures) following a surgical procedure; they can be toothed or non-toothed and are generally fine-tipped, short forceps. Gillies forceps are also commonly used when suturing the skin. The tip is relatively fine, but this forceps is slightly longer than an Adson. A Kocher forceps is a heavy-toothed instrument normally used for clamping or holding tissue, but also other materials used during surgery. It is used in many disciplines including orthopedics, general surgery, and gynecology.

Various types of strong-toothed forceps are used by orthopedic surgeons and gynecologists when grasping large chunks of tissue. Examples of strong-toothed forceps include Russian, Lane, and Jean forceps (Figure 4.21). A Russian forceps is considered less traumatic when used surgically than other toothed forceps and is used by some gynecologists when suturing (stitching) tissue. Bayonet forceps, so called because they are shaped like a knife on the end of a rifle, are normally used in small surgical spaces (Figure 4.22); they are angled so that the surgeon can see around the forceps into the space.

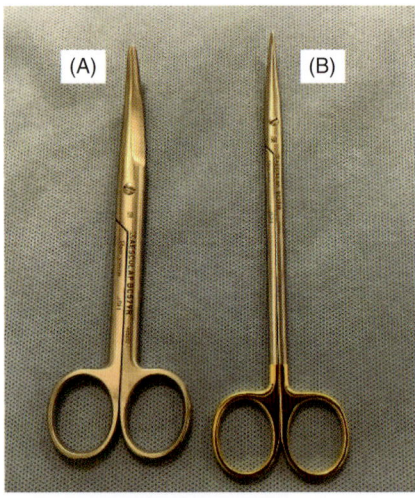
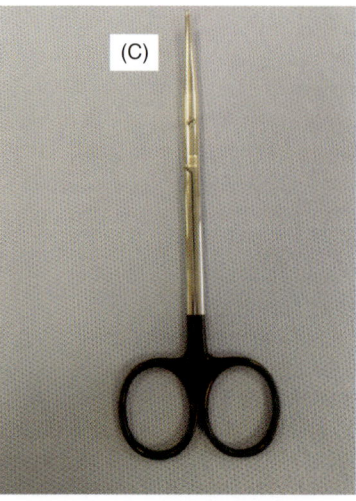

Figure 4.14 Various types of surgical scissors. (A) Mayo curved scissors. (B) Mayo straight scissors. (C) Dissecting SuperCut scissors. Note the specially designed razor-sharp upper blade edge that cuts effortlessly through tissue (black handles). (D) Angled micro scissors. (E) Potts vascular scissors.

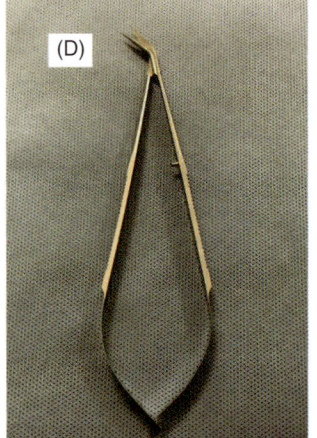
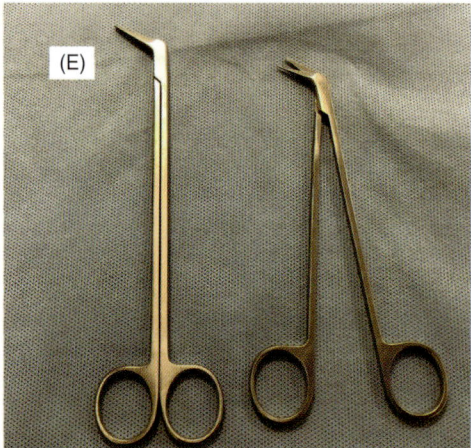

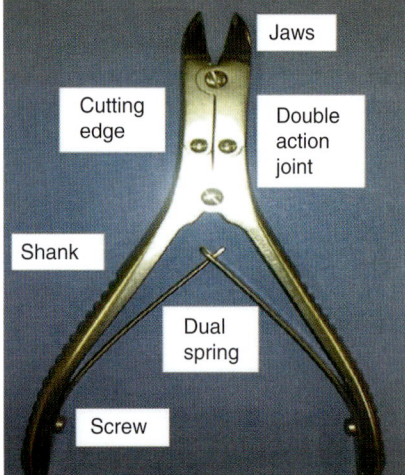

Figure 4.15 A double-action bone cutter (also known as a rongeur or nibbler).

Bayonet-shaped forceps are used in neurosurgery and ear, nose, and throat surgery.

An example of a diathermy forceps is shown in Figure 4.23. These are used to cauterize (burn or freeze) blood vessels in order to stop bleeding quickly; "diathermy" specifically refers to the local production of heat at the tip of the forceps. These types of forceps are available in various lengths and have various shaped tips at the working (patient) ends. An electric source is connected at the surgeon's end of the instrument for heating purposes. Diathermy forceps are covered with insulation (usually a plastic coating) to protect the surgeon while in use. Examples of various other commonly used types of forceps are shown in Figure 4.24. Lane tissue forceps are used to grasp tough tissues and are often used in orthopedics and gynecology. Babcock forceps are designed to fit around a specific structure and to cause minimal or no damage to tissue; they are used in various disciplines (e.g. to grasp the appendix). Vulsellum forceps are used to grasp the cervix when doing a dilation and curettage (surgery to remove tissue)

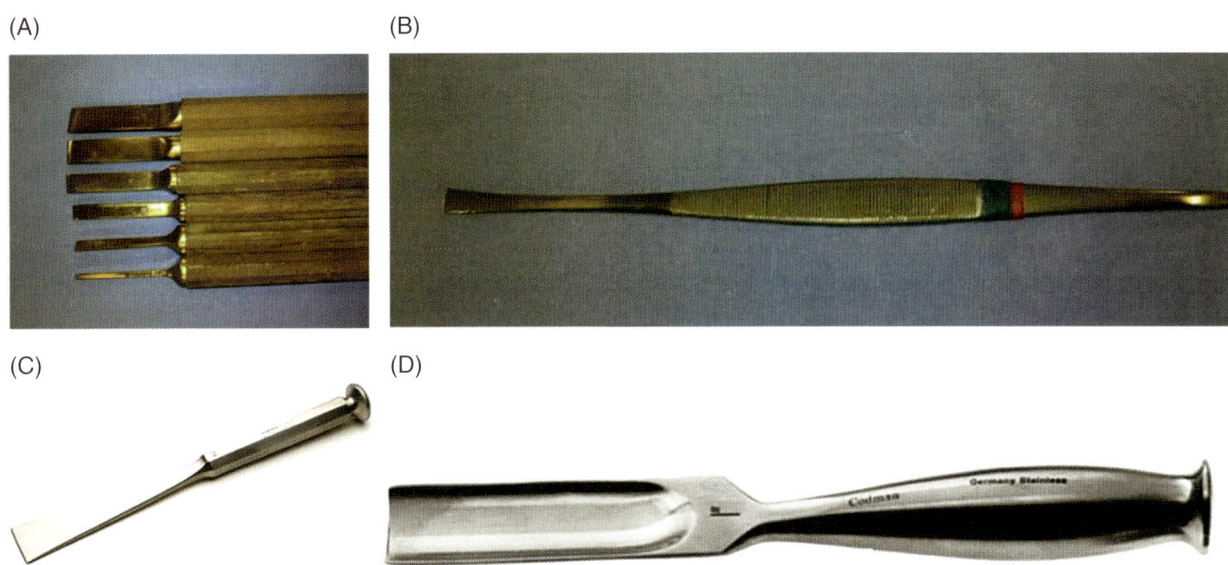

Figure 4.16 Other types of instruments used to cut into or from bone. (A) Osteotomes; (B) a Freer periosteal elevator; (C) chisel; (D) bone gouge.

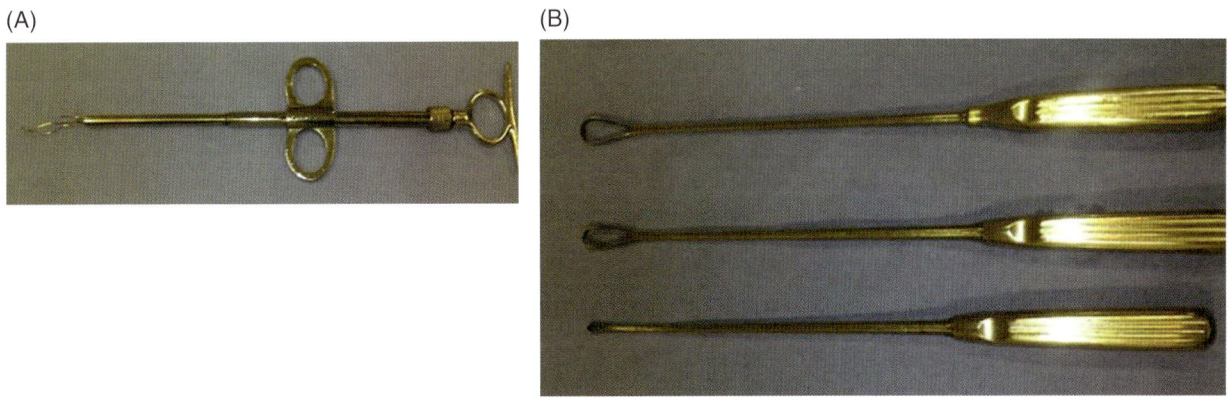

Figure 4.17 Other types of sharp dissectors. (A) Tonsil snare; (B) types of uterine curettes.

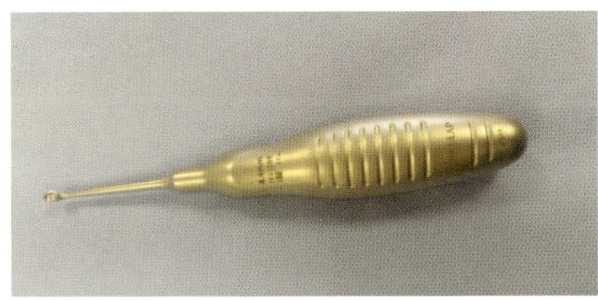

Figure 4.18 Volkmann's bone curette.

or a vaginal hysterectomy. They are strong-toothed forceps. Green Armytage forceps are used during cesarean sections to grasp the uterus and can be used to clamp its bleeding vessels.

Bone holder forceps (Figure 4.25) are specific types of heavy grasping forceps used to stabilize bone tissue, especially when reducing a fracture (fixing a broken bone, where "broken" is the same as "fracture," to its pre-injury position).

A further example is the Wrigley forceps that are used to assist with the delivery of a baby (Figure 4.26). The forceps are applied gently around the baby's head, allowing safe delivery. There are different types and designs of delivery forceps, but Wrigley forceps are most often used during a cesarean section.

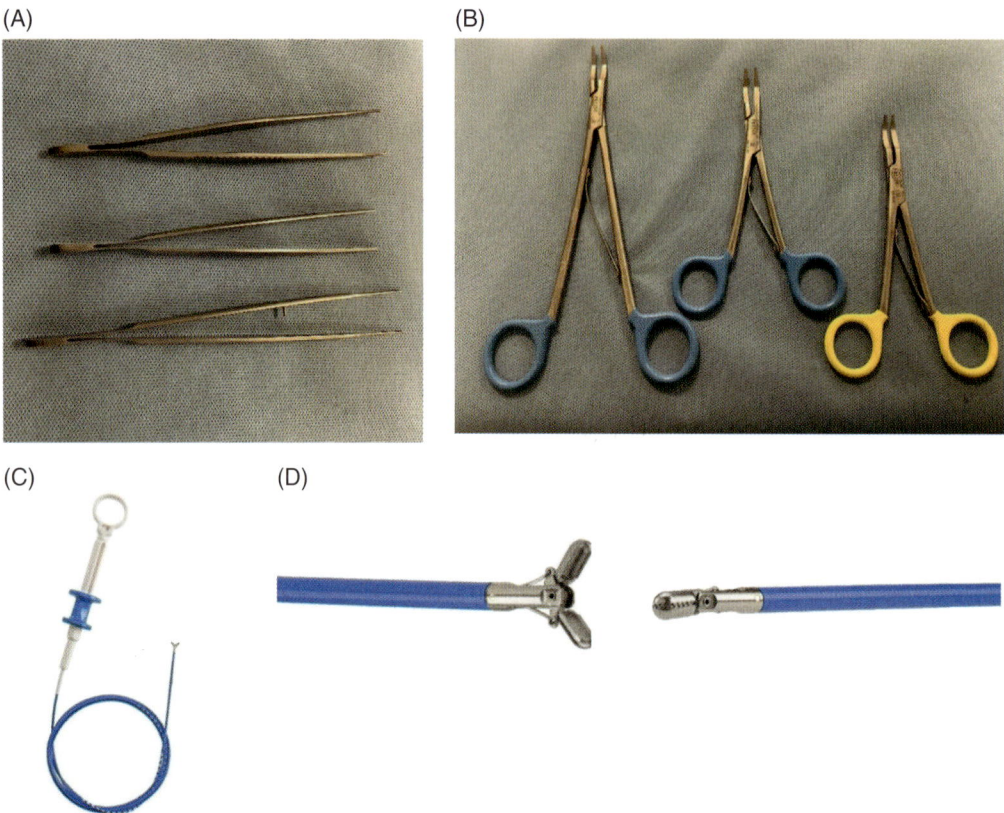

Figure 4.19 Various types of forceps. (A) Dissecting forceps; (B) clip applier forceps; (C) single-use biopsy forceps used during polypectomy; (D) a close-up of biopsy forceps in open and closed positions.

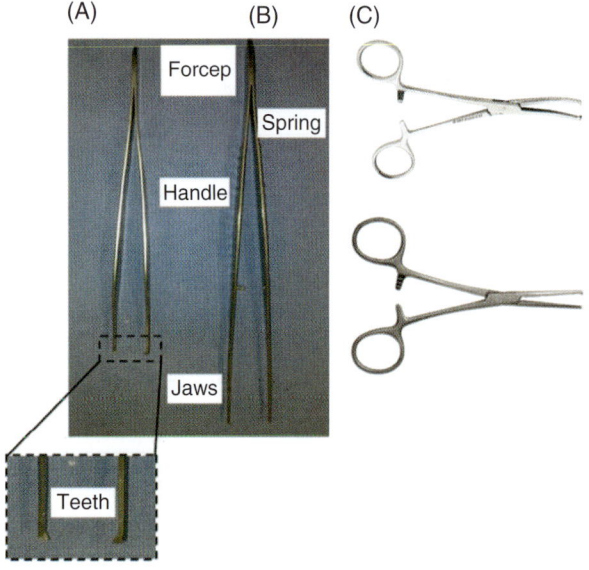

Figure 4.20 Examples of (A) Adson; (B) Gillies; and (C) Kocher curve (shown over straight example) forceps.

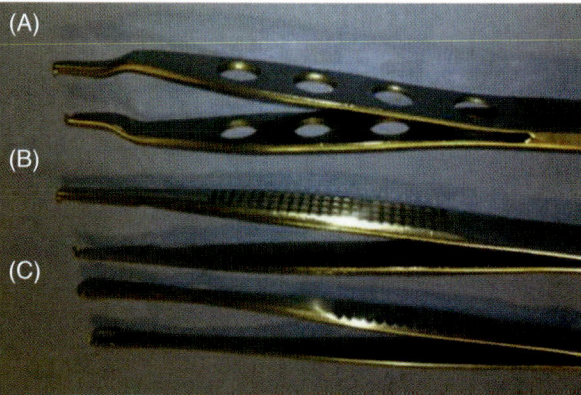

Figure 4.21 (A) Russian, (B) Lane, and (C) Jean forceps.

In addition to holding and manipulating tissues, certain types of forceps are used to hold various objects that assist in a surgical procedure. Sponge- or swab-holding forceps are examples (Figure 4.27). These are used to grasp swabs

Figure 4.22 (A) Bayonet-shaped diathermy forceps, shown (B) being used in a procedure.

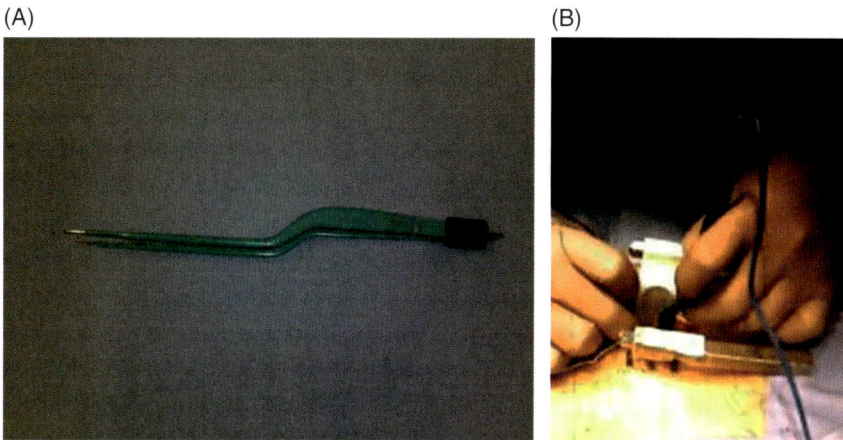

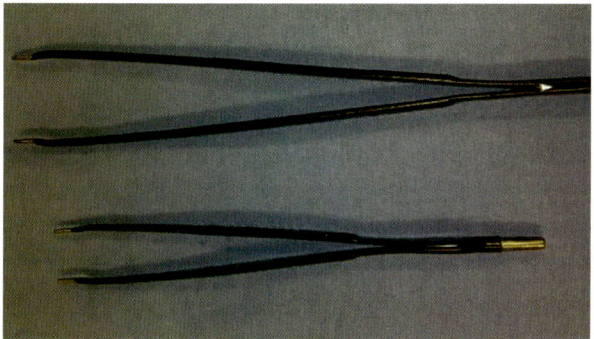

Figure 4.23 Long and short, non-toothed diathermy forceps.

or sponges immersed in antiseptic to disinfect the skin (pre-operative preparative; see Chapter 3, in the section on surgical procedures) just prior to the surgeon making an incision.

Common types of towel clips are used to secure items and drapes within the sterile field (Figure 4.28). As reusable devices, they are often forgotten post surgery and mistakenly thrown away with disposable drapes.

Instruments used for clamping and occluding

These types of instruments are used to apply pressure to a structure, clamp a structure, or close or block a passage ("occlude," as in the case of hemostats and their use on blood vessels). Some will crush tissue and others are non-crushing. The type of instrument used will depend on the patient's anatomy, the type of operation, the location of the surgical site, and the surgeon. The various parts of a typical clamping/occluding device are shown in Figure 4.29.

Hemostatic forceps are clamps designed to stop a blood vessel from bleeding (Figure 4.30). They normally have serrations (grooves in the surface) on both jaws. The serrations can run across the jaws or down their length. There are a number of different types of these forceps; each instrument is designed to clamp blood vessels and tissue in different areas of the body.

An example of a crushing clamp, where the serrations run down the length of the instrument, is a Maingot (Figure 4.31). It is used to clamp the uterine pedicle during a hysterectomy (surgical removal of the uterus); the forceps are placed straight on either side of the uterus (womb) and used to clamp down on the associated blood vessels.

Other types of clamps include various types of blood vessel ("vascular") clamps. There are two types of vascular clamps, those that partially occlude and those that totally occlude. Vascular clamps have different jaw designs (Figure 4.32):

- Cooley-type jaws have a double row of finely serrated teeth arranged in opposing rows.
- DeBakey-type jaws have two rows of finely serrated teeth on one blade and one row on the opposing blade to provide a triangular grip.
- Dardick-type jaws have a three or two vascular teeth configuration, and a flatter, more flexible blade.

Instruments used for exposing and retracting

Retraction refers to pulling or holding back. Retractors are crucial instruments for providing adequate working space and visualization of the operative site for the surgeon, by keeping an incision through the skin open and exposing underlying tissue. Equal forces of traction (grip or pulling power) and counter-traction are actually needed to hold the incision open correctly; damage may result from mismatched retractors, causing tissue healing problems.

Handheld retractors are designed to hold open a wound or to pull a structure (such as an internal organ) aside so the surgeon can reach the various internal anatomies (Figure 4.33). The Langenbeck retractor was designed by German surgeon Bernhard von Langenbeck, originally for urological procedures. Today it is used for plastics, general, and urological procedures.

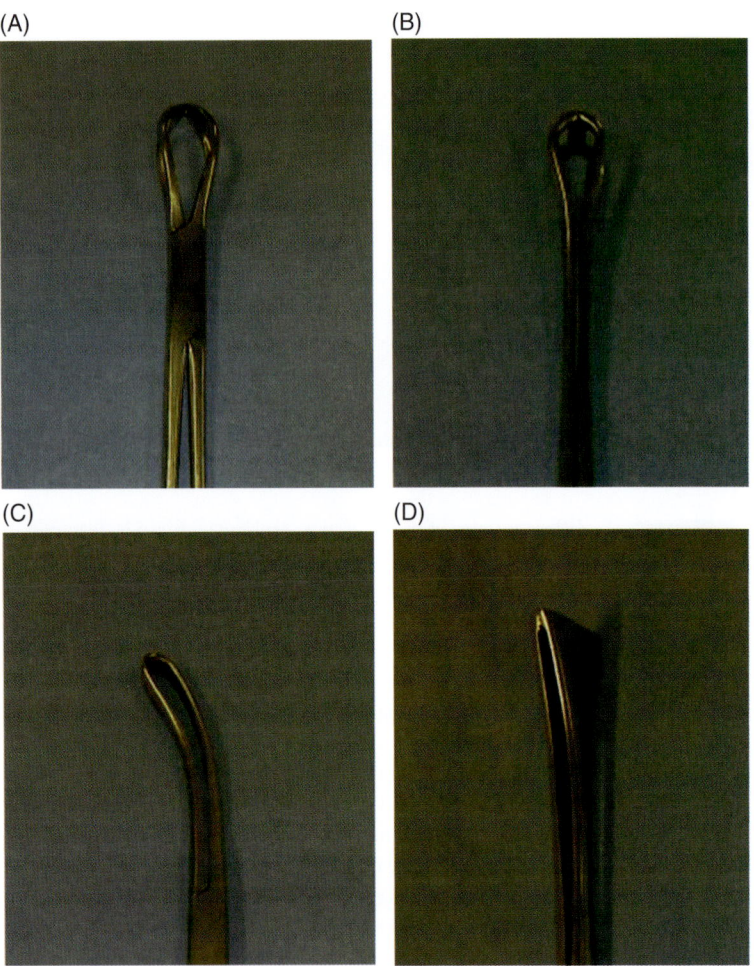

Figure 4.24 Other types of forceps, with their patient-end tips shown. (A) Lane tissue; (B) Babcock; (C) Vulsellum; (D) Green Armytage forceps.

Other examples of widely used retractor designs are Czerny and Doyens. Deaver, Kelly, and Morris retractors are particularly used in abdominal surgery. These are handheld retractors that are normally held by the surgeon's assistant.

Malleable retractors can be bent into whatever shape is required. They are made from different materials and can be used anywhere in the body, particularly with soft tissues such as in the abdomen or even the mouth. They are available in different shapes, widths, and lengths (Figure 4.34). Simple hooks are also used for retraction (Figure 4.35). Hooks can be sharp or blunt, single or double. They are often used to retract skin, nerves, and tendons. Self-retaining retractor designs are retractors that can be placed into a wound to spread and hold it open on its own, in contrast to the handheld retractors already discussed. There are a variety of shapes and sizes of self-retainers, all used in different areas of the body (Figure 4.36).

A final example of a commonly used retractor is the Balfour retractor, which is used to keep an abdominal wound open. It can be used on its own or with the Doyens retractor, which attaches to the Balfour (Figure 4.37). The Doyens is normally used in conjunction with the Balfour when doing surgery on organs in the pelvic cavity. The Balfour typically has three screws that are loosened and tightened during surgery (note, this is a concern as these can be easily lost during processing or even surgical use). The Doyens retractor can also be used on its own as a handheld retractor (Figure 4.37).

Instruments used for suturing or stapling

Suturing and stapling are two methods used to close ("ligate") a wound or cut into a tissue. Suturing (stitching) is done using a needle and suture material (thread made of materials such as silk, nylon, and polypropylene) (Figure 4.38), while stapling uses a U-shaped piece of wire.

Different devices are used to assist with suturing and stapling. Common examples are needle holders, used during suturing. Needle holders are designed to be used with curved suture needles (Figure 4.39) and with specific needle and suture sizes. They lock the needle in a manner that allows the surgeon to push the needle and associated suture through the tissue. Needle holders are available in many different lengths and have different types of tips (Figure 4.39). The tips of the holder can be thick or thin, they can have tungsten carbide inserts, and the pattern on the jaw can vary. Tungsten carbide is much stiffer than steel so it grips the needle well and does not wear out as quickly as steel.

Staplers (or clip appliers) are used to insert staples (clips; Figure 4.40). Ligaclips are commonly used staples in general and vascular surgery that can be used to clip any tissue. There are different types and sizes of clips (depending on what type of tissue is being stapled) and these are also available as disposable items. The correct clip applier must be used with a particular clip – they often have color-coded ring handles, where the color on the applicator will match up with the color of the packaging of the clip. Automated clip systems are available and are often single-use, disposable devices.

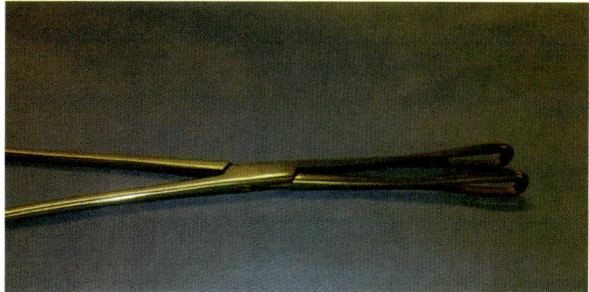

Figure 4.27 Sponge/swab-holding forceps.

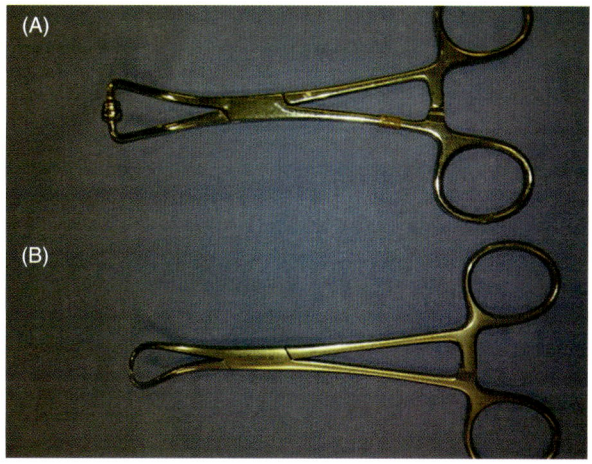

Figure 4.28 (A) Backhaus towel clamp has a blunt tip and is ideal to use to secure a disposable drape. (B) Linen drapes are often secured with the pointed tip towel clamp.

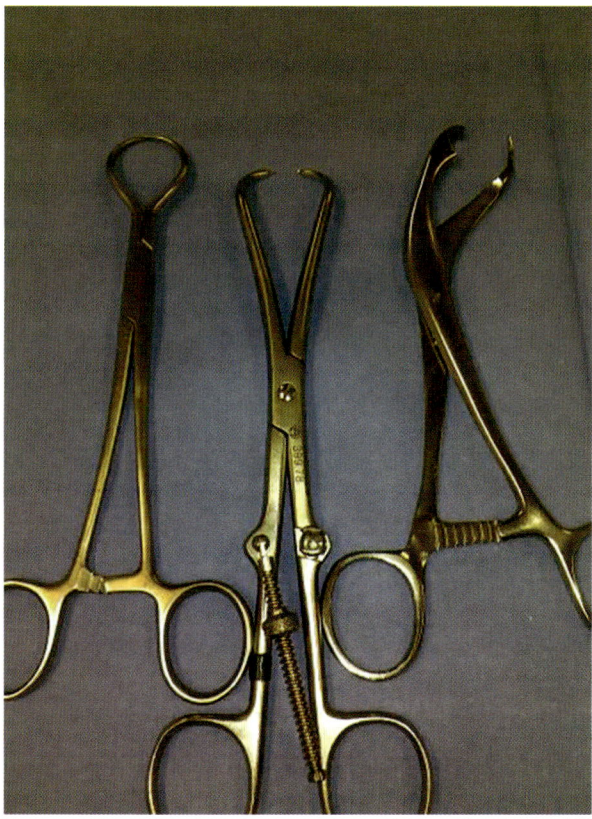

Figure 4.25 Various types of bone holder forceps.

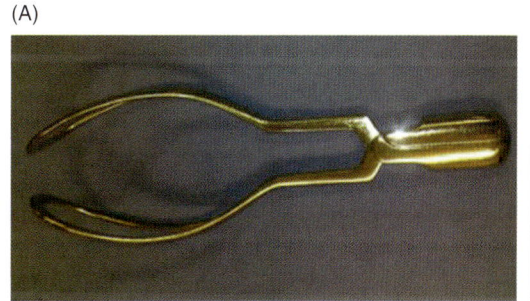
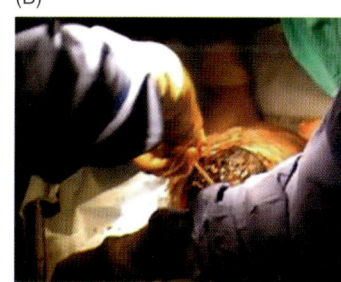

Figure 4.26 (A) Wrigley forceps and (B) their use during childbirth.

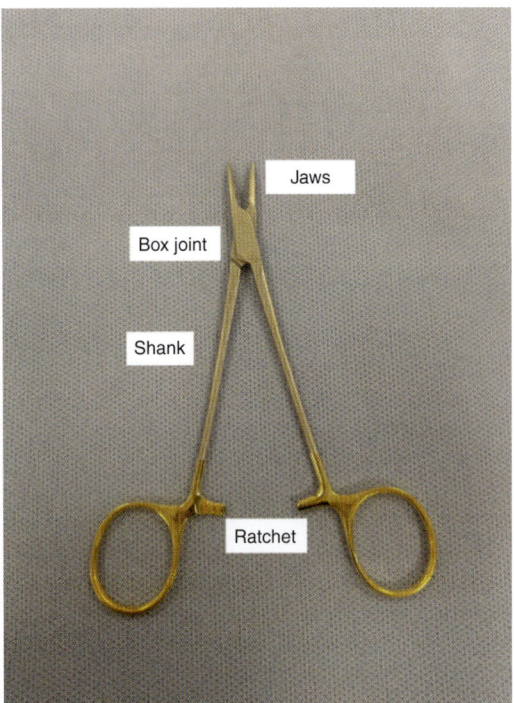

Figure 4.29 Various parts of a needle holder, shown as an example. The inserts of the jaws are made of tungsten carbide, as indicated by the gold handles. Note the ratchet that is designed to allow a locking-and- release mechanism. Needle holders grasp suture needles.

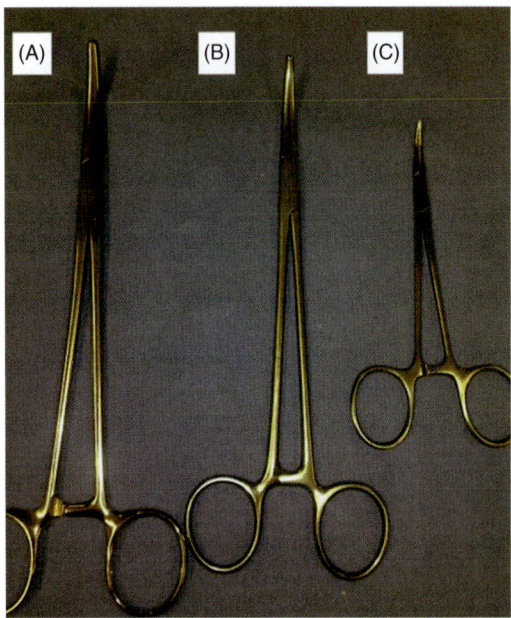

Figure 4.30 Various types of hemostatic forceps ("hemostats"). (A) Artery; (B) Birkett; (C) mosquito.

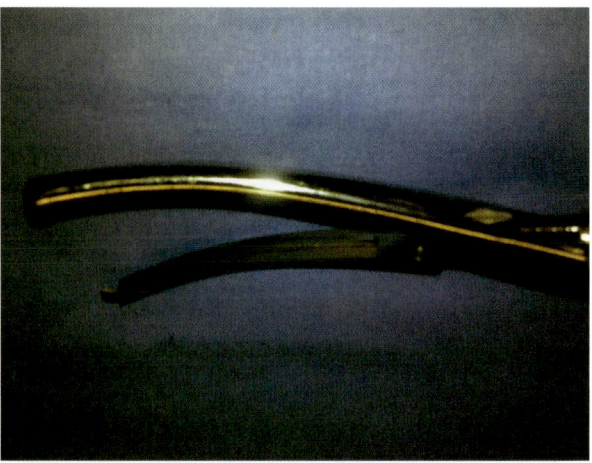

Figure 4.31 The patient end of a Maingot clamp.

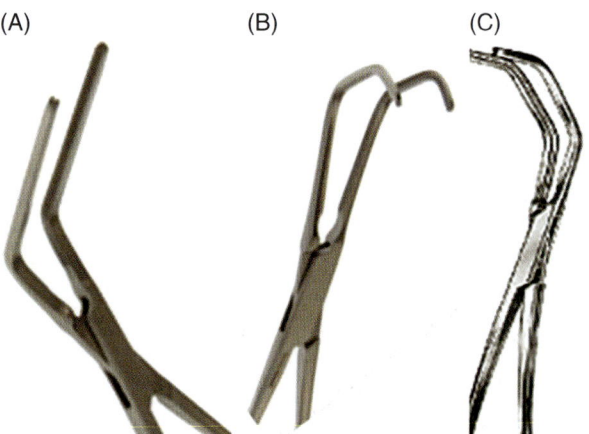

Figure 4.32 Examples of vascular clamps, with types of jaws shown. (A) Cooley type; (B) DeBakey type; (C) Dardick type.

Instruments used for general viewing

Specula are retracting instruments that are used during operations or examinations on the external openings of the body, including the ear, mouth, eye, nostril, rectum, and vagina, allowing better view of the internal structures. The shape of the speculum generally corresponds to where and how it is used, with examples shown in Figure 4.41. Endoscopes are a more complicated type of viewing instrument. These are used for both viewing and diagnostic and surgical procedures. They are considered further in a dedicated section later in this chapter.

Instruments used for suction and aspiration

Various types of tubular suction devices are used to connect to a vacuum source to aspirate (suck up) various body fluids (such as blood) or other liquids that can be present during the

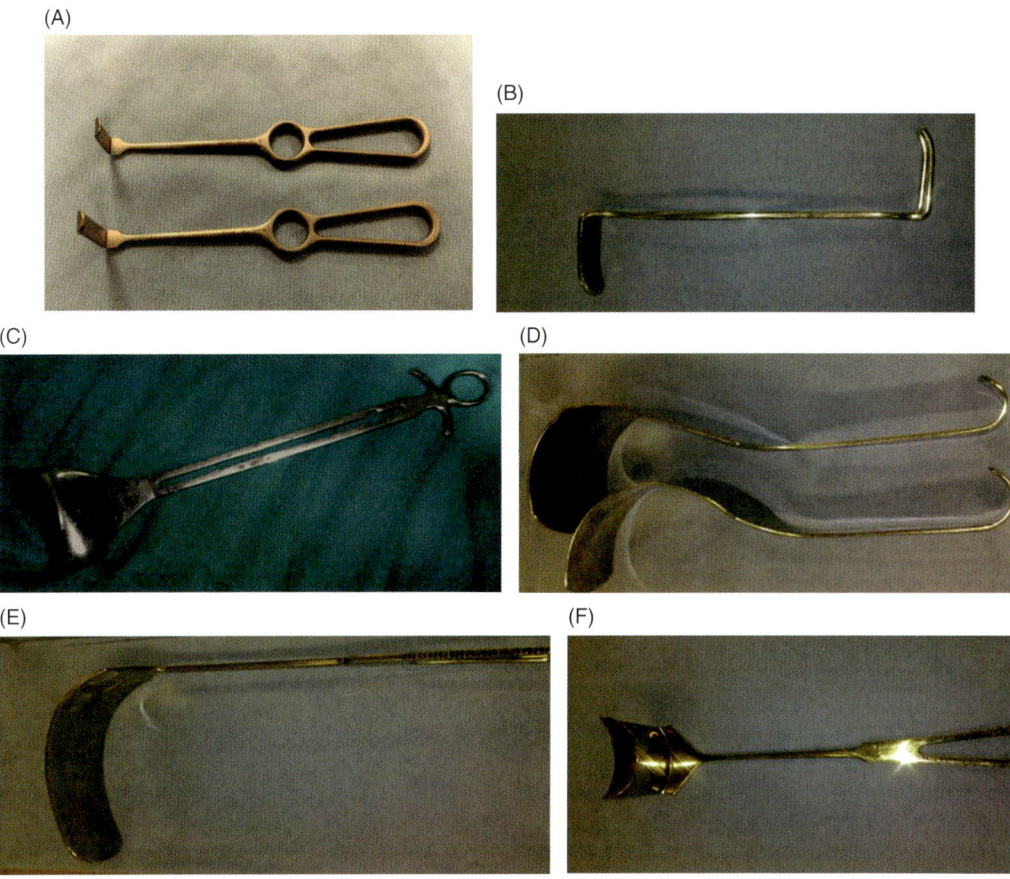

Figure 4.33 Various types of retractors. (A) Langenbeck; (B) Czerny; (C) Doyen; (D) Deaver; (E) Kelly; (F) Morris.

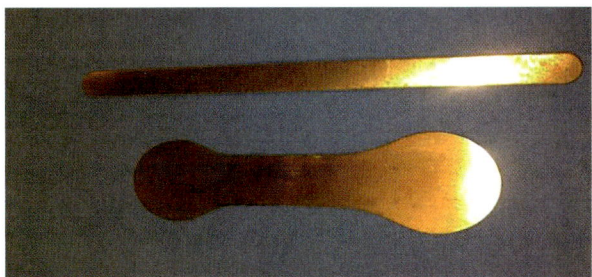

Figure 4.34 Malleable copper retractors used in the mouth.

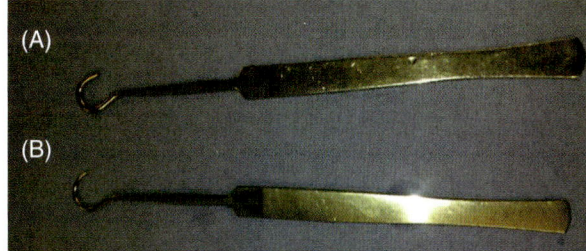

Figure 4.35 (A) Blunt and (B) sharp hooks.

surgical procedure. There are many shapes and sizes of suction devices, again each designed to be used in specific areas of the body and to suck up different volumes of fluid (Figure 4.42).

The Yankauer suction nozzle was originally designed to be used by the surgeon when operating on the throat, but it is now often used for abdominal surgery as it has a large bore to suck away fluid. A pool suction nozzle is designed with a cover to stop any soft tissues (such as the intestines) being accidentally sucked up into the tube, thus causing damage. It is very useful when sucking up large volumes of fluid in the abdomen.

Similar instruments are used to irrigate a wound or area under surgery, such as a simple syringe/needle or more complicated systems such as those in flexible endoscopes (see the section on endoscopy) and dental water line units.

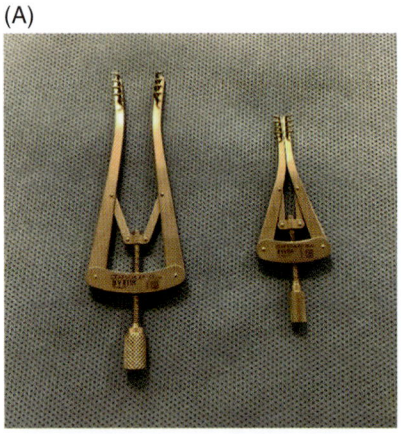

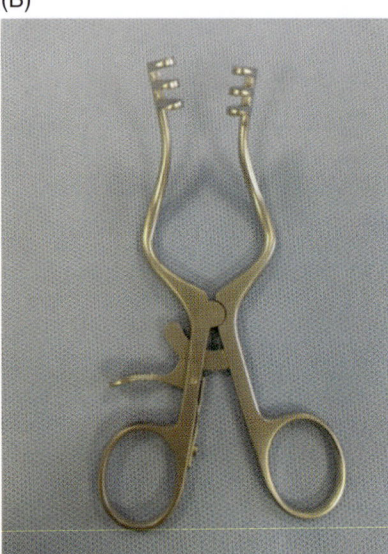

Figure 4.36 Examples of self-retaining retractors. (A) ALM; (B) Weitlaner.

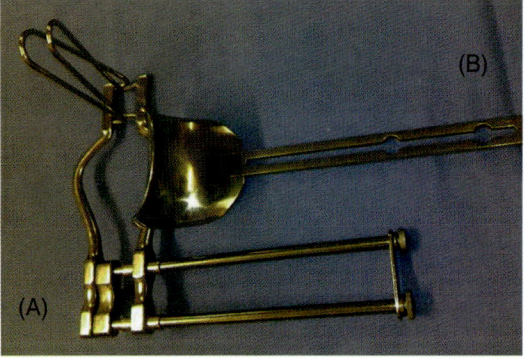

Figure 4.37 (A) A Balfour retractor with screws attached and associated with (B) a Doyen retractor.

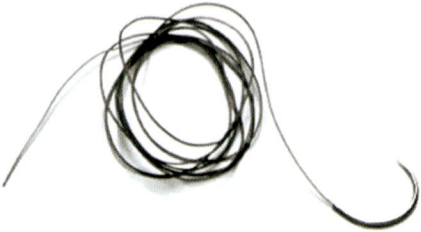

Figure 4.38 A needle and suture, used for suturing.

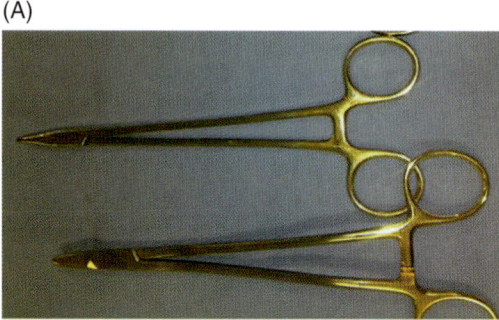

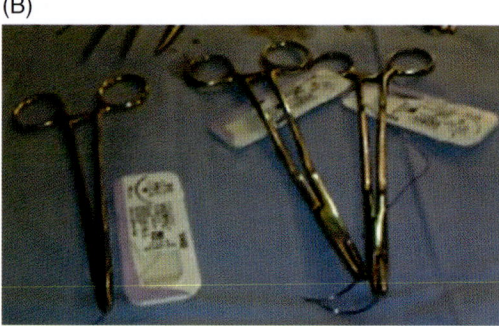

Figure 4.39 Types of needle holders. (A) DeBakey; (B) Thompson-Walker, with needles/sutures.

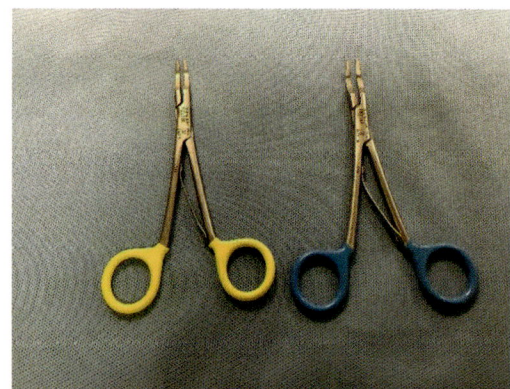

Figure 4.40 Clip appliers.

Figure 4.41 Types of specula. (A) Nasal; (B) vaginal; (C) anal.

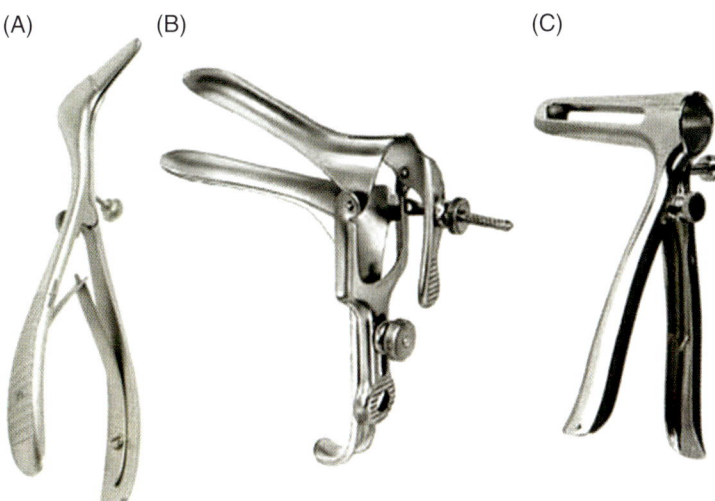

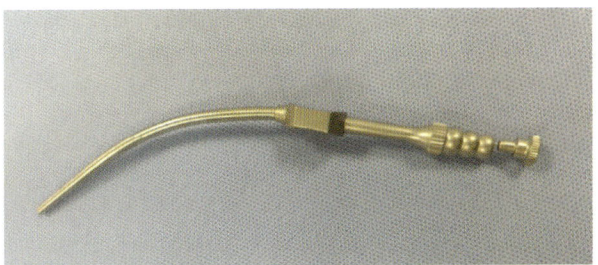

Figure 4.42 Suction nozzle.

Instruments used for dilation

Dilators are used to enlarge or open up various orifices or ducts during surgery (Figure 4.43). The tissue is expanded by starting with a smaller size and then increasing to wider sizes until the surgeon is satisfied that the anatomy has been dilated enough.

Instruments used for measuring or positioning

Various instruments can be used for measuring during surgical procedures, such as simple rulers, trial sizes, depth gauges, and calipers. A depth gauge (Figure 4.44), for example, is used to measure the length of a hole drilled into bone so the surgeon knows what length of screw to insert during an orthopedic procedure. A caliper is a device used to measure the distance between two sides of an object (Figure 4.45).

In addition, various devices are used for surgical positioning, with one of the more advanced examples being instruments used in stereotactic surgery (Figure 4.46). This makes use of a computer-based locating system to identify and operate on relatively small targets inside the body, such as in the brain. These and similar procedures can be assisted with X-ray or tomography computer systems to directly visualize the target tissue.

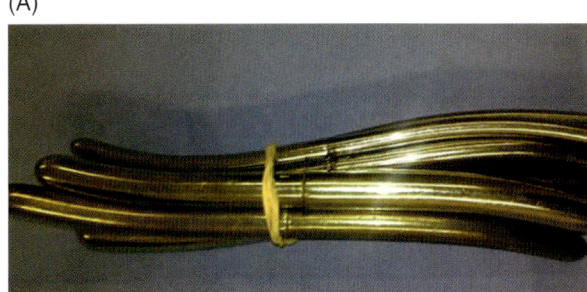

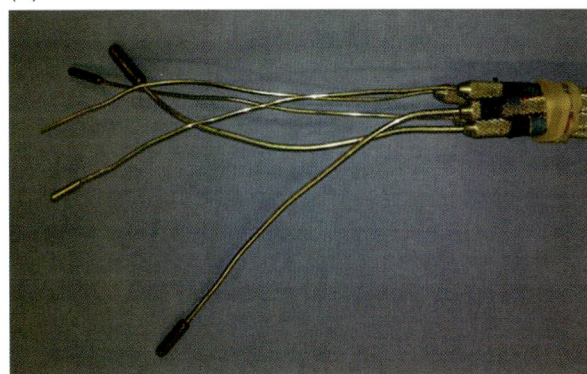

Figure 4.43 Examples of dilators used in surgery. Sets of (A) Hegar uterine and (B) Bakes gall duct dilators.

Powered instruments/tools

Powered devices can operate on electricity, batteries, or high-pressure air. They can often be complex instruments, associated with a variety of accessories. Due to the presence of electronic

88 Decontamination and Device Processing in Healthcare

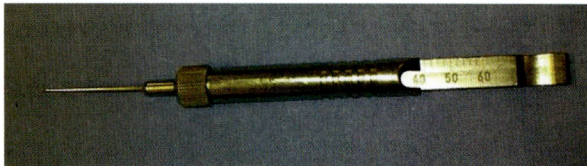

Figure 4.44 A surgical depth gauge.

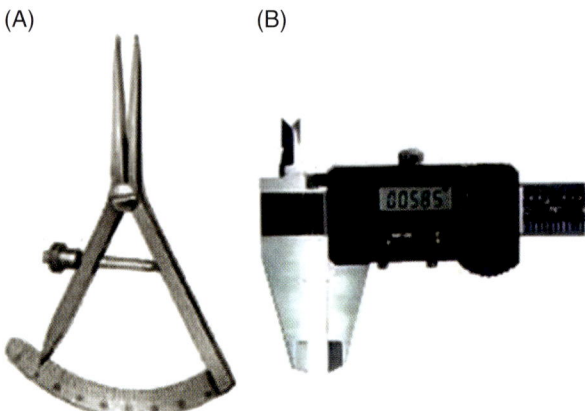

Figure 4.45 Examples of (A) manual and (B) digital calipers.

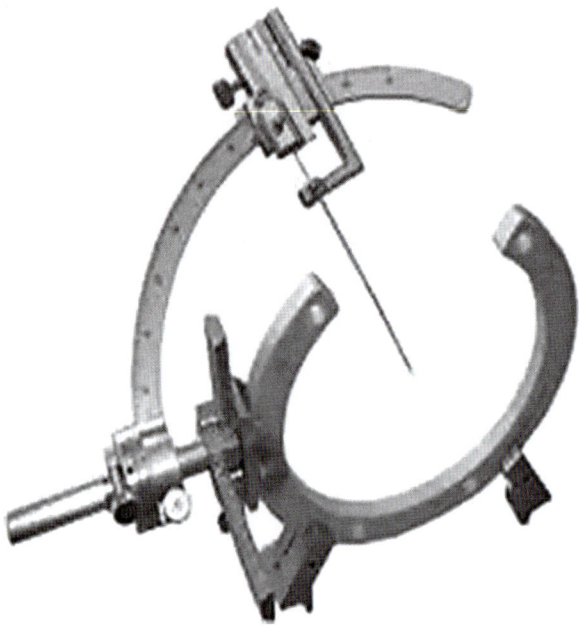

Figure 4.46 An example of a frame-type device used on the head for stereotactic surgery.

components, they may require special handling during the decontamination process, such as manual wiping or putting through a gas sterilization process. Examples are shown in Figure 4.47. It is very important to follow the manufacturer's instructions carefully when disassembling, reassembling, and decontaminating these instruments.

Other miscellaneous surgical instruments

There are many other miscellaneous types of devices that are used for surgery. Examples are mallets, which are generally used in orthopedics to hammer with (into bone). There are various sizes and types of mallets, with heavy mallets being used for strong, hard bones (Figure 4.48). Another example is a chisel (used with a hammer).

Other types of surgical devices include surgical bone screws and bone plates used in orthopedic surgery (Figure 4.49). These are often provided in sets, as a mixture of single-use (e.g. screws and pins) and reusable (e.g. forceps, depth gauges, etc.) devices, and are also frequently on loan to a hospital or clinic. Although some of the devices provided in the set are single use, the surgeon will only use a number of these during a procedure, while the remainder are processed along with the other reusable devices. They provide much debate in decontamination and infection prevention/control discussions, as they are typically a mixture of single- and multiple-use devices, are often heavy sets (as is typical of many orthopedic sets), and are passed from hospital to hospital. The topic of loan sets is discussed further in Chapter 15.

Microsurgery

Microsurgery is a general term used for surgery that is done with the aid of a microscope, a device used to magnify, by a series of lenses, an area of the body or indeed any small object to view its structure. Microsurgery is used extensively in plastic (reconstructive) surgery as well as neurosurgical, ophthalmological, and cardiovascular surgery. The procedures done with a microscope include replantation (reattachment of a part of the body), transplantation (transfer of one tissue/organ/body part from one subject to another), and LASIK laser-assisted in situ keratomileusis) eye surgery. These specialty procedures often require the most delicate and complicated surgical instrumentation, to allow access and manipulation of small tissues and organs. These include electrosurgical bipolar forceps, Frazier suction tubes, aneurysm clip appliers, curettes, and cranial clamps and screws. Examples of these instruments are shown in Figure 4.50.

Micro instruments are designed to be used when operating while looking through a microscope and are specially designed so that they do not obscure the surgeon's vision during such procedures. These are fine, delicate instruments and must be handled with the utmost care.

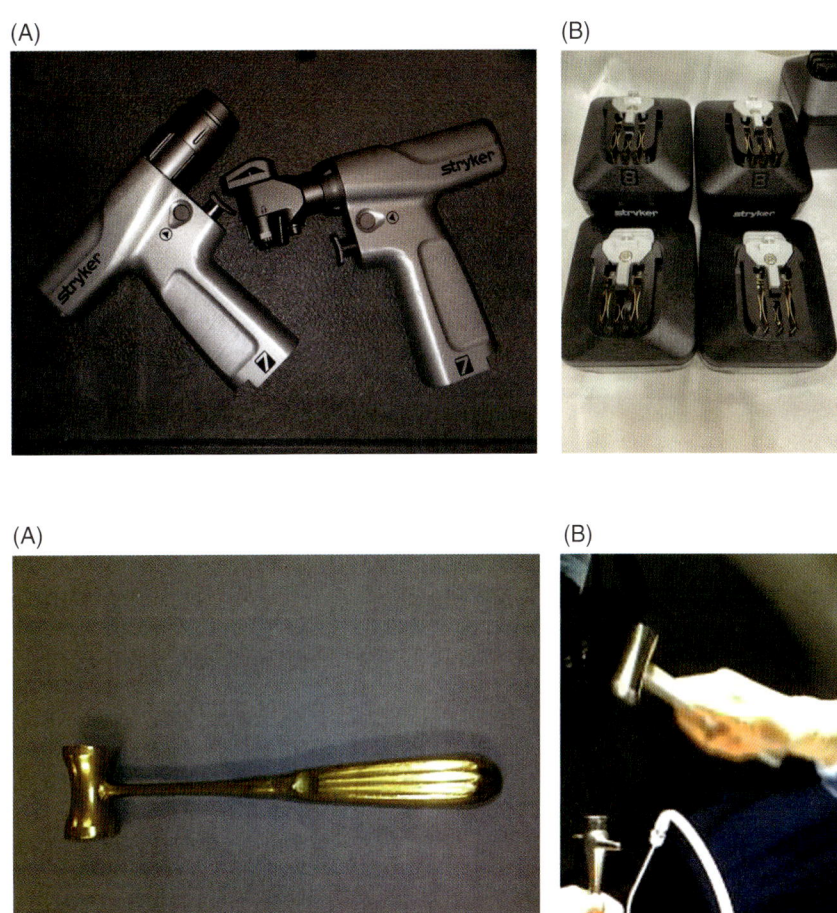

Figure 4.47 Examples of powered instruments. (A) Orthopedic handpieces; (B) reusable battery packs.

Figure 4.48 (A) A surgical mallet, (B) being used during orthopedic surgery.

Devices used in dental surgery

There are typically three different sets of instruments used in oral and maxillofacial surgery: simple extraction sets, surgical extraction sets, and biopsy sets. Other instruments will include those used for minor procedures, observation, and probing, such as dental mirrors, suture scissors, forceps, suction tips, and so on. An example of a typical extraction set is shown in Figure 4.51.

There are examples of some specific dental devices in Figure 4.52. Many of these devices are similar to those used in general surgery, described in the preceding sections, such as retractors, probes, and forceps. An example is a dental syringe that is used to inject local anesthetic (usually provided in a glass cartridge) into a patient.

Endoscopes

Endoscopes are advanced, sophisticated types of viewing devices serving both a diagnostic and a therapeutic role. The word endoscopy is derived from the Greek *endon*, meaning "within," and *scopeo*, meaning "examine" (see Chapter 3, in the section on endoscopic procedures). Endoscopy therefore refers to any procedure to look inside the body, for medical, diagnostic, and surgical purposes. Endoscopes are the dedicated medical devices for performing an endoscopic procedure. They are most usually inserted into the body through existing orifices, such as the mouth and rectum, but in certain cases small incisions ("holes") may be made so that otherwise inaccessible body areas may be examined. One way in which the various types of endoscopic procedures may be defined is based on the area of the body where they are performed, as discussed in detail in Chapter 3.

In the early days endoscopes were used only as diagnostic tools to examine, evaluate, and diagnose the normal physiologic and pathologic conditions of the body. These include investigation of benign or malignant tumors, suspect lesions, sites of infections, and other pathology. Alongside the diagnostic benefits, endoscopes' design and structure have now

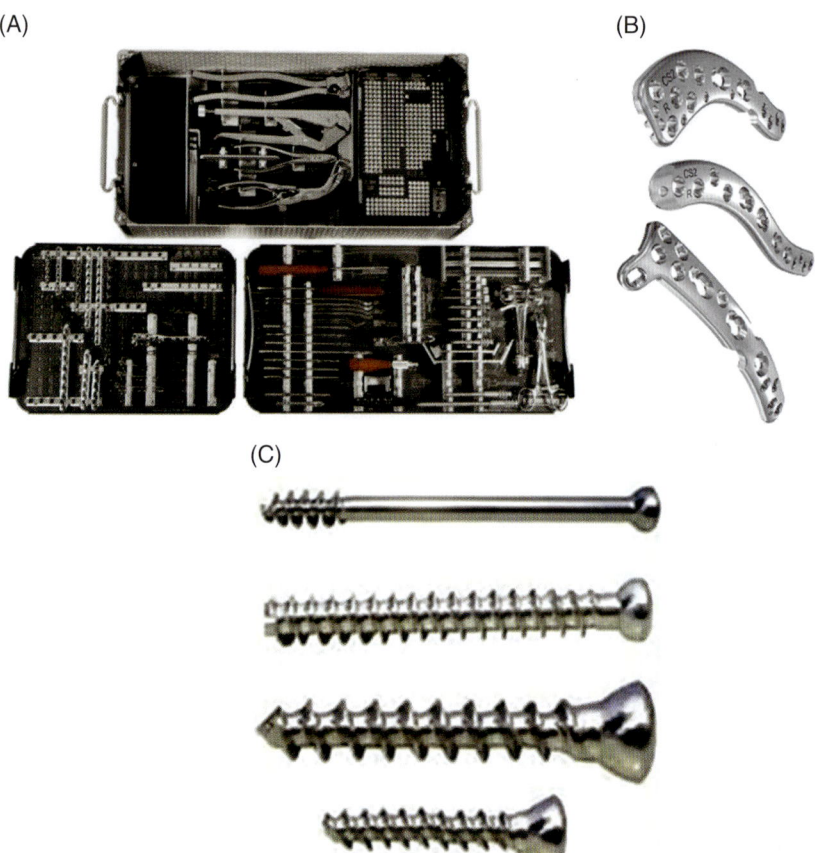

Figure 4.49 Example of a mixture of single-use and reusable devices, in this case an orthopedic instrument and screw set. (A) The instrument set; (B) bone plates; (C) orthopedic screws.

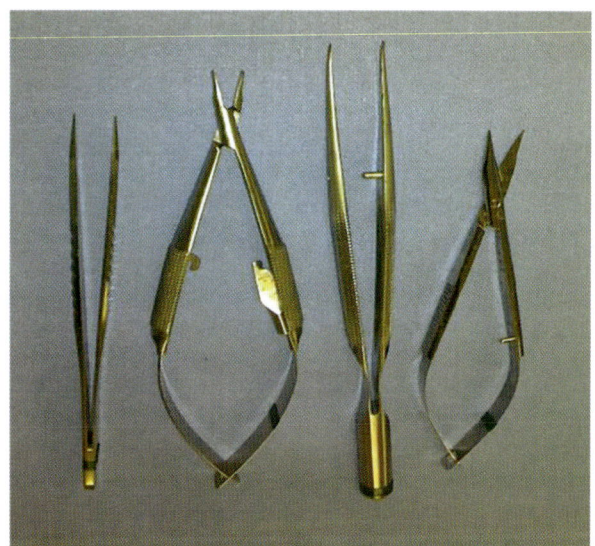

Figure 4.50 Examples of microsurgical instruments, including needle holder, tying forceps, and scissors.

advanced to allow for variable surgical interventions, both minor and advanced. For example:
- Obtain a biopsy, the removal of tissue for microscopic study to detect the presence or extent of a disease, i.e. malignancy.
- Perform cytology tests, in which a specific-purpose brush is passed through the channel of the endoscope to collect tissue cells for analysis.
- Treat internal tissue bleeding with cautery (diathermy) instruments.
- Further advanced surgical procedures, formerly using open techniques, typically in the abdomen, or even in the thoracic cavity to treat critical heart and lung conditions.

A few typical examples of endoscopic procedures are bronchoscopy (used in the respiratory system including the pharynx or throat, the larynx or voice box, the vocal cords, the trachea, the bronchi, and the lungs), which has been a great asset in the diagnosis of lung cancer and other respiratory diseases; cystoscopy, for the investigation of the urethra, bladder, and prostate disease; and colonoscopy, for procedures in the colon (large intestine), including as a routine screening test for colorectal cancer (a type of cancer that affects the colon or rectum).

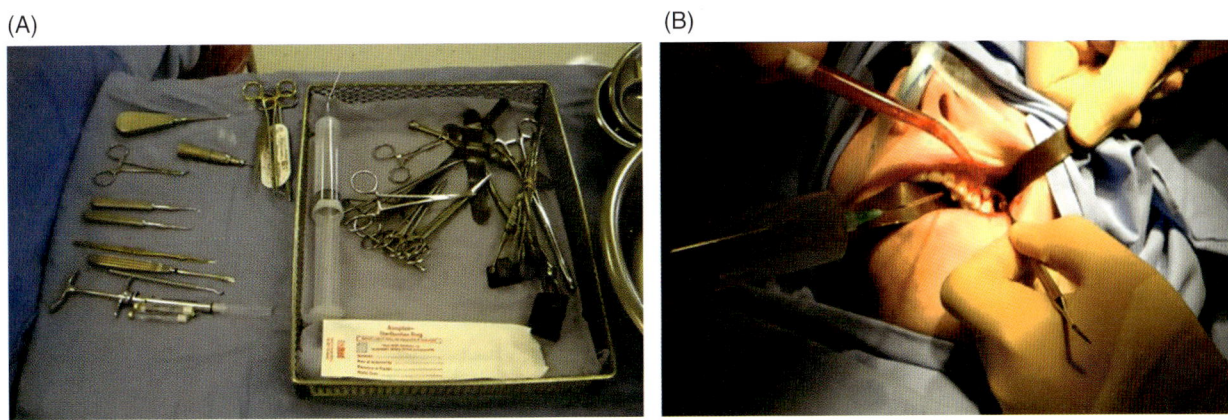

Figure 4.51 An example of (A) a dental extraction (wisdom tooth) instrument set and (B) its use in a procedure. Note in the procedure a suction tube (top left), syringe (bottom left), retractor (top right), and probe (bottom right).

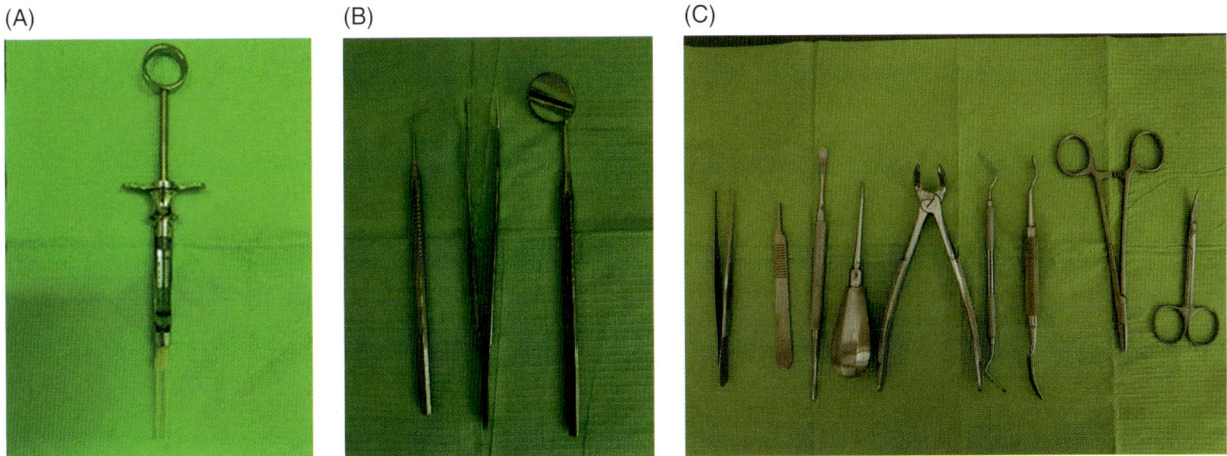

Figure 4.52 Examples of dental surgery devices. (A) Dental syringe with anesthetic glass cartridge and single-use injection needle. (B) Dental examination set comprising explorer, tweezers/forceps, and mirror. (C) Surgical extraction set.

As a clinical note, at the time of writing colorectal cancer is the third most common cancer worldwide, accounting for approximately 10% of all cancer cases, and is the second leading cause of cancer-related deaths globally, according to World Health Organization. It affects older individuals, with the majority of cases occurring in people aged 50 and above. Various studies show that screening methods including colonoscopy can significantly reduce its incidence and mortality rates.

Endoscopes vary greatly in terms of design, construction, materials, and intended use. They can be rigid, semi-rigid, or flexible in design, simple or complex in structure, critical or semi-critical based on risk of infection, diagnostic or therapeutic in application. In recent years single-use endoscopes have also emerged and are available for various applications.

In addition to being very expensive devices to purchase (hence there is usually a limited inventory for specific models in service), endoscopes are extremely delicate and are often associated with expensive repairs. A good understanding of their anatomy, function, as well as proper care and handling during clinical use and decontamination is essential to maintain the endoscope in optimum condition. Attention is particularly required with the decontamination process, because it requires some unique procedures compared to other reusable medical devices (see in Chapter 15 in the section on endoscopes).

No matter the type of endoscope, they all have similar design characteristics, being essentially a rigid or flexible tube with knobs to allow maneuver of its tip, a lens assembly, and a light source that allows the surgeon to see directly or project the image on a monitor. They contain either a lens system, a video system, or both; a fiberoptic cable for providing light; an internal channel(s) for irrigation, suction, or passing accessories; and a channel for insufflation of air within a cavity. Being flexible, semi-rigid, or rigid refers to their design: rigid devices are constructed of rigid (inflexible) materials and flexible devices are designed to be more supple (in particular those parts that are placed into the patient). They can be designed to allow for direct viewing through an eyepiece on the endoscope (as shown for the rigid devices in Figure 3.2 in Chapter 3) as well as through a video system viewing images on a monitor (a flexible video endoscope is shown in Figure 3.2, where part of the device is introduced into the patient, part is attached to a control and supply system, and a central part is held and managed by the operator).

Rigid endoscopes are the oldest types of endoscope. They are available as reusable, disposable, or a combination and are used frequently in many surgical endoscopic applications in MIS procedures, typically in an operating room environment. Common examples include those used for procedures on the joints (arthroscopes), abdomen (laparoscopes), chest (thoracoscopes), bladder (cystoscopes), and ear, nose, and throat (rhinoscopes, nasopharyngoscopes), to name a few. Examples are shown in Figure 4.53.

Rigid endoscopes are often mistakenly considered to be simple in structure, whereas in reality they are complex, delicate, and fragile instruments, as susceptible to damage as any other device. They feature the following basic components: a solid body that joins everything together, an imaging interface, a light guide beam interface, and an eye end nozzle (distal tip). Therapeutic endoscopes further consist of an operating/work channel and an irrigation channel. In more detail:
- The body (insertion tube) is typically a solid, airtight and waterproof metal tube that contains the lenses that transmit the image and the fiberoptics that transmit the light. Its outer surface, which is referred to as the shaft, is very thin and is available in a large range of external diameters, from 1 to 12 mm. It generally does not bend. During clinical use it is often covered by a sheath, which may be reusable or disposable and provides a barrier between the endoscope and the patient.
- The eyepiece is the proximal, surgeon's end of the endoscope body. Originally it was designed for direct use with the eye, allowing ocular vision into the various internal human body structures. Today it is more often used to fit a camera head via an optical "coupler" and through that to a video monitor (Figure 4.54). The eyepiece houses a focus ocular lens that retracts the image at the distal tip (patient end) and magnifies it into an easily viewed image.

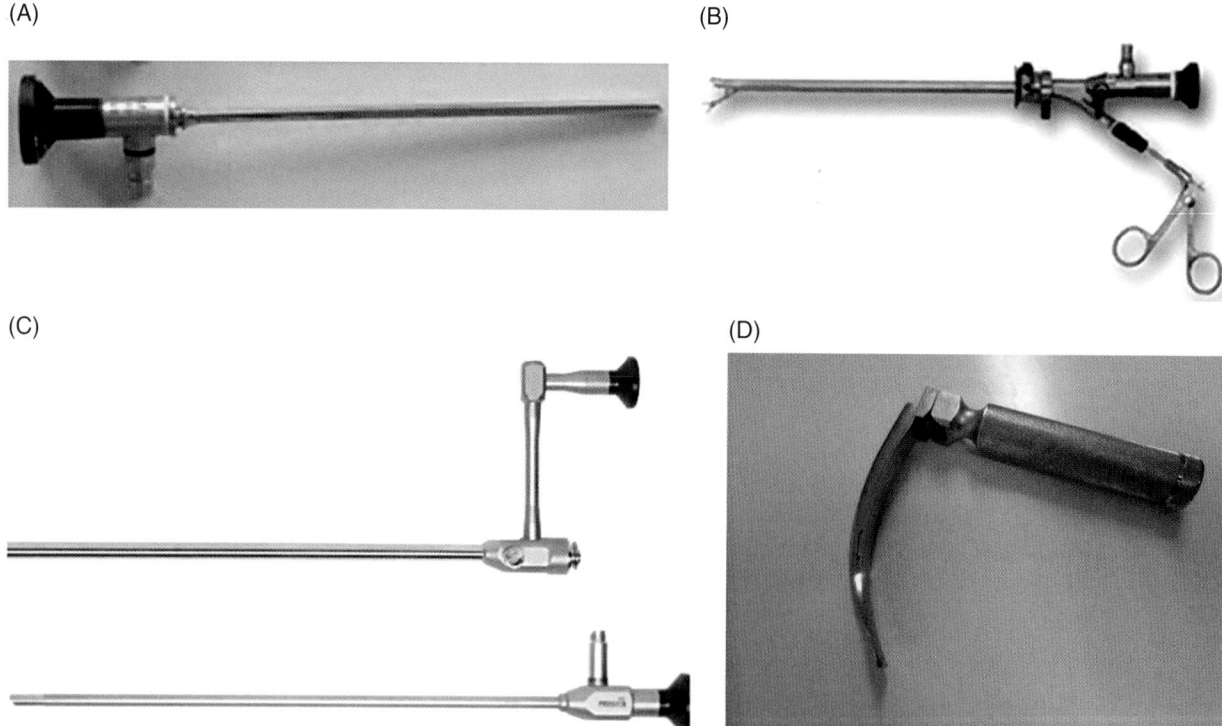

Figure 4.53 Types of rigid endoscopes. (A) Arthroscope; (B) cystoscope, with an associated device; (C) two types of laparoscopes; (D) laryngoscope.

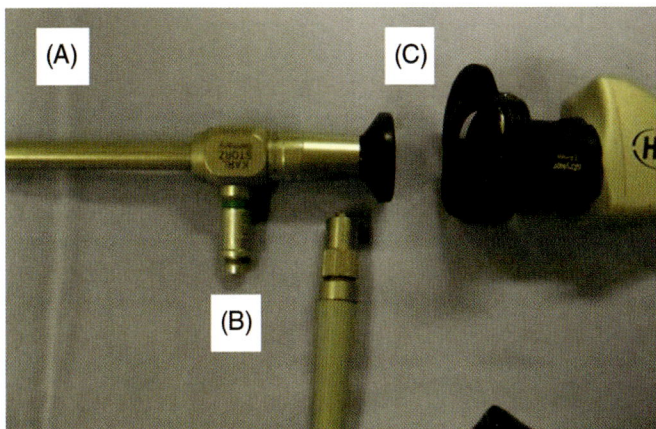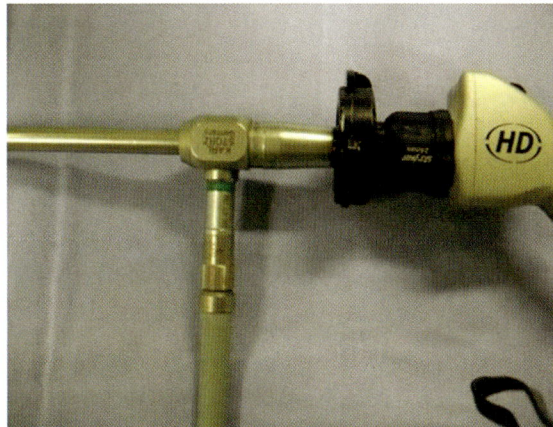

Figure 4.54 Example of assembly of a rigid endoscope (surgeon end shown), on the left disassembled and on the right assembled. (A) Rigid endoscope; (B) light cable (and attachment site, light post, on the device); (C) camera (attaches to the device eyepiece).

- The distal tip of the endoscope is the house of an objective lens that forms the image at the surgical field.
- A series of internal glass lenses comprising precisely aligned lenses and spacers form the optical chain. The optical element of a rigid endoscope is called a telescope. The endoscope can be forward viewing (0 degrees) or angled (10–120 degrees) to allow visualization out of the axis of the telescope. Some of the factors that determine the optical quality of a rigid endoscope include viewing angle, depth of field, magnification, image brightness, image size, and others.
- A light post and fiberoptic system. Light is delivered throughout the endoscope through fiberoptic bundles, which are situated around the outside of the lens housing running down the entire tube.
- Bridges and adapters connect to the telescope and cannula (lumen) opening (if present), and allow for the introduction of accessories (e.g. Figure 4.53) and the application of electrosurgical energy to resect or coagulate tissue. Channels in rigid endoscopes, or within associated devices utilized as part of the procedure (such as trocars), are used for the placement of accessory instruments (such as forceps) and are often used when doing certain types of endoscopic procedures like arthroscopies or laparoscopies (with an example given in Figure 4.53).

A specific note should be made about rigid laryngoscopes, which are one of the most common types of rigid endoscope and are used to expose and view the larynx to facilitate endotracheal intubation. These endoscopes have a fiberoptic disposable or reusable blade that is available in different sizes, may be curved or straight, and connects to the laryngoscope's handle (Figure 4.55). They do not generally have any associated channels.

The ongoing transformation of surgery and the introduction of newer methods, such as RAS, continues to advance the development of rigid endoscopes dramatically.

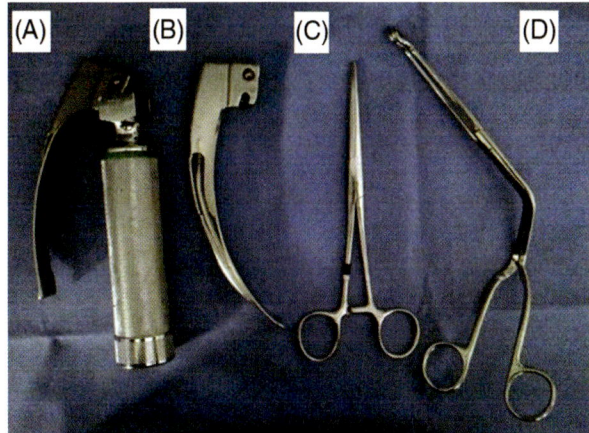

Figure 4.55 A typical laryngoscopy set. (A) Laryngoscope; (B) laryngoscope blade; (C) artery forceps; (D) Magill forceps.

Many types of rigid endoscope are also available in a flexible form, based on where they are used (such as cystoscopes and bronchoscopes). Flexible devices are often preferred because they can flex and bend when introduced into the patient, as well as for viewing and manipulation during the surgical or medical procedure. This is important in introducing the endoscope into natural orifices of the body, such as in the mouth (for gastroscopy and bronchoscopy) and the anus (during colonoscopy).

In general, flexible endoscopes have much longer tubing and they are designed for inspection, sampling (e.g. taking a biopsy), and even advanced surgical procedures. Flexible endoscopes are particularly useful for viewing the inside of the stomach, duodenum, and intestines, where the endoscope may have to pass a long distance into the body and around the twists and curves of the alimentary canal. Examples of flexible endoscopes are shown in Figure 4.56.

The main parts of a flexible endoscope are shown in Figure 4.57. They are extremely complicated in design and are divided into three sections: the control section, the insertion section, and the connector section. Each manufacturer may use different terminology for similar parts, thus it is important to refer to the instruction manual for more information. To describe the design in detail:

• A control handle/head/body that houses components necessary to regulate the functions of the endoscope while in operation by the surgeon or a specialized endoscopist (Figure 4.58). Various switches, including angulation and brake knobs (to maneuver the tip and allow navigation) and electrical switches (to enable taking pictures and video operation), feature on this part of the endoscope. Depending on the type of endoscope several procedure valves ("buttons") are also present: the suction and air/water valves are used to cover and activate the corresponding ports/channels; and the biopsy valve covers the working/instrument port/channel, often referred to as the "biopsy channel" because the biopsy forceps is the single most common instrument to run through that channel. Except for the biopsy valve, the rest may be reusable or single use. Reusable valves ought to undergo decontamination, just as endoscopes do. Finally, it should also be pointed out that valves are specific to the type and model

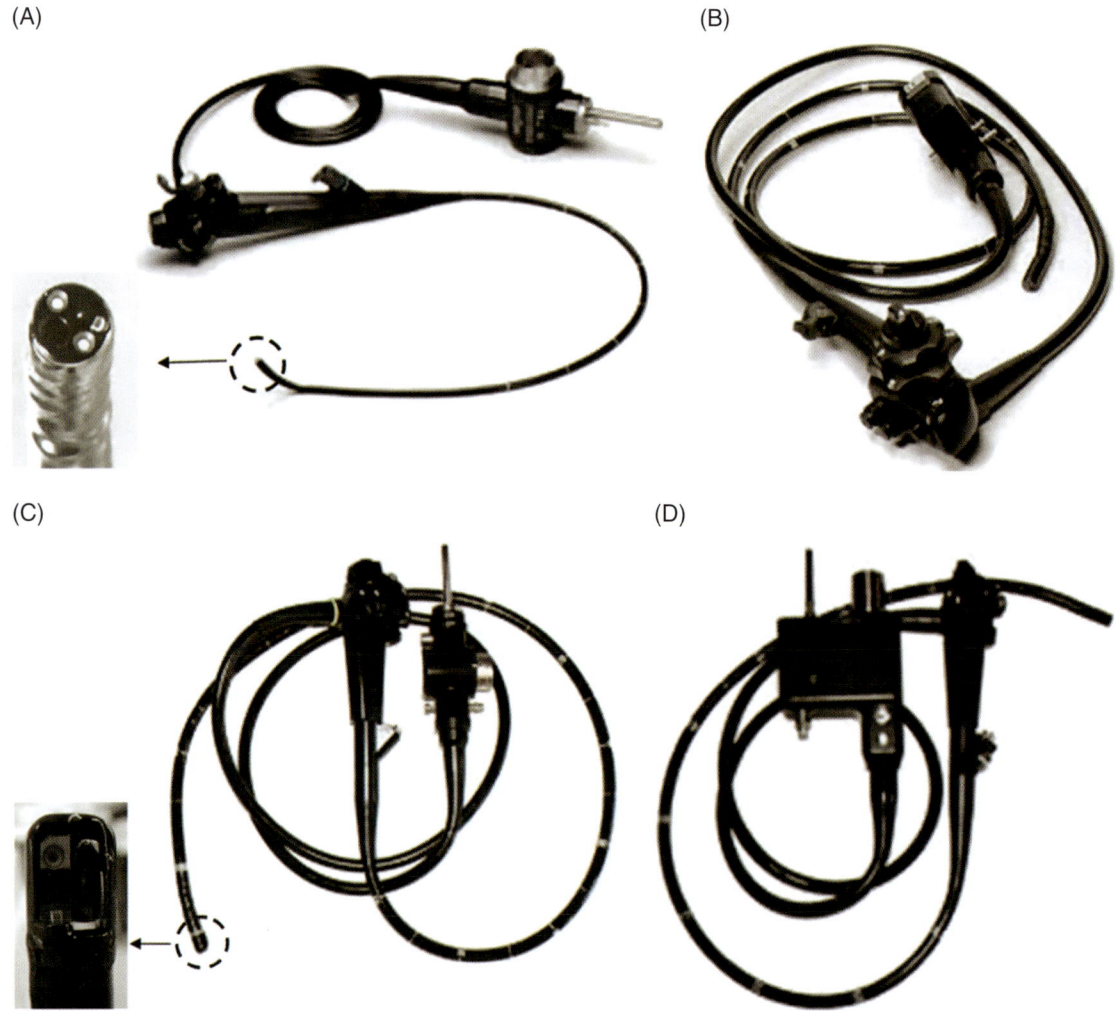

Figure 4.56 Types of flexible endoscopes. All devices shown are video endoscopes. (A) Bronchoscope (with a view of the end of the scope showing the end of a channel and light source); (B) colonoscope; (C) duodenoscope (with a view of the side-viewing end of the scope); (D) gastroscope.

of endoscope. Examples of the various valves are shown in Figure 4.59.
- The insertion tube is the flexible portion of the endoscope that is inserted into the patient. Graduated white marks act as reference points during the procedure (Figure 4.57).

Throughout the length of the insertion tube internal channels are present, as well as fiberglass optic bundles carrying light from the light source to the internal structure, or image bundles carrying the image from the tip of the device to the image interface part and the monitor. Various wires enclosed in an insulated mesh jacket also run the length of the entire insertion tube and allow the device to be angulated during the procedure. An outer sheath covers this mesh. The length of the insertion tube can vary greatly depending on the application of the endoscope. On the upper section of the insertion tube at the juncture with the control head a rubber tension relief boot supports the connection between rigid components and

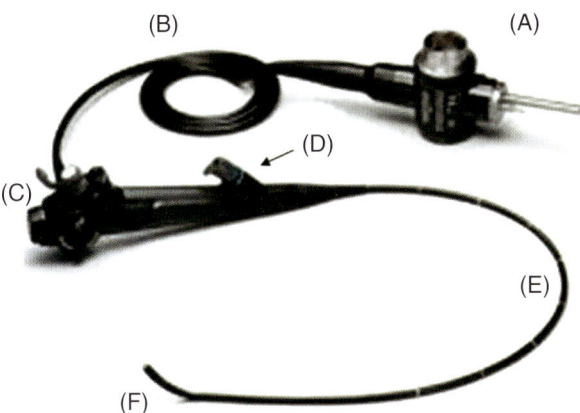

Figure 4.57 The main parts of a flexible endoscope. (A) Light guide connector (the device can include air and/or air/water connectors, attachment to a light source/video system, suction system. and even other gas supply systems such as carbon dioxide). (B) Light guide cable. (C) Control handle/head/body, which controls the functions of the device and features openings to various ports, switches, and valves. (D) Biopsy/instrument port (if present, allows accessories to be inserted through the device and into the patient). (E) Insertion tube, gradually marked, and at its end (F) the distal tip (including a section known as the bending rubber, which can be controlled by the endoscopist during a procedure).

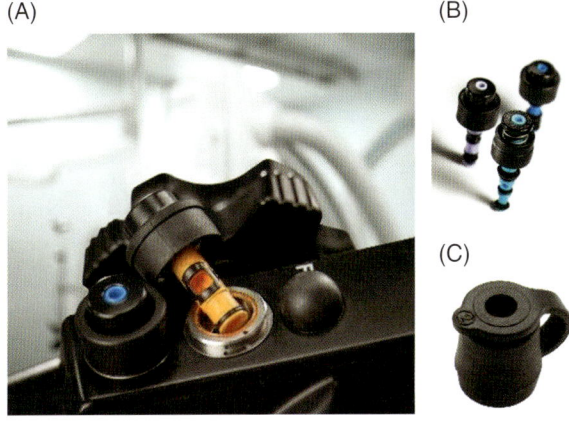

Figure 4.59 Examples of various single-use procedure valves. (A) Suction valve; (B) air/water valves; (C) biopsy valve. Courtesy STERIS Corporation 2024. All rights reserved.

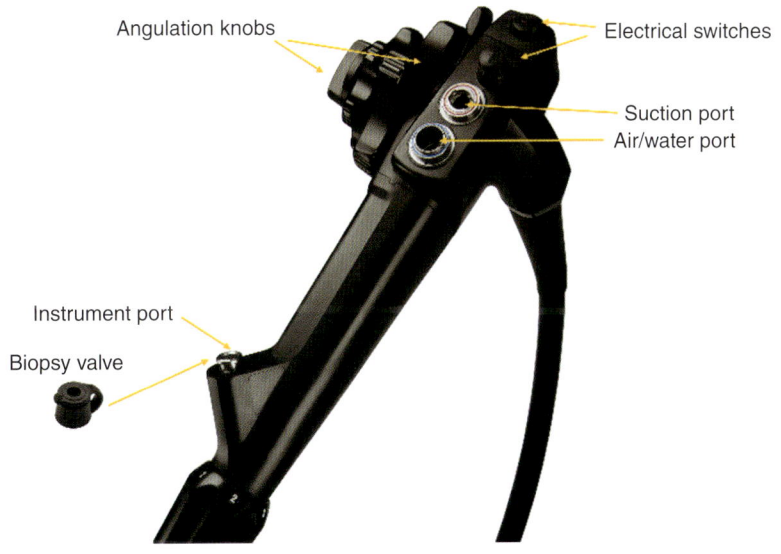

Figure 4.58 Zooming in on the control handle/head/body of a flexible endoscope and its housing components necessary to regulate the functions of the endoscope.

flexible parts. The insertion tube additionally features a bending section that the endoscopist can move to operate the control knobs, for example to position the distal tip. The bending rubber section is the most manipulated and angulated section of the entire endoscope, hence it tends to be often damaged and repaired.

- The distal tip is the insertion tube's farthest point from the control handle/head/body. It may be simple or complex and face forward or sideways, depending on the procedure. It contains the objective lens(es) and the light lenses, and it also houses the terminal ends of the different channels. Video endoscopes also feature a camera chip, the charge-coupled device (CCD) that converts the light image into an electronic signal for viewing on a monitor. An air/water nozzle and an auxiliary water-jet nozzle may also be present. In the case of a duodenoscope, which allows for additional side viewing of body areas adjacent to the duodenum, a special component, the elevator, is present at the distal tip. This is unique to this type of device (shows in Figure 4.56). Instruments passed through the working channel of the duodenoscope can be raised or lowered by this elevator and positioned in a manner that enables access into the bile and pancreatic duct openings. It is also very interesting to note, because ineffective cleaning of this has been associated with numerous well-publicized endoscopy-associated infections.
- There is an internal series of channels, which in simple terms are lumens running from one end of the endoscope to the other with an on/off procedural valve. Flexible endoscopes can vary in design, from very simple when they do not contain any internal channels and are used only for visual examination to very complex ones that contain dual instrument channels to allow two accessories to be used simultaneously. At the time of the writing flexible endoscopes may have up to seven separate and/or interconnected channels, such as the suction/instrument (biopsy), air/water, auxiliary water (or water-jet force), and elevator guidewire ("alberran") channels. All channeled flexible endoscopes have at minimum a suction/biopsy system. The suction channel is used to suction away water and debris and always merges with the instrument channel. The instrument channel is used to deliver instruments, for example biopsy forceps (see the section on instruments for cutting and dissecting) to the procedure site. The instrument channel is usually the largest operating channel, varying greatly in diameter and length. The water/air channel is used to introduce water or air, respectively, to enhance visualization. The auxiliary water jet or forward water-jet channel pushes water outward to irrigate the procedure site and improve visibility. It is usually an independent channel. Typically, therapeutic endoscopes will have an auxiliary water-jet channel.
- A light source (connected to the control head via the light guide cable) assists in inspecting internal areas. The light source

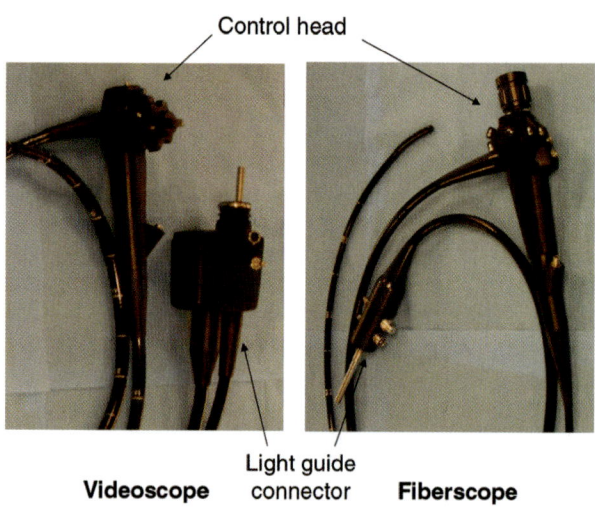

Figure 4.60 Examples of control heads and light guide connectors of flexible video- and fiberscopes.

connectors vary in design depending on the manufacturer and connect to a light source. Light is transmitted by optical fibers. The light guide connector end may also allow connection to air, water, and suction sources, as well as to a video system.

Based on the method of sensing and transmitting images, flexible endoscopes are also classified into two types: fiberscopes and videoscopes (Figure 4.60). In a fiberoptic endoscope, the image is carried from the distal tip of the endoscope to an eyepiece at the control handle/head/body via bundles of optical glass fibers. In a video endoscope, the image is transmitted electronically to a video monitor from the distal tip of the endoscope where it is "sensed" by a CCD chip. Similar to rigid endoscopes, a camera head may be attached to the eyepiece of a fiberscope to produce an image on the electronic sensor, which is then displayed on a monitor or other display device. Modern cameras can provide 3D images in high definition (HD) and offer a vision of the operative field comparable to open surgery.

In many cases, flexible and rigid endoscopes use a variety of other devices/instruments during a procedure to access internal tissues and operate (Figure 4.61). These include separate devices used as part of the procedure, such as light and suction source instruments, injection and aspiration needles, trocars, snares, forceps, irrigation catheters, coagulating electrodes, cytology brushes, retrieval nets, and many more; others are specific parts of the device, such as the procedural valves that were mentioned earlier. Each of these accessories is specific for the procedure and the type of endoscope. These accessories to the procedure may be reusable or single use,

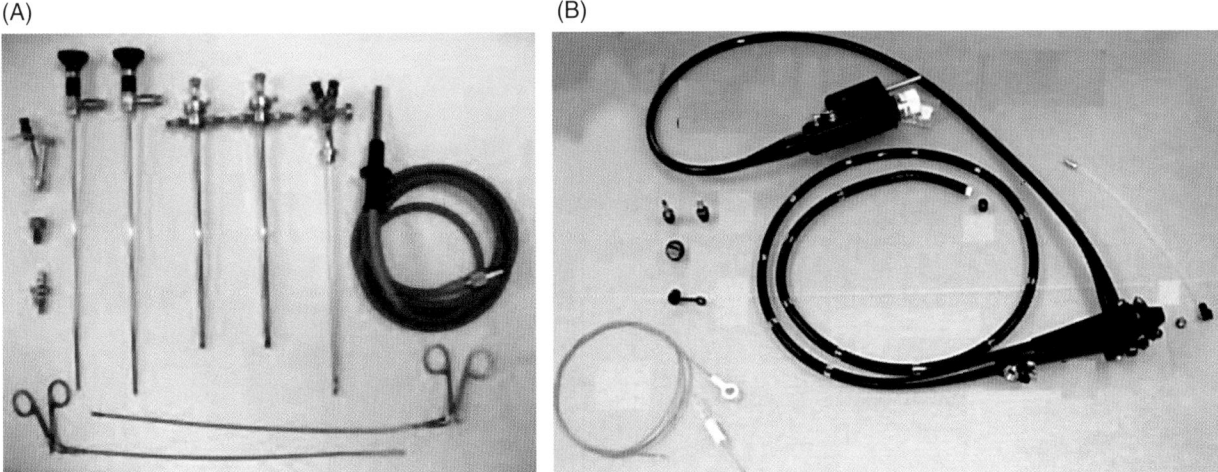

Figure 4.61 Sets of endoscopes used in procedures. (A) Cystoscopic procedure (cystoscopy) and (B) flexible endoscopy (showing biopsy forceps on the left) sets of devices.

and may vary in size, configuration, and intended use. Reusable accessories, just like the endoscopes themselves, should be checked thoroughly for function and integrity before and after each use.

Future applications of flexible endoscopy include advances in the imaging systems, newer endoscopes with "self-drive" capabilities, and enhancement of targeted therapeutics that allow for more elaborate procedures. Endoscopic ultrasound (EUS) or echo-endoscopy, for example, is a relatively recent procedure in which endoscopy is combined with ultrasound to visualize the lining and the wall beyond the respiratory and digestive tract and obtain detailed images of the nearby internal organs and adjacent structures such as the lungs, pancreas and liver, and lymph nodes. In this case, the generic types of bronchoscope and/or gastroscope are modified so that an ultrasound probe is built in at their distal tip. When combined with a procedure called fine-needle aspiration (FNA), EUS allows for a therapeutical approach that is an alternative to exploratory open surgery.

Also falling within the spectrum of flexible endoscopy is the application of NOTES (natural orifice transluminal endoscopic surgery), a technique whereby the abdominal cavity is entered through the gastrointestinal tract using a natural orifice (mouth, anus, bellybutton, etc.) as an inlet. In such cases the flexible endoscope – that is, an upper endoscope or a colonoscope – and its associated accessories have been modified to allow for their microsurgical use. Cholecystectomy (removal of the gall bladder), splenectomy (removal of the spleen), and other historically open or MIS laparoscopic procedures are now performed efficiently in this revolutionary approach. The potential of NOTES has gained widespread attention in the clinical community and further advances in this area continue taking place, enabling for example vaginal natural orifice transluminal endoscopic surgery (vNOTES).

Robotic-assisted surgery

Robotic technologies have grown substantially in the last few decades and have been adopted steadily in a variety of industries, enabling greater flexibility, increasing productivity, and improving safety. Healthcare has also embraced the opportunity to use robotic applications in order to enhance the patient experience: they assist in surgery and diagnosis, aid in training for medical professions, and serve for therapeutic use in applications such as rehabilitation. Besides patient care, robotics are also often an integral part of wider solutions, such as in the logistics of running large hospitals, for instance using automated guided vehicles (AGVs) to deliver medication, disinfect surfaces, and so on.

RAS is used to perform many types of complex procedures with more precision, flexibility, and control than is possible with conventional techniques and was mainly developed to overcome the limitations of MIS. The surgeon is still the one who performs the surgery but with the aid of a computerized robotic system that at minimum consists of a console and a patient cart; instead of directly moving the instruments in the operating field, the surgeon uses ad hoc controllers (i.e. joysticks, pedals, etc.) and software to manipulate the instruments, which are attached to stationary or mobile, single or multiple robotic arms (also known as articulated robots, which are meant to emulate the functions of a human arm).

The console is supplied with an HD, 3D view of the operating space. The computer translates the surgeon's movements for the robotic system to carry them out on the patient, thereby allowing enhanced dexterity, greater precision, a better view of the surgical site, and ergonomic comfort, improving overall performance. During the procedure, the surgeon may stand next to the patient and maintain a direct view of the surgical field, or stand away behind a console or even distantly, not physically in the OR but instead located in a remote area encompassing telesurgery (remote surgery using wireless networking) approach. Despite the numerous clinical benefits of RAS, progress is still to be made in reducing operative times and associated costs, as well as accelerating the learning curve of surgeons and other healthcare professionals involved in the execution of such a novel approach.

RAS is applied today in various surgical specialties, such as general surgery, urology, gynecology, orthopedics, and cardiac and thoracic surgery, and is already considered a "standard of care" clinical option for procedures on prostate glands and uteruses. The robotic prostatectomy is an excellent example of the benefits of RAS. It is essential to note that robotic technologies are also used with other specialties, such as in the field of spinal surgery and neurosurgery to aid in navigation and increase the accuracy of screw placement, as well as to mitigate much of the harmful radiation exposure to which the patient and the surgical team are subjected. In fact, the first records of RAS being performed date back to 1985, when an industrial robotic arm, the PUMA 200, was modified to perform a CT-guided brain biopsy in a neurosurgical procedure. Since then, enormous progress has been made and many innovative platforms have been introduced, including the multi-armed da Vinci surgical system by Intuitive Surgical, which is the predominant robotic system globally (Figure 4.62). The Versius robot from CMR Surgical comprises a set of independent small arms, each with its own base. The Hugo™ RAS system by Medtronic, a portable, modular system available as one-arm or three- and four-arm configurations, and many others are in development.

Examples of various robotic systems are shown in Figure 4.63. These robotic arms resemble the human arm but provide a wider range of maneuver. Versius, for example, has three joints, corresponding to the shoulder, the elbow, and the wrist, holding a 3D HD endoscope/camera and versatile instrumentation that can be interchanged while maintaining a sterile field. In general, traditional instruments such as forceps, staplers, graspers, needle drivers, clip appliers, energy tools, and others intended for use in MIS have been engineered to fit in these arms, although they end up with much more complex designs and mechanics. One big modification is around the tip of these instruments, which is articulated up to 360° so that they can be fully wristed. A typical robotic instrument comprises a part that attaches to the robotic arm, a long

(A)

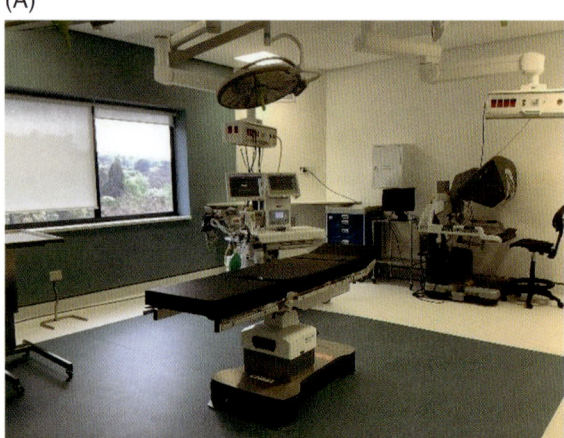

(B)

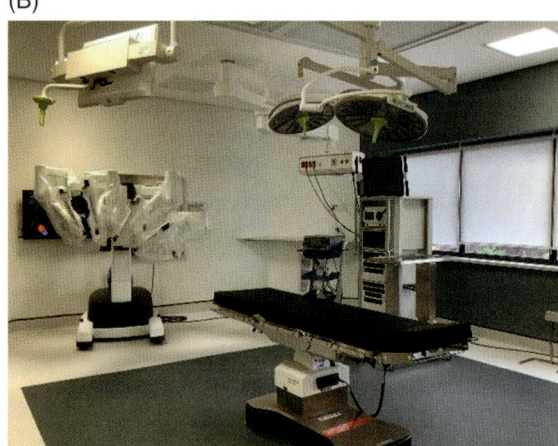

Figure 4.62 Da Vinci robotic system. (A) A surgical table with the surgeon da Vinci robotic console. (B) The da Vinci patient cart with three robot arms.

insulated shaft that contains cables and wires, a wrist that articulates based on the impetus of the surgeon's hand and finger movements, and an active tip that may be a cautery, jaws, scissors, and so on (Figure 4.63).

Due to the presence of multiple articulation points controlled by various wires and pulley systems, in addition to the use of newer types of substrates that may require specific treatment, robotic instruments pose a big challenge during the decontamination process. Following the manufacturer's IFU is critical and may require an involved process, including numerous manual steps during cleaning, use of specific-purpose accessories such as wash racks, or dedicated cleaning and sterilization cycles developed and validated only for this type of instrument. Another restrictive consideration is that some of the RAS system manufacturers design the associated

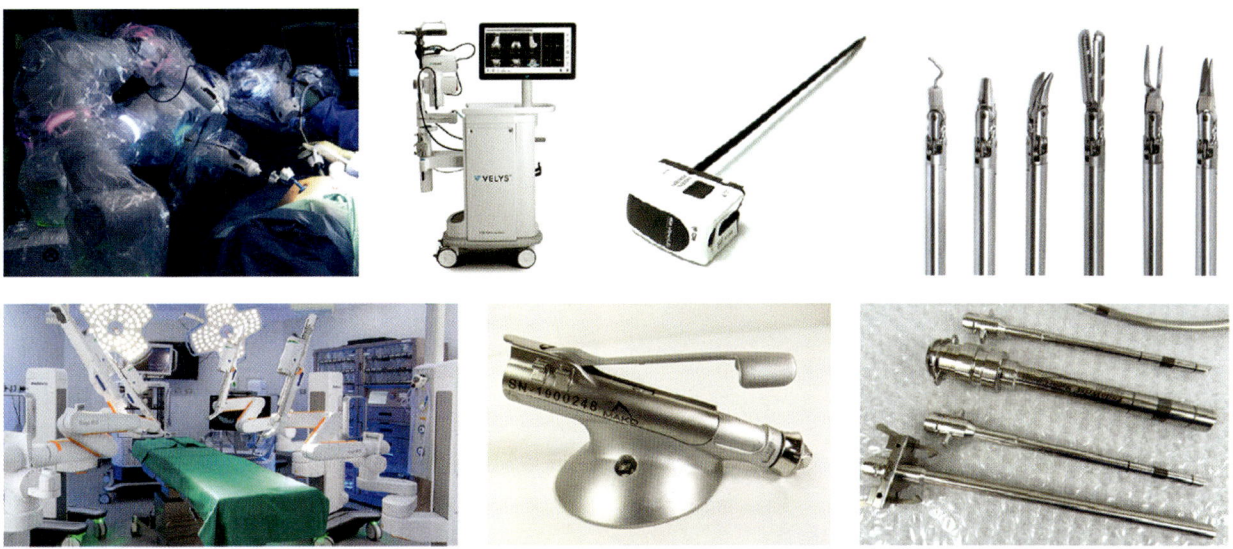

Figure 4.63 Examples of various types of robotic surgical devices and associated instruments.

instruments with usage and processing limits. Besides the increased costs for the facility required to purchase new devices regularly, there is a high risk of continued reuse beyond the prescribed limits, which may lead to instrument failure or even compromised patient cases, unless meticulous caution is taken to track uses.

As robotic technologies continue to evolve and AI is integrated, RAS will also expand and become more efficient, flexible, and autonomous, resulting in better patient outcomes.

Tattooing

Medical tattooing exists to reconstruct perceived deformities and conceal a condition or the effects of a treatment. Although tattooing is conducted in a wide variety of non-clinical settings, many of the devices or instruments that are used for these procedures are considered critical as they may penetrate the skin and may come into contact with the blood. A typical example is a reusable tattoo gun, with an example given in Figure 4.64. The gun handle and other associated parts of the device may be disposable or reusable.

Miscellaneous devices used medically

There are various types of generally, non-critical medical devices that are used for basic patient monitoring and/or diagnosis (with examples shown in Figure 4.65). A number of common examples are discussed in this section.

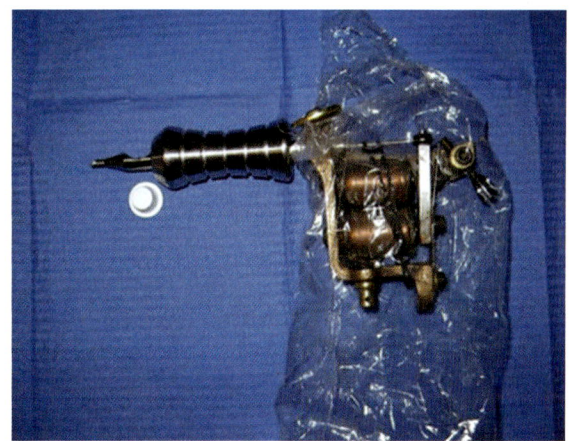

Figure 4.64 A tattooing gun and handle.

Blood pressure monitors

A blood pressure monitor is a non-invasive blood pressure–measuring device. There are various types of blood pressure apparatus, including the older mercury gravity manometer and more modern gauge or electronic monitors. The most widely used devices (Figure 4.65) consist of an arm cuff connected to a source of pressure (manual or automated) and a pressure gauge (manual or digital).

Reflex hammer

A reflex hammer is a medical instrument to test deep muscle-tendon reflexes. There are several types of hammers, usually constructed to resemble a metal disk that have a rubber

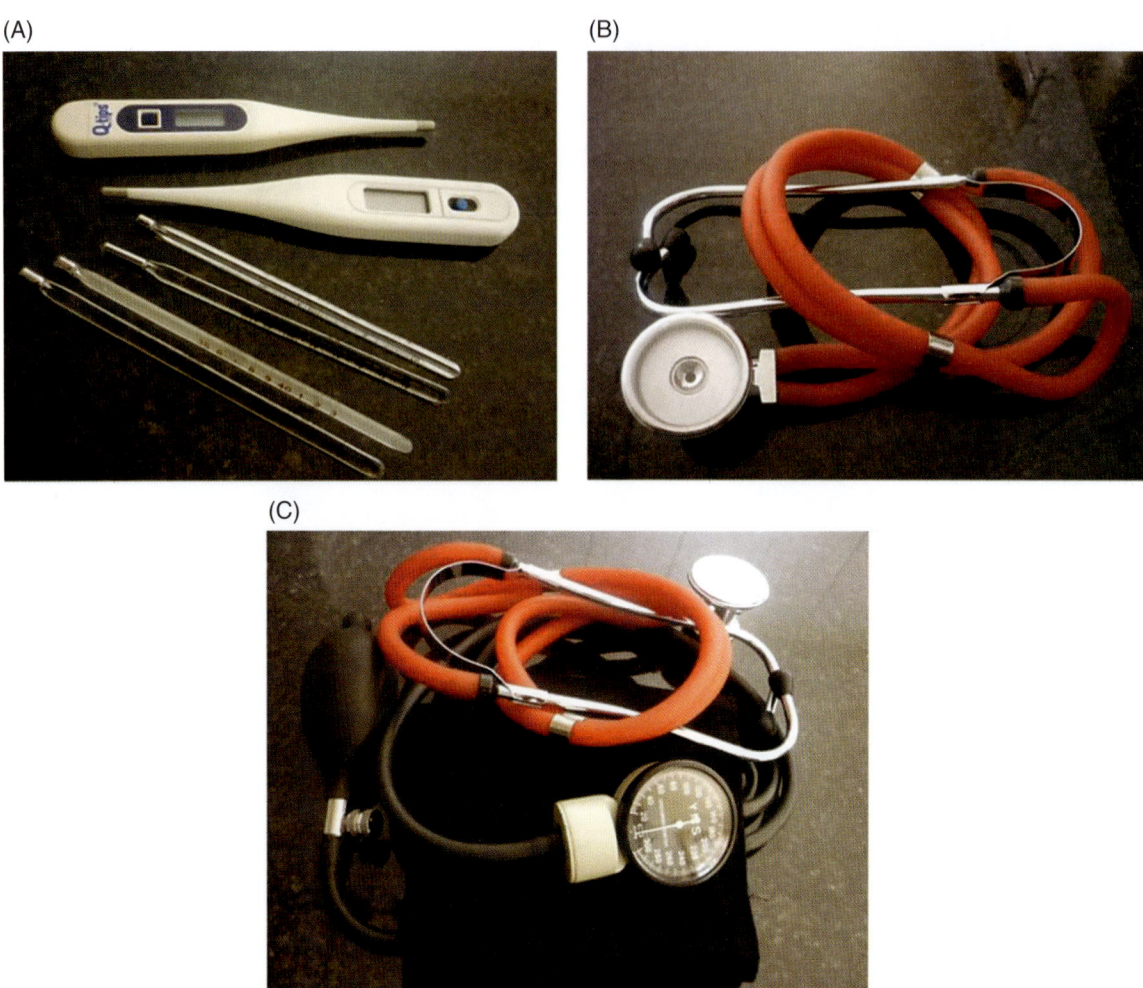

Figure 4.65 Examples of commonly used devices for routine medical use. (A) Thermometers;, (B) stethoscope; (C) manual blood pressure monitor.

bumper attached to them, itself attached to a stem with a tapered edge that may be used to test reflexes, for example by scratching the underside of the foot.

Medical thermometers

Medical thermometers are used to measure body temperature. There are several, external places on the body where temperatures can be measured and many different types of thermometers (Figure 4.65). An oral thermometer is used in the mouth and under the tongue, or in the crease of the armpit. A rectal thermometer is similar to an oral thermometer, but differs in that the metal bulb on the end is wider. An ear thermometer is a digital device designed to fit into the ear canal. The most commonly used thermometer is made of glass, with a narrow metal bulb at the end with a small ball of mercury or colored (red) alcohol inside it. There is a temperature range on the side where the temperature is registered. The mercury/alcohol rises as the temperature rises. Most thermometers come in both Fahrenheit and Celsius scales. Digital varieties of both oral and rectal thermometers are also available. Thermometers are generally provided with a disposable plastic sheath that covers the end to take a temperature.

Stethoscopes

A stethoscope is used to listen to sounds produced inside the body. It is used primarily to listen to the lungs, heart, and intestinal tract. It is also used to listen to blood flow in certain areas and heart sounds of developing fetuses in pregnant women. Stethoscopes vary in their design and material. Most are made of Y-shaped rubber tubing comprising two flexible rubber tubes running from a valve to the earpieces (Figure 4.65). The valve also connects the tubes to a "chestpiece," allowing sound to enter the device at one end, which can be either bell-shaped or a flat disk for higher frequencies, and then travel up the tubes and through to the earpieces. Most modern stethoscopes are designed for use with both ears. Single stethoscopes are designed for use with one ear and differential stethoscopes allow comparison of sounds at two different body sites. Electronic stethoscopes, which electronically amplify tones, are also available.

5 Microbiology and infection prevention/control

Microbiology is the study of microscopic organisms ("microorganisms"). *Mikros* is the Greek word for small and therefore microbiology is the study of small, living forms. It is an interesting science, including the study of many types of organisms that can be beneficial as well as detrimental to our lives and health. In this chapter we are particularly concerned with those microorganisms that can do us harm and cause ill-health or disease. A "disease" is a disorder of the structure or function of the body and is usually associated with specific signs and symptoms. An "infection" is a type of disease caused by microorganisms, which are collectively referred to as "pathogens" or disease-causing microorganisms. Examples of some of the prominent pathogens (or pathogenic microorganisms) are given in Table 5.1. An infection occurs when a pathogen is allowed to grow on or within a host (e.g. the human body), possibly leading to detrimental effects (or disease). It is important to note that many microorganisms can live on and in the body with no ill effects and in some cases are important to its normal functioning. The natural and healthy interrelationships between microorganisms and our bodies are an area of active research, on which we continue to evolve our understanding.

Infection prevention and control (IPC) is the science, discipline, and practices that reduce or prevent the transmission of infectious agents and control their further spread, such as in the case of an outbreak. An outbreak is a sudden increase in the numbers of cases of an infection or disease over what is expected in a defined setting or group in a specified time that may put others at risk. IPC aims to minimize the risk of healthcare-acquired infections (HAIs) among patients, visitors, and healthcare workers wherever healthcare is provided. HAIs pose significant challenges to patient safety, contributing to increased rates of morbidity (being unhealthy for a particular disease or situation) and mortality (the number of deaths that occur in a population) and imposing substantial financial burdens on healthcare systems. It is essential to ensure that healthcare facilities are maintaining high standards of IPC to safeguard the well-being of patients and staff. Proper cleaning, disinfection, and sterilization of reusable medical devices are essential for effective IPC in healthcare settings.

Microorganism types

The microbial world: an introduction

The microbial world is very diverse and is only briefly described in this section. In the introduction to Chapter 2 the different types of cells and their components that make up the human body were discussed. In general, many similar structures make up the microbial world, but they are not directly visible to us and require a powerful microscope (a magnification instrument) to observe them. For example, if you measure across the head of a typical sewing pin it is about 1 mm in diameter and the end of a human hair about 10 times less (0.1 mm); you can just about see these with the human eye. Then you can estimate that the average number of cells or microorganisms across the head of a pin could be:

- 100 human cells (~0.01 mm per cell).
- 100 yeast cells (~0.01 mm per cell).
- 1000 bacteria (~0.001 mm per cell).
- 100,000 small viruses (~0.00001 mm per virus).

These organisms vary in size and structure. Some are multicellular, similar to humans, where different cell types join together to make up the various parts (organs) of the organism. These include the helminths and are commonly known as microscopic "worms." Others are unicellular (single, individual cells), but of the same essential structure as a human cell (known as "eukaryotes", including fungi and protozoa) or a different and smaller type of cell structure (known as "prokaryotes" such as bacteria). It was thought for many years that cell structures, although varied, were the basis of life. But microbiology also includes viable but non-cellular forms such as viruses and prions that can be more simply composed of molecules such as nucleic acids and proteins. In the following sections, each of these classes of microorganisms is considered

---

Decontamination and Device Processing in Healthcare, Second Edition. Gerald McDonnell and Georgia Alevizopoulou.
© 2025 John Wiley & Sons Ltd. Published 2025 by John Wiley & Sons Ltd.

Table 5.1 Examples of microbial pathogens and their associated diseases.

Microorganism type	Microorganism	Associated disease(s)[1]
Prion[2]	PrP^{res}	Creutzfeldt-Jakob disease (CJD) and variant CJD (vCJD), diseases particularly associated with the nervous system and loss of brain functions
Viruses	Hepatitis B	Hepatitis, an inflammation leading to liver damage and possibly liver cancer
	Human immunodeficiency virus (HIV)	Primary cause of acquired immune deficiency syndrome (AIDS), a disease affecting the immune system, with increased vulnerability to other infections
	Norovirus (previously called the "Norwalk agent")	Acute infection (also known as gastric flu, tummy bug, and stomach flu) of the gut leading to diarrhea and vomiting
	Coronaviruses (such as the SARS-CoV-2 virus)	Coronavirus disease (COVID-19), typically a respiratory illness but often associated with multiple health effects
Bacteria[3]	*Staphylococcus aureus*	Causes skin (and wound), gastrointestinal, and respiratory tract infections MRSA (for methicillin-resistant *S. aureus*) is a type of *S. aureus* that has developed resistance to certain types of antibiotics
	Escherichia coli	While it is a normal inhabitant of the gut, certain strains can cause severe infections of the intestinal and urinary tracts
	Mycobacterium tuberculosis	Tuberculosis, mainly a disease of the respiratory tract, but can also infect other parts of the body
Fungi	*Aspergillus niger* or *braziliensis*	Causes mainly respiratory tract infections ("aspergillosis")
	Candida albicans	Candidiasis, infections of the skin, mucous membranes, and blood
	Candida auris	Candidiasis, often hospital acquired by patients with weakened immune systems Can demonstrate multiple drug resistance
Protozoa	*Cryptosporidium parvum*	Cryptosporidiosis, a form of acute diarrhea
	Acanthamoeba castellanii	Infections of the skin and eyes (keratitis)
	Plasmodium falciparum	Malaria, a disease of red blood cells and the liver
Helminths ("parasitic worms")	*Wuchereria bancrofti*	Elephantiasis, where worms get lodged in the blood or lymphatic system
	Ascaris lumbricoides	Ascariasis, infection of the lung and intestine (often associated with poor hygiene)

[1] For information on the structure and functions of the various systems of the human body, refer to Chapter 2.
[2] Prions are not strictly considered as "living," but are often considered under microbiology as they are transmissible and infectious like other microorganisms.
[3] The scientific names of all organisms including microorganisms are written either in italics or underlined, such as Staphylococcus aureus or *Staphylococcus aureus*. Viruses are an exception to this rule.

in further detail. It should be noted that microbiology is a progressive science, with new types of microorganisms being discovered continually. Their description, classification, and our knowledge of the types of diseases they may cause or be associated with form an area of ongoing research.

Prions and other infectious proteins

Prions are widely accepted to be infectious proteins. Proteins are one of the major biochemical molecules that make up life (see Chapter 2); they play an important role in the structure and function of cellular and non-cellular life. In cells, they are constantly being made, used for specific functions, and then broken down. In certain types of diseases, some protein types appear not to be degraded by normal cellular processes, accumulate, and therefore precipitate in various organs of the body. In prion-associated diseases such a protein is known as PrP^C, which is normally found in human and animal cells. The protein appears to play a role in the normal functions of neurons (as part of the nervous system), but the extent of its activity continues to be a subject of research. Like other proteins, it is made and broken down over time by the cell, but in rare cases it changes its shape into a different form (known as PrP^{res} or similarly as PrP^{Sc} or PrP^{TSE}), which is not degraded by the cell (Figure 5.1). In such cases, PrP^{res} can induce normal PrP^C to also change shape and then further accumulate in the cells, leading to cell damage/death and the appearance of the disease over time. These effects are seen particularly in the nervous

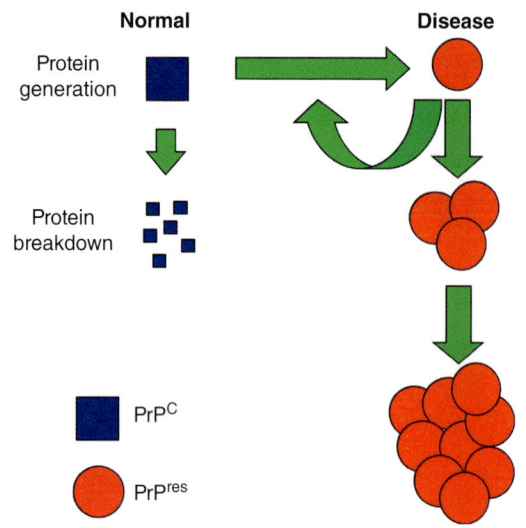

Figure 5.1 The prion theory. The accumulation and precipitation of protein lead to the development of disease.

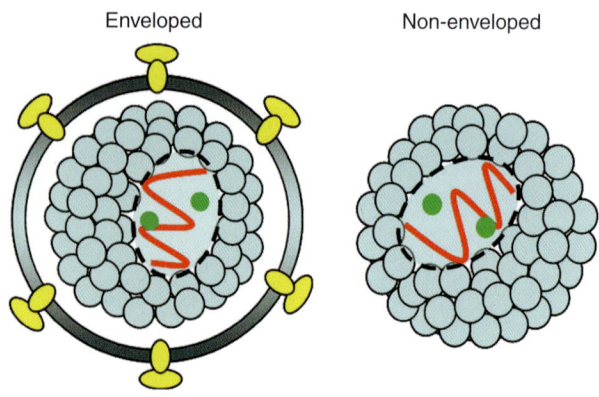

Figure 5.2 The basic structure of viruses. Viruses display a wide range of structures but can be classified into two main types: enveloped and non-enveloped. In non-enveloped viruses the central nucleic acid (often associated with proteins) is surrounded by a capsid (protein) structure that is unique to the specific virus type/strain. This basic structure is the same for enveloped viruses but is surrounded by an external, lipid-based envelope.

system (see Chapter 2), where the dead nerve cells are not replaced, unlike other types of essential cells in the body. Over time, the cumulative damage to the nervous system causes gradual and irreversible loss of body functions and eventually death. The exact reasons for the changes in protein shape are not known, but in about 10% of cases there is a genetic cause and certain prion-based diseases can therefore be inherited. The remaining 90% of cases appear sporadically and randomly with no known cause.

Prions are unusual infectious agents as they appear to be composed of protein alone without any detectable DNA or RNA, unlike other types of life forms. They were previously called "slow viruses," but are now known to be quite distinct from viruses in composition and structure. For these reasons they are not strictly considered as "living," but are self-promoting and infectious. Research is continuing to further define the nature of these agents, as it appears that other factors that are yet to be defined are involved in the initiation and progression of protein precipitation/deposition and therefore disease.

Prions are implicated in a group of rare diseases known as transmissible spongiform encephalopathies (TSEs). These include the animal diseases scrapie (in sheep) and bovine spongiform encephalopathy (BSE) (in cattle), human diseases such as Creutzfeldt-Jakob disease (CJD) and a similar disease known as variant CJD (vCJD). Variant CJD in humans has been known to be due to the same agent as BSE in cattle. These diseases, once diagnosed, are always progressive, invariably fatal, and with no known treatments. Prion diseases are transmissible via injection, ingestion, and transplantation of contaminated nervous tissues (such as the brain) and through improperly decontaminated reusable devices such as those in brain surgery. Prions are generally highly resistant to common chemical and physical methods of disinfection and sterilization. There is continuing research into the potential of other prion-like misfolded and precipitated proteins being the cause of (or at least implicated in) other diseases such as Alzheimer's disease.

Viruses

Viruses are sub-microscopic and relatively simple forms of life that are obligate parasites. While they do not resemble any typical prokaryotic or eukaryotic cell, they possess typical structural features of their own and vary in size and shape. A typical viral particle (virion) consists of an internal DNA or RNA genome surrounded by a protective protein shell or "capsid." Certain types of viruses contain a second lipid-containing coat or "envelope." Viruses with only the capsid are termed "naked," non-enveloped, or "hydrophilic." The other category is termed enveloped or "hydrophobic" (Figure 5.2). In general, enveloped viruses are less stable to environmental conditions and more susceptible to chemical and physical agents when compared to the non-enveloped ones.

This classification is generally used to differentiate between virus types and as a guide to their resistance to various chemical and physical disinfection/sterilization methods. Non-enveloped viruses consist of an inner compartment that holds the DNA or RNA (the nucleic acid specific for that virus type), but can also include various types of structural or other associated proteins. This is surrounded by a protein coat (the capsid), also unique to the virus type, which can protect the virus from damage. Although these structures may sound relatively fragile, they are the opposite and the most difficult viruses to inactivate. They tend to have tight structures that render them often resilient to inactivation. Examples include the poxviruses, parvoviruses, rotaviruses, hepatitis A virus, and coxsackieviruses.

Enveloped viruses have the same essential structure as that described for the non-enveloped types but also have at least an additional, external envelope that is lipid based and can contain various types of proteins. For some enveloped viruses, these envelope-based proteins can play important roles in how the viruses attack and take over host cells. A common example is influenza virus, a member of the orthomyxovirus family. Influenza virus causes a respiratory disease known as flu, with typical symptoms including fatigue (feeling tired), headache, fever (increased temperature), and cough. These viruses have been associated with various pandemics (avian flu, Spanish flu, and swine flu). A pandemic is an infectious disease that spreads worldwide and affects many people over a wide geographic region, as opposed to an epidemic that would occur in a smaller region/area. These viruses are classified based on two types of surface proteins that are involved in infecting human cells: H for hemagglutinin and N for neuraminidase, therefore classified for instance as influenza H1N1 or H5N1. Other examples of enveloped viruses include human immunodeficiency virus (HIV, a type of "retrovirus" that causes acquired immune deficiency syndrome, AIDS), severe acute respiratory syndrome (SARS) viruses (e.g. SARS-CoV-2, the cause of the recent COVID-19 pandemic), hepatitis B virus, Ebola virus, herpesviruses, and measles virus. Because the external envelope structure plays an important role in the ability of such viruses to infect cells, damage to these structures can prevent the virus from causing disease and for that reason they are found to be much more sensitive to inactivation. This can often cause confusion, as viruses such as HIV are widely known to be particularly difficult to treat in infected patients but are actually relatively easy to inactivate on exposed surfaces (even by drying alone under some conditions). At the same time, these viruses are most often associated with various types of human fluids such as mucus and blood, which can prevent them from contacting a disinfection or sterilization method; this is an important perspective for safe decontamination of not only these viruses but all other microorganisms and is an important concept in decontamination practices.

In some classification systems a third group of viruses can also be differentiated, based on their having moderate resistance to disinfection/sterilization, essentially being non-enveloped although with features like enveloped viruses and presenting greater resistance to enveloped viruses, but less than other non-enveloped viruses. Important examples are the adenoviruses, which can cause a variety of conditions such as respiratory, eye, and intestinal (diarrheal) diseases.

Examples of the various structures of viruses are shown in Figure 5.3. They can range in diameter from ~20 nm (e.g. parvoviruses and polio virus) to ~400 nm (typical of the poxviruses such as vaccinia). Different types of viruses can infect (and therefore can cause disease in) a wide variety of cell types, including human, animal, and plant cells as well as bacteria. For example, viruses that live in bacteria are known as bacteriophages; these are used for various laboratory investigations (e.g. to test disinfectants as they are considered difficult to inactivate) and have even been used as alternatives to antibiotics to treat bacterial infections. Some of the most widely known human diseases caused by viruses are summarized in Table 5.2. It is interesting to note that in addition to diseases typically associated with virus infections, such as inflammation, tissue damage, and so on, some viruses have also been associated with cancer; examples include specific types of human papillomaviruses (HPVs) that are the most common cause of cervical cancer in women (and can be routinely monitored during a procedure known as a Pap smear).

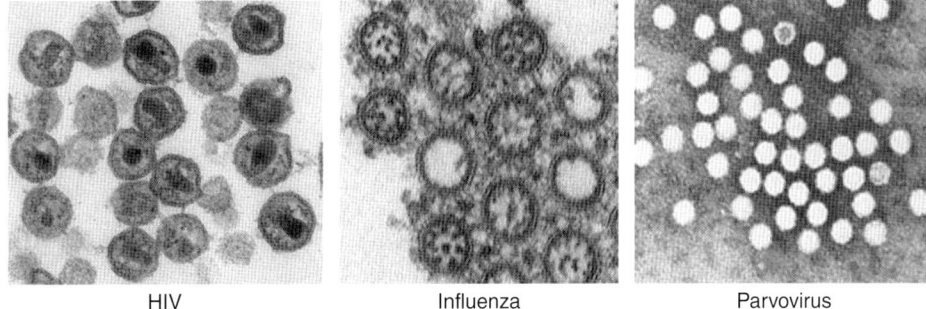

Figure 5.3 Examples of the variety of viral structures. These examples are not shown to scale and special (electron) microscopes are used in order to directly observe them, due to the small size of the viruses.

Table 5.2 Examples of human diseases caused by viruses.

Virus name	Family	Type	Associated diseases
Human immunodeficiency virus (HIV)	Retroviridae	Enveloped	AIDS (acquired immune deficiency disease)
Influenza virus	Orthomyxoviridae	Enveloped	Influenza ("flu")
SARS-CoV-2 virus		Enveloped	Respiratory disease, including the COVID-19 pandemic
Varicella zoster virus	Herpesviridae	Enveloped	Chicken pox, shingles
Hepatitis B virus	Hepadnaviridae	Enveloped	Hepatitis
Measles virus	Paramyxoviridae	Enveloped	Measles
Orthopoxvirus monkeypox	Poxviridae	Enveloped	Mpox ("monkeypox")
Adenovirus	Adenoviridae	Non-enveloped	Pharyngitis, conjunctivitis
Papillomavirus	Papillomaviridae	Non-enveloped	Warts, cervical cancer
Parvovirus	Parvoviridae	Non-enveloped	Fifth disease
Poliovirus	Picornaviridae	Non-enveloped	Poliomyelitis

In addition to being enveloped or non-enveloped, viruses are often classified and named based on other criteria such as the type of nucleic acid (DNA or RNA), the shape of the virus, and type of disease they cause. An example is a series of viruses that are the most common cause of liver inflammation (the reaction of the liver to infection or damage), known as the hepatitis viruses. These are recognized by their alphabetic names such as hepatitis A, B, C, D, and E. Although all these viruses have similar names, they do vary in their effects during an infection and are also structurally distinct. For example, hepatitis A is a non-enveloped virus (therefore considered to have higher resistant to disinfection), while hepatitis B and C are both enveloped (and therefore more sensitive to disinfection).

Further consideration of hepatitis B virus and HIV should be given here as they are both known to be transmitted through blood and other bodily tissues; for this reason, they are often referred to as blood-borne pathogens and are an important consideration for anyone working with patient-contaminated materials such as reusable devices. Other examples of viruses that are often highlighted as being blood transmitted include hepatitis C virus and hemorrhagic fever viruses (e.g. Ebola virus), as well as other types of microorganisms (bacteria, protozoa, and fungi). These diseases are transmissible and healthcare workers have a significant risk of being infected when not taking the correct precautions. Therefore, an important principle in IPC and in decontamination practices is to regard all blood (or indeed any bodily fluid/tissue) as potentially infectious. Standard precautions are required in these cases to minimize disease transmission; in device decontamination these include the use of personal protective equipment (PPE) and vaccination (immunization). PPE consists of clothing and/or equipment worn to protect a worker from spillages, splashing, and so on. Typical examples include the use of gloves, eye protection, and face masks.

Vaccination (or immunization) refers to taking a vaccine to reduce the risk of developing a serious disease. One of the most important historical findings in microbiology was that previous exposure to a given type of pathogen could render a person "immune" from infection and disease via any subsequent exposure to the same or closely related pathogens. A simple solution was to prepare samples of the pathogen (or parts thereof) that were damaged, modified, or even dead; these are referred to as vaccines, and when introduced into us allow our bodies to generate a reaction and resistance to those agents as part of the response of our immune system (Chapter 2). Vaccines are now available for a wide range of diseases, including viral ones. This includes the MMR vaccine for measles, mumps, and rubella, and the series of COVID vaccinations, including COVID booster shots. They are unique to specific microorganisms and in some cases are specific to certain strains of virus types (as in the case of seasonal flu vaccines). Healthcare workers are also recommended to take a hepatitis B vaccine (usually given over a course of three injections) that is widely available. This is considered a very effective and safe vaccine, but it can only protect against the virus causing hepatitis B and not against other viruses such as HIV. It is important to note that these practices do not completely prevent transmission or progression, but when used correctly they can reduce this risk to a greater safety level. Further consideration of IPC measures and standard precautions is provided later in the chapter.

Viral diseases can often be difficult to treat, as they generally require specific identification to recommend applicable drugs for the type of virus implicated. Examples of antiviral drugs include oseltamivir (commonly known as Tamiflu®), specifically against influenza viruses, and ribavirin, more generally used to treat a wide range of RNA-containing viruses such as measles, mumps, and hepatitis C viruses. Viruses can develop resistance to such drugs over time, rendering the drug often ineffective against the new form of the virus; this is a common concept in the treatment of all microbial diseases and is considered in more detail in the following section.

Bacteria

Bacteria (or bacterium in the singular form) are a class of microorganisms that have a prokaryotic, unicellular (one-celled) structure. They are probably the most studied types in microbiology. They are classified in many ways, such as by their appearance when examined under a microscope (e.g. shapes, staining characteristics), how they grow (e.g. biochemical reactions, ability to use oxygen (or not) to grow), or various structural characteristics (lipids and more recently by their genetic nature). Their basic structure is shown in Figure 5.4, but like viruses they present with a wide range of structures, shapes, and sizes, which can even change over time.

Bacteria are often classified as being "Gram positive" or "Gram negative." This is based on a very simple staining

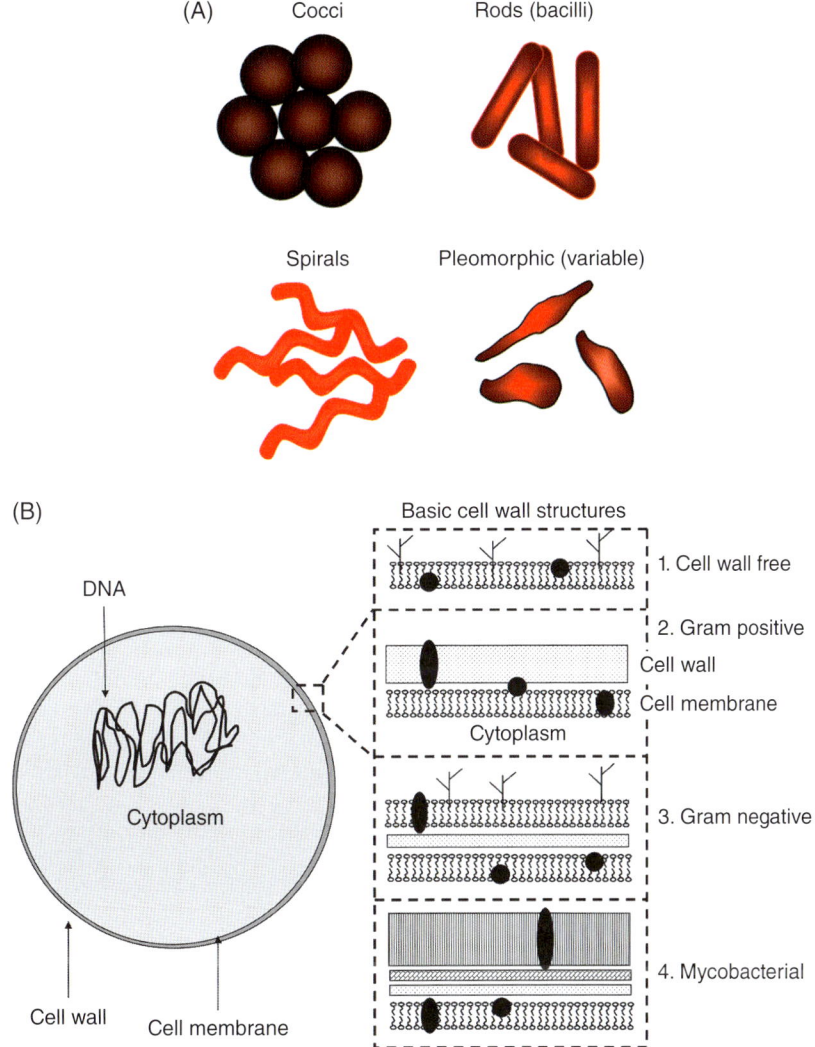

Figure 5.4 The basic structure of bacteria. (A) Examples of bacterial shapes. (B) A representation of a typical bacterial cell is shown on the left, consisting of the interior cytoplasm (the genetic material DNA is shown), surrounded by a cell membrane and an outermost cell wall. A cross-section of various types of cell wall structures is shown on the right, highlighting the cell membrane and cell wall in the Gram-positive example. In this case the majority of the cell wall is made up of peptidoglycan (a peptide-polysaccharide); it also exists as a smaller section in Gram-negative and mycobacterial cell walls but not in cell wall free bacteria.

method; stains are essentially dyes or pigments that are used to visualize bacteria (and other types of microorganisms) under the microscope. The Gram staining method was described by Hans Christian Gram, a Danish scientist, in 1884. The method can differentiate between two types of bacteria, based on the outer, cell wall structure (Figure 5.4). In Gram-positive bacteria, the cell wall is composed mostly (up to 90% in some cases) of a net-like structure known as peptidoglycan (a polysaccharide-peptide structure). In Gram-negative bacteria this is quite different, consisting of a small layer of peptidoglycan (~10%), an area known as the periplasmic space, and an outer lipid membrane structure. In the staining method, two dyes are used first (crystal violet followed by iodine to give a purple color) that stain the peptidoglycan layer, followed by a quick alcohol wash that can remove the dyes; Gram-positive bacteria will retain most of the dyes but Gram-negative bacteria will lose them quickly (are "destained"). The final step is to restain the bacteria with another dye (safranin or fuchsin) that will color them pink or light red. Overall, when examined under a microscope, Gram-positive bacteria will appear purple and Gram-negative pink/red. It is at this stage that bacteria can also be examined for their shapes: cocci (circular), rods (bacilli), or spirals are the main examples (Figure 5.4). In this way bacteria are often referred to as "Gram-positive rods," "Gram-negative cocci," and so on. This is, however, an oversimplification as the staining method can vary depending on the person performing the procedure, the exact method used, how the bacteria are examined under the microscope, and even the bacteria themselves (e.g. if they are freshly grown, as microbiologists would say "cultured," or an older culture). Some bacteria are known to be particularly Gram variable, meaning that some individual cells will stain purple while others in the same group look pink. Similarly, many types of bacteria will show a variety of shapes when stained (known as pleomorphic, meaning of different shapes/sizes).

Bacteria also vary in their requirements for growth and multiplication. An example is their ability to grow only in the presence of air ("aerobic"), in the absence of air ("anaerobic") and under both conditions ("facultative"). Some bacteria can grow under what we would refer to as extreme conditions (e.g. less than 4°C, higher than 50°C, or in the presence of high concentrations of salts), under conditions with few nutrients (e.g. types of bacteria from the genus *Pseudomonas* or other "pseudomonads" can grow in high-purity water systems with minimal available nutrients), and, similar to viruses, some only multiply in other cells (e.g. of the genus *Rickettsia* and *Chlamydia* that grow in human cells, and *Bdellovibrio* in bacterial cells).

When bacteria find themselves in the right environment, including the right nutrients, temperatures, and so on, they can begin to grow, divide, and multiply. They do this by a process known as binary fission, where one cell divides to give two identical "daughter" cells. Under optimum conditions for that bacteria type, this process can happen very quickly (e.g. for *Escherichia coli* this can be ~20–30 minutes) or very slowly (*Mycobacterium tuberculosis* can take up to 15–24 hours). In the case of *Escherichia coli*, one bacterium alone can rapidly multiply to give thousands in only a few hours under the right conditions. They will continue to multiply until these optimal conditions are no longer available. At this stage bacteria can demonstrate a wide range of reactions that help them survive. These include slowing down their multiplication rate and metabolism to conserve energy, production of various types of enzymes and chemicals to protect them from damage and scavenge resources, the production of surface structures that make them mobile, and the production of external protective mechanisms. As an example of a protective structure, many bacteria produce what is referred to as a capsule, which is a protein or carbohydrate-based (polysaccharide) structure that is formed over the bacteria to protect it and therefore help it to survive. Capsules can prevent drying (which can kill a lot of bacteria), prevent the interaction of chemicals (such as drugs and disinfectants), and protect bacteria from the human body's defense mechanisms (the immune system, as described in Chapter 2). Bacterial communities can also protect themselves in a similar way by producing what is known as a biofilm or simply a community of cells (discussed in more detail later in this section).

Probably the most extreme change that has been described in bacteria in relation to adverse environmental conditions is a process known as sporulation. This is a remarkable process, where an actively growing cell decides to fundamentally change its structure to produce a dormant form of itself. These dormant forms are known as "spores" (or more correctly in bacteria as "endospores" due to the method by which they are produced, from within the original cell; endo- for internal). They are not only dormant (non-metabolizing or non-active) forms of bacteria but have been radically changed in structure to make them highly resistant to various types of chemical and physical inactivation methods. It is for this reason that they are considered one of the hardest types of microorganism structures to kill and are used to test sterilization methods. Only certain types of bacteria have been described that produce spores, with typical examples being bacteria belonging to the groups known as *Geobacillus*, *Bacillus*, and *Clostridium*. Not all spores are the same in structure or in resistance to inactivation. For example, spores of the bacteria *Geobacillus stearothermophilus* are very heat resistant, requiring temperatures in excess of 115°C for inactivation; they are also highly resistant to most types of but not all chemicals. Notable exceptions are the spores of *Bacillus atrophaeus* that are less resistant to wet heat, but more resistant to ethylene oxide (a gas used for sterilization) and dry heat. Spores of *Clostridium* are

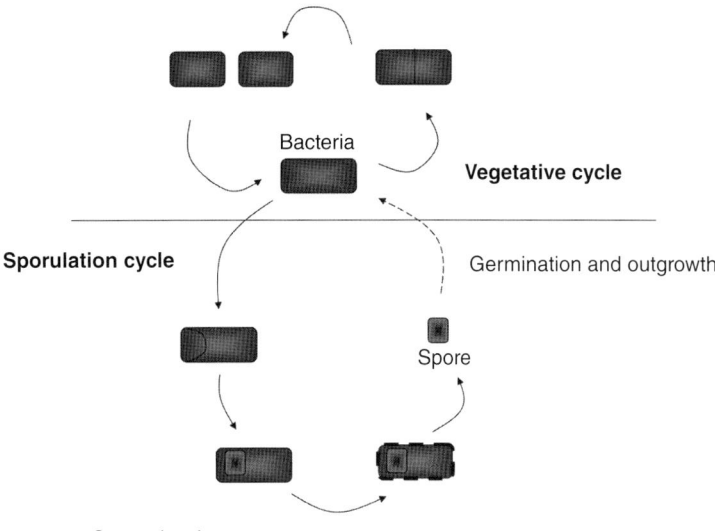

Figure 5.5 An overview of the sporulation process in bacteria.

generally much more sensitive to heat and chemicals than those of *Bacillus* or *Geobacillus*. Due to their high resistance to disinfection and sterilization, the spores (endospores) formed from these types of bacteria are used to develop and routinely test sterilization methods. Examples include the use of *Geobacillus stearothermophilus* spores for steam and hydrogen peroxide gas sterilization processes and *Bacillus atrophaeus* spores in ethylene oxide sterilizers. These are further discussed in Chapters 11 and 14.

It is worthwhile considering the sporulation process in bacteria in further detail, as a remarkable example of what some bacteria are capable of (Figure 5.5). During vegetative growth, the bacterial cell is continually sensing its environment and will adapt its growth rate and metabolism. When these conditions become limited, the bacteria can decide to sporulate (produce a spore). During the process the cell commits itself totally to this process, producing only one spore for each bacterium cell. During development, part of the cell is separated with a complete copy of the DNA molecule and various layers are built around the spore to protect it. The internal compartment of the spore is further dried out and different types of chemicals and proteins are deposited. Their function is to protect the DNA from damage, but also to provide nutrients later when the spore decides to grow again. Sporulation is considered complete when the final spore is released from the cell and the cell dies. Bacterial spores can survive for years, if not decades in some cases, in dormant form. This can include extremes of temperature, dryness, and the presence of chemicals at concentrations that would normally kill vegetative cells. They are in a dormant stage but monitor their environment for any changes that will allow them to regrow. When these conditions are favorable, including temperature, presence of nutri-

ents, and so on, the spore reactivates. Reactivation is in two phases, known as germination and outgrowth, to eventually provide a vegetative cell identical to the original cell that made the spore, which can then proceed to multiply as before in the vegetative cycle (Figure 5.5).

Although bacteria are unicellular, they commonly live together as groups of their own type (as they have multiplied together) and/or with other microorganisms. The way they grow and multiply alone often ensures that they are connected if not in very close proximity to each other. There are various terms used to describe these populations of bacteria, such as biofilms and microbiomes. A microbiome is a relatively more recent term in microbiology that describes a population or community of microorganisms in a given environment. Examples of microbiomes include within the oral cavity (mouth), the lower intestine, and the skin, all populated by various types of bacteria and other microorganisms that co-exist. Today it is known that these communities of microorganisms are often beneficial to us, for example by preventing other bacteria from attacking us to cause infection, and their importance or impact in human health is an area of active research.

A biofilm is defined as a community of microorganisms (either single or multiple types). They have been particularly described as developing on or with various types of surfaces/interfaces, especially in the presence of water or liquid-contacting surfaces (such as water pipes and indwelling catheters that are often used in hospitalized patients). Despite their traditional and well-known association with wet surfaces, "dry" biofilms on environmental surfaces have also been described in more recent years and are sometimes considered controversial. Bacterial biofilms have been well studied, with notable examples including *Pseudomonas aeruginosa*, *Staphylococcus aureus*, *Staphylococcus epidermidis*, *Mycobacterium* species (e.g. *M. fortuitum*), and *Legionella pneumophila*. Biofilms are also developed by fungi, with an important example being *Candida albicans* (fungi are discussed later in this chapter). In addition to the individual bacteria or fungi that develop into biofilms, many other types of microorganisms can live within biofilms.

Biofilms can have many negative impacts, such as causing pipework damage ("biocorrosion"), blockages, and, more importantly for our discussion, bacterial infections. Biofilms are a common source of bacterial contamination and infections from indwelling medical devices, incorrectly processed devices (e.g. flexible endoscopes), devices that remain within us for extended periods of time such as contact lenses, catheters in the blood system and urinary tract, and implants or prostheses (an artificial replacement for a body part such as a hip or joint). Other sources include water, water-handling systems, or medical devices that use water, which when not maintained correctly can quickly become overgrown by biofilms. Such biofilms are a concern as they are hard to remove from surfaces and difficult to disinfect/sterilize. They form at or on surfaces by a series of steps (Figure 5.6). First, the bacteria will attach or be associated with the surface and begin to multiply; as they multiply and develop, the bacteria begin to produce a matrix not dissimilar to the capsule material described earlier, which is polysaccharide in nature. This is often referred to as "slime" as it typically has a slimy appearance. A good example of this is along the surface of teeth, where the slime material is actually a biofilm based on bacteria such as *Streptococcus mutans*. It is this structure that is difficult to remove from surfaces and protects the bacteria in the biofilm from attack by drugs, detergents, and disinfectants. It is also in this form that bacteria can produce a variety of chemicals and enzymes that can damage surfaces. As the biofilm further matures, other bacteria, viruses, and protozoa can become associated with the biofilm, growing/dividing within the matrix, surviving within it, or even living off it (as a food source). This relationship between bacteria of various kinds and other microorganisms is an area of active research, such as understanding communication, hierarchical structures, and disruption mechanisms. Further, parts of the biofilm can become loose and dissociate from the original biofilm to develop elsewhere. Overall, biofilm can be a source of contamination and therefore infection in medical institutions, especially when related to water, fluids, and other liquids. It is particularly resistant to chemical disinfection but also physical removal during cleaning, which can make decontamination inefficient.

Examples of various types of disease-forming bacteria are given in Table 5.3. Bacteria are named based on various groups that are similar in structure and genetic type; the group (or what is specifically called the "genus") name is given first and the specific branch of the group (known as a species) is given next. The names of bacteria should always be italicized or underlined, as is the case for *Mycobacterium tuberculosis* or <u>Staphylococcus aureus</u>. They can also be referred to as particular varieties (known as sub-species, strains, isolates, or types). As an example, *Staphylococcus aureus* (or *S. aureus* for short and often referred to as *Staph. aureus*) is a well-known bacterium that can cause various types of diseases such as wound infections, skin infections (carbuncles, pimples, and impetigo), pneumonia, and toxic shock syndrome. The genus is *Staphylococcus*, species *aureus*, and an example of a sub-species is *S. aureus* subsp. *aureus* N315. *S. aureus* Newman and ATCC 6538 are other examples of strains or isolates. American Type Culture Collection (ATCC) refers to a culture collection of microorganisms from which various types of bacteria and other microorganisms can be purchased; these strains are considered standard strains and are specified in various antimicrobial test methods for disinfectant testing purposes. Other examples of culture collections include the United Kingdom National Culture Collection (UKNCC), China Center for Type Culture Collection (CCTCC), Collection de l'Institut Pasteur (CIP), and All-Russian Collection of Microorganisms (VKM). A very common series of strains are known as MRSA, for methicillin-resistant *Staphylococcus aureus*, referring to strains of *S. aureus* that have developed resistance to some drugs (antibiotics, such as the b-lactams including methicillin) that used to very effective against these types of bacteria. Other more recent examples include the carbapenem-resistant

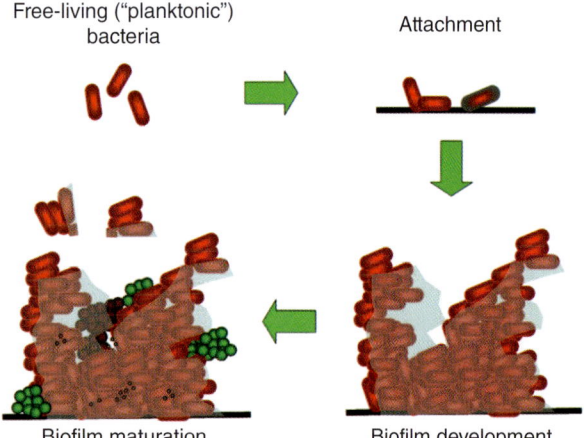

Figure 5.6 Biofilm development: free-living bacteria attach or become associated with a surface, which allows them to begin to divide and develop a biofilm, with production of a polysaccharide-based matrix that protects them from the environment and from removal, including the effects of drugs, detergents (used in cleaning chemistries), and disinfectants. As the biofilm matures, other bacteria, protozoa, and viruses can become associated, grow, and even feed on the biofilm. Parts of the biofilm can become dissociated from the matrix, being released and free to form other biofilms.

Table 5.3 Examples of human diseases caused by bacteria (pathogenic bacteria).

Bacteria name	Features	Associated diseases
Mycoplasma pneumoniae	Cell wall free, pleomorphic	Pneumonia (inflammation of the lung) and other respiratory diseases
Chlamydia trachomatis	Gram-negative cocci or rods; only grow inside host cells ("obligate intracellular pathogens")	Infections of the eye and genital tract. Other species such as *C. pneumoniae* can cause pneumonia
Staphylococcus aureus	Gram-positive cocci	Wound and surgical site infections; impetigo (a skin infection), toxic shock syndrome, gastroenteritis (inflammation of the stomach/intestines). Antibiotic-resistant forms, such as methicillin-resistant *S. aureus* (MRSA), are a particular concern as they are more difficult to treat due to their resistance to the drugs (antibiotics) used to control them
Enterococcus faecium and Enterococcus faecalis	Gram-positive cocci	Commonly found as part of the normal types of bacteria in the human intestine, but can be infectious such as in wounds and in the urinary tract. Some strains are also highly resistant to antibiotics, such as the vancomycin-resistant *Enterococcus* strains
Streptococcus pyogenes	Gram-positive cocci	Pharyngitis ("strep sore throat"), impetigo, scarlet fever, otitis media (middle ear infection, "ear-ache," but also commonly caused by another species called *S. pneumoniae*, a common cause of bacterial pneumonia)
Clostridioides (or Clostridium) difficile	Gram-positive rods. *Clostridioides* and *Clostridium* species only grow in the absence of oxygen ("anaerobic")	Diarrhea and intestinal perforation (leaking of the intestine contents into the body). Other species can cause wound infections such as *Clostridium tetani* (tetanus) and *Cl. perfringens* (gangrene)
Neisseria gonorrhoeae	Gram-negative cocci	Gonorrhea (commonly referred to as "the clap") is a sexually transmitted disease shown by a discharge from the sex organs and can lead to a variety of complications; treated in the past with drugs such as penicillin, but many strains are now resistant to such antibiotics
Enterobacteriaceae, such as Escherichia coli, Salmonella enterica, and Klebsiella pneumoniae	A family of Gram-negative rods	Many are associated with diarrhea and gastrointestinal infection, such as *Escherichia* and *Salmonella*. *E. coli* is also a leading cause of urinary tract infections and meningitis (in neonates or young children). *Salmonella enterica* causes typhoid ("enteric fever"), an aggressive gastrointestinal disease. *Klebsiella pneumoniae* and other species are common causes of infections in hospitals such as in wounds, pneumonia, and urinary tract infections
Pseudomonas aeruginosa	Gram-negative rods	Can cause of range of opportunistic infections (infections in individuals who are more susceptible than normal, e.g. due to an existing infection or damage to part of the body or being "immunodeficient," where the body's ability to fight an infection is compromised). Examples include wound infections, pneumonia, and urinary tract infections
Mycobacterium tuberculosis	Gram-positive rods; also referred to as "acid-fast" due to other staining methods used to differentiate them from other bacteria	Tuberculosis; there is another similar form known as "bovine" tuberculosis that can occur in humans and animals caused by *Mycobacterium bovis*
Mycobacterium leprae	Gram-positive, acid-fast rods; do not grow under normal microbiology laboratory growth (culture) conditions and only in certain animals (armadillos)	Leprosy or Hansen's disease, which is a disease of the nerves (peripheral) but presents with skin lesions
Corynebacterium diphtheriae	Gram-positive rods; they have a cell wall similar to *Mycobacterium*, but are not acid fast	Diphtheria, an upper respiratory tract disease associated with a sore throat and other complications; once considered very common, the overall occurrence is low due to the diphtheria vaccine; the vaccine is usually given as part of a combined vaccine for three bacterial diseases, known as DPT, for *C. diphtheriae*, *Bordetella pertussis* (pertussis or whooping cough), and *Clostridium tetani* (tetanus)

strains of Gram-negative bacteria, or carbapenem-resistant Enterobacteriaceae, such as *Klebsiella pneumoniae* or *E. coli* strains. There is more on antibiotics later in this section.

What makes certain types of bacteria good for us while others are bad and can cause disease? Even similar types of bacteria can cause different effects or diseases. Remember that not all bacteria can or want to do harm to a host (human, animal, plant, or other organism). The ability to cause disease is based on two considerations: the host and the bacterium (or any other microorganism for that matter). There are many factors that can influence this relationship. Host factors include the patient's age, their health, genetic predispositions, if they are on certain types of drugs, if they have an existing disease, use of devices in parts of the body (such as in the urinary tract and through the skin into the bloodstream), and so on. Examples of the effects of drugs or medications include antibiotics (since they are often used to treat an infection they may also kill many of the other bacteria that may be preventing infection from other microorganisms), chemotherapeutic agents (e.g. for cancer treatment), and immunosuppressive drugs. In all these cases, patients on these types of drugs can be more susceptible to getting infections. Patients can be immunocompromised due to existing bacterial, viral, or other infections; HIV has already been discussed as a virus (see the previous section) that affects the human immune system causing it not to work well and predisposes an infected individual to a variety of bacterial, fungal, and other infections that they would normally be able to fight off (leading to AIDS). In healthcare environments, considering their function to treat people with injuries, illness, and disease, it should be no surprise that patients there will be more susceptible to infections.

Epidemiology is the study of the various factors that affect health, illness, and disease in populations. This not only applies to infectious diseases but also other illnesses such as cancer and the influence of various other factors on public health (such as smoking, eating habits, etc.). Epidemiology studies the rates of diseases; in the study of infectious diseases there are two commonly used rates relating to morbidity and mortality. Morbidity refers to a disease or illness, where the morbidity rate is the number of cases of a particular disease in a population over time. Mortality refers to death due to an illness or disease, where the mortality rate is the rate of death from a particular disease/illness in a population over time. The study of epidemiology is closely linked with the practice of IPC, which is considered later in this chapter.

The other consideration is the bacterium (or microorganism) itself. In this regard, two terms that are useful to define are pathogenicity and virulence. They both refer to the ability of a microorganism to cause disease. A pathogen is a disease-causing microorganism and virulence is a measure of how aggressive a pathogen is to be able to cause disease. Some bacteria can cause mild diseases even when present at high numbers, but others are more virulent even when present at low numbers. One measure of virulence is the LD_{50}, which can be defined as the dose of a microorganism that can be given to cause death in 50% of cases (usually determined in experimental animals and estimated for humans).

Pathogens can be considered over two extremes: those that always cause a disease (examples include bacteria like *Neisseria gonorrhoeae* and *Treponema palladium*, which cause the sexually transmitted diseases gonorrhea and syphilis, respectively) and those that only cause infections under special, opportunistic conditions ("opportunistic pathogens"). In the first case these bacteria may be considered aggressive pathogens that cause disease on contact, over time, with humans or animals. Opportunistic bacterial pathogens are considered poorer pathogens, rarely if ever causing disease in healthy persons, but under the right situations (such as in sick patients) they can cause disease. An example is *Staphylococcus epidermidis*, which is actually found as a major component of the normal bacteria that live on the skin, but within a patient who is immunocompromised it is often implicated in infection, particularly when related to skin or mucous membrane contact such as with indwelling catheters. Many bacterial pathogens are considered to have pathogenic potentials between these extremes and are referred to as facultative pathogens; important examples are *Escherichia coli* and *Staphylococcus aureus*, and these can vary depending on the specific strain. The capability to cause disease is due to having various types of virulent factors that contribute to allowing microorganisms to invade humans (e.g. through the lungs, intestine, or skin), evade the immune system, and damage the host.

One of the most important virulence factors in bacteria is the production of toxins. Toxins are various types of proteins or polysaccharides that are produced or released from bacteria that have a direct toxic effect in the body. Examples are given in Table 5.4. There are two main types: exotoxins, which are produced and released by the bacteria, and endotoxins, which are a structural component of the outer, cell wall structure of Gram-negative bacteria. Exotoxins, depending on their structure, have been shown to have a variety of effects that cause host cell damage and death; the disease effects that we see include rashes on the skin, vomiting, paralysis, and diarrhea (Table 5.4). Most exotoxins are proteins. In some cases, where the exotoxin is no longer produced by the bacteria, they are no longer pathogenic. Also, some of these exotoxins are heat stable, so even though the bacteria are inactivated by heat, their exotoxins can remain in water or on a surface to elicit their toxic effects. Endotoxins are different in that they are part of the outer cell wall structure (Figure 5.4) of Gram-negative bacteria such as *E. coli* and *Pseudomonas*. They are high-molecular-weight complexes that contain lipopolysaccharide (LPS, a lipid and polysaccharide structure), proteins, and phospholipid. As a structural part of bacteria they are not

Table 5.4 Various types of toxins produced from bacteria and their effects in humans.

Bacteria	Toxin(s)	Effects
Exotoxins *Streptococcus pyogenes*	Erythrogenic ("pyrogenic") toxin	Cause the red skin rash during scarlet fever, as well as fever and other complications during infection
Escherichia coli	Variety of toxins including LT, ST, verotoxin, and the shiga toxin	LT and ST cause intestinal cells to lose fluid/electrolytes, leading to diarrhea; LT is considered heat sensitive and ST is heat resistant. Verotoxin also leads to diarrhea, but by a different mechanism. The shiga toxin is produced by specific strains known as *E. coli* O157:H7, but the original source of the toxin is from *Shigella dysenteriae*; in both cases it prevents protein synthesis in cells, which leads to diarrhea and other effects
Vibrio cholerae	Cholera toxin (Ctx)	Similar to the *E. coli* LT toxin, it causes intestinal cells to lose fluid/electrolytes, leading to diarrhea
Clostridium tetani	Tetanus toxin	Inhibits communication between nerve cells leading to paralysis
Bacillus cereus	Emetic toxin (ETE), diarrheagenic enterotoxin[1] (Nhe), and hemolytic enterotoxin[1] (HBL)	The emetic toxin (which is heat stable) causes vomiting, being the first sign of disease; this is followed by the diarrheal toxins Nhe and HBL (both heat sensitive) due to the loss of fluids from intestinal cells
Clostridioides (or *Clostridium*) *difficile*	Toxin A/toxin B	Causes intestinal cells to die, leading to bloody diarrhea
Corynebacterium diphtheriae	Diphtheria toxin (Dtx)	Inhibition of protein synthesis leading to cell death
Endotoxins Gram-negative bacteria such as *Neisseria meningitidis*, *E. coli*, and *Pseudomonas aeruginosa*	Endotoxin or lipopolysaccharide (LPS)	These molecules are an important part of the structure of the outer membrane of Gram-negative bacteria; they can be released (in small amounts) during growth of the bacteria, but more importantly when they are damaged or killed. Endotoxins can be heat stable (even by boiling or by steam); they are toxic by stimulating the immune system leading to a variety of effects, including fever (increased body temperature), changes in blood cells, shock, and even death (depending on the level)

[1] The term enterotoxin is often used to describe an exotoxin that is produced by bacteria and has an effect in the intestine.

generally released by the bacteria, but when the cell is damaged or is killed (due to the effects of the body's immune system, antibiotics, or disinfectants/sterilants), endotoxins can be released. At accumulative levels they can have dramatic effects in patients. Endotoxins are known to causes a cascade reaction in the immune system, leading to fever and more serious effects (depending on the dose), such as organ failure and even death. They are also known to be heat resistant (e.g. to boiling, although they can be inactivated by steam or dry heat sterilization under some conditions).

In addition to toxins, other virulence factors include the production of enzymes (urease, collagenase, and lipases as examples), production of capsules or biofilms (as protective mechanisms), ability to bind and penetrate host cells or structures associated with cells (e.g. collagen), and ability to survive within cells for extended times (e.g. *Mycobacterium tuberculosis*). A further interesting virulence factor of importance today is the ability of bacteria to develop resistance to antibiotics. Antibiotics are a group of drugs that kill or inhibit the growth of bacteria; this is an important definition, as antibiotics are only generally effective against bacteria and should not be used for other purposes such as to treat viral infections. Since the first antibiotic was discovered (penicillin in 1928), they have become widely used both to prevent bacterial infections (as with the practice of giving antibiotics before invasive surgery, referred to as antibiotic prophylaxis) and to treat them. In many cases they have become abused, such as not being used correctly (at the right dose for the right amount of time), being used with diseases that are caused by viruses, or as growth promoters in animal feeds. Examples of some of the most widely used antibiotics today to treat bacterial diseases are given in Table 5.5.

Antibiotics have very specific mechanisms of action against bacteria. As an example, the β-lactams such as penicillin and methicillin inhibit the ability of bacteria to produce the structure of peptidoglycan, a major part of the cell wall structure (Figure 5.4). This is important because since the effects are specific to the target bacteria and not human cells (e.g. human

Table 5.5 Examples of groups/types of antibiotics.

Antibiotic group[1]	Examples
β-lactams and cephalosporins	Penicillin, flucloxacillin, amoxicillin, methicillin Cephalosporins are closely related to the β-lactams and include ceftazidime
Glycopeptides	Vancomycin, teicoplanin
Aminoglycosides	Streptomycin, kanamycin, neomycin
Quinolones, fluoroquinolones	Nalidixic acid, ciprofloxacin

[1] Antibiotic groups are usually classified based on their chemical structure. They often have official names as well as commercial/trade names. Many antibiotics are naturally occurring, such as penicillin that is isolated from the fungus *Penicillium chrysogenum*; others have been chemically synthesized.

cells do not have peptidoglycan), antibiotics can be used to treat infections at low doses within the body without any significant toxic effects (in most cases) against human/animal cells. Naturally, penicillin itself is not equally effective against all types of bacteria, being particularly effective against Gram-positive bacteria; other β-lactams such ampicillin and amoxicillin have much greater activity, including against Gram-negative bacteria, despite having similar chemical structures. This is a natural phenomenon, where the normal structure of bacteria does not allow access of the antibiotic to its site of activity or has other means of making them insusceptible to the antibiotic. Mycobacteria are an example of this, where specific antibiotics have been identified or developed as being effective against mycobacteria due to their natural resistance to other antibiotics, predominantly due to their unique cell wall structure (Figure 5.4).

Bacteria can be very resilient and as antibiotics are used (or abused) they can develop mechanisms of resistance to those antibiotics with dramatic consequences. This is not surprising, as their mechanisms are so specific that bacteria can use a variety of ways to overcome their effects. For example, bacteria can change the structure of the antibiotic target so that it no longer reacts with the drug, produce enzymes that break down the antibiotic so that it is no longer effective, or use specific proteins that act as cellular pumps to expel the antibiotic from where it needs to be present to have its effect. In some cases these are unique mechanisms that have been developed by specific bacterial strains, and in others the factors responsible for resistance can be transferred to other bacteria, even different genera and species. In all these cases, the ability to survive the presence of the antibiotic allows the strain to survive even in the presence of antibiotics, an important virulence factor, and therefore to cause disease more readily in patients. Well-cited examples of antibiotic-resistant bacteria include methicillin-resistant *Staphylococcus aureus* (MRSA, which despite the name is resistant to the β-lactams and cephalosporins and is a leading cause of healthcare-acquired infections); vancomycin-resistant *Enterococcus* (*Enterococcus* are naturally resistant to many antibiotics and vancomycin is often used to treat enterococcal infections); multi-drug-resistant and even extensively drug-resistant *Mycobacterium tuberculosis* (TB; resistant to many and even most of the specific antibiotics that are used to treat mycobacterial infections); and carbapenem-resistant Enterobacteriaceae such as *Klebsiella pneumoniae* and *Escherichia coli*, which are often associated with high rates of morbidity and mortality.

Overall, antimicrobial resistance threatens the effective prevention and treatment of an ever-increasing range of infections caused not only by bacteria but also by other microorganisms such as viruses and fungi. This can occur over time, and particularly on exposure to antimicrobials such as antibiotics. In these situations, patients may no longer respond to medicines, making infections harder to treat and increasing the risk of disease spread, severe illness, and death.

As a final consideration, there is also a large, separate group of microorganisms that are considered prokaryotes and are similar to bacteria but are actually quite distinct. They are known as the archaea and include a wide variety of groups and types. Examples include genera such as *Halobacterium*, *Methanococcus*, and *Thermococcus*. They have been of interest scientifically as they have been identified to live and grow in a variety of extreme environments on earth, such as hot springs, where humans and other forms of organisms could not survive. Interestingly, they have not (or have rarely) been associated with human or animal disease, and so are not further considered here, but there is speculation on potential links to disease.

Fungi

Fungi are a group of cell-based microorganisms but have a different basic cell structure to prokaryotes (such as bacteria) and are known as eukaryotes. Eukaryotes (or eukaryotic cells) are larger and more structurally organized cells than prokaryotes. They include fungi, protozoa, helminths, and human, animal, and plant cells, but their exact structure and how they are organized internally or together will vary significantly.

Fungi are a large collection of microorganisms that are found everywhere in the environment (air, food, water, surfaces, etc.); they are therefore found as surface contaminants (e.g. in dust and in the air). Despite their diversity, it is estimated that we have only truly identified less than one-tenth of the various types of fungi that are present in the world. From a medical perspective, most fungi are not known as serious pathogens, but many are opportunistic or facultative pathogens (see the previous section for discussion on pathogenicity). They are, however, often associated with product spoilage (such as in foods or liquids) and are widely used for industrial purposes (for making bread, cheese, wine, and as a source of drugs like antibiotics, while large-growth forms such as mushrooms are themselves edible fungi). Specific examples include the yeast known as baker's or brewer's yeast that is officially called *Saccharomyces cerevisiae*; *Rhizopus stolonifer*, a type of mold that is also known as black bread mold due to its common furry black growth on bread; and *Penicillium roqueforti*, which is the "blue" in blue cheese. Fungi are therefore officially named in a similar way to bacteria, with the genus followed by species name always in italics or underlined (*Saccharomyces cerevisiae* or Saccharomyces cerevisiae); various sub-species and strain types/numbers can also be defined after the genus/species name in a similar way to bacteria. Microscopic examples of fungal structures are shown in Figure 5.7. The cells are more organized intracellularly (as typical eukaryotes) and are surrounded by a fungal cell wall; the basic fungal cell wall structure is similar to that of bacteria, consisting of an inner cell membrane attached to an outer cell wall, but the cell wall consists of various types of polysaccharides, with internal fibrils of cellulose or chitin that give the cell wall a rigid structure. These structures are generally more resistant to inactivation than many types of bacteria.

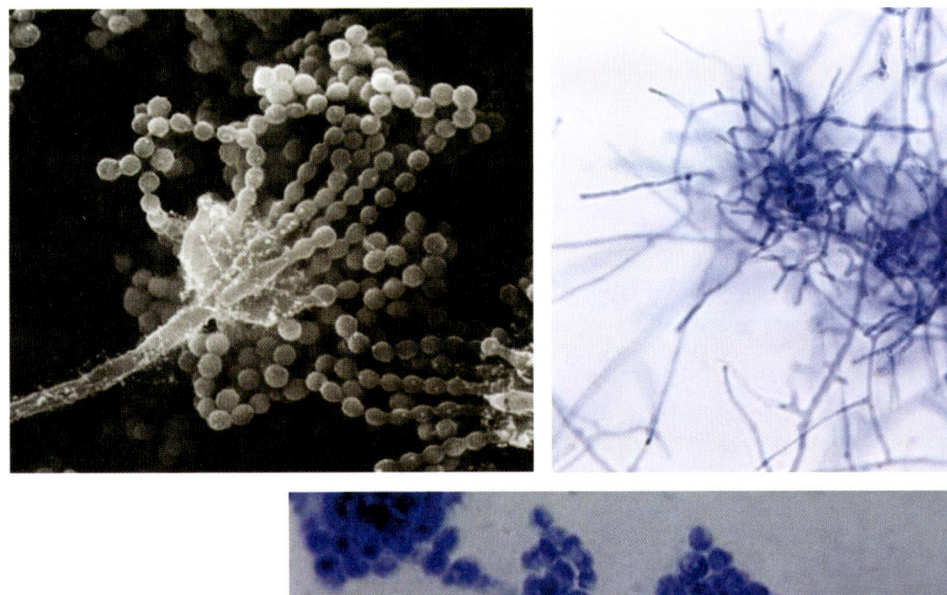

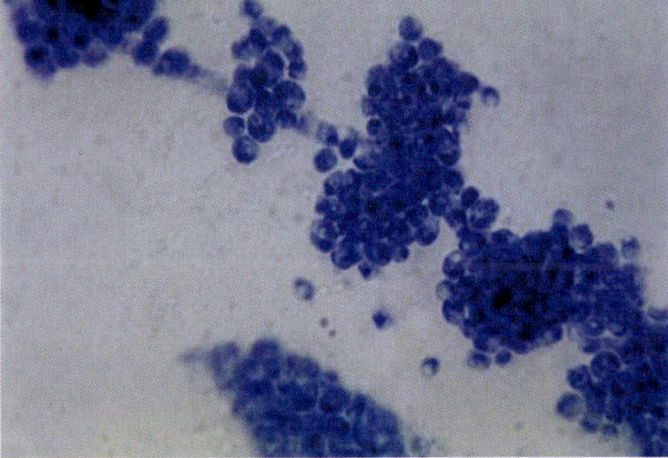

Figure 5.7 Microscopic examples of fungi, including filaments of cells and spores.

Fungi are classified into two groups based on how they grow: filamentous fungi (also known as molds) and unicellular forms (known as yeasts). Filamentous fungi typically grow together as long filaments (lines of cells connected to each other), while yeasts are generally unicellular (grow as individual cells; Figure 5.7); some fungi are found to present in both ways when examined (known as dimorphic) and depending on the conditions they are exposed to during growth.

In addition to cell division, fungi reproduce in two main ways, depending on the specific species: by the production of asexual and/or sexual spores. Similar to bacteria, they can grow vegetatively by cell division. For molds, when the cells divide they may not separate and form the long, filamentous lines of cells (called hyphae); these filaments form a loose net-like structure typical of mold growth on surfaces (known as mycelia; Figure 5.7). Many yeast divide by cell division (like bacteria, to give two identical cells) and/or by budding, where a small part of the cell "buds" off to form a small cell. *Candida* is an example of typical dimorphic yeast that can grow vegetatively in both ways (as filaments or as one-cell forms). In addition to vegetative growth, fungi also reproduce by producing spores, but in mechanisms quite different to those described in bacteria. Spores can be produced in two ways: sexual and asexual. Asexual spores are produced directly from fungal cells by budding and generally develop together in specialized structures typical of the fungal type (e.g. within conidia or sporangia). Sexual spores are produced when two cell types of the same fungus, known as male and female forms, join together and develop to make the dormant spore forms. These spores can also be contained within specialized structures (such as ascospores within an ascus); these structures are often used microscopically to identify the type of fungus under laboratory conditions. Overall, the structures of the various types of fungal spores have not been studied in detail, but they are generally considered more resistant than vegetative fungi cells and much less resistant than bacterial spores; the ascospores of *Aspergillus*, as an example, are widely considered one of the most resistant forms of fungi to disinfection.

Fungi have been traditionally classified based on how they grow on culture media in the laboratory and how they appear microscopically (including the types of spores and how these are produced); more recently, classification systems are based on genetic techniques.

Table 5.6 Fungal pathogens and their respective diseases.

Fungus type	Diseases
Molds	
Aspergillus fumigatus	Aspergillosis
	Symptoms include cough, chest pain, breathlessness, and fever
	Many allergic reactions (with similar symptoms) are due to reactions of the immune system to fungal spores including *Aspergillus*
Mucor indicus	Mucormycosis is used to describe rare but serious infections caused by *Mucor* and *Rhizopus*
	Disease is most often associated with the lungs, sinuses, and sometimes in serious cases the brain
	These infections are generally only encountered in immunocompromised hosts
Trichophyton rubrum	Commonly known as a dermatophyte (as well as other *Trichophyton*, *Microsporum*, and *Epidermophyton* species) as they are often implicated in skin and nail infections in animals and humans
	Examples include athlete's foot (an itchy, scaling infection typically reported between the toes, medically referred to as tinea pedis) and ringworm (dermatophytosis)
Stachybotrys chartarum	A green-black mold often associated with buildings that have been flooded, allowing the mold to grow; often referred to as "sick-building" syndrome, associated with a series of symptoms similar to allergies, including irritation of the eyes, nose, and throat, but also leading to other complications
Yeasts	
Candida albicans	By far the most common fungal infection in humans, particularly in immunocompromised or hospitalized patients
	Infections are often associated with the oral and genital cavities, commonly referred to as thrush
	More serious infections (where the yeast becomes disseminated around the body) are frequently reported in hospitalized patients
	These diseases are generally known as candidiasis
Cryptococcus neoformans	Cryptococcosis, most often as lung-based infections, but similar to other fungi can lead to a variety of serious effects in immunocompromised patients
Histoplasma capsulatum	Infections often reported in the lungs, but symptoms/health effects can vary and be disseminated

Minor fungal infections in humans can be rather common, such as thrush in the oral or genital cavities and athlete's foot/ringworm as skin-based infections. Serious infections of their own accord in healthy individuals are rare, but can be severe in immunocompromised or sick patients. Examples of pathogenic fungi and their associated diseases are given in Table 5.6. *Candida albicans* is an important example that can be found in the oral or genital cavities with no ill effects, but in some cases can lead to mild infections such as thrush; it can lead to more serious infections in immunocompromised individuals, such as blood infections. *C. albicans* and other *Candida* species are leading causes of bloodstream and urinary tract infections in hospitalized patients. Other fungal species that are often implicated in infections, particularly in hospitalized patients, include *Aspergillus* and *Cryptococcus*, while in the general population infections and complications due to molds such as *Trichophyton* (also known as tinea infections) and *Stachybotrys* are common (Table 5.6).

Fungi can cause disease due to the many pathogenic or virulence factors similar to bacteria (as described earlier). Examples include the production of toxins, known as mycotoxins, the presence of protective capsules on their external surface, their ability to survive and spread through the environment, cell surface binding capabilities, immune system interference, and their intrinsic resistance to disinfection and even biofilm formation. Mycotoxins are produced by many types of molds and are not considered as potent (dangerous) as some bacterial toxins; despite this they can have significant health effects. It is widely known, for example, that some mushrooms are poisonous when eaten, due to the presence of these toxins, and in many countries the levels of mycotoxins in foods are required to be controlled. Other mycotoxin examples include the aflatoxins (in *Aspergillus* species, some of which are carcinogenic, referring to their ability to cause cancer in humans/animals), ochratoxins, and citrinins.

There are a variety of drugs that can be used to treat fungal infections, generally known as antifungal drugs. They are often specific in their activity against fungi, and in some cases are only effective against certain types of fungi, due to unique targets in fungal structures (such as the production of specific molecules for their cell walls). Examples include amphotericin B and terbinafine. Similar to antibiotics and bacteria, the use of these drugs has also led to the development of resistance in some fungi with similar clinical implications (requirements to use higher concentrations that are often toxic to patients or inability to control the infection).

Protozoa

Protozoa are a further group of unicellular (one-celled) eukaryotic microorganisms, but are distinct from fungi. Protozoa and another group of eukaryotes known as the helminths (see the following section) are often referred to as "parasites," although strictly speaking a parasite is defined as any microorganism able to live on and cause damage to its host (human, animal, plant, microorganism, etc.). Similar to fungi, protozoa are considered abundant and many species remain to be described (as well as any potential health effects). They can be found in a variety of environmental sources and are often associated particularly with water and even in the air. They are further sub-divided into four groups: sporozoans, ciliates, amoebae, and flagellates, based on their microscopic structures. Protozoa have not been as widely studied as bacteria and have been even less studied from a disinfection point of view. A summary of some of the more important protozoal pathogens and their associated diseases in given is Table 5.7. These include *Plasmodium falciparum* (the cause of malaria), *Cryptosporidium parvum* and *Giardia lamblia* (important causes of diarrheal disease), and *Acanthamoeba* species (eye infections). As can been seen from these names, protozoa are classified and designated in a similar mechanism to bacteria and fungi.

Many protozoal diseases are associated with poor water quality. They can be transmitted through contaminated water but also through other means, including flies. An example is *Trypanosoma brucei*, a flagellate causing a disease known as sleeping sickness that is transferred through tsetse flies and is commonly described in sub-Saharan Africa. The tsetse fly is considered a "vector" for the microorganism, where a vector can be any living agent (human, animal, fly, microorganism, etc.) that transmits an infection. Vectors are commonly used to describe various types of flies/insects that transmit infection, including the mosquito as a vector for the malaria parasite, *Plasmodium falciparum* (Table 5.7). In a similar way, any disease that is transmitted by an animal is known as a zoonosis or zoonotic disease, such as rabies (the rabies virus in dogs and other animals), anthrax (the bacteria *Bacillus anthracis* in cattle), and toxoplasmosis (the protozoa *Toxoplasma gondii* through contaminated meat or cat feces).

Protozoa present with a variety of vegetative (actively growing) forms, including what are known as trophozoites (e.g. sporozoites; Figure 5.8). They reproduce in a variety of ways depending on the specific type, including by cell division and by other sexual/asexual mechanisms. These vegetative structures can vary in sensitivity to disinfection, due to their individual structures and various protective mechanisms, but of note is their ability to form dormant, resistant forms of themselves that are known as cysts or oocysts. Examples of cyst-forming protozoa include *Giardia* and *Acanthameoba* species, while *Cryptosporidium* and *Plasmodium* species produce what are known as oocysts. These structures can survive various extreme environmental conditions such as drying and the presence of chemical disinfectants, allowing them to be disseminated through water and the air. *Cryptosporidium* oocysts have been described as highly resistant to chemical disinfection,

Table 5.7 Protozoa and associated diseases.

Protozoa type	Diseases
Sporozoans *Cryptosporidium parvum*	Cryptosporidiosis Transmitted through contaminated water, even in cases where the water has been disinfected (e.g. chlorinated) due to the resistance to the oocyst form of the protozoa to chemical disinfection treatments Disease most commonly presents with diarrhea, although can lead to other complications in immunocompromised patients
Plasmodium falciparum	Malaria, a widespread disease in tropical and sub-tropical regions of the world, carried from person to person by female mosquitoes (a type of fly) through infected blood Malaria is a leading cause of disease and death worldwide; other species of *Plasmodium* also cause milder forms of the same disease It is a disease of the blood, affecting particularly the red blood cells, where typical signs of the disease include anemia (low levels of red blood cells, which limits the carriage of oxygen through the blood) and repeated cycles of coldness followed by fever, shaking (known as "rigor"), and sweating; in severe cases this can lead to coma (loss of consciousness similar to a deep sleep) and death
Ciliates *Balantidium coli*	Balantidiasis, a diarrheal disease, which is often transmitted through pigs (in many cases where it shows no ill effects but causes disease in humans), via contaminated water or foods
Amoeba *Acanthameoba castellanii*	Diseases include eye infections (amoebic keratitis) and encephalitis (inflammation of the brain) They are generally considered as opportunistic pathogens
Flagellates *Giardia lamblia*	Giardiasis, a disease of the lower intestine in humans but also other animals and birds Disease outbreaks are commonly associated with contaminated water and foods (e.g. where the foods are rinsed with water) The disease usually presents with diarrhea, often explosive, but generally short-lived
Trypanosoma brucei (also known as *T. gambiense*)	Sleeping sickness (African trypanosomiasis), a common disease in Africa that presents as fever, swollen lymph nodes, confusion, and periods of fatigue/tiredness and the opposite, insomnia The protozoa are transmitted through flies (specifically tsetse flies) and human contact (e.g. blood transmission).

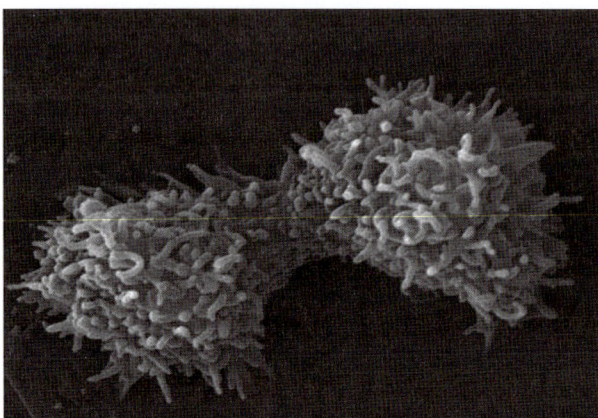
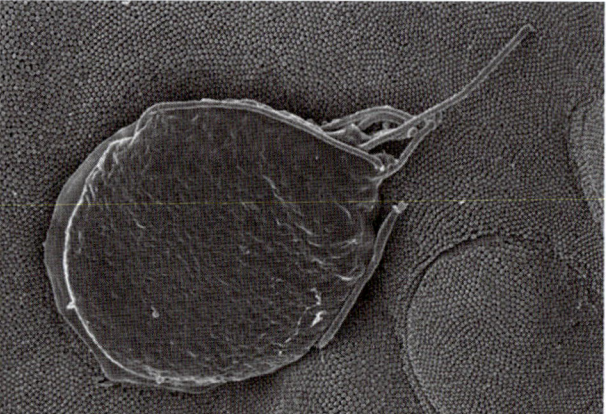
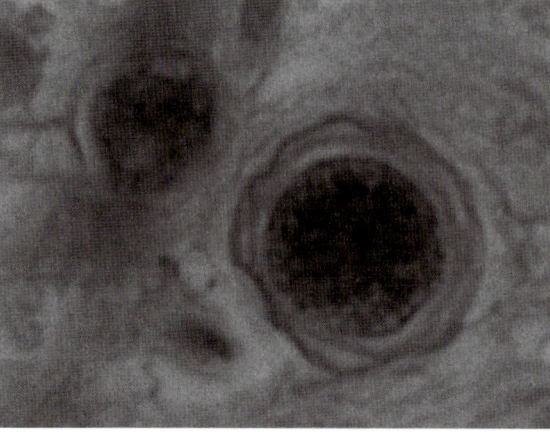

Figure 5.8 Examples of various types of protozoal structures.

surviving concentrations of chlorine typically used for the preparation of potable (drinking) water.

Protozoal infections can be controlled or prevented by various types of drugs, such as chloroquine (against malaria), and, interestingly certain types of antibacterial drugs (antibiotics), such as metronidazole and tetracycline. Chloroquine is often prescribed to prevent malaria transmission (medically this is an example of prophylaxis, which is defined as a measure taken to prevent a disease or infection), although in recent years there have been increasing reports of *Plasmodium* strains showing resistance to this drug.

Helminths

Bacteria, fungi, and protozoa are all unicellular microorganisms at their basic structures, where each individual cell has the ability to grow alone or to develop into communities but retaining the ability to grow on their own. Helminths (also known as parasitic worms) are multi-cellular, eukaryotic microorganisms. They are similar to animals and humans in that they have an organized cell structure of various organs and systems not dissimilar to those described in animals/humans; these structures are required for survival. Other examples of multi-cellular organisms are the arthropods, such as flies, fleas, and lice. Externally, helminths are surrounded by a tough layer, known as a tegument or cuticle (equivalent to skin in animals/humans but more protein based), with internal organization such as a digestive system (including intestines), reproductive system (testes and ovaries), attachment organs, and even primitive brain organs. They can be further sub-divided into three groups based on their structures (Figure 5.9): tapeworms (cestodes), flukes (trematodes), and roundworms (nematodes). The tapeworms and flukes are often grouped together as platyhelminths, due to their flat structures, while the nematodes are more rounded, thread-like structures. Similar to other types of microorganisms, it is believed that only a small proportion of the various types of helminths that exist have been described. Although many require microscopy to observe them (especially when in

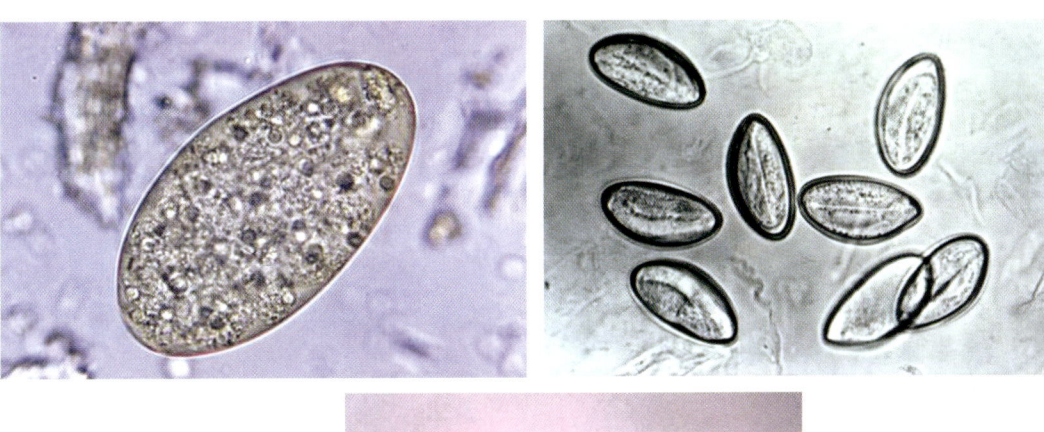

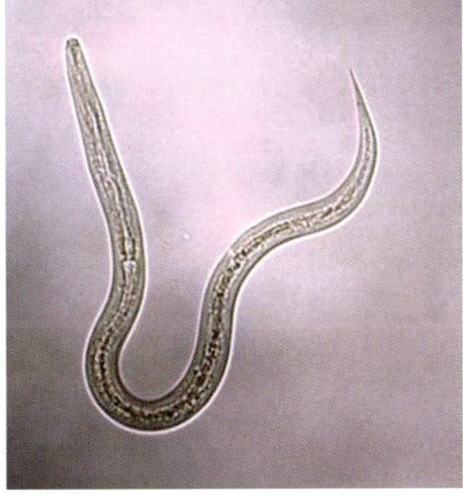

Figure 5.9 Examples of various types of helminth structures. Helminths grow in life cycles that can show various different structural forms during the cycle, such as eggs/cysts (dormant forms), larvae, and worms/flukes (adult forms).

egg or cyst form), others can be very visible by normal sight, as in the case of some of the larger worms in this group; examples include the adult worm forms (called giant roundworms) of *Ascaris lumbricoides* that can grow up to typical lengths of 35 mm and up to 4 mm in thickness. They are often associated with water, food (especially meat), and environmental surface contamination.

Helminths develop in life cycles, where they grow through different physical stages: an adult form (worms/flukes), larvae (that can have various stages), and eggs/cyst (dormant forms). *A. lumbricoides*, for example, is introduced into humans via the oral route and in its eggs can survive the acidic conditions in the stomach; on passing through the duodenum (the part of the digestive system between the stomach and the small intestine) the egg can then produce larvae that can attach to the intestinal wall and enter the blood system. Interestingly, the larvae are carried to the heart, liver, and eventually the lungs to develop; they can then be reintroduced into the intestine (by coughing and swallowing), where they can mature as adult worms to produce new eggs in the intestine that get released into the environment through the digestive system. During disease, typical symptoms can include vomiting, diarrhea, and coughing, but other effects can lead to more serious disease presentation. The eggs can survive for many years in the environment until introduced into a new host. The eggs/cysts are produced sexually in helminths; they have male and female forms, although the worms themselves can be considered "bisexual" (developing into specific male or female forms, reproducing between two worms) or hermaphroditic (both male and female systems, and reproduction in the same worm).

Similar to protozoa, the structures and protective mechanisms of helminth eggs/cysts have not been studied in detail, but they appear to have protective lipid, protein, and polysaccharide (e.g. chitin) layers that help them resist not only drying and to a certain extent heat, but also various types of chemicals such as those used for disinfection. They are parasites as they live on animals and humans, and can be present asymptomatically (not causing any obvious symptoms, which is a benefit to the host and the parasite), but can also cause damage to their hosts (often intestinal-related diseases/symptoms; Table 5.8). Examples include diseases such as schistosomiasis often associated with contaminated water, leading to intestinal disease, and elephantiasis, a disease of the lymphatic system (Table 5.8). Unfortunately, immunocompromised patients can have more serious helminth diseases that can lead to death.

Investigations of and medical treatments for helminth infections are limited, with most serious diseases being seen in various parts of Africa, South America, and Asia. Emphasis is on preventing helminth transmission, usually by improving water quality or removing vectors for the helminths (such as water snails to prevent *Schistosoma* transmission). Infections

Table 5.8 Helminths and associated diseases.

Helminth type	Diseases
Wuchereria bancrofti	Elephantiasis, a roundworm (nematode) infection that is spread by the mosquito
	The disease is also known as lymphatic filariasis, where the worms become lodged in the lymphatic systems (typically in the legs) leading to a build-up of fluid, causing the limbs to swell
	It is a common disease in tropical and sub-tropical areas
Schistosoma mansoni	Schistosomiasis (also known as bilharzia) is a common trematode (fluke) disease in Asia, Africa, and South America associated with contaminated water (as water snails are an important host in addition to humans)
	This species of *Schistosoma* causes an intestinal disease
	Infected humans present with various signs, such as abdominal pain and diarrhea
Enterobius vermicularis	Enterobiasis (or pinworm/threadworm infection) is usually associated with itching in the anal area and is particularly prevalent in children
	These nematodes are usually transmitted in egg form by hands, food, or water contamination
	Not considered a serious pathogen
Ascaris lumbricoides	Ascariasis, the most common helminth infection in humans
	These roundworms can grow up to 35 cm in length, are often found in the intestine, and are known as giant worms
	They can cause serious disease and even death in immunocompromised humans, presenting a variety of effects, such as in the intestinal tract (vomiting, diarrhea) and other systems (the lungs and coughing)
Taenia saginata	The beef tapeworm causes taeniasis in humans and is transmitted through infected meat (beef)
	These worms can grow up to 5 m in length
	Infections are generally asymptomatic (no obvious symptoms)
	More serious complications can occur when they proliferate, such as constipation, abdominal pain, and diarrhea

can be treated using deworming methods to aid in expelling the worms, or by injuring or killing them; examples of such drugs include ivermectin and praziquantel. Interestingly, although often considered controversial, helminths have been used therapeutically to help in the control of immune system-related disorders (such as inflammatory bowel disease, asthma, eczema, and hay fever). The theory is that helminth infections help the immune system react correctly (prevent overreaction) on exposure to agents such as pollen and dust that trigger such reactions.

An introduction to infection prevention and control

Public health is an important subject to all of us individually, to our families, and to the communities in which we live. As a science, the study of public health may be defined as preventing diseases, prolonging life, and promoting health. Within this definition, a disease may be defined as any effect that impairs/harms the body's normal function and therefore influences our health (in mild, moderate, or even severe ways). Diseases can be infectious (such as those caused by bacteria and viruses) or non-infectious (as with certain types of cancer, effects of drug abuse, stress, chemicals, etc.).

Examples of public health efforts to reduce disease in populations include improving drinking water quality (chemical and microbiological), campaigns to stop smoking (due to the associated risks of cancer and other health effects), washing of hands, and good waste collection and disposal/treatment. These efforts can have significant effects on our health and well-being, ranging from major efforts within populations (water treatment, waste control) to personal choices, cultures, and practices (washing our hands and deciding not to smoke). Epidemiology is part of the science of public health, being the study of the factors involved in disease and the control of such diseases. Specialists in this area are known as epidemiologists and they investigate the rates of various diseases in populations as well as the effects of preventative measures in reducing these rates. Epidemiology allows scientists to recommend various evidence-based practices that have been shown to have a significant impact in reducing the rates of diseases.

The analysis and control of infectious diseases form an important part of this science; they not only affect public health but have wider implications in certain high-risk groups such as in those who are younger, older, infirm, in hospital, immunocompromised, or with underlying diseases. Infection prevention and control (IPC, also commonly referred to as "infection control") is the discipline concerned with preventing the spread of microorganisms and the infections they can cause; it can be considered a branch of epidemiology, both in scientific investigations as well as in its practical application.

IPC is a practical, evidence-based approach for preventing patients, health workers, and the public from being harmed by avoidable infections. It can affect all aspects of healthcare, in both acute and community settings. Effective practices require well-structured programs with well-defined actions at all levels of the healthcare system, including policymakers, facility managers, health workers, and those who access health services. Evidence-based best practices for IPC provide guidelines and guidance to healthcare providers to ensure that safe, quality care is provided to patients, visitors, healthcare providers, and in the healthcare environment.

It is useful to distinguish between "prevention" and "control." Prevention strategies are employed to prevent microorganism transmission, mainly from spreading from one person to another, from one part of our body to another, from animals/insects, from the air, and from surfaces; examples include hand washing (antisepsis) and surface disinfection. They can also include measures that prevent disease even if the microorganism is transmitted, which is the concept behind vaccination. Vaccination is defined as the intentional introduction of microorganisms (usually modified or parts of the microorganism) into the body to allow the development of immunity (or resistance) to the development of infection with that microorganism; this is discussed in further detail later in this section.

Control strategies may be differentiated as those used to control and manage an infection when it has happened, with a typical example being the use of anti-infective drugs such as antibiotics and preventing transmission to others by isolating infected patients. It is important to note that these practices are not only important to the patient but also to those caring for or visiting the patient. These definitions are, of course, not strict, as sometimes the same practices are used in both cases, for prevention and control, depending on the situation. In addition to these measures, IPC personnel are also involved in many other aspects such as investigating the sources of infection outbreaks, managing outbreaks, and studying the effects of various preventative and/or control measures. Experts in this area may be known by a variety of terms, such as infection control practitioners, infection preventionists, specialists, infection control nurses or doctors, clinical microbiologists, or epidemiologists.

When IPC practices are used consistently, the transfer of HAIs can be prevented in healthcare settings. This section offers a brief introduction to IPC, including the different strategies that are used. These directly affect device decontamination practices, as they are important infection prevention strategies within healthcare facilities. These basic principles are considered:
- Microorganisms are everywhere.
- Sources of contamination.
- The role of IPC.

- Basic IPC strategies.
- The processing role in IPC.

Microorganisms are everywhere

Earlier in this chapter we learned about the various types of microorganisms, the places they can be found, and the types of diseases they can cause. An important concept to remember is that microorganisms are invisible to the eye. If we were able to see them directly, we would be suitably impressed by the variety and number of these microorganisms naturally on our bodies, in the air, and on various surfaces that we touch. But we are unable to detect them with the human eye. Most of us would have an instant reaction to seeing a single insect on our skin, and would vigorously react if a swarm of insects was present on a surface that we wanted to use; this is despite the fact that many (though admittedly not all) insects are harmless. At the same time, the way we would react could depend on how dangerous we view the insert to be, such as a relatively harmless housefly compared to a biting or stinging insect (such as wasps or mosquitoes). In this case we have the benefit of seeing the danger. This is not applicable with microorganisms, and in particular pathogenic microorganisms that can cause infectious disease.

In some cases and settings there could be thousands or millions of microorganisms on a surface, while in others there may be few to none. But we may not be able to know their impact and the harm they may cause to our health. Therefore, it is also good to remember when working in healthcare facilities (such as hospitals or clinics) that have a higher risk of contamination or infection transmission that one should always assume that microorganisms are everywhere, and that they can do harm. As an example, consider touching a heavily contaminated surface with your hands and then using those hands for eating or rubbing an eye; you can quickly understand how easily transmission can occur. This is an important consideration when surfaces are contaminated with blood or other bodily fluids, which should always be assumed to include pathogenic microorganisms. This concept allows us to introduce two further terms: standard precautions and blood-borne pathogens.

Standard (also in the past known as "universal") precautions are a set of measures designed for the care of all patients in every healthcare setting, whenever relevant. This is regardless of a person's diagnosis or presumed infectious status, in order to reduce the risk of transmission of microorganisms from both recognized and unrecognized sources. These sources of potential infection include blood and other bodily fluids as secretions or excretions (excluding sweat), non-intact skin or mucous membranes, and any equipment or items in the care environment that are likely to become contaminated. Standard precautions must be implemented at all times within healthcare and community settings. This can include consideration of the level of interaction between the healthcare worker and patient, and the anticipated level of exposure to blood and/or bodily fluid. Elements of standard precautions include:

- Hand hygiene.
- Respiratory hygiene/cough etiquette.
- Use of PPE, such as gloves and masks.
- Aseptic technique and safe injection or sharp handling practices.
- Safe management (and processing) of devices, equipment, and laundry.
- Waste management.

Blood-borne pathogens are important in these situations and are defined as disease-producing microorganisms spread by contact with blood or other contaminated bodily fluids from an infected person. Notable examples of blood-borne pathogens are HIV and hepatitis B viruses (see the section on viruses). We do not need to know if the patient is infected; the patient or those caring for them may not even know at the time of care. We automatically assume that blood and bodily fluids from others pose a risk. Other bodily fluids and tissues can also be contaminated with pathogens or by cross-contamination with blood. Therefore, standard precautions for blood-borne pathogens are generally adopted with all body tissues and fluids. Devices and equipment used in surgical and medical procedures should always be considered contaminated and handled appropriately. It is recommended to follow the same precautions whether devices, items, and equipment are visibly contaminated with blood or not.

Sources of contamination

Contamination can mean many things depending on your perspective; for the purposes of our discussion we are primarily concerned with microbial contamination. Microbial contamination is defined as the presence of microorganisms, such as bacteria, viruses, and so on. They may be present at high or low numbers, and may vary in type and risk of infection. Contamination does not necessarily mean infection, and infection does not mean disease. Contamination can also include many other materials such as patient tissues and fluids (often referred to as "soil"), but also chemical and even radioactive contaminants.

As discussed in Chapter 1, decontamination is defined as the removal of contaminants to specified levels or a process to render a surface/object safe for reuse. Depending on the situation this may include microorganisms or other materials that could remain on the surface (living, non-living, chemicals, proteins, radioactivity, etc.) that could do harm. In this section we focus on microorganisms and microbial contamination, which are the focus of infection control and prevention. Microorganisms are everywhere and can be transferred to an individual, including a hospitalized patient, by a variety of mechanisms that are summarized in Figure 5.10. At the center

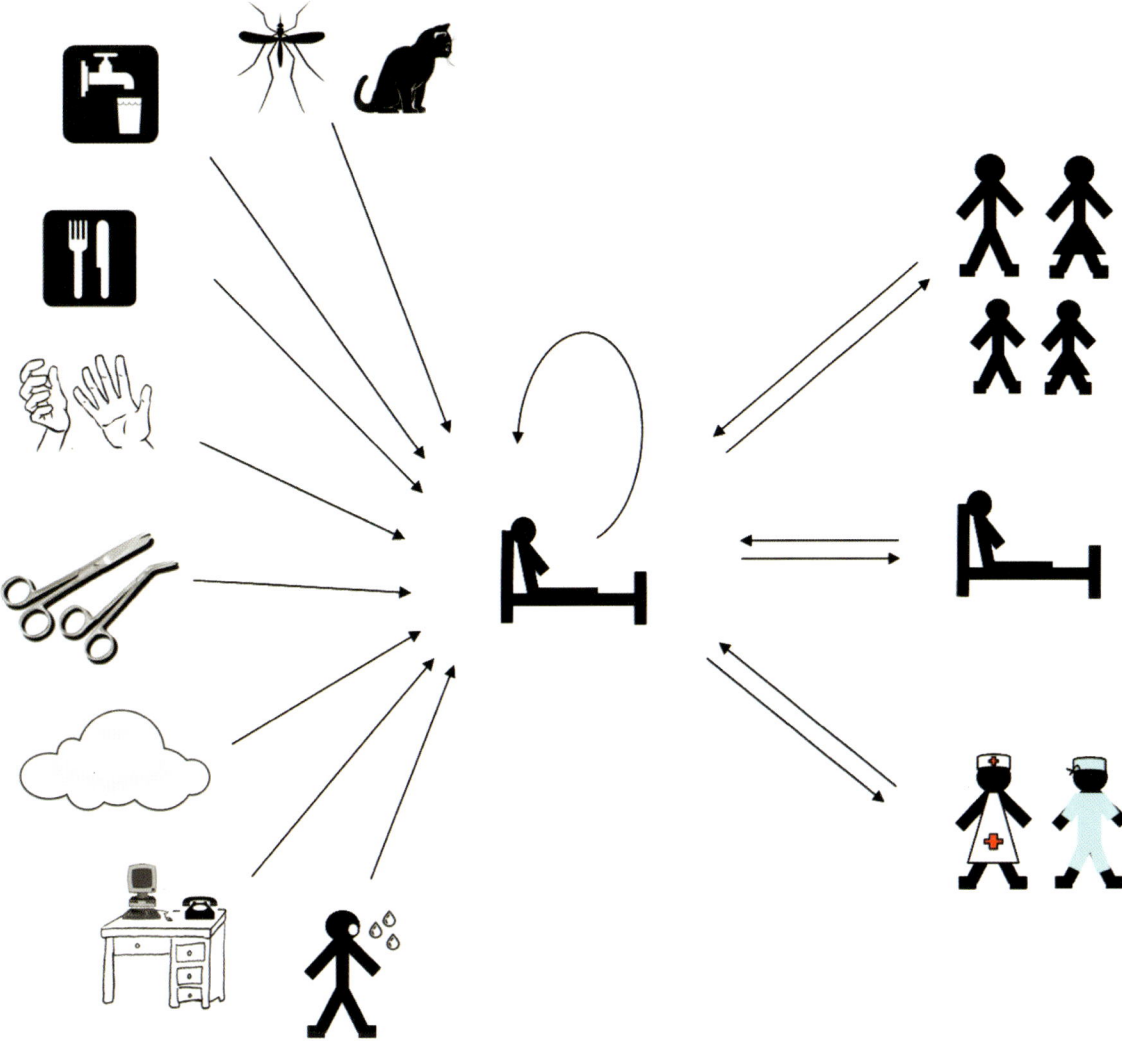

Figure 5.10 Sources of microbial contamination. From the top left this includes animals/vectors, water, food, hands, devices/instruments, air/gases, general surfaces, and droplets. The patient can be contaminated from these sources and can also be the source of contamination. In a healthcare facility the same applies to visitors, other patients, and healthcare staff (shown on the right).

is the patient and it is important to consider that patients themselves can be the source of microorganisms; patients may arrive at a healthcare facility already carrying or infected with a pathogen. They may therefore develop an infection, for example by scratching a wound, from microorganisms they already carry that would normally have caused them no harm. While in a facility there are many sources of pathogens (shown on the left of Figure 5.10). Major sources can include contaminated hands of healthcare workers (doctors, nurses, assistants, etc.) or visitors, surfaces (importantly high-touch surfaces), aerosols (e.g. coughing) or even the air itself, and reusable medical devices. Other sources include foods, water, and animals/insects. These sources are not unique to healthcare facilities and apply to our daily lives, with many of these risks being reduced by practical public health measures (see the following sections). Remember, the risks of infection are higher in many healthcare facilities because the patient may be more sensitive to developing an infection (immunocompromised), due to having other illnesses, undergoing therapies for other diseases (e.g. chemotherapy for cancer), or having serious wounds due to injury or surgical procedures. As the patient can be contaminated by a variety of sources, the patient can also be the source of contamination to other patients, facility staff, and visitors (shown on the right of Figure 5.10).

The role of infection prevention and control

The primary role of IPC is to put procedures and practices in place to reduce the risks of microbial, in particular pathogen, transmission. This is not only directed at reducing the risks to patients, but is equally important for the protection of facility staff and visitors. It is therefore a quality standard for any facility and, like any quality standard, requires constant support and maintenance.

The overall responsibility for IPC at any facility is the hospital manager, director, or management team. Infection control and prevention should interact closely with the various facility departments and their staff, ranging from operating rooms and wards to decontamination facilities and staff, waste disposal, facility maintenance, pharmacy, and even finance. It is important to point out that infections are not only a significant cause of morbidity (disease cases) and mortality (death due to diseases) in healthcare, causing distress to patients and their families, but can also lead to considerable costs due to increased hospital stay, additional treatments required, specialized patient handling, repeated surgery, and so on. This can be avoided by ensuring practical and active IPC measures.

The organization of IPC within a facility will vary in size, depending on the facility. It can range from a single individual (typical of small clinics and practices) to large infection control teams (especially in larger hospital groups). What is recommended is that responsibility is designated for establishing, maintaining, and ensuring the practice of various policies and procedures. Designated staff can typically involve specialists such as infection control nurses, epidemiologists, consultant microbiologists, infection control officers, decontamination department managers, and so on. Their expertise can include infectious diseases, medical microbiology, nursing, prescription practices, and IPC practices. In larger facilities it is typical to have a designated infection control team and/or committee, with the head of such a group being represented at the upper levels of hospital management. It is important to remember, particularly in healthcare facilities, that *everyone* is responsible for ensuring that IPC policies are safely applied, not only those who are in direct contact with a patient. The best procedures and practices can be in place but if they are not adhered to, they will have no impact; success is dependent on people and their training. Examples of the various procedures and practices that are employed are further discussed in the next section, with emphasis on the processing of reusable devices wherever they are used in a facility.

While the primary role of IPC practitioners is to put procedures and practices in place to minimize microbial transmission, their day-to-day role will include:

- Ensuring facilities and equipment are available to staff and patients (e.g. washer-disinfectors, sterilizers, and hand-washing facilities).
- Ensuring that policies and procedures are being followed.
- Advising on any infection concerns within the facility.
- Developing and maintaining procedures and guidelines as required by clinical practice.
- Monitoring the rates of infections (surveillance) and identifying any problems (e.g. outbreaks). An infection outbreak may be defined as an occurrence of a disease (infection) at a higher rate than would otherwise be expected at a particular time and place. Outbreaks of infections may be within a small group at a single facility or can impact thousands of people across the world. They may also be referred to as epidemics (affecting a particular region, such as part of a country or of a continent, including a number of countries) or pandemics (where the outbreak spreads across the world). Examples include the outbreak of a bacterial or viral disease in a hospital leading to ward closures or the recent COVID-19 pandemic. IPC specialists can play an important role in ensuring that any infection outbreaks that occur are rapidly investigated and controlled.
- Monitoring the correct use of anti-infective chemicals (e.g. antibiotics) used to control infections (as either preventative or treatment measures).

Infection control and prevention strategies

As already stated, IPC specialists are responsible for establishing policies and practices to reduce the risks of infection and cross-infection. Examples of measures that are part of this goal, including in healthcare facilities, are summarized in Table 5.9. This is not an exclusive list but includes most of the important interventions that involve various decontamination methods, such as cleaning, disinfection, and sterilization. Other examples can include the prudent use of antimicrobials (such as antibiotics) and correct patient handling procedures.

A familiar example should be hand disinfection, a practice that is often cited to be one of the most significant yet simple ways to reduce microorganism transmission. The skin, and particularly the hands, is naturally colonized with a variety of resident and transient microorganisms (see Chapter 2) and it is the carriage of various types of microbial pathogens that causes the most concern in healthcare workers and in the transmission of contamination. Reducing the level of microbial contamination is an important IPC strategy to reduce the risk to patients and staff. Hand disinfection (a form of antisepsis or disinfection of the skin or mucous membranes) can include hand washing (using water and soaps, including antimicrobial soaps) and hand rubbing (which does not use water, typical examples including 60–80% alcohol-based products that are rubbed into the skin and allowed to dry). Hand or skin disinfection can be used routinely for personal hygiene (e.g. before eating or after using the toilet, where non-antimicrobial soap and water is actually sufficient) but also in clinical practice before and after patient contact (e.g. by nurses and doctors

Table 5.9 Examples of infection control and prevention measures.

Sources of contamination	Infection prevention and control measures
Reusable devices, instruments, and equipment	Cleaning, disinfection, and/or sterilization as applicable to the device type Inspection and maintenance
Single-use, sterile devices	Best practices in storage (e.g. temperature, humidity, preventing damage to packaging) Aseptic technique in handling Correct practices in patient use (insertion, maintenance, and removal) of catheters, surgical implants, needles, etc. Methods to prevent accidental needle or sharp injuries Technologies to reduce the attachment or growth of bacteria on surfaces
Wound care	Wound cleanliness, dressing and maintenance Wound closure (suturing) Antibiotic or antimicrobial use
Droplet/air/gas	Isolation rooms and associated precautions Air-handling systems including filtration Masks, eye protection, wound protection
Soiled textiles, liquids, and various single-use instruments (e.g. needles, sharps, etc.)	Cleaning, disinfection, and/or sterilization Examples include laundry cleaning and disinfection, waste disposal and incineration
Environmental surfaces, such as tables, chairs, and bedrails	Cleaning Disinfection
Hands and skin	Hand washing (with water) Hand rubbing (without water, e.g. with alcohols) Glove use Surgical scrubbing
Food	Hand washing Glove use Correct storage (at cold temperatures) Appropriate handling
Water	Sanitization (e.g. chlorination, ozonation, UV treatment) Disinfection (of water and/or water lines) Filtration
Animals/insects	Limit or exclude contact De-infestation (e.g. spraying) Pest control

tending to a patient, including before surgery), handling instruments that have been used or before they are used on patients, or in preparation of an area of skin for incision during a surgical procedure (referred to as part of pre-operative preparation). While compliance with hand washing prior to surgical intervention is considered high, it may be surprising to note that compliance with general hand disinfection practices in caring for patients is lower. Studies have shown that this can vary from 16% to 81% compliance; these rates may often be lower in non-patient contact areas, but may be important to personal health, as is particularly the case in decontamination areas. It is also important to note that hand washing or hand rubbing is often not done correctly to ensure that all areas of the hands are properly cleaned (Figure 5.11).

Further examples that will be familiar are the use of gloves (non-sterile or sterile, depending on their use), disinfecting surfaces, and the use of specialized air-handling or isolation rooms. Gloves are widely used to present a physical barrier, not only to microorganisms but also in handling of chemicals (e.g. during manual cleaning or disinfection practices). They are designed for different uses and these are typical examples in clinical practice:

- Vinyl (polyvinyl chloride, PVC) gloves are used for general low-risk or housekeeping activities.
- Natural rubber (latex) gloves can be used for high (microbial) risks such as handling blood or blood spills, but are also commonly associated with allergic reactions that can even be severe in some cases (latex allergy).

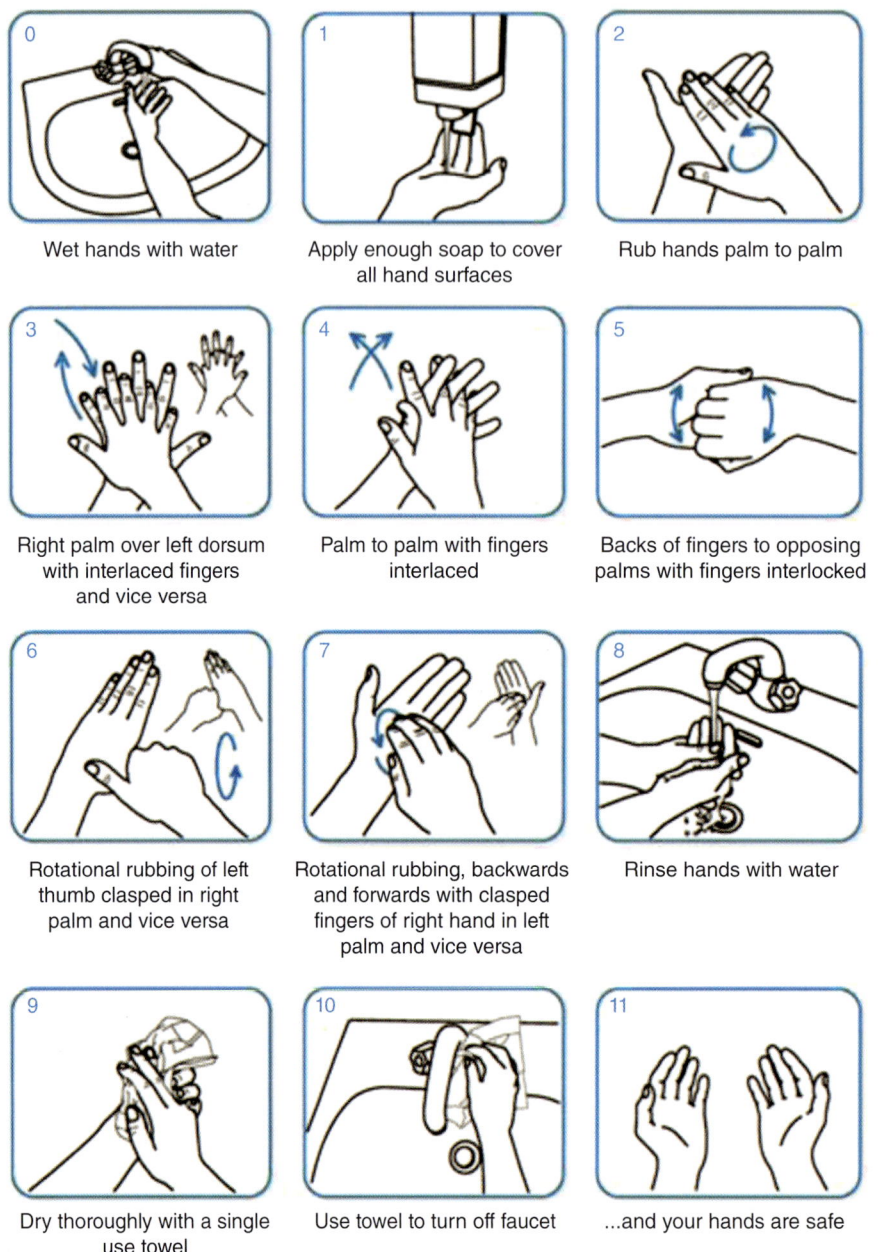

Figure 5.11 A recommended hand-washing technique with water to ensure that it is done correctly. Note: when using a hand-rubbing (alcohol-based) product, only steps 1–7 should be followed as water is not necessary.

- Nitrile (acrylonitrile) gloves can provide good biological and chemical barrier functions and are often used as a safer alternative to latex or when using chemicals.
- Neoprene (polychloroprene) gloves are also generally used due to their good biological and chemical barrier capabilities.

Gloves can also be provided pre-packaged and sterilized, for use with, on, or in a patient (e.g. during surgery), or non-sterile, as well as powdered or non-powdered. In instrument cleaning (manual) applications it is generally recommended that gloves should be worn that have chemical and microbial barrier properties (such as natural rubber, nitrile, or neoprene gloves), but other types of gloves may be recommended for particular applications, such as the handling of certain types of chemicals (e.g. chemical-resistant gloves such as heavy-duty neoprene-coated gloves) and for handling hot surfaces (e.g. autoclave gauntlets made out of chemical polymers known as aromatic polyamides that are thermal resistant).

Surface disinfection is widely used to reduce the levels of microorganisms that may be present on a surface, be they work areas, patient contact surfaces, or reusable surgical instruments. Examples of surface disinfectants include alcohols, bleach solutions (preparation of sodium hypochlorite that release chlorine, an efficient antimicrobial chemical), iodophors (which provide active iodine), and products containing a variety of other antimicrobials (such as phenolics and quaternary ammonium compounds). These antimicrobial chemicals are also known as microbicides (or sometimes as biocides) and are considered in further detail in Chapter 6.

It is typical for all these strategies to be used together in a hospital or clinical situation. None of them on their own will completely reduce the risk of cross-contamination to a patient or member of staff. An example is in the surgical theater, where surgical implants and instruments are provided clean and sterilized, surgeons and staff usually follow strict routines for hand washing (surgical scrubbing) and use of pre-sterilized gloves, an air-handling system is employed to keep the microbial population in the air low (e.g. using air filters such as high-efficiency particulate air or HEPA filters), various surfaces are frequently disinfected and the patient is prepared by skin disinfection (at the proposed site of intervention), and gowns are used. For surgery, a series of best practices are used in the preparation of the patient, precautions during surgery itself, and procedures following surgery that help reduce infection risks and other complications. It is equally the case that if one of these practices is compromised, such as rigorously washing the hands, putting on gloves, and then touching various contaminated surfaces prior to handling a patient, contamination can readily transfer and could cause an infection. Therefore, a common term that is used in IPC practices is a "care bundle"; this refers to a collection of between three and six IPC practices that are specified to be used collectively, reliably, and continuously to significantly reduce the risk of infection. An example of a surgical site infection (SSI) bundle, to reduce the risk of a patient getting an infection, could include ensuring the following:

- Skin preparation including skin disinfection and avoiding hair removal (or damage to the skin).
- Administration of prophylactic antibiotics, where a dose of antibiotics is given immediately before surgery to a patient to reduce the risk of getting a bacterial infection.
- Maintaining the patient's body temperature at normal throughout the operation (excluding certain types of procedure such as cardiac interventions).
- Hand washing and glove use in surgical staff.
- Conducting device cleaning, disinfection, inspection, and/or sterilization practices (when applicable).
- Aseptic technique during the handling of materials and procedures during surgery.

This care bundle includes a number of the strategies outlined in Table 5.9, but also the use of prophylactic antibiotics to prevent infections that could happen during or after the surgical procedure (e.g. from the skin, hands, or even the surgical instrument) and correct peri-operative (during surgery) care of the patient.

A further important strategy in IPC, as well as for public health in general, is disease surveillance. Surveillance can be defined as monitoring of the occurrence and distribution of infections within a facility, area, or population. By surveying the rates of infection, strategies can be investigated to reduce infection rates, outbreaks can be rapidly identified, and steps taken to control the outbreak. The incidence rates of HAIs can vary for many reasons, including due to the methods of surveillance as well as the impact of various IPC strategies in place from hospital to hospital, area to area, and country to county. Typical average rates worldwide may be in the range of 2–19% of admitted patients to hospitals who may present with an HAI. These can lead to significant costs, increased length of hospital stay, stress, and further patient complications. These rates are quite significant considering that a further estimated average of 10% of these cases may lead to death. Therefore, efforts to reduce the rates of HAIs in a hospital and targeting areas for reducing these rates are important strategies for IPC staff.

Role of device processing in infection control and prevention

Processing or decontamination personnel play an important role in IPC strategies, specifically in reducing the risk of SSIs and device-associated infections (DAIs). These infections can occur by the introduction of microorganisms via the use of instruments and devices used for various patient procedures, including non-invasive and invasive, such as endoscopic investigations and surgery. DAIs can be defined as being always associated with a device and its use on a patient as the source of infection. In general, from epidemiology investigations, the rates of DAIs are considered relatively low and are infrequently reported in medical literature when best practices in device processing or aseptic handling are employed; despite this, there are many examples of infections and infection outbreaks that have been linked to the inadequate cleaning, disinfection, and/or sterilization of a variety of instruments. In the majority of cases this can be associated with the improper application of important cleaning, disinfection, and/or sterilization steps as defined in international standards, guidelines, and manufacturer's instructions for use. It is generally agreed that many cases of infection (or other patient complications such as toxicity or immune reactions) are never reported or adequately investigated, so while these rates may be considered low they remain significant and, most importantly, preventable. SSIs may be due to the use of a device (and therefore may be also DAIs), but not always; other sources of infection may be from the patient's own skin (this is the leading cause), contamination of a wound following a surgical procedure (e.g. from contaminated gloves or hands), or from the environment (e.g. present in the air). In many of these cases it is difficult to identify a cause and investigators rarely have the time to investigate these cases in full detail.

The infection prevention role of associates performing decontamination should be considered in two parts: protecting themselves and co-workers, and protecting the patient.

Protect yourself and co-workers

In any IPC consideration, the objective is to reduce a known source of risk of cross-contamination. This not only applies to the safety of patients, it is also important that these risks should be reduced to those working in decontamination facilities. Remember, as discussed earlier, microorganisms can be everywhere and you will not see them. In clinical use, it is good practice to handle any contaminated surface (whether contamination is visual or not) as if it poses a risk to your health. To reduce any risks, a series of types of PPE can be used that are based on the various strategies outlined earlier. Examples of these are summarized in Table 5.10.

It is typical for a number of these preventative measures to be applied together, in particular in areas with higher risks, as in the case of manual cleaning of contaminated instruments. The exact policies on the use of PPE will vary from facility to facility, and further guidance is given on the recommended minimum requirements in further chapters of this book. Many of these protective methods apply not only to microbial risks but equally to chemical risks (Chapter 6). There are two further points that should be considered:

- PPE should be provided by an employer and is recommended for your personal protection. Do not underestimate its value or its impact on your health. If any recommended PPE method is difficult to use correctly or causes pain/discomfort, it is important that this is not ignored and is highlighted to management and/or the policy is reviewed. In most parts of the world it is a legal requirement to provide a safe working environment and that is an important part of any decontamination facility.
- PPE is only as good as the person using it. Correct training on the use of PPE is essential and should be periodically reviewed. As examples, nose/mouth masks will only be effective if used correctly, and eyeglasses or safety goggles will provide only partial protection if they do not fit well or do not have side shields.

Protect the patient

The primary purpose of any decontamination or processing facility is to ensure that a reusable device is safely returned for further clinical use (Chapter 1). The instrument or device can be heavily or lightly contaminated with microorganisms and the various steps of cleaning, disinfection, and/or sterilization are designed to reduce the risks of transferring these organisms to another person to a minimum (if not to an absolute) level. The various processes and practices associated with cleaning, disinfection, and sterilization are outlined in further detail in this book. It is sufficient to highlight at this point that any lapses

Table 5.10 Examples of personal protective equipment that can be used to reduce the risks of microbial cross-contamination.

Personal protective equipment (PPE)	Risk reduction
Gloves	Prevent hand contamination that could lead to cross-contamination or direct penetration through the skin or associated wound Heavy-duty gloves may protect the hands from accidental sharp object risks Objects that pose a risk to glove tearing (e.g. jewelry) should be avoided
Hand washing or hand rinsing	Reduces the risk of hand contamination in a cleaning area (e.g. on touching a contaminated surface) or cross-contamination on handling instruments after they have been reprocessed General good personal hygiene
General surface disinfection	Reduces the levels of microbial contaminants on a surface in high-risk areas, such as around a manual cleaning sink
Instrument cleaning/disinfection	Reduces the levels of microbial contaminants on surfaces to make them safe for handling/packaging for further sterilization
Face masks	Reduce inhalation or swallowing risks from air or droplets generated during manual cleaning
Protective/safety glasses or goggles	Reduce the risks of introduction of microorganisms (and chemicals) into the eyes from air or water droplets generated during manual cleaning The eyes are particularly at risk from chemical and microbial exposures
Aprons, overalls	Protect clothing from contamination that could be transferred outside a designated area and even to the home

or failures in these practices can have a significant and often dramatic effect on patient health and well-being. Put yourself in their shoes: it is the duty of every processing associate, staff and management, to ensure that these risks are reduced, if not eliminated.

Establish a policy and ensure it is followed

Processing practices can vary from place to place, depending on facility, regional, and even cultural requirements. This variability can be acceptable due to historical requirements, but in each case the facility should have a written policy of what is expected to be done. The policy should reflect the established practices that are expected to be performed and therefore should be clearly and practically written. Such policies make it clear to management and staff what is expected and safe for the patient; individual modifications to the policy (e.g. skipping a step, fast-tracking, etc.) are unacceptable unless approved by an authorized manager and such situations should always be documented. Documenting such situations is a simple and effective way of ensuring that a change in facility policy has been authorized and that those authorizing the change are held responsible for it. Once a policy is in place it can then be periodically reviewed and modified as required by changing guidelines/standards, hospital management, and infection prevention/control needs. Remember, the presence of a decontamination policy itself does not mean that the policy is being faithfully applied in the facility. So training, frequent retraining, and competency assessments are essential to ensure that staff are aware of the policies and understand how to conduct their jobs safely and effectively.

6 Chemistry and physics

Chemistry is the study of chemicals and chemical reactions. It is the basis for all living and non-living things, including forms of life (humans, animals, plants, microorganisms, etc.), surfaces or liquids we touch and see, and the air around us. In chemistry living and non-living things are referred to as matter. As described in Chapter 2, the human body is like an encyclopedia, with chemistry and the essential elements of chemistry (the elements) providing the words or essential building blocks for the various body structures (Table 6.1). These same elements, although a larger range of them, make up or are the source of all non-living materials around us: air, water, radioactivity, rocks, and so on, including the world itself and indeed the universe as we know it. In this chapter we consider in further detail the basics of chemistry, since it is essential for our understanding of how cleaning, disinfection, and sterilization work. The study of chemistry is closely linked to physics, which is the study of matter (or nature) and how it behaves. This includes concepts such as energy, the structure of elements/atoms, radiation (including light), temperature, pressure, and so on; these are also basic concepts that are considered further in this chapter.

The elements (also known as atoms) are the essential building blocks of chemistry. They can be further sub-divided into other parts (such as electrons, protons, and neutrons), but this is beyond the scope of this book and it is not necessary to consider further, apart from mentioning that electrons and protons also make up electricity. Based on these simple structures, there are at least 94 naturally occurring elements in the world (but when other unstable elements are considered there are over 100) that have been described and these are generally organized, based on their complexity, into what is known as the periodic table (Figure 6.1). Examples include carbon (C), oxygen (O), and nitrogen (N); they can be referred to by their full name (e.g. gold and silver) or their abbreviated name/symbol (e.g. Au and Ag, respectively).

These elements can exist on their own (e.g. gold, silver) or combine together to form molecules (e.g. H_2O, the chemical symbol for water, made up of two hydrogens and one oxygen).

A molecule is therefore made up of two or more atoms with the following examples: O_2 (the oxygen molecule, being made up of two atoms of oxygen), N_2 (the nitrogen molecule), and NaCl (sodium chloride, table salt). NaCl is a stable molecule, but when it is dissolved in water (by mixing it) it does sub-divide into its elemental forms as charged particles that are known as ions: the ions of NaCl are Na^+ (a cation, as it has a positive charge) and Cl^- (an anion, as it has a negative charge). Ions are often unstable and can be very reactive. In the introduction to anatomy (Chapter 2, introductory section), we discussed the fact that only six types of elements make up the different molecules that form life: carbon (C), hydrogen (H), nitrogen (N), oxygen (O), sulfur (S), and phosphorus (P). But there is a much wider variety used naturally in nature and artificially. Examples include a group of antimicrobial chemicals that are known as the halogens and include chlorine (Cl) and iodine (I); further examples are synthetic polymers (these are long molecules) that are widely used such as plastics (e.g. nylon and polystyrene), and molecules like ferric oxide (Fe_2O_3, commonly known as rust, where Fe is the symbol for iron) and calcium carbonate ($CaCO_3$, a major component of water hardness or scale).

The study of chemistry can be further sub-divided into various disciplines. A common example is organic chemistry, which considers any molecule that is based on carbon, and the other discipline of inorganic chemistry, which considers all non-carbon-based chemistry. This simple differentiation is useful, but strictly speaking does not mean that all carbon-containing chemistries are "organic" and all those that are non-carbon are "inorganic." However, these are exceptions, and a simple example is a group of chemicals known as carbonates, such as calcium carbonate ($CaCO_3$) and sodium carbonate (Na_2CO_3), which are considered as inorganic (since they do not contain carbon with hydrogen). Biochemistry (the branch of chemistry concerned with chemicals and processes that occur within living organisms) can be considered part of organic chemistry, as life is carbon based and biochemists specifically study chemical processes and structures in

---

Decontamination and Device Processing in Healthcare, Second Edition. Gerald McDonnell and Georgia Alevizopoulou.
© 2025 John Wiley & Sons Ltd. Published 2025 by John Wiley & Sons Ltd.

Table 6.1 Chemistry is the basis of living and non-living materials (known as matter), with the elements forming the essential building blocks. In this case the structure of the body is broken down to these elements in an analogy to an encyclopedia.

Structures	Encyclopedia analogy	Examples
Systems	Volume/section	Nervous, respiratory, digestive, and cardiovascular systems
Organs	Chapters	Stomach, heart, kidney, liver, brain
Tissues	Sub-chapters	Epithelial, muscular, nervous, connective tissues
Cells	Paragraphs	Nerve, muscle, skin, blood cells
Molecules	Words	Water (H_2O), proteins, carbohydrates, lipids, nucleic acids
Atoms/elements	Letters	Carbon (C), hydrogen (H), oxygen (O), nitrogen (N)

living organisms. Other branches of chemistry include pharmacology (study of chemical drugs), physical chemistry (study of physical properties of atoms), analytical chemistry (study of obtaining, processing, and communicating information about the composition and structure of matter), and radiochemistry (study of radioactive materials). It is interesting to note that radioactivity is produced from special types of elements known as radioactive isotopes; these are unstable elements (naturally occurring or artificially generated) that release radiation over time to become more stable. Although a detailed understanding of radioactivity and its properties is not necessary, it is important to note that radioactivity is often used for medical procedures (nuclear medicine). Examples include the use of radioactive isotopes for medical imaging (to view internal parts of the body, such as during positron emission tomography or PET) and for cancer radiotherapy. Widely used radioactive isotopes include technetium (^{99}Tc or Tc-99m), iodine (123 and 131), and thallium (201). In some cases these may require special consideration in device decontamination (Chapter 13, in the section on types of workplace safety hazards).

Solids, liquids, gases, and plasmas

The most commonly known states of matter are solids, liquids, and gases (we will also discuss the so-called fourth state of matter, plasma). All molecules can assume various different states depending on the energy available; an example of energy is thermal energy (measured by temperature) and electromagnetic energy, from ultraviolet (UV), X-ray, or gamma (γ) radiation. Temperature is an important source of energy (thermal energy), used not only to increase how quickly chemical reactions work (e.g. for cleaning and disinfection applications with chemicals) but also as a reliable method on its own for disinfection (e.g. hot water over 65°C) and sterilization (in the form of steam, but also dry heat at temperatures over 115°C).

Let us consider the effect of temperature on a common molecule: water (H_2O). The three forms shown in Figure 6.2 are ice (solid), water (liquid), and steam (gas). Solids will have a defined (or maintain their own) shape (in the case of water, ice crystals), liquids adopt the shape they are put into (e.g. in a glass), and gases have essentially no shape (not restrained). Water likes to be in a liquid form, an essential component for life and covering over 70% of the world's surface. The liquid form is generally present under ambient conditions of temperature and pressure, atmospheric pressure; the influence of pressure is considered in further detail later in this section. If the temperature of water is reduced below 0°C ("degrees Celsius") or 32°F ("degrees Fahrenheit"), it forms a solid, ice. The freezing (liquid to solid) or melting (solid to liquid) point of water is therefore 0°C. (Note: for conversion between various different methods of measuring temperature, see the section on common chemical measurement methods.) If the temperature is increased (above 100°C or 212°F) it forms a gas, known with water as steam. Therefore, the boiling (liquid to gas) or condensation (gas to liquid) point of steam is 100°C, under normal atmospheric pressure conditions. In this case, steam is also referred to as a "vapor," a gas that can readily return to being a liquid (e.g. by reducing the temperature). As shown in Figure 6.2, true steam (as a gas) is invisible (at the point of exiting the kettle), but what is generally seen is actually "condensed" steam, a mixture of steam (gas) and water (liquid). This is an important concept in considering steam sterilization (Chapter 11, in the section on steam (moist heat) sterilization). Other examples of water in a mixture of gas and liquid forms that are visible are fog, mists, and clouds. Another example of a liquid that forms a gas or vapor similar to water is hydrogen peroxide, also used as a liquid and as a gas/vapor for disinfection and sterilization (Chapters 9 and 11). Essentially, all other forms of matter can form similar phases depending on their chemistry. It is important to remember that not all forms of matter exhibit the same phases under the same conditions. As an example, carbon dioxide (CO_2, not to be mistaken for CO, carbon monoxide, a poisonous gas) forms a gas under normal, ambient conditions (temperature and pressure); CO_2 is breathed out through our lungs as a waste product from the body. For CO_2 to form a solid the temperature must be reduced to −78°C. The associated words used to describe

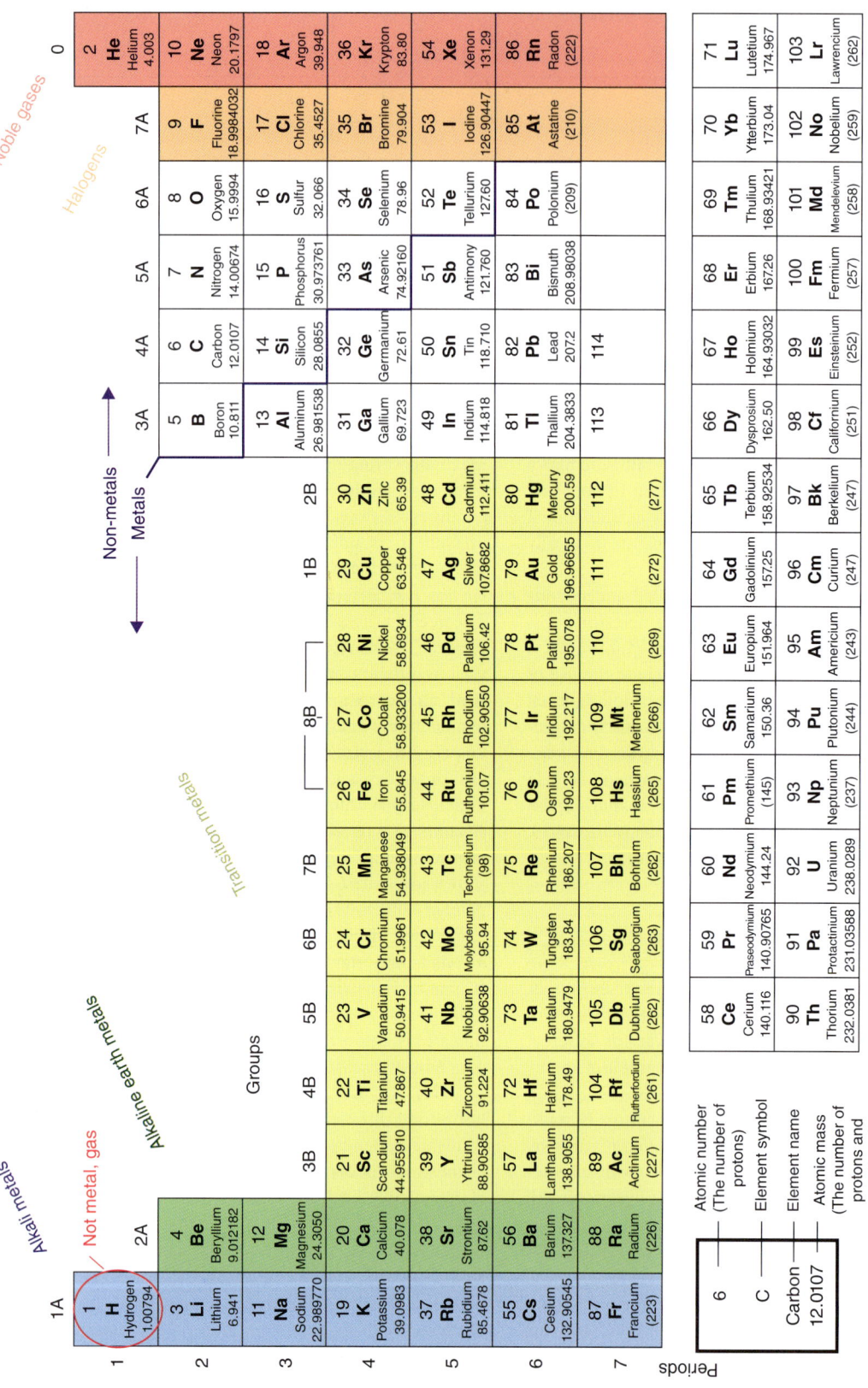

Figure 6.1 The periodic table of elements.

Chemistry and physics   133

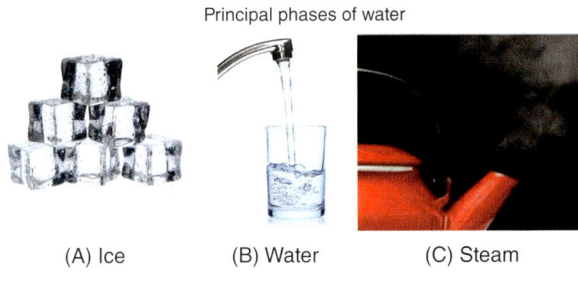

(A) Ice (B) Water (C) Steam

Figure 6.2 (A–C) The three principal forms or phases of water commonly found. As energy increases (e.g. by temperature), the phase changes from one to another (i.e. from ice to water to steam). Note that, contrary to common belief, true steam (as a gas) is invisible (just at the point of exiting the kettle), but what is generally seen is "condensed" steam, a mixture of steam (gas) and water (liquid). This is an important concept in considering steam sterilization (Chapter 11, section on steam (moist heat) sterilization). Sources: (A) pabijan / Adobe Stock; (B) Juri / Adobe Stock; (C) jStock / Adobe Stock.

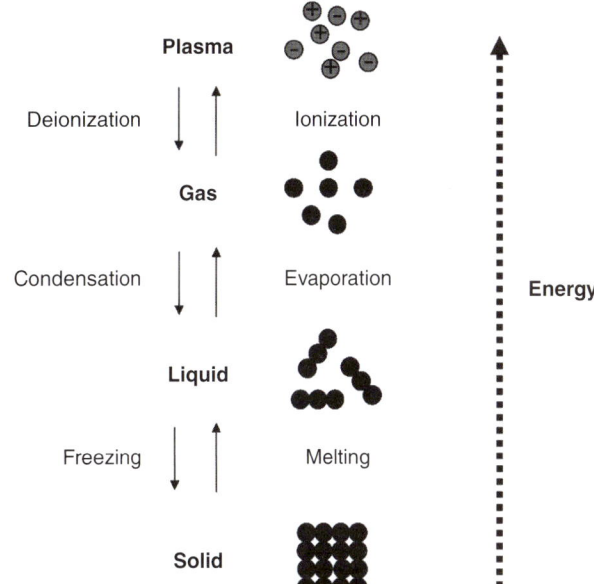

Figure 6.3 Phase (or state) changes of matter. As energy increases the phases change from solids to liquids, gases, and plasmas, and vice versa. Various other terms can be used to describe these changes in phase, for example evaporation can also be described as vaporization or boiling, and in some cases a phase can be skipped, such as in a phase change known as sublimation, where a solid can go directly into a gas. Note that the release of energy during the condensation of steam (gas) to water (liquid) is responsible for the antimicrobial efficiency of steam sterilization (see Chapter 11, the section on steam (moist heat) sterilization).

the conversion between the different phases of matter are summarized in Figure 6.3.

In discussing solids, liquids, and gases, constant reference is made to "ambient" conditions of temperature and pressure. This is important and it is the basis of one of the groups of "laws" of chemistry: the gas laws. The gas laws define relationships between the volume, temperature, pressure, and concentration (amount) of a gas. Examples include Boyle's Law (the specific relationship between the pressure and volume of a gas) and Charles' Law (the specific relationship between the temperature and volume of a gas). They can be all be defined mathematically, but in simple terms if you have a fixed amount (concentration) of any gas in a fixed volume (the area or space in which the gas is contained), there is a direct relationship between the temperature and the pressure: as the temperature increases the pressure decreases and vice versa. Pressure refers to a force applied to a surface. A high pressure suggests a greater force, while a low pressure indicates less force. Pressure is measured in a variety of ways, but specifically as the force applied to a specific size of surface (e.g. psi: pressure per square inch; mmHg: millimeters of mercury, where the pressure applied acts on mercury in a confined area; atm: atmospheres; and the correct international measurement of pressure is Pa: Pascal). For more discussion on weights and measures see the section on common chemical measurement methods. Therefore, if we continue to consider water, at atmospheric pressure (sea level) at about 100,000 Pa (also given as 100 kPa, where k is kilo or 1000) water is a liquid between 0 and 100°C, below which it forms ice and above which it forms steam. But if the pressure changes, so do these ranges (Figure 6.4).

At lower pressures, also referred to as being under a vacuum (where the lower the pressure the "deeper" the vacuum), steam is formed at lower temperatures and at higher pressure (under pressure) steam is formed at higher temperatures. For example, in Figure 6.4 for water, at 101 kPa pressure (which is atmospheric pressure at sea level) steam will form at 100°C, but at about 47 kPa steam forms at 80°C and at 200 kPa steam forms at 120°C. In this way, higher temperatures can be achieved with steam as the pressure increases, which is the basis for a steam sterilization process (Chapter 11).

Finally, let us consider plasma. A plasma is essentially a gas that has been further energized (or ionized; Figure 6.3). In its true form the gas is energized to break apart the molecules that make up the gas into sub-parts (ions and other reactive species), which basically makes the molecules and elements unstable. Therefore, let us again consider water (H_2O) as an example. As the energy is increased, ice (H_2O in solid form) will turn to water (H_2O in liquid form), then steam (H_2O in gas form), then into water plasma (essentially H and O, although the various species formed will vary to include OH, OH^-, O_2^-, and H^+). When the energy used to make the plasma is removed, the elements will rapidly recombine to form the starting gas (e.g. H_2O), but also other molecules

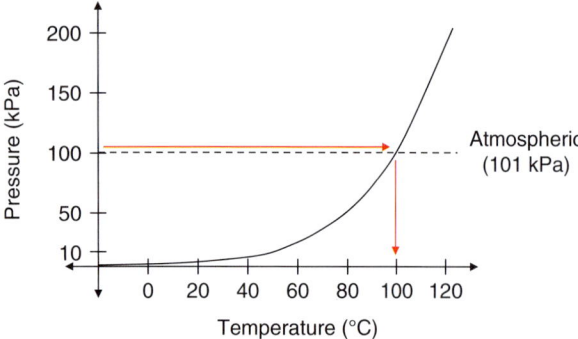

Figure 6.4 The relationship between temperature and pressure. The relationship shown is specifically for water and would vary in temperature/pressure ranges depending on the molecule or matter being considered. The line in the graph represents the point at which gas (steam) is made at a given temperature and pressure; an example is given in red, where at 101 kPa pressure (which is atmospheric pressure at sea level) steam will form at 100°C. At lower pressures steam is formed at lower temperatures and at higher pressures steam forms at higher temperatures.

(O_3: ozone and H_2O_2: hydrogen peroxide) may form as well as releasing energy (e.g. released as UV light; see the section on light, radiation, and the electromagnetic spectrum).

Mixtures, formulations, and solutions

Solids, liquids, and gases can range in their chemical composition; they can be used on their own (e.g. pure water) or as mixtures. A mixture may be defined as a combination of two or more chemicals into one. The air is an example of a mixture of gases, consisting of approximately (in chemistry this is given as the symbol ~) 78% nitrogen, 21% oxygen, and a range of other gases at much lower amounts (e.g. carbon dioxide, CO_2). It is not quite as simple as that, however, with various other components being present, such as water and various particles (e.g. dust, pollen, and microorganisms). Important examples of liquid and solid mixtures that are used in processing are various types of cleaning or disinfection formulations. A formulation is a mixture of chemicals and can be further defined as a combination of ingredients, including active and inert ingredients, into a product for an intended use. Examples of the various chemicals used in such liquid formulations and the reasons for their use are given in Table 6.2.

It was stated at the opening of this section that solids, liquids, and gases can range in their chemical composition, with some, like pure water (just containing H_2O), being used on their own. It is important to note that water is rarely pure, but is found to have a range of different chemical, microbial, and other contaminants present (Table 6.3; water is discussed in further detail in Chapter 15).

Many chemicals dissolve into water to give a homogeneous (or uniform) mixture that is known as a solution. As an example, take a glass of water and then add common salt (NaCl) to it: the salt will dissolve into the water to give a solution of salt in water. A solution is therefore a homogeneous mixture of two or more chemicals into one. In our example of salt in water, as you continue to add more salt you will eventually reach a point where the water cannot take (or dissolve) any further salt (this is referred to as being saturated or full). If you increase the temperature more salt can be dissolved, but it will fall out of the solution as you reduce the heat; similarly, if you boil the water, the water is removed as steam and the salt will be left behind. Also note that in the example of water there are other components that are not dissolved (not in solution), but are just floating (or "suspended") in the water (Table 6.3).

Note that the terms mixture, formulation, and solution are often used interchangeably to mean similar things, but they do have different chemical definitions (provided earlier).

Weights, measures, and other physical considerations

Units of measurement are used to define quantity (amounts) in chemistry, physics, mathematics, and the sciences in general. We use them in our daily lives, with examples being weights, volumes, and lengths. Some of the more important units are described briefly in this section.

A variety of methods of measurement are used, with the two major systems being imperial and metric. Imperial system units of measurement include pounds (lb) and inches (in), while equivalent units in the metric system are grams (g) and meters (m). Most countries around the world have adopted the International System of Units (SI) as their official units of measurement, which is based on the metric system. Exceptions for example are the United States, where imperial measurements are still widely used, and in the United Kingdom, where the SI system has been adopted but is used in parallel with the imperial system. For the purpose of simplification, SI units are used throughout the book but reference is given to the imperial system (or other widely used units) when considered applicable. In this section, units of measurements from the two systems are introduced. In addition, to convert from one unit to another some mathematical conversion factors are given, but these are not exclusive and may be more readily converted using many of the internet-based conversion sites (such as www.onlineconversion.com).

The basic metric units of measurement are summarized in Table 6.4. It is quite a long list, although there are some that we will use more frequently than others, such as those for temperature (C or K/°C or °K), weights (grams, g), volumes (liters, L), and pressures (pascals, Pa).

Table 6.2 Various different chemical components used in formulations for cleaning and disinfection.

Chemical type	Examples[1]	Formulation use
Water	–	Dissolving other chemicals (for this purpose, water is considered chemically as a "solvent")
Surfactants	Ionic surfactants, amphophilic surfactants	Aid in dissolving and dispersing materials such as soil, including lipids that do not mix with water Assist in cleaning and can have some antimicrobial activity
Chelating agents (or chelants)	EDTA, DTPA, NTA	Bind elements (in particular "heavy" metals) such as calcium and iron By binding they cannot react or interfere with the desired chemical action and can therefore optimize activity (including soil breakdown and damage/inhibiting effects when present in water)
Solvents	Water, alcohols	Dissolving other chemicals or materials
Bases	NaOH, KOH	Make solutions more alkaline and also break down organic materials (by basic hydrolysis)
Acids	Acetic acid, citric acid	Make solutions more acidic and also dissolve inorganic materials
Corrosion inhibitors	Hexamine, benzotriazole	Protect against corrosion (damage) on surfaces
Microbicides (or biocides)	Quaternary ammonium compounds, phenolics, glutaraldehyde, hydrogen peroxide	Microbicides are antimicrobial chemicals and are used to kill (in disinfectants/sterilants) or inhibit (preserve, as preservatives) microorganisms Some may also be used for hydrolysis (soil breakdown)
Enzymes	Proteases, lipases	To break down organic molecules such as proteins and lipids (enzymatic hydrolysis; see the section on cleaning chemistries)

[1] Note: specific chemicals can be given different names (official, trade, descriptive, etc.) and it is usual to abbreviate them to make them easier to refer to. An example is the chemical EDTA, which stands for ethylenediaminetetraacetic acid but also edetic acid, Hampene, or Versene™.

Table 6.3 Examples of various common components that can be found in water. Some components are dissolved (or in solution) in water, while others are suspended (floating in or on water).

Component	Examples
Water	Pure water (H_2O)
Dissolved components	
Inorganic materials	Calcium (Ca), magnesium (Mg), chlorine (Cl_2)/chloride (Cl^-), silicates (molecules with $SiO4^{-4}$), sodium (Na), nitrates (molecules with NO_3^-), iron (Fe)
Organic materials	Pesticides and herbicides, for example trihalomethanes, trichlorethylene, and polychlorinated biphenyls (PCBs)
Gases	Oxygen (O_2), carbon dioxide (CO_2)
Suspended components	
Inorganic materials	Calcium carbonate ($CaCO_2$), clay, silt, silica
Organic materials	Endotoxins, proteins, fats, oil
Microorganisms	Bacteria, viruses, protozoa

One of the benefits of the metric system is that it is based on factors of 10. In the system a prefix can be placed before the unit to make it more practical to write or describe. A summary of some of the most widely used prefixes is given in Table 6.5. These prefixes are based on multiples or divisions of 10 and include terms such as kilo- (e.g. kilogram or kg) and centi- (e.g. centimeter, cm). For example, 1 kg is equal to 1000 g, also written mathematically as 10^3 g; counting the number of zeros, so 10^0 is 1, 10^1 is 10, and so on, and 10^{-1} is 0.1 (in some countries given as 0,1), 10^{-2} is 0.01, and so on. Note that such mathematical terms are also used widely in microbiology, where 10^6 is 1 million or 1,000,000 of, say, a bacteria or

Table 6.4 The SI (metric) units of measurements and other units commonly used.

Quantity	Unit		Other measures
	Name	Symbol[1]	
Area	Square meter (metre)	m²	Acre, square foot
Chemical amount[2]	Mole	mol	
Flow (of volume)[3]	Cubic meters (metres)/second	m³/s	Gallons per hour, cubic feet per minute
Frequency	Hertz	Hz	
Length	Meter (metre)	m	Foot, inch, mile
Mass/weight	Gram	g	Ounce, pound, ton
Power	Watt	W	Horsepower, calorie per second, BTU/min
Pressure	Pascal	Pa	Bar, atmosphere (atm), millimeters of mercury (mmHg), Torr, pounds per square inch (psi)
Speed	Meters (metres)/second	m/s	Miles per hour, knots
Temperature[4]	Kelvin	K	Celsius (C), Fahrenheit (F)
Time[5]	Second	s	
Volume	Cubic meter (metre) or liter (litre)	m³ or L	Cubic inch, gallon, pint, ounce, teaspoon

[1] Any capitalized symbols for units are correctly written as such.
[2] Chemists consider the "amount" of a chemical as different to its weight or volume, referring to "moles" of a chemical.
[3] The symbol / in this context means "per," as in cubic meters per second.
[4] Kelvin (K) is used but not as widely as Celsius (C) or Fahrenheit (F). Note that in both cases they are often referred to as "degrees" of that unit (°F or °C).
[5] A second is the SI unit, but unlike other SI measures it follows the traditional convention of 60 seconds in a minute (min), 60 minutes in an hour (hr), and 24 hours in a day.

Table 6.5 Commonly used prefixes in the SI/metric system for units of measurement. For example, 1 kg is equal to 1000 g but is also written mathematically as 10^3 g, counting the number of zeros and where 10^0 is 1, 10^1 is 10, etc. Also, in divisions of these units, counting the number of decimal places (or numbers after 0.), so 10^{-1} is 0.1, 10^{-2} is 0.01, etc. Therefore 10^{-2} g is 0.01 g and 10^{-3} g is 0.001 g.

Prefix symbol[1]	Name	Factor	Example
Unit multiples			
k	kilo-	10^3, thousand	kg, kilogram
M	mega-	10^6, million	Mm, megameter
G	giga-	10^9, billion	GL, gigaliter
Unit divisions			
c	centi-	10^{-2}, hundredth	cm, centimeter
m	milli-	10^{-3}, thousandth	mm, millimeter
μ	micro-	10^{-6}, millionth	μg, microgram

[1] Any capitalized symbols for units are dcorrectly written as such.

virus population. The more correct term is 1×10^6, where 2×10^6 is 2 million and 10×10^6 is 10 million, or more correctly written as 1×10^7.

A further benefit of SI units is that they are standardized internationally, whereas in older systems some weights and measures could vary in their specific quantity depending on the country of origin (for example, the US and UK gallon and ounce represent different measures/weights in each country).

Thankfully it is now normal process for product suppliers providing instructions on weights and measures to give any local and widely used units in addition to the metric/SI units, to minimize any misunderstanding. Some common conversion factors are provided in Table 6.6 for reference.

As a final consideration, let us look briefly at dilution and dissolution. Diluting is mixing a concentrated liquid product with water to give the intended product concentration for a

Table 6.6 Conversion factors for common units of measurement. Note that it may be more convenient to check with an expert or use simple conversion tools online.

Measurement	Conversion factor
Length	1 foot (international) = 1/3 yard = 12 inches = 0.305 meter 1 m = 100 cm = 1000 mm
Weight	1 stone = 14 pounds (lb) = 6.35 kg 1 ounce (oz) = 28 g 1 kg = 1000 g
Pressure	1 Torr = 1 mmHg = 133.3 Pa 1 psi = 6.89 kPa; 1 atm = 101 kPa; 1 bar = 100 kPa 1 kPa = 1000 Pa Note: atmospheric pressure (at sea level) is ~101.3 kPa = 1 atm = 760 Torr or mmHg = 1 bar
Temperature	1°C = 33.8°F = 274 K. But unlike the other factors, you cannot simply multiply to get the correct conversion. To convert between the two major units (C and F) use: °C = (°F−32)/1.8 °F = °C × 1.8 = 32
Volume (of liquid)[1]	1 gallon (imperial) = 160 fluid ounces (fl oz) = 4.546 L 1 gallon (US) = 128 fl oz = 3.785 L 1 L = 1000 mL = 1000 cm^3 (therefore 1 mL = 1 cm^3)

[1] Note: the conversion of the volume of liquid using non-metric units may be different depending on whether it is the volume of a solid/liquid and on where you live (e.g. a "gallon" in the United States can be a dry or liquid gallon and both are different to the imperial gallon).

given application (e.g. for cleaning or disinfection). In chemical use it is important that the instructions for diluting a product are closely followed to prevent waste of the product (if too much being used for the application), where damage can occur (again, if too much product is used), or where the product is not going to be effective (too little product is used or "under-dilution"). Instructions are normally given on a product label and/or instructions as a certain volume or weight of a product mixed with a volume/weight of water. Examples include:

- g/L: weight of the product (liquid or solid) in a liter of water. For example, 1 g/L (one gram per liter) is 1 g in a final volume of 1 liter of water, which is the same as 50 g/50 L if making up a final desired volume of 50 L.
- mL/L: volume of the product in a volume (liter) of water. For example, 10 mL/L is made up by taking 10 mL of the product and adding water until you make 1 L (i.e. 10 mL product +990 mL water).
- %: percent, being a weight or volume in 100 mL of water, such that 1% is 1 mL in a final volume of 100 mL (i.e. 1 mL + 99 mL water). In this case it is common to see terms such as v/v and w/v, referring to volume in a volume or weight in a volume. As an example, 1% v/v would mean measuring a volume of 1 mL and adding 99 mL of water; in the case of w/v the weight of a product is added to water to give a final volume of 100 mL.

In all cases it is important that the liquid product is well mixed to ensure it is diluted correctly. Dissolution is where a solid product is added to water. In certain situations a product is given in two parts, which are mixed together (sometimes, but not always, including water) for the desired product; in these cases the chemical product may require a reaction time to be ready for use and will always require adequate mixing to ensure the product is correctly prepared. Overall it can be quite complicated, but remember these rules: follow the manufacturer's written instructions on how to prepare chemistries for their desired use; and if you do not understand the instructions, ask for assistance.

The pH scale: defining acids and bases

Chemists use a variety of ways to study and analyze chemicals and solutions. One such measurement is known as pH, which is a measure of how acidic or alkaline a liquid or solution is. The strict chemical understanding of pH is that it is a measure of the hydrogen ion (H^+) concentration in a solution, but this can be a bit complex. What it is important to understand is that the pH scale ranges from 0 to 14 (Figure 6.5) and that all liquids will fall somewhere on this scale. The mid-range of the scale is at 7, at which a liquid is considered "neutral," while the more acidic the liquid the lower the number ("strong acid") and the more alkaline (or basic) the higher the number ("strong alkali/base").

An example of a neutral liquid is drinking water (if it is correctly provided), which is generally in the neutral range (pH 6–8). Another is blood, which is generally circulated in the body at a pH of about 7.4 (this can also be referred to as

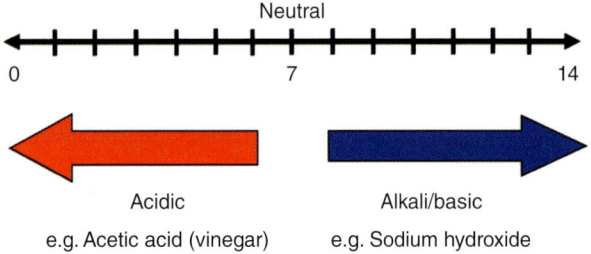

Figure 6.5 The pH scale. Note: it is correct to write the p in lower case and the H in upper case. Neutral is to the center (pH 6–8) of the range, with acids to the left (<6) and alkali (or bases; >8) to the right. At lower levels of pH liquids are considered more acidic and at higher levels of pH they are considered more alkaline/basic.

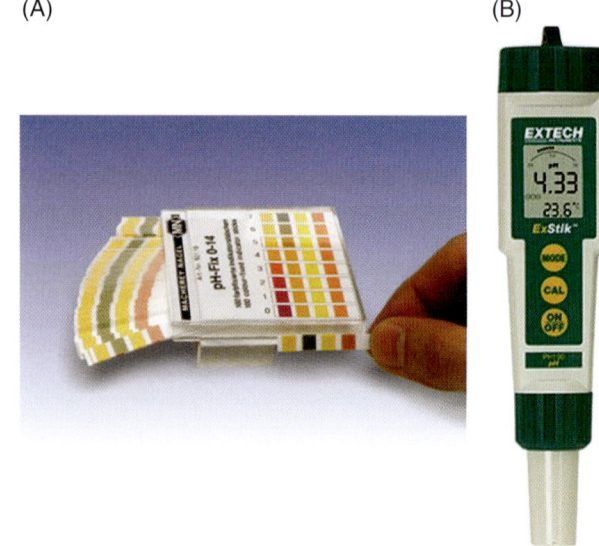

Figure 6.6 Examples of methods used to measure pH. (A) pH paper and its associated color chart (where the color developed on placing the paper into the solution is matched to the chart); (B) a pH probe, which is placed into the solution and gives a digital readout of the pH.

being slightly alkaline). As liquids are measured to be more acidic (<6) or alkaline/basic (>8), they are considered more aggressive on surfaces. Some common types of acids are vinegar (which is a dilute or watered-down version of an acid known as acetic acid, which has the chemical formula CH_3COOH or is also written as $C_2H_4O_2$), orange juice, and lemon juice, composed of citric acid, $C_6H_8O_7$, and ascorbic acid (vitamin C), $C_6H_8O_6$. Hydrochloric acid (HCl) is produced by the body in the stomach, which gives the stomach contents an acidic pH to aid in the digestive process (see Chapter 2). Examples of alkaline liquids are bleach solutions (a mixture of a chemical known as sodium hypochlorite, NaOCl, in water) and many types of liquid soaps and detergents. It should be noted that the difference, for example, between a solution of pH 6 and pH 5 is larger than it seems because it is what is referred to as a "log" scale. A log scale means that for every 1 unit increase or decrease in pH the actual scale is 10 times different; therefore, an acid at pH 2 is 10 times more acidic than at pH 3 and 100 times than at pH 4.

Acids and bases are used for a variety of decontamination purposes, including cleaning, disinfection, and sterilization; however, it is unusual to see them used as just pure acids or bases. Examples of a pure acid solution would be dilutions of hydrochloric acid, citric acid, or peracetic acid. These acids are particularly good at dissolving inorganic salts (e.g. calcium carbonate, a major component of water hardness or "scale"; see Chapter 15, the section on water quality and purity), and peracetic acid is an efficacious antimicrobial chemical (see Chapter 9, the section on peroxygens). Although they could all be used for cleaning and disinfection purposes, they would also be considered damaging to many device materials. It is for these reasons that they are used in combination with other chemicals in formulations, which are designed to give the benefit of the acid but minimize the negative effects. Similarly, alkalines such as sodium hydroxide (NaOH) and potassium hydroxide (KOH) are extremely good for breaking down and removing organic materials (e.g. proteins) from surfaces, therefore they would be efficient cleaners (in removing blood and other materials from surfaces after surgical procedures); but they are also considered aggressive and are optimally used in formulations for the same reasons. Another common use of pH in formulation is to help other chemicals be efficient for their desired use. An example mentioned earlier is in bleach solutions; bleach is a mixture of sodium hypochlorite in water, where the hypochlorite provides or releases chlorine for its antimicrobial properties. Solutions of peracetic acid are used for antimicrobial purposes, where although the pH of a peracetic acid solution on its own is very low (<pH 2), in typical disinfectants and sterilants it will be closer to a neutral pH; in this way they are less aggressive on surfaces, but still are effective at killing microorganisms. Acidic pH is an important condition for the optimization of the efficacy of some hydrogen peroxide–based disinfectants. A common term used to describe this is a "buffer," itself a type of chemistry that is used to control the pH to its desired level.

The pH of a solution can be conveniently measured using pH paper (which changes color when placed in the solution and is compared to a color chart to match the pre-defined pH level) or using a handheld probe (Figure 6.6). Note that the pH can vary depending on the temperature; therefore, it is common for pH measurement to be conducted at an ambient temperature (~20°C) or for the temperature to be stated with the pH measurement.

Other common chemical measurement methods

The variety of techniques that chemists use to study and analyze chemicals and solutions help them determine what types ("qualitative") and how much ("quantitative") of various chemicals are present in each sample of a gas, liquid, or solid. Therefore, as an example, in a chemical analysis of a water sample one could say qualitatively that there was carbon and chlorine present, but quantitatively there was 240 and 20 mg/L, respectively. Analytical chemistry is the use of these techniques to study chemical composition. Several further examples of these methods are now discussed in brief, with particular emphasis on methods you may come across in use in, or being conducted for, a processing department.

Sampling
A sample is simply a small amount of any solid, liquid, or gas taken for analysis (e.g. a water sample). There are two important considerations in sampling that should be understood. The first is that the analysis of a sample is only as good as the person taking or collecting the sample; if, for example, a water sample is taken in a dirty bottle (remembering that chemical dirt may or may not be visible to the eye), it will be contaminated and give a wrong result when analyzed. The second is that any sample taken is only representative at the time it was taken. A typical example is with water: most facilities will have two sources of water, hot and cold, and the chemical quality of both can change even over a day, and considerably over a year.

Titration
Titration is a quantitative method to determine the concentration of a chemical/type of chemistry in a sample. It is also known as "volumetric analysis." In a typical titration a defined, known chemical (a "reagent," since it reacts) is added to the sample being analyzed to react with it (e.g. to change its pH, which can give a color change in the presence of a dye not dissimilar to those used for pH measurements; see the section on the pH scale: defining acids and bases). By then adding a measured amount of another chemical, in this example to change the pH to a certain point to allow a color change, the final amount of this chemical added is related to the original amount of the chemical being analyzed. Examples of the use of titration in water analysis include the measurement of water hardness and chlorine levels (Figure 6.7).

Conductivity
Conductivity is a quantitative method used to measure the ability to conduct electricity (specifically electrical conductivity or EC, as the term can also refer to heat or even sound

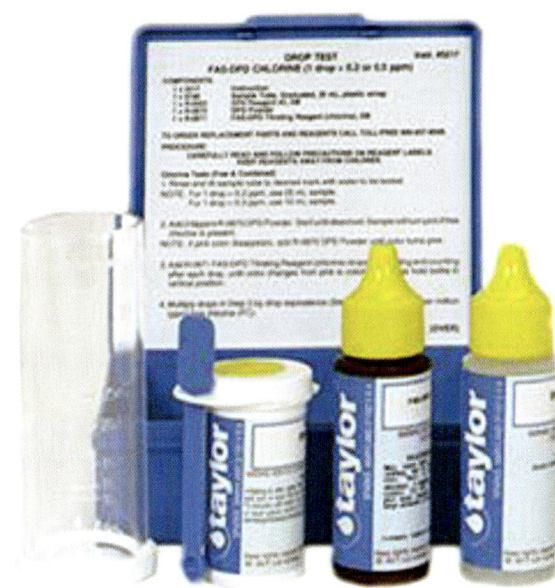

Figure 6.7 Example of a titration kit for chlorine analysis.

conductivity). It is measured in microSiemens per centimeter (μSi/m or μSi m^2), but is often also given as millimhos per centimeter (mmho/cm). It is a simple, but indirect, method for estimating the amount of various types of charged contaminants in a sample (particularly metals such as iron, copper, and silver, and other elements like chlorine and silicates). A good example is the conductivity of water, where the higher the measured conductivity the greater the level of charged chemicals present. An example of a conductivity meter is given in Figure 6.8. Conductivity is often directly compared to another analysis method, total dissolved solids (TDS).

Total dissolved solids
TDS is the measurement of all organic and inorganic substances in a liquid. A simple way of thinking about this is to take a water sample and boil off all the water, with whatever remains being the TDS. This will include various elements (calcium, iron), suspended molecules (phosphates, nitrates), and other materials. It is therefore a measure of all chemicals in a sample (given as mg/L) and can be estimated in relation to EC, as the more chemicals present the greater the conductivity. It is typical for a conductivity probe to be used to estimate both conductivity (in μSi/m) and TDS (in mg/L).

Total organic carbon
In its simplest terms, total organic carbon (TOC) is the measure of the amount of organic carbon present in a sample. It is generally used to estimate the quality of a sample, in particular water cleanliness, and for surface cleaning evaluation. Carbon

molecules are the basis for any type of human, plant, animal, and even microbial contamination, but also other chemistries that can be present, such as herbicides, detergents, and some disinfectants (e.g. phenols and aldehydes). Note that TOC only gives the total amount of organic carbon present, not any further information on the exact types or sources of carbon.

Inductively coupled plasma mass spectrometry

Measurements such as conductivity and TOC are gross estimates of chemicals that can be present and are not very specific. Inductively coupled plasma mass spectrometry (ICP-MS) analysis is an example of a very specific measurement method. It is capable of determining the types and amounts of metals and non-metals (i.e. sulfur, phosphorus, chlorine, bromine, etc.) present in a sample even at extremely low concentrations. It is beyond the scope of this book to describe the exact method, but it includes preparing the sample and then introducing it into a specific machine for the analysis.

Light, radiation, and the electromagnetic spectrum

One branch of chemistry and physics is the study of light. "Light" is actually more than what we see with our eyes, which is known as "visible" or white light. In technical terms it refers to the electromagnetic spectrum (Figure 6.9).

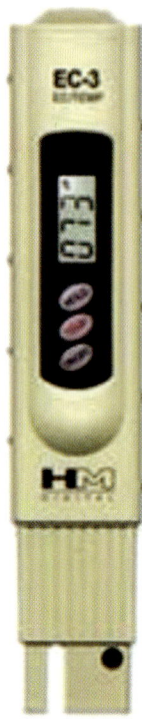

Figure 6.8 Example of a handheld conductivity meter.

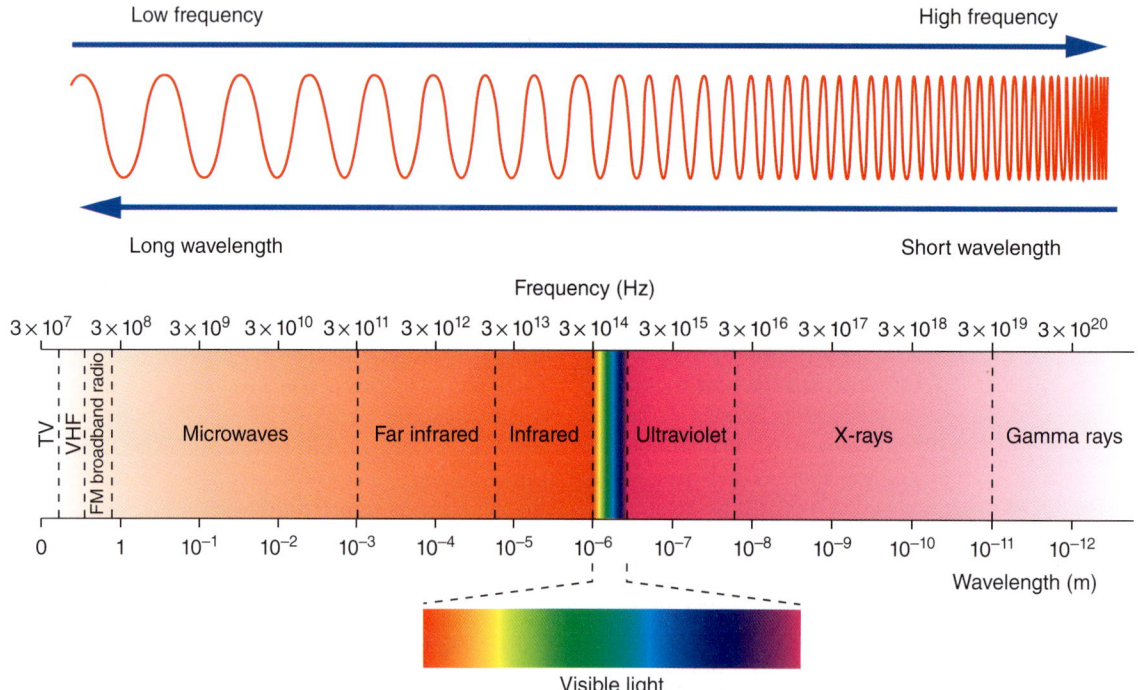

Figure 6.9 Various forms of light or the electromagnetic spectrum. As you move from left to right, the energy level associated with the type of light (or "frequency") increases. The shorter the wavelength, the greater the energy.

Various forms of light are used for antimicrobial purposes, including microwaves and infrared (IR), both as methods of heating, and UV, X-rays, and γ-rays (which can be used for antimicrobial purposes due to their higher energy levels; Figure 6.9). Microwaves, IR, and UV light can be used indirectly or directly as disinfection methods in hospitals and other clinical facilities. X-rays and γ-rays are not commonly or practically used in such facilities for such applications, but are used for industrial disinfection/sterilization (e.g. for single-use devices that are provided pre-sterilized to a hospital); as antimicrobial technologies, they are not considered further in this book.

Safety considerations

Various types of chemicals are used in clinical facilities, including those for cleaning, disinfection, and sterilization. They are designed to disrupt, remove, damage, breakdown, and/or inactivate various materials (or soils) that remain on a device surface from patients after surgical, medical, or dental use. It should therefore not come as any surprise that these chemicals can and usually are also dangerous to human health, as we are made up of the same types of basic molecules. As a general statement, all chemicals can do you harm under the right conditions. Some of these are obvious, such as strong acids and alkalis (see the section on the pH scale: defining acids and bases), which can give a direct, quick, and even serious burn when placed on the skin. Others will be more subtle, with some extreme cases leading to increased allergic reactions (sensitization), toxic effects or damage over time, and carcinogenicity ("cancer-causing," where a carcinogen is a cancer-causing agent/chemical). Even chemicals we take for granted can lead to problems, for example common table salt (NaCl) when taken at high doses in your diet can be damaging to your health. The lesson to learn from this discussion is to respect the use of chemicals and take the necessary precautions to limit your exposure to them.

Concerning chemical safety there are at least three considerations:
• Personal safety.
• Patient safety, which can be associated with chemicals remaining on a device surface (e.g. not being rinsed away) or that could damage the device.
• Environmental safety, which is becoming a growing concern internationally.

Personal safety is the responsibility of each employee to ensure that chemicals are correctly handled, but also the responsibility of supervisors/managers to ensure that their employees are aware of any safety risks and have been given the correct training and equipment to minimize those risks. Note that this may not apply only to those working in each area but also to visitors in the area, as many chemical accidents happen to those in the vicinity of someone using a chemical.

There are four steps to consider in establishing and maintaining good personal safety practices when using chemicals:
• Identify and understand the chemical risks in each area. Good sources are product labels, manufacturer's safety data sheets (SDSs), etc.
• Decide what precautions are necessary (e.g. ventilation, eye or face protection, monitoring systems).
• Introduce and train on any procedures or control mechanisms to prevent or control exposure.
• Ensure that procedures/measures are used and are maintained (e.g. by auditing).

It is good practice (if not a legal requirement in most countries) for safety information to be provided with each chemical product. This is usually provided with the product label; note that a product label can include what is physically written on the product (the attached label) but also any other accessory information such as additional instructions for use, the SDS, and technical literature.

The label (in all its parts) is an excellent source of information, but many of us pay little attention to the detail provided. It can provide information on how the product should be used (e.g. correct dilution or not diluted but ready for use), any safety risks/symbols, storage and disposal considerations, and any immediate steps (or first aid) that can be taken on exposure (e.g. eye/skin contact or accidental swallowing). As labeling requirements vary from country to country, the label itself may not actually provide all the correct safety information; in these cases it is recommended to request further information from the supplier or even to change suppliers/products. Internationally, for example, there is a series of standardized warning symbols that can be used to recognize certain health risks associated with a product (Figure 6.10).

In general, the most effective ways to reduce the risks associated with any chemical in use are training, using personal protective equipment (PPE), and periodic auditing of areas to confirm that safety practices are being followed in that department. Training is the first step, to allow any chemical user to understand their risks and for them to appreciate how PPE or other safety precautions can reduce those risks. PPE includes equipment such as gloves, safety glasses or goggles, face shields, and disposable aprons (Figure 6.11; see Chapter 13). Note, for example, that safety glasses are usually designed to protect the eyes from splashes from the front as well as from the sides.

The final step is safety auditing. Auditing can be defined as an evaluation or review of practices based on established procedures. When safety policies and procedures are put in place it is important to review over time that they are being followed. Audits can be defined at intervals, in cases where they are expected or, more beneficially, unexpected; they help establish

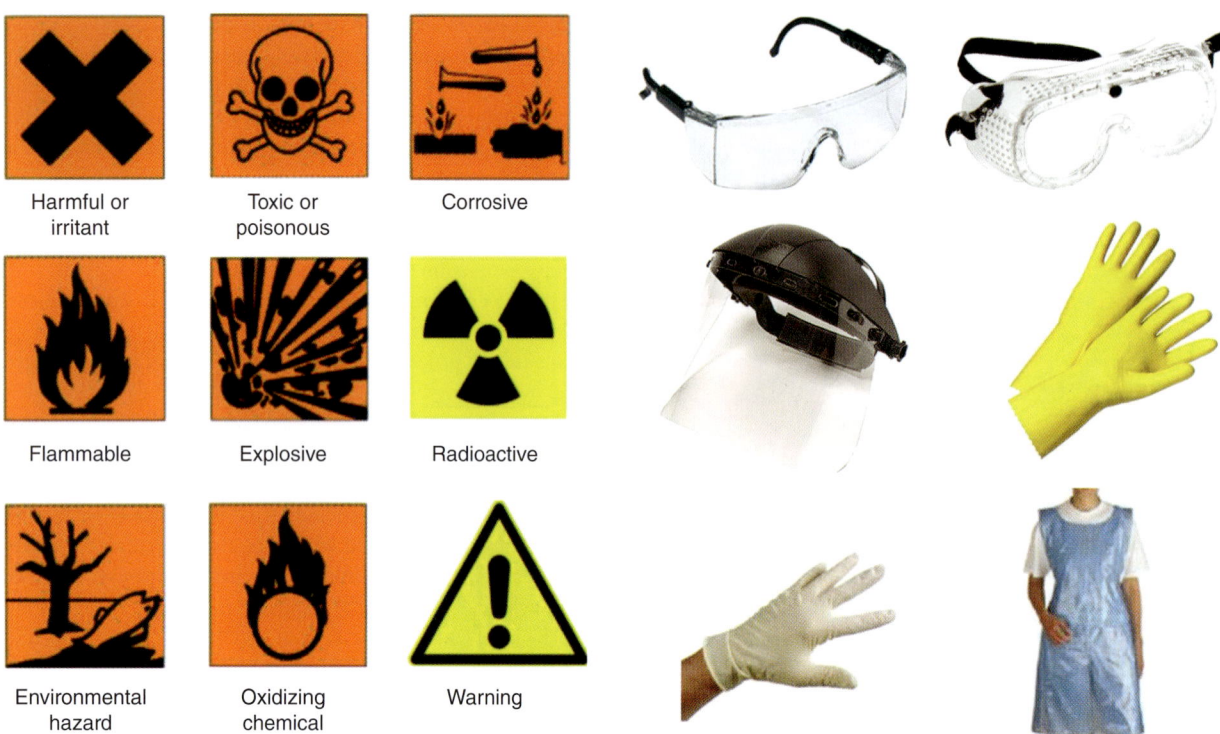

Figure 6.10 Some examples of widely used internationally standardized chemical safety warning symbols.

Figure 6.11 Various types of personal protective equipment (PPE).

that safety is important in an area and that staff/management are committed to it.

Specific chemicals may require further and even tighter controls. Examples include the use of various types of gases such as ethylene oxide (for sterilization; see Chapter 11) or aldehyde-based liquid disinfectants like glutaraldehyde (see Chapter 9). Ethylene oxide gas, for example, is considered flammable/explosive at concentrations of ~3% gas in air, can be lethal at 800 ppm, and is considered a carcinogen (cancer causing) on exposure over time. For this reason, reasonably tight controls and monitoring systems are strongly suggested in areas using the gas for sterilization.

In addition to personal safety, there are chemical risks to patients and to the environment. Patient chemical risks should be minimized by correct use and removal of chemicals used for processing or maintaining the device. Patient risks will include direct and indirect safety concerns. A direct concern is where a chemical is mistakenly used and left on a device prior to the use in/on a patient; in these cases, toxic effects can be observed in the patient, leading to health consequences. Examples can include overuse of the chemical (e.g. not diluted correctly) and inadequate rinsing (to remove the chemical after use). Many chemical disinfectants, for example, require multiple cycles of water rinsing (sometimes up to five to six rinses in fresh water each time) to adequately remove toxic residues of the chemistry. Indirect effects are due to damage by the chemical to the device; this damage, over time, can lead to problems in the safe use of the instrument on a patient.

Environmental safety in the use of chemicals is a growing concern internationally, with many countries putting greater restrictions on the types of chemicals that can be used. The main concern lies with those chemicals that are not easily broken down in the environment and can therefore lead to accumulation or other issues in environmental sources (such as water, the air, and plants/animals).

How to choose and use a chemical product

In deciding to use any chemical or chemical-containing product, there should always be three considerations: safety, compatibility, and efficacy. Safety has been addressed in the section on safety considerations, and includes safety for the person using the chemical, for the patient, and for the environment. Compatibility is the ability of the chemical to be used on a device and the materials it is made from without any significant damage. This is discussed separately in this section.

Device compatibility is an important aspect: a chemical has little benefit if it is used for its intended purpose but also damages/destroys the device. This can be a difficult area to address as it may vary depending on the chemical, its formulation, the temperature, or even the pressure used. Equally, it can vary depending on the various types of metals, plastics, glass, adhesives, and so on in a device. Compatibility (or more specifically the opposite, incompatibility) can be obvious to the eye in many cases, but may not be in others and may only show an impact over time. If plastics or adhesives are thermo-sensitive (sensitive to heat) they will obviously be damaged if the device is heat disinfected or steam sterilized, rendering them unfit for future use. An example includes rusting of stainless steel devices (formed from the reaction of iron, which is in stainless steel, with oxygen, to form a red-brown color, chemically known as ferric oxide); rusting forms where there is existing damage (scratching, wear and tear) on the device surface that allows for oxygen to react with exposed iron and can develop over time until we can see it. This leads to corrosion of the device. Note that the physical signs of rusting can be removed (see Chapter 15) but not the underlying damage. Device and chemical/process manufacturers are a good source of information regarding device compatibility.

Efficacy (or effectiveness for a given task) is the main reason a chemical product is used, such as for cleaning, disinfection, sterilization, or other uses (e.g. lubrication that allows the devices to be correctly used). It is important to remember that chemical products vary considerably in formulation, despite even having similar main, active ingredients; therefore, close inspection should be made of product claims to ensure that they are used correctly and are fit for purpose. For example, it would not be good practice to use an antiseptic product that has been developed and labeled for use on the skin (e.g. chlorhexidine- and iodine-based products used for surgical hand washing prior to surgery by operating room staff) for cleaning devices following their use in a surgical procedure. Equally, the presence of the chemical or chemical product alone may not ensure efficacy if it is not used with the right process conditions: time, temperature, concentration, and so on. These conditions should be defined by the product manufacturer and specified in the labeling provided with the product.

Although safety, compatibility, and efficacy are essential to consider, there are other requirements, many of which may be specific to each facility depending on its local, regional, and/or country-specific requirements. These include that a chemical product has been registered or approved for use in a given country or regional area, that the product is cost effective, and whether it can be routinely used for the given application (e.g. reasonable contact time). All these considerations are important in choosing the right chemical product for specific stages in device processing.

Introduction to cleaning and accessory chemistries

Cleaning is the removal of contamination (or "soil") from an item to the extent necessary for its further processing and its intended subsequent use. It is usually enabled using a cleaning chemistry, in addition to physical and other process effects such as spraying, brushing, flushing, or temperature control. Further, detailed consideration is given to cleaning in Chapter 8. In this section a brief introduction is made to the types of chemistries that are used for cleaning, as well as different types of accessory chemicals (e.g. for lubrication or to aid in drying) that are used during processing.

Patient soil

The target for cleaning is the removal of patient soil, which can be made up of a variety of components, including organic and inorganic materials from the patient or chemicals used during the procedure (e.g. gels, lubricants, cements, etc.; Table 6.7). The primary contaminant found on reusable devices following surgical or endoscopic use is protein, from contact with patient tissues (Chapter 2), but many other contaminants can be present depending on how the device was used.

Classification of cleaning chemistries

Cleaning chemistries can be classified in two main ways: based on the main types of active chemicals that are present and/or how they are used during processing. First and foremost, cleaning chemistries are formulations of chemistries for their intended use. They can include the main active ingredients such as enzymes, alkalis, and acids, but also other components that combine together to aid in the cleaning process.

Let us first consider the classification based on how they are used. The same product can often be used for multiple

Table 6.7 Examples of various components of soil found on devices following use on/in patients.

Organic materials	Inorganic materials
Blood, mucus, feces, urine	Salts, such as NaCl
Tissues, such as those in skin, muscles, etc.	Metals, including iron
Proteins, carbohydrates, lipids/fats, lipopolysaccharides[1]	Other elements and molecules, such as calcium and iodine
Microorganisms such as bacteria, viruses, and fungi	Cements (used in orthopedic procedures)
Gels and lubricants	

[1] A lipopolysaccharide is a molecule that includes a lipid ("lipo") and polysaccharide (carbohydrate) part.

purposes, for instance for transport, manual or pre-cleaning, and automated cleaning. Cleaning chemistries can be used or designed for:

- Point-of-use treatment and transport: these can include liquids, foam-, or gel-based products that limit soil on devices from drying while being transported to a defined area for processing. In addition to preventing drying, these products may also inhibit the growth of bacteria and fungi, protect the device from damage (due to the presence of soil), and initiate the cleaning process.
- Pre-cleaning or manual cleaning: used directly at the point of use (e.g. at or adjacent to a surgical site) or in a defined processing area for manual cleaning, usually in a sink or basin. They are also used in ultrasonic baths to aid in the ultrasonic cleaning process (Chapter 8).
- Automated cleaning: used in a washer or washer-disinfector machine for cleaning (Chapter 8).
- Accessory cleaning: specific chemistries used to remove certain soil components, such as acid cleaners to remove rusting or dissolve water hardness accumulation, or used for a particular accessory application such as neutralization (where some high alkaline products used for cleaning need to be returned to a neutral pH, despite being drained and rinsed), lubrication (applied particularly to moving parts to allow the device to operate correctly and smoothly), and drying aids (to speed up the drying process following cleaning disinfection).

As stated earlier, patient soil can include a variety of complex materials such as blood, various tissues, lipids/fats, proteins, and so on. These can be difficult to remove by water alone, as only some will be water soluble or immiscible ("hydrophilic," meaning water loving) while others will be water insoluble ("hydrophobic," meaning water hating). Cleaning chemistries provide different ways to aid in the removal of such soils when used in combination with the right cleaning process conditions (e.g. temperature and time). These include:

- Hydrolysis: the breakdown of larger molecules into smaller molecules that are easier to remove by cleaning. Hydrolysis can be achieved in some cases by heat alone, but is most effective in cleaning processes that use acids, bases, and various types of enzymes (see the section on enzyme-based cleaners).
- Solubility: the ability to be dissolved (or go into solution; see the section on mixtures, formulations and solutions). The chemical being dissolved is called the "solute" and it is being dissolved into the "solvent." Water, for example, is a great solvent for many chemicals such as salt (NaCl, the solute).
- Wetting: the ability to spread over a surface. By wetting, a cleaning product can contact a greater surface area and improve interaction with surfaces/materials that may be hydrophobic ("water hating"). Surfactants (see the section on mixtures, formulations and solutions) are both good wetting and emulsification agents.

- Emulsification: a substance/liquid to be dispersed (in small, fine droplets) within another liquid. This allows for soils to be mixed with water that would normally be repelled by water (such as a lipid in water emulsion). The soils are dispersed (suspended) not dissolved (solubilized), thereby they can be removed with water-based processes.
- Dispersion: for one component to be mixed with another (but not dissolved). Examples include emulsions/emulsification.
- Chelation: binding elements (in particular "heavy" metals such as calcium and iron; see the section on mixtures, formulations, and solutions). Such heavy metals can interfere with the cleaning process and have other negative effects on device surfaces.

Other chemicals that can be found in cleaning chemistry formulations are considered in the section on mixtures, formulations, and solutions.

Cleaning chemicals can also be classified based on the type of chemistry, or indeed the main mechanism of hydrolysis, that is used for their cleaning activity. They are:

- Enzyme-based chemistries.
- Non-enzyme-based chemistries, including acid, neutral, or alkaline/basic chemistries.

It is important to note that these terms are not exclusive: enzymatic chemistries can be used at acid, neutral, or alkaline conditions. Also, a cleaning formulation can include further mixtures, where, for example, enzymes may be present as one mechanism but also a non-enzyme-based hydrolysis mechanism may be in place as a separate mechanism.

Enzyme-based cleaners

In the introduction to Chapter 2 the four basic types of molecules that make up the structures of the variety of cells found in our bodies were discussed: proteins, lipids, carbohydrates, and nucleic acids. Proteins are important because they play essential roles not only in the structure of cells but also in their function. A group of proteins involved in these functions are known as "enzymes." An enzyme is a protein molecule that speeds up a chemical reaction (but is not changed in the process); they are therefore examples of catalysts, any chemical that can speed up a chemical reaction. Enzymes are thus often referred to as biological catalysts. They are responsible for making and breaking down different parts of the cell over time, including the variety of proteins, lipids, carbohydrates, and nucleic acids that exist. For example, when we eat food it is the variety of enzymes (as well as chemicals) found in the digestive tract (Chapter 2) that break down the food into smaller parts, which then allows the body to adsorb them into the blood system for use around the body. It is the ability of some of these enzymes to break down these molecules (known as "substrates") that makes them useful for cleaning purposes. A description of how enzymes work is given in Figure 6.12.

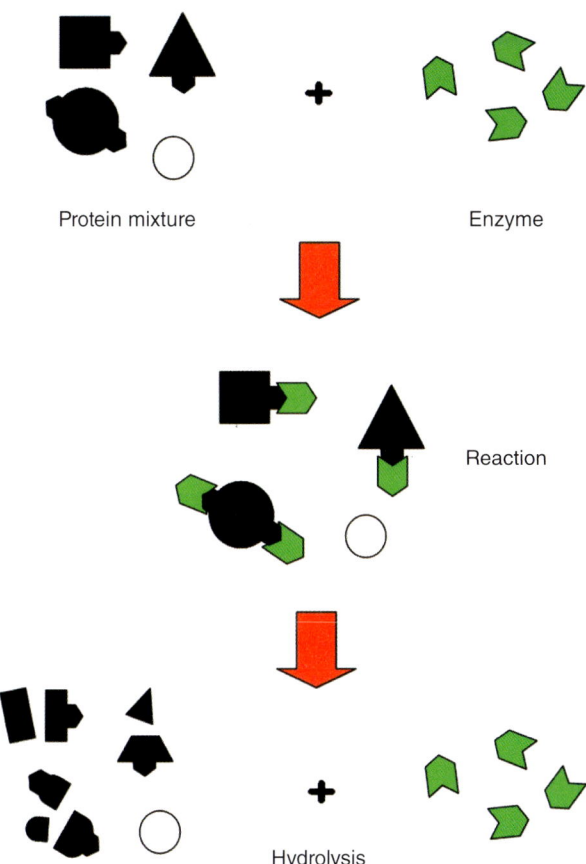

Figure 6.12 The mechanism of action of enzymes. Note: target molecules (e.g. proteins or lipids) are only broken down if they react with the enzyme and the enzyme remains unchanged after the reaction.

Table 6.8 Various types and examples of enzymes commonly used for cleaning purposes.

Enzyme type	Target substrate[1]	Example
Protease	Protein	Alcalase, savinase, properase
Carbohydrases		
Amylase	Amylose, a type of carbohydrate	α-amylase, purastar
Cellulase	Cellulose, a type of carbohydrate found in plants	Fungal cellulose, Cellusoft®
Lipase	Lipids	Lipolase

[1] The "substrate" is the material on which an enzyme acts.

For an enzyme to act it first must be able to recognize a target on the molecule; this target is called an active site. When the enzyme binds, it causes a breakdown in the structure of the molecule, releasing the enzyme. The enzyme remains unchanged (and can proceed to react with other molecules), while the original substrate is broken down into fragments. Some enzymes are very specific in how they work, only being effective against some types of target molecules, "substrates," while others have a wider range of activity. Generally, those with a broader range of activity are used for cleaning purposes.

Enzymes are further classified depending on the types of molecules that they target. Some of the more common types are given in Table 6.8. In general, they are named by adding the suffix "-ase" to the type of substrate they attack, for instance proteases refer to enzymes that attack proteins and lipases attack lipids. In the case of proteases, note that these enzymes are proteins themselves but break down other types of proteins. This is due to differences in their structure. It is also important that although enzymes such as proteases and lipases used in cleaning applications can react with a wide range of substrates, there may be many types of proteins and lipids that are not affected by these enzymes (as shown in Figure 6.12). Enzymes are also given commercial names by companies that manufacture them as well as official names that describe their type of enzymatic function.

As biological catalysts, enzymes are not only specific in their mechanisms of action but their optimal activity is very dependent on how they are used, with specific variables such as:

- Contact time and enzyme concentration (or right amount/quantity of enzyme). They need to be present and have the time to penetrate and react with soils to be effective.
- Temperature: enzymes are very sensitive to the effects of temperature, with each type of enzyme having an optimum range in which they work best. Lower temperatures would make them less efficient, higher temperatures stop them from working.
- Other conditions are required for them to be "active," such as the correct pH range (acid, alkaline, or neutral conditions), which will be specific to the type of enzyme.

Non-enzyme-based cleaners

Non-enzymatic cleaning formulations can be used on a variety of other chemical methods to remove and/or hydrolyze soils. These various components have been discussed in the section on classification of cleaning chemistries. Chemicals that hydrolyze soils when used correctly in formulation can include oxidizing agents (e.g. sodium hypochlorite, a source of chlorine, hydrogen peroxide, and peracetic acid), acids, alkalis, and other specific chemicals (such as urea). In general, unlike enzymes, these chemical agents are considered less specific in their mechanisms of action. Oxidizing agents are not widely used for cleaning applications in healthcare facilities but have been used successfully in some parts of the world. More commonly used chemicals are acids and alkalis/bases. Acids and bases have been previously discussed in the section on the pH scale: defining acids and bases. Their specific applications as cleaning mechanisms are further discussed in this section.

Acid-based cleaners are considered to have a pH of <7 and are moderately acidic (pH 4–7) or strongly acidic (pH <4). They are used for the removal (dissolution) of inorganic materials such as various types of salts. Specific examples include the removal of hardness (such as calcium carbonate, $CaCO_3$; "descaling") or rust (ferric oxide, FeO_2) deposits that can build up or form on instrument, washer-disinfector, sink, and steam sterilizer surfaces. Acid cleaners are also used as neutralizers following cleaning with some types of high-alkaline cleaners, where high-alkaline conditions are returned to a neutral pH before proceeding with further reprocessing.

Alkaline/basic chemistries are formulated to have pH levels of >7, ranging from being moderately alkaline (pH 7–10) to highly alkaline (pH 10–14). They are particularly effective at removing organic materials, including proteins and lipids, from surfaces. A variety of types of alkalis can be used in these products and they work by assisting in the removal as well as the hydrolysis of soils. In general, the higher the pH the more aggressive the product will be on surface and soil removal, but this is not always the case and will depend on the product label. Moderate- and high-alkaline products are widely used for manual and particularly automated cleaning processes.

Other types of chemicals are used for cleaning purposes, to aid in the physical removal of soil from a surface although without necessarily causing hydrolysis on the soil. They include various types of detergents and solvents, as examples of solubilization/dispersion/emulsification agents. Others are used to control the effects of poor-quality water (such as using chelating agents to control calcium ions that can interfere with the cleaning process) to ensure the formulation is effective. As stated before, these are used in combination with or without hydrolysis chemicals in cleaning formulations.

Introduction to antimicrobial (disinfection/sterilization) chemistries

A wide variety of chemicals are used for their antimicrobial purposes. Some of these are used as drugs (or anti-infectives) to treat infections in or on patients, such as antibiotics (these are specific drugs against bacteria and some types of fungi), antifungals, and antiviral drugs. But an even wider range of chemicals are used for antiseptic, disinfection, and sterilization applications. These chemicals are commonly known as "biocides," "microbicides," or in certain areas of the world may be called pesticides (a pest being another term to include microorganisms). They are used due to their ability to inhibit (-static activity, such as bacteriostatic and fungistatic) and/or kill (-cidal, such as bactericidal and viricidal) various types of microorganism. The science of microbiology has already been discussed in Chapter 5 and includes various types of infectious/disease-causing agents such as prions, viruses, bacteria, fungi, protozoa, and helminths. This section will discuss the various types and uses of chemical biocides in microbial control.

Classification of microbiocides

Microbiocides can be classified based on their primary mechanisms of action (i.e. how they kill microorganisms), their specific chemical type, and how they are used in healthcare applications. A summary of their primary mechanisms of action (how they kill) and chemical types are given in Table 6.9.

The basic chemical types include groups of elements known as the "halogens," with examples including chlorine and iodine, and molecules such as the aldehydes, alcohols, phenolics, and peroxygens. These chemicals are rarely used on their own but are combined with other components in liquid-, gel-, or foam-formulated products (such as liquid disinfectants) and/or as part of defined processes (e.g. gases used for disinfection and/or sterilization such as ethylene oxide, hydrogen peroxide,

Table 6.9 Examples of the basic types of chemicals (biocides) used for antimicrobial purposes. These are classified based on their major mechanisms of action against microorganisms and their chemical type.

Mechanism of action	Chemical types	Examples
Structure disruption	Surfactants	Quaternary ammonium compounds, anionics
	Biguanides	Chlorhexidine, polyhexamethylbiguanide (PHMB)
	Metals	Copper, silver
Oxidizing agents	Halogens	Chlorine, iodine
	Peroxygens	Peracetic acid, hydrogen peroxide, chlorine dioxide, ozone
Cross-linking/ coagulating agents	Aldehydes	Glutaraldehyde, formaldehyde, ortho-phthaldehyde (OPA)
	Alkylating agent	Ethylene oxide
	Phenolics	2-phenylphenol, cresols, triclosan
	Alcohols	Ethanol, isopropanol

and formaldehyde). For many of these biocides it is unknown exactly how they work against microorganisms and their various components, but they may be considered to be generally toxic/damaging to microorganisms. Some, such as the surfactants (in particular a group of biocides known as quaternary ammonium compounds, QACs, also known as QUATs) specifically target the cell membranes (Chapter 5) of bacteria and fungi, leading to disruption of their structure and function. Others, such as glutaraldehyde and formaldehyde, react with various proteins found on the surface of microorganisms and can cause them to "cross-link" (or attach to each other), therefore losing their essential functions. These examples are simplified in that each individual type of microbiocide will range in its ability to inactivate microorganisms. Consider, for example, the QACs: there are many different types (chemical structures) of QACs and other types of surfactants available that have a range of antimicrobial activities; they are often used in combination with each other and/or with other types of microbiocides to give maximum antimicrobial effects. Further, the activity of a microbiocide on its own can be dramatically enhanced (or even the opposite, made less effective) by various different formulation effects (see the section on mixtures, formulations, and solutions). This discussion highlights that the antimicrobial activity of any antiseptic, disinfectant, or sterilant will not only be based on the microbiocides present, but on the overall activity tested with the product or process. It will also be based on how the product/process is used and controlled, as discussed in the section on how to choose and use a chemical product.

The various types of microorganisms were discussed in Chapter 5; they range in sizes, shape, surface structure, and so on. As introduced in Chapter 1 (in the section on the decontamination process), they range in structure and resistance to inactivation by physical (e.g. with steam) or chemical means (Figure 6.13).

Further discussion of Figure 6.13 is required. First, this list is only given as an example and will vary depending on the type of microbiocide or biocidal process. It is generally considered that bacterial spores are the most resistant to microbiocides and that mycobacteria are some of the more resistant forms of vegetative bacteria (see Chapter 5 in the section on bacteria). Viruses also range in microbiocide resistance, with the non-enveloped viruses (such as polio and parvoviruses) being highly resistant and the enveloped viruses (hepatitis B, HIV, and SARS-CoV-2, the virus responsible for the COVID-19 pandemic) being very sensitive to disinfection (Figure 6.13 and Chapter 5, the section on bacteria). Second, it may not always be taken for granted that if antimicrobial activity is shown for one type of microorganism (e.g. bacterial spores), all other microorganisms listed under this type will be sensitive to the same disinfectant; in some cases this will be true and in others it may not. Third, this list is given as an estimate and does not reflect other factors that may affect the resistance of any microorganism to a chemical microbiocide, such as the clumping of microorganisms and presence of soil/interfering substances that protect them from the biocide. These and other factors will affect the ability of a disinfectant or even a sterilization process to be effective.

Microbiocides may also be classified based on how they are used. In healthcare applications they are defined as being used for antisepsis, disinfection, preservation, and sterilization. Note that in some regions antiseptics are referred to as skin disinfectants. Essentially, antiseptics are unique types of disinfectants that are used on the skin or mucous membranes. A brief summary of these applications is given in Table 6.10 and these are discussed in further detail later in the final sections of this chapter.

In considering their practical use, microbiocides are often restricted to certain applications. For example, not all microbiocides could be used as antiseptics (on the skin and mucous membranes) in that they need to be effective against certain types of microorganisms (e.g. bacteria and enveloped viruses) but at the same time cause minimal damage or irritation to the skin; examples of microbiocides used in antiseptics include triclosan, chlorhexidine, some QACs, iodine, and various types of alcohols. A much wider range of microbiocides are used for disinfectant purposes, particularly when used on a variety of surface materials (metals, plastics, etc.). These include alcohols, phenolics, aldehydes, and oxidizing agents. These microbiocides and biocidal products will range in activity and are often sub-divided into three types based on their antimicrobial activity: low-, intermediate-, and high-level disinfectants (Figure 6.14).

Low-level disinfectants are generally effective against enveloped viruses and various forms of vegetative bacteria. Intermediate-level disinfectants are considered effective against a wider range, including fungi, non-enveloped viruses, and mycobacteria. High-level disinfectants are effective against all of these microorganisms, including bacterial spores (although for sporicidal activity they may require longer contact time and/or special exposure conditions). In all cases this is in line with their definition as disinfectants: to reduce the level of microorganisms to a safe level. Other traditionally used terms, such as fumigants, pasteurizers, and sanitizers, are also considered as disinfectants; in many countries these terms are defined for particular applications and/or to be able to kill certain types of microorganisms. In some cases following disinfection there may be no viable microorganisms present, but in others there may be; complete inactivation of all and every type of microorganism is not assured. The final, higher level of inactivation is sterilization, which is the complete inactivation of all microorganisms. Sterilization provides the highest level of microbial control assurance. In practical application, sterilization can only be achieved with a limited

	Microorganism types	Examples
More difficult to kill ↑	Bacterial spores	*Geobacillus stearothermophilus, Bacillus atrophaeus, Bacillus cereus, Clostridium difficile*
	Mycobacteria	*Mycobacterium tuberculosis, Mycobacterium avium, Mycobacterium leprae, Mycobacterium chelonae*
	Non-enveloped viruses	Poliovirus, papillomavirus, parvovirus, rhinoviruses (common cold)
	Fungi	*Trichophyton, Aspergillus, Candida albicans*
	Gram-negative bacteria	*Pseudomonas, Escherichia coli, Salmonella, Acinetobacter baumannii, Klebsiella pneumoniae*
	Gram-positive bacteria	*Staphylococcus aureus, Streptococcus pyogenes, Enterococcus*
Less difficult to kill	Enveloped viruses	Human immunodeficiency virus (HIV), herpes virus, hepatitis B virus, influenza virus

	Microorganism types	Examples
More difficult to kill ↑	Prions	Creutzfeldt-Jacob disease (CJD), scrapie
	Dormant microorganisms Bacterial spores Protozoal oocysts/cysts Helminth eggs	*Geobacillus stearothermophilus, Clostridium difficile* *Cryptosporidium, Giardia* *Ascaris, Schistosoma*
	Mycobacteria	*Mycobacterium tuberculosis, Mycobacterium avium*
	Small, non-enveloped viruses	Poliovirus, papillomavirus, parvovirus, rhinoviruses (common cold)
	Dormant fungi (spores)	*Aspergillus, Penicillium*
	Helminths Protozoa	*Cryptosporidium, Giardia* *Ascaris, Schistosoma*
	Fungi Molds Yeasts	*Aspergillus, Penicillium* *Candida*
	Gram-negative bacteria	*Pseudomonas, Escherichia coli, Acinetobacter*
	Large non-enveloped viruses	Adenovirus
	Gram-positive bacteria	*Staphylococcus aureus, Streptococcus pyogenes*
Less difficult to kill	Enveloped viruses	Human immunodeficiency virus (HIV), influenza virus

Figure 6.13 Resistance levels of microorganisms to inactivation. Traditionally the list of microorganisms is often given as in the upper section, but the lower section is an extended list that has been updated based on microbiology research. Note that this is only given as a guide: the resistance level will vary depending on the product/process being considered.

Table 6.10 Classification and examples of various types of biocides based on how they are used. Note: the range of biocides that can be used for each application is not exclusive, for example some antiseptics are also used for disinfection and vice versa.

Biocide application	Definition	Biocide examples
Antisepsis	Reduction or inhibition of microorganisms on the skin or mucous membranes	Alcohols, iodine, chlorhexidine, triclosan
Disinfection	Antimicrobial reduction of microorganisms	Alcohols, chlorine, hydrogen peroxide, peracetic acid, glutaraldehyde
Preservation	Preventing the multiplication of microorganisms	Acids, formaldehyde, phenolics
Sterilization	Defined process used to render an item completely free from viable microorganisms	Ethylene oxide, formaldehyde, hydrogen peroxide, ozone

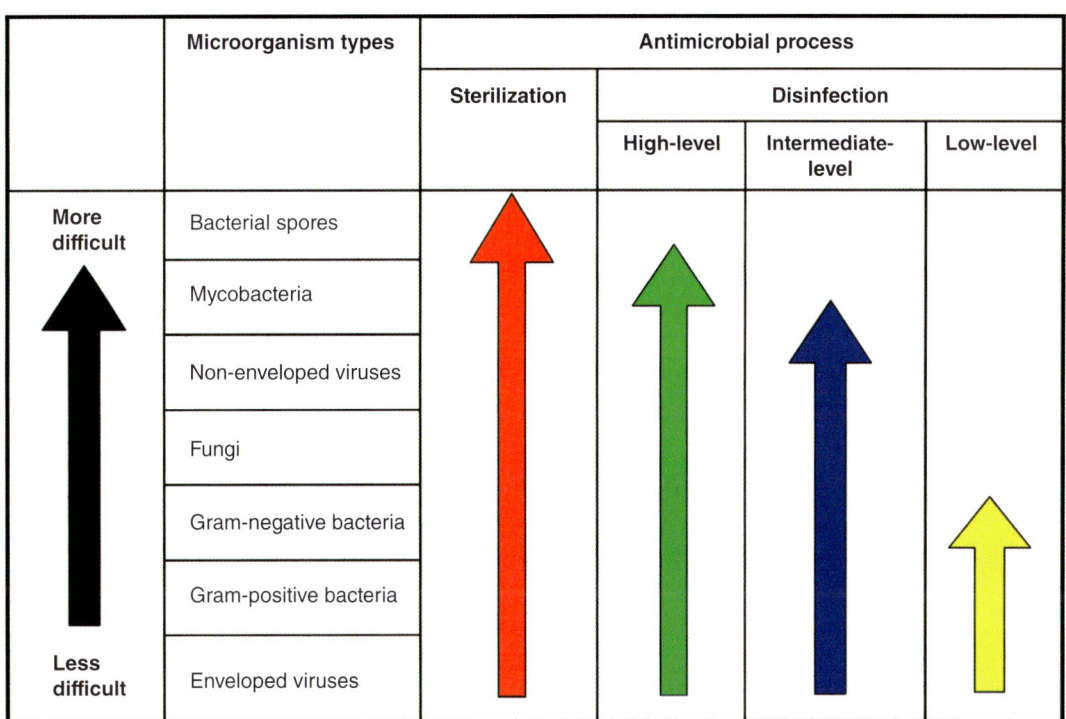

Figure 6.14 Definition of various levels of disinfectants, based on their activity against different types of microorganisms.

number of microbiocides that have been shown to inactivate all types of disease-causing microorganisms. These include microbiocides, such as ethylene oxide, formaldehyde, and hydrogen peroxide, all used for sterilization in gas form. Heat-based mechanisms (including the use of hot water or steam) are also widely employed.

Antiseptics

Antisepsis is the reduction or inhibition of microorganisms on the skin or mucous membranes. Products used as antiseptics are also known by a variety of other terms such as hand washes, hand rubs, antimicrobial soaps, pre-operative preparations, surgical scrubs, tinctures, and mouthwashes. Hand hygiene is one of the simplest yet most effective methods of reducing the transmission of microorganisms in healthcare facilities.

Antiseptics are sub-classified in a variety of ways to include:
• Products that are used with or without water. Examples include antimicrobial soaps that are used to wash the hands or skin with water and those that are simply applied or rubbed into and left on the hands or skin. Examples of rub-in or leave-on antiseptics include alcohol-based gels and foams, antiseptic creams, and mouthwashes.

- Products used for defined healthcare applications. Examples include antiseptic hand washes/hand rubs (also known as hygienic hand disinfectants and healthcare personal hand washes) for routine use in many environments, pre-operative preparations (used to disinfect the skin prior to a surgical procedure, such as antiseptics based on iodine and chlorhexidine), surgical scrubs (used to disinfect the hands of surgeons and other peri-operative personnel prior to surgery, particularly iodine- and chlorhexidine-based products), and products for wound treatment (e.g. iodine and hydrogen peroxide). In many countries specific tests are required to ensure that they meet specific efficacy requirements for these particular purposes.
- Types of antimicrobial biocides that are used in these products, such as triclosan, iodine, alcohols, chlorhexidine, and even combinations thereof.

A summary of the most widely used biocides in antiseptics is given in Table 6.11, but it is important to highlight that products containing these biocides can range considerably in antimicrobial activity.

In processing facilities we are primarily concerned with the use of hand washes or hand rubs to reduce the risk of carrying contamination out from a cleaning area (e.g. on touching a contaminated surface) or on handling instruments (recontamination) after they have been processed (cleaned and/or disinfected). Good hand hygiene in these cases will particularly reduce these risks to our own and the patient's health.

There are three important considerations for antiseptics: efficacy within a typical time of application, how gentle they are on the hands, and that they are used correctly. The typical time taken to routinely disinfect the hands, for example, is 5–10 seconds, but a typical time for surgical scrubbing is 3 minutes (depending on the product). These products should therefore be designed to provide maximum efficacy within the minimum recommended (and practical) application time. Antimicrobial hand-washing products (used with water) in such situations can have the added advantage of the physical removal of various microorganisms from the skin by the washing process alone, in addition to any antimicrobial effect. Irritation from the use of antiseptics is a common complaint, with the majority of healthcare workers reporting problems at some time. Having a product that is rapidly effective but at the same time non-irritating is a difficult balance given the disadvantages of the various types of biocides that can be used for antisepsis (Table 6.11). In general, if a product is, or is even perceived to be, irritating it will not be used; therefore the choice of an antiseptic product that is acceptable to staff is

Table 6.11 Major types of biocides used in antiseptic products. Note that the specific antimicrobial efficacy and any negative effects will vary from product to product. Most antiseptics are considered low- to intermediate-level disinfectants (see the section on antiseptics).

Biocides	Antimicrobial effects[1]	Negative effects[1]	Comments
Alcohols; ethanol, isopropanol (IPA), and n-propanol	Bacteria, fungi, some viruses, mycobacteria	Can cause skin drying and irritation	Hand-rubbing products Typical recommended concentrations are at 60–80% alcohol Products often use chemicals to prevent the alcohol from drying too quickly, therefore increasing its activity Effects can vary depending on the alcohol used and type of fungi/virus in particular
Chlorhexidine (CHG)	Bacteria, mycobacteria, and some viruses (particularly enveloped) Inhibits fungi	Irritation has been reported	Used for skin washing and in combination with alcohols as a skin rub Can remain on the skin following washing to give a residual activity (prevent growth of bacteria) Often used for high-risk applications such as surgical scrubs
Iodine and iodophors	Bacteria, fungi, viruses, mycobacteria	Irritation has been reported and can cause staining	Iodine in alcohol (tinctures) is rarely used today Iodophors (e.g. PVPI) are iodine-releasing agents that release active iodine on demand
Triclosan	Bacteria (particular Gram positive) and some viruses (enveloped) Inhibits the growth of fungi and mycobacteria	Environmental stability	Widely used due to its low irritation but is more limited in its antimicrobial activity (product specific)

[1] Refer to the product manufacturer regarding specific product claims on efficacy, safety, and irritation.

an important decision in any healthcare facility. Finally, the correct antiseptic technique is important (as highlighted in Chapter 5 in the section on infection control and prevention strategies) to ensure that the product can be effective all over the surfaces of the hands.

Disinfectants, including preservatives

Disinfection is the antimicrobial reduction of microorganisms. The various levels of disinfection (high, intermediate, and low) have been defined based on their ability to inactivate certain types of microorganisms (Figure 6.4). Disinfectants are used to disinfect water, the air, and various surfaces, including work areas, patient contact surfaces, and reusable surgical instruments. A further use of microbiocides is for preservation, to prevent the multiplication of microorganisms in products or even in water (an example is the use of chlorine for water disinfection). Preservatives, as microbiocides, are widely used in products such as liquids and other formulated products, including cleaning chemistries and antiseptics themselves. In such cases they may not, and are not intended to, inactivate microorganisms, but will prevent the growth of bacteria (bacteriostatic) and fungi (fungistatic) over time, which are often associated with product spoilage. Examples of such microbiocides include a group of biocides known as the parabens, alcohols, and the QACs.

There is a wide variety of microbiocides used for various disinfection purposes. They are also classified in a number of different ways including:
- Type of chemical biocide (e.g. aldehyde and phenolic based).
- How they are supplied for use (e.g. concentrates, liquids, solids, or even gases).
- How they are used in healthcare facilities (such as device/instrument disinfection and general surface disinfection).

Some of the most widely used microbiocides for disinfection in healthcare facilities are summarized in Table 6.12 with consideration of chemical types. Most of these are used in liquid form, including their direct use alone on surfaces (such as prepared concentrations of alcohols and hydrogen peroxide), but more commonly in formulation with other chemicals. These include bleach solutions (preparations of sodium hypochlorite that release chlorine, an efficient antimicrobial chemical), iodophors (which provide or "release" active iodine), phenolics, QACs, aldehydes (e.g. glutaraldehyde), and oxidizing agent-based formulations (such as those based on hydrogen peroxide, peracetic acid, or chlorine dioxide). They can be provided in a variety of forms: as concentrates or in dry form (diluted in water for use as recommended by the manufacturer), activated products (two components mixed to prepare the disinfectant for use), ready-to-use products (liquid disinfectants provided in spray bottles, for example, for immediate use requiring no activation or dilution), and biocide-impregnated wipes.

There are also a limited number of biocides that are used either on their own or as formulations for air/surface disinfection; these are known as fumigants (for fumigation), where the disinfectant is provided as a fog/mist or gas into a general area for disinfection. Examples of fumigants include hydrogen peroxide mists or gas/vapor and formaldehyde gas processes. A further group of biocides are used to integrate into various surface materials, to provide "antimicrobial surfaces"; examples include the specific use of silver-, triclosan-, and copper-containing materials.

Close attention should be paid to the instructions (label) provided with disinfection products to ensure optimal activity (including recommended dilutions and preparation methods when applicable, recommended contact times and how long they can be used for, and their "shelf-life") and to understand any safety risks in using the product (see Chapter 9). Some general considerations include:

- Only use disinfectants for their intended and labeled use, for example a general surface disinfectant should not be used on patient instruments and vice versa.
- *All* chemical disinfectants will be negatively affected by the presence of soil, although some are considered more sensitive than others. These negative effects can include loss of activity, loss of microbial protection (and therefore lack of activity), and fixing of patient material to surfaces.
- They will vary depending on the product formulation/process, biocide(s) being used, and the level, type, and extent of soiling, as examples. As a general rule, disinfectants work better on cleaned surfaces compared to soiled surfaces, but some products are labeled to be used for combined cleaning (wiping) and disinfection.
- Always prepare and use disinfectants according to their label claims or to written instructions provided by the manufacturer. Failure to do so can lead to efficacy and safety risks. Consider, in particular, any recommended preparation method, handling procedures, exposure method, and any limitations on how long they can be used (shelf-life).
- For diluted products, always use the correct and recommended dilution; more highly or less concentrated products can have more negative than positive effects.
- Never mix chemicals unless they are designed for mixing; the consequences can be quite serious including toxic gas formation and explosive risks.
- All disinfectant products can do harm to human health and all necessary precautions should be used, in particular the use of PPE (see the section on safety considerations) and other safe handling recommendations.
- If you are unsure about the efficacy and safety recommendations for a product, seek advice from someone in authority. It is better to be safe than sorry.
- In some applications, such as disinfecting instruments, it may be necessary to remove any residual disinfectant that

Table 6.12 Major types of biocides used in disinfectant products. Note that the specific antimicrobial efficacy and any negative effects will vary from product to product.

Biocides	Antimicrobial effects[1]	Negative effects[1]	Comments
Alcohols; ethanol and isopropanol (IPA)	Bacteria, fungi, some viruses, mycobacteria, some cyst forms	Flammability risks. Can be damaging to some surfaces	General surface and device disinfectant (usually low and intermediate level) in the 60–90% alcohol range. Fast drying, used for disinfection and drying applications. Efficacy against fungi and viruses can vary. Not effective against bacterial spores
Aldehydes: glutaraldehyde, orthophthaldehyde (OPA), and formaldehyde	Bacteria, fungi, viruses, most mycobacteria, and bacterial spores	Difficult to rinse away residues prior to patient use. Only use in areas with correct ventilation due to toxic risks. Strong odor and irritating. OPA can cause surface staining	Widely used for high-level disinfection of flexible endoscopes and other devices. Glutaraldehyde is significantly more effective against bacterial spores than OPA. Formaldehyde is generally only used in gas form and rarely for disinfection in healthcare
Halogens: iodine and chlorine	Bacteria, fungi, viruses, mycobacteria, bacterial spores, protozoal cysts. In some cases prions	Can be damaging on surfaces, particularly at higher concentrations on metals. Strong odor and irritating	Can be used for rapid low-, intermediate-, and high-level disinfection. Chlorine (as bleach or sodium hypochlorite solutions) is widely used for environmental surface and water disinfection. Not widely used on instruments/devices
Peroxygens: hydrogen peroxide, peracetic acid, chlorine dioxide, and ozone	Bacteria, fungi, viruses, bacterial spores, protozoal cysts. In some cases prions	Can be damaging to some surfaces. Strong odor (particularly peracetic acid) and irritating	Used as (or in) liquids and in gas form, for various levels of disinfection and in some cases sterilization, including environmental surfaces and on reusable devices/instruments. Gas and liquid forms can differ in activity and safety characteristics
Phenolics: cresols, 2-phenylphenol, and 2-chlorophenol	Bacteria, fungi, viruses (especially enveloped and variable against non-enveloped)	Can be damaging to some surfaces. Often strong odor. Residue can have toxic effects	Used for low- and intermediate-level environmental disinfection, with little to no activity against dormant forms, including bacterial spores. Can be acid, neutral, or alkaline in formulation
Quaternary ammonium compounds (QACs or QUATs): cetrimide, benzalkonium chloride, and cetylpyridinium chloride	Bactericidal (particularly Gram-positive bacteria and vary in activity against Gram-negative bacteria), enveloped viruses, some fungi, and mycobacteria (some formulations)	In diluted products, water quality can affect activity. Can damage some surfaces	Used for low- and intermediate-level environmental disinfection, with little to no activity against dormant forms, including bacterial spores. Often used for combined cleaning and disinfection activity due to their surfactant nature

[1] Refer to the product manufacturer regarding specific product claims on how these should be used, their efficacy, safety, and irritation potential (see the section on how to choose and use a chemical product). Antimicrobial activity and negative effects can vary depending on how the biocide is used.

is on or in the device prior to use on a patient. This is particularly true with the disinfection of instruments/devices (Chapter 9).

Disinfectants can also be classified depending on their specific healthcare (device) use. A useful and widely employed example of such a classification is the Spaulding classification, named after E.H. Spaulding and developed during the 1950s–1960s (see Chapter 1). This classification is based on the risk of infection to a patient on the use (or reuse) of a device or indeed any surface. The greater the risk to a patient, the greater the level of antimicrobial activity that should be applied. The different levels of antimicrobial activity were introduced previously (summarized in Figure 6.14) as sterilization and high-, intermediate-, and low-level disinfection. According to the Spaulding classification, these are recommended in the following situations (with examples given in Figure 6.15):

- Critical devices: these present the highest risk to a patient as they enter (or could enter) a normally "sterile" area of the body and therefore require sterilization (complete inactivation of all microorganisms). Sterile areas of the body are the bloodstream and the various internal organs (with the exception of the intestinal tract) and therefore sterilization is the standard applied to most surgical devices, be they single use or reusable. Sterilization methods include steam, dry heat, and chemical sterilization (Chapter 11).
- Semi-critical devices: these are devices that may only contact mucous membranes or non-intact (broken) skin, such as laryngoscope blades, rectal specula, and some types of flexible endoscopes. It is also suggested that such devices should be sterilized, if practical before patient use, but at a minimum they should be subjected to high-level disinfection, which should eliminate most viruses, bacteria (particularly mycobacteria), fungi, and in some cases bacterial spores (although this may require long exposure times). Typical biocides widely used in high-level disinfectants include glutaraldehyde, ortho-phthaldehyde (OPA), hydrogen peroxide, chlorine dioxide, and peracetic acid. Note that in some countries the term "sterilant" is used, often in combination with high-level disinfectants; a sterilant should *not* be confused with sterilization. A sterilant, in these cases, should have the ability to kill all forms of microorganisms to particularly include bacterial spores and generally requires longer contact times according to approved label claims. This is distinct to sterilization, which is a defined and controlled process to provide sterility (see Chapters 9 and 11).
- Non-critical or low risk devices: where intact (non-broken) skin is contacted such as stethoscopes, sinks, general work surfaces, etc. It is recommended that such surfaces/devices be treated either with disinfectants that have a low or intermediate level of disinfection or even in some cases just by cleaning alone (to physically remove soil and microorganisms). Examples of biocides used in low/intermediate disinfectants are QACs, phenolics, and alcohols.

Although this classification can in most cases be easily applied in a healthcare facility, it is good practice to establish and maintain a facility policy regarding disinfection and sterilization practices. This policy should be developed and maintained in close interaction with surgical, medical, and particularly IPC staff. This is important not only in the classification of the various devices/instruments used in clinical practice but also in consideration of what types of disinfection and sterilization products/processes should be used in each case. A good source of information is the device manufacturer; it is a requirement for the device manufacturer to provide detailed instructions on cleaning, disinfecting, and (if required) sterilization of reusable devices (e.g. in conformance to ISO 17664-1 and ISO 17664-2 on information to be provided by the manufacturer for the processing of healthcare products). In some countries disinfection products require strict regulatory (governmental) approval before they are allowed to be used (e.g. in the United States by the Food and Drug Administration for any disinfectant used on a device and by the Environmental Protection Agency for any environmental disinfectant; in Australia by the Therapeutic Goods Administration); in other regions there may be self-regulation by the companies that provide individual products (as in the case of the European Union). In all cases it is important that any disinfectant is chosen based on the efficacy and safety requirements of the facility (see Chapter 9).

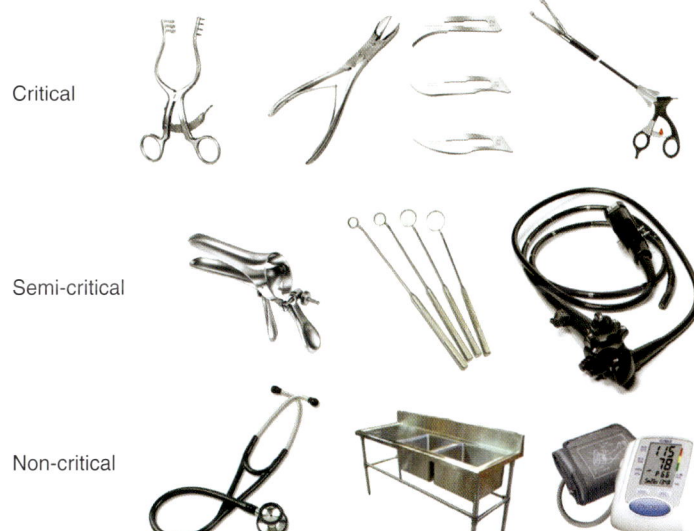

Figure 6.15 Examples of typical critical, semi-critical, and non-critical devices according to the Spaulding classification. It is important to note that the device classification may vary depending on its use on a patient; for example, a normally non-critical device will be considered critical if for some reason it is used in a sterile area of the body (e.g. during many surgical procedures) and vice versa.

Chemical sterilization

Unlike disinfectants, there are only a limited number of microbiocides used for sterilization applications. This is primarily due to the fact that the minimum criterion for sterilization is to be able to inactivate all forms of microbial life, including bacterial spores; only a limited number of biocides can be practically used for this purpose. In addition to being able to inactivate all microorganisms, chemical sterilization processes are also required to meet strict process definition requirements (such as sterility assurance levels, a concept further discussed in Chapter 11). At this time it is sufficient to know that the ability to kill all microorganisms is only one of the starting requirements for a microbiocide to be used in a defined sterilization process. In addition to efficacy requirements, the other considerations of safety and compatibility should also be evaluated. In many cases chemical sterilization is only recommended when steam sterilization cannot be used (e.g. with heat-sensitive devices or materials), but this is not in any way a rule. All systems are controlled under defined process control conditions, as a requirement for any sterilization process. A brief summary of the major types of chemical sterilization processes is given in Table 6.13.

Table 6.13 Examples of sterilization processes using chemical biocides.[1] The exact process (times, temperatures, gas concentrations, etc.) and specific advantages/disadvantages will vary considerably depending on the product/sterilizer design. Each sterilization process/product should be considered individually (see Chapter 11).

Chemical	Typical process	Comments
Ethylene oxide (ETO or EO) gas	Load humidified and heated (using low-temperature steam[2]), gas distributed, held for an exposure time, and then residual gas flushed ("aerated") from the chamber/load using pulses of low-temperature steam	Many loads may require additional aeration following a cycle to ensure all gas residuals are removed Processes are well described, and the gas is very penetrating, but can require long exposure/aeration times EO is toxic and explosive at low concentrations, requiring tight safety monitoring
Hydrogen peroxide gas	Air/water is removed from the chamber/load under low pressure, load exposed to repeated phase of peroxide gas introduction, exposure and removal, and then removed at low pressure	Rapid cycle times, with loads ready for immediate use Certain materials (e.g. liquids, paper) are restricted from use Gas process is penetrating Peroxide gas can be toxic, but has a good safety and environmental profile
Hydrogen peroxide gas plasma	Air is removed from the chamber/load under low pressure (sometimes with plasma generation assistance), load exposed to repeated phases of peroxide gas introduction, exposure and removal followed by plasma generation (to remove liquid/gas residues). and then aerated at low pressure (sometimes assisted by plasma generation)	Rapid cycle times, with loads ready for immediate use Certain materials (e.g. liquids, paper) are restricted from use Gas process can be penetrating Peroxide gas can be toxic, but has a good safety and environmental profile
Formaldehyde gas	Similar to EO, where load is pre-conditioned with steam (heating and humidity) and gas distribution, exposed for sterilization, and then aerated using steam/low-pressure pulses	Most loads require additional aeration following a cycle to ensure gas residual removal Processes are well described, and the gas is very penetrating, but requires long exposure/aeration times Gas is toxic and requires strict safety monitoring
Ozone gas	Load is pre-conditioned humidity and ozone distribution, exposed to repeated phases of ozone gas introduction, exposure and removal under low pressure for sterilization, and then aerated under low pressure	Minimum chemical requirements (ozone made from oxygen and water) Cycle times are longer than peroxide but shorter than EO processes Can be damaging to certain types of materials
Peracetic acid liquid formulation	Devices exposed to a peracetic acid-based formulation at a specified temperature range and time, followed by water rinsing	Rapid process Can only be used for devices that can be immersed in water and devices should be used immediately after sterilization (no storage)

[1] There are other biocides (e.g. chlorine dioxide, other types of gas plasma) that have been described for sterilization purposes, but at the time of writing these were not commercially available.
[2] Low-temperature steam is made by decreasing the pressure at which the steam is provided into the sterilization chamber; this is ruled by the gas laws and is the same concept that allows high-temperature steam to be made under increased pressures.

Until recently the most widely used systems were those based on ethylene oxide gas and, to a much smaller extent and only in certain countries, formaldehyde gas. In both cases the antimicrobial activity is optimized by ensuring that the load placed into the sterilizer is correctly humidified and heated prior to and during gas exposure. However, these systems have become more rarely used. A growing number of alternative chemical sterilization processes have been developed, such as those based on hydrogen peroxide gas (with or without the assistance of plasma generation), ozone gas mixtures, or even liquid peracetic acid formulations (Table 6.13). These systems vary in their design and process systems and are considered in further detail in Chapter 11.

7 Point-of-use treatment and transport

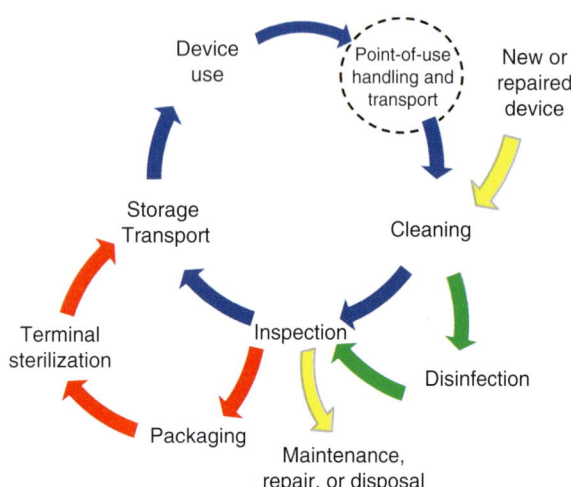

Processing of medical devices has been commonly thought of as a process that begins at some central location, such as a central services department (CSD), when the reality is that it starts (or ought to start) where the device was most recently used clinically. These areas can practically be anywhere in the healthcare facility where a device is used on a patient, and are currently referred to as the "point of use" (POU). This term is now consistently used globally in many standards and guidelines that address the care and handling of medical devices pre-operatively, intra-operatively, and post-operatively by clinical and technical staff. In surgery, POU care of devices starts with the entrance into the operating or procedure room and ends with their departure for processing.

During the procedure devices need care, for example they may be wiped or lumens flushed with sterile water to remain functional while in use. They are also handled with caution to avoid any risks of damage. All devices should be protected from mechanical shock (being dropped, striking other devices, etc.) and stress (bending, being placed under heavier devices, etc.). Staff should not drop or handle devices roughly during procedures or while returning them to their trays at the end of a procedure. The tips of delicate and sharp medical devices should be protected at all times to avoid unnecessary damage or accidental injury to those handling them. Post-procedure care continues with any POU treatment (formerly known as "pre-cleaning") and provides a foundation for successful processing. It has been scientifically investigated and published that soil drying on or in devices significantly increases the cleaning challenge, including the risk of biofilm development, and increases the risk of cleaning endpoints not being achieved (Chapter 6), particularly in device areas that have restricted access. Keeping devices moist at the POU is a requirement and it cannot be overlooked or neglected. In some facilities devices will be handled and processed directly in the operating or procedure room. Best practice dictates that reusable medical devices are ideally transported to a separate dedicated area to be processed (Chapter 1). These areas may be adjacent to the procedure area, at a remote location within the hospital (e.g. a central sterile services department, CSSD), or even at a completely different facility (e.g. a "super-center" or off-site processing center).

A frequently asked question is who is responsible for any POU treatment. In a surgical environment this is usually the peri-operative staff. In other situations it can be designated nursing or other specific staff (e.g. in a dental clinic). The most appropriate answer, though, is that it requires teamwork between any central area and the clinical personnel at the POU. Handoff communication about the care, treatment, and condition of devices is part of this teamwork. This chapter discusses the care and handling of devices directly post procedure and their subsequent safe transport to the designated processing area.

Decontamination and Device Processing in Healthcare, Second Edition. Gerald McDonnell and Georgia Alevizopoulou.
© 2025 John Wiley & Sons Ltd. Published 2025 by John Wiley & Sons Ltd.

Post-procedure sorting

It is good practice post procedure for all reusable devices to be sorted, separated, and accounted for. This is important for several reasons:

- To ensure that all the devices are present and not mislaid during the procedure. It is unfortunately not an uncommon occurrence for devices to mistakenly remain in a patient following a surgical procedure, which poses a significant risk to their health.
- To keep reusable devices in designated sets for processing together and subsequent reuse.
- To inspect the devices for any signs of damage and make a note of any repair or disposal of devices for biomedical or designated decontamination staff.
- To allow for traceability of individual devices or device sets in any case where infection prevention/control (IPC) would desire to know on whom or with whom these devices have been used. This has become a particular concern in many parts of the world with the risks associated with many types of transmissible diseases (e.g. Creutzfeldt-Jakob disease (CJD); see Chapter 5, the section on prions and other infectious proteins, and Chapter 15, on devices known or suspected to be contaminated with prion material).

Sorting is primarily a manual process and may be assisted by using device checklists, either paper based or in electronic format. These checklists are used to perform pre- and post-procedure counts and may often also function in ensuring that devices are counted back on arrival at the processing facility. They may well be the same ones used when assembling a device set in a tray/container prior to sterilization (Chapter 10). Electronic tracking and traceability systems may also be used for this purpose, close to a surgical area or within a designated processing facility (for further details see tracking and traceability in Chapter 14). Only trained personnel should sort contaminated items from any procedure areas.

Note that during a procedure a variety of disposable materials, single-use devices, reusable devices, linens/coverings, and other materials (solids and liquids) may have been used (Figure 7.1). All materials and devices should be considered unsafe to handle without following standard precautions (always assume they are potentially contaminated with infectious materials) and should be handled, collected, and delivered by skilled trained staff wearing the appropriate protective clothing in accordance with relevant safety policies and procedures. It is recommended to always wash hands thoroughly after handling such used equipment – even if protective gloves have been worn during handling.

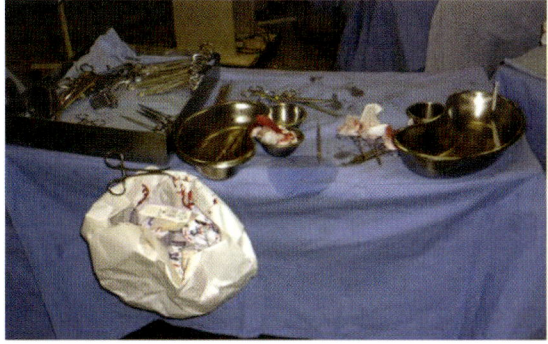
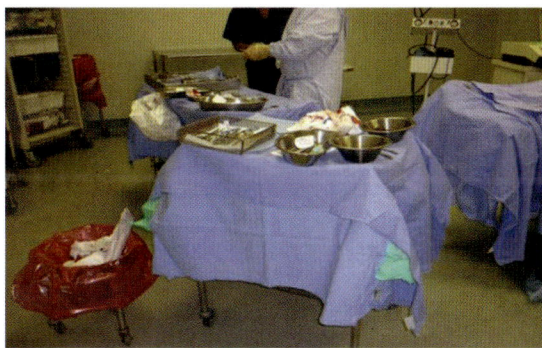
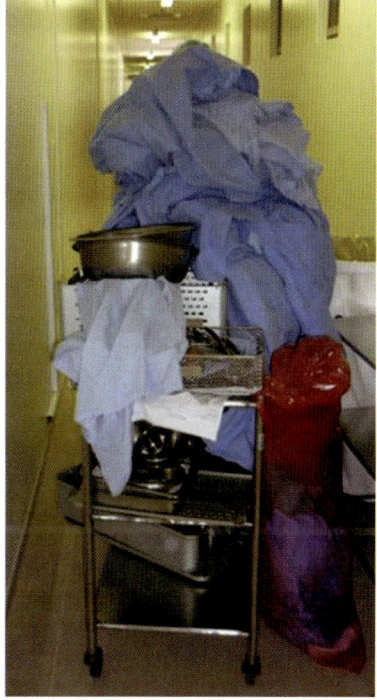

Figure 7.1 A typical range of disposal and reusable items following a surgical procedure. The picture on the right is an unfortunate bad example of how devices and materials are not sorted or correctly transported for processing.

All reusable devices should be separated from soiled linens and disposable items at the POU. It is considered good practice that these devices are then placed into leak-proof, puncture-resistant containers for transport, and clearly labeled as being biohazardous, to allow easy identification that the contents are contaminated. This includes all devices, particularly within a set, whether they appear to be used or not, as they are all considered contaminated and a possible source of microorganisms.

Care should be given in the handling of any sharp devices, single use (disposable) or reusable. As discussed in Chapter 4 under surgical instrument types and description, various types of sharp instruments are used for cutting and dissecting, including disposable needles and blades. Consideration should be given to safety and risks of sharp accidents to the person responsible for sorting and also to those subsequently involved or at risk of contact during transport and decontamination. This highlights the recommendation for using hard, puncture-resistant containers for transport. Therefore, any single-use sharps (e.g. blades and needles) should be removed and discarded at the POU. Care should be taken not to inadvertently discard any associated reusable devices. In many cases, the blades or needles are single-use devices but are mounted onto reusable holders or handles during use (e.g. "BP holders" with surgical blades). Disposable needles and blades must be removed and disposed of in appropriate puncture-resistant sharps containers at the POU, prior to transportation. It is the responsibility of the user or designated staff to remove all blades from reusable handles so as not to endanger others. Examples of blade-removal techniques are given in Figure 7.2.

Other general considerations on handling reusable devices post procedure include:
- Arrange devices to minimize any risks of damage to them or harm to staff. Device stacking, in particular placing heavier items on top of lighter devices and when transporting sensitive devices (such as endoscopes), should be avoided.
- Follow any manufacturer's guidelines regarding safety, disassembly, and POU treatment.
- Remove and dispose of any disposable parts or components.
- Remove and correctly discard any associated liquids used with the device as part of the procedure.
- Note and preferably inform any designated processing staff about damaged devices requiring disposal or repair.
- Inform processing staff of any known missing or additional reusable device components noted during the count.

Reusable linens remain widely used worldwide; they are also considered contaminated following many medical or surgical procedures (Chapter 15, the section on surgical and medical laundry). Therefore they should be treated in many ways like reusable devices: separated, sorted, and safely transported for decontamination (usually in a defined laundry facility, which may be part of or separate to a device decontamination site). Reusable devices should *never* be washed with laundry items. Chemicals and processes used in laundry processing may not be suitable for devices. Devices that may become hidden in soiled linen can also injure unsuspecting laundry workers, may be inadvertently discarded as waste, and may also cause damage to the linens.

Any single-use devices, liquids, and materials (such as disposable drapes and linens) should be separately disposed of according to established policies at or near to the POU. These are usually discarded directly into hazardous waste bins or liquid-waste disposal containers (if known to be contaminated) and collected for incineration or other similar safe disposal policy. As already highlighted, particular consideration should be given to the presence of any sharp materials.

Special consideration should also be given to the safe disposal or transport of materials (including devices) that have been used with radioactive or cytotoxic chemicals. Radioactive chemicals are often used for medical procedures (nuclear medicine; see Chapter 6 under light, radiation, and the electromagnetic spectrum). Examples include the use of radioactive isotopes for medical imaging and for cancer radiotherapy (see Chapter 3). Widely used radioactive chemicals ("isotopes") are technetium (99m), iodine (123 and 131), and thallium (201). Cytotoxic chemicals (or drugs) are chemicals used for medical purposes for the treatment of various conditions such as autoimmune diseases (e.g. arthritis) and cancer ("chemotherapy"); cytotoxic ("cell-toxic") refers to their ability to control the growth of or kill cells. Examples of cytotoxic drugs used for cancer chemotherapy include cisplatin, cyclophosphamide, doxorubicin, and vincristine. Some of these chemicals are short-lived (degrading safely, naturally, and quickly, e.g. over a few hours), while others are not. In both cases, special handling procedures may be required. In such situations, a facility policy should be in place to ensure that any waste or processing is handled safely to reduce any risks to staff or subsequent patients.

Other associated and fixed surfaces in the operating or procedure room area, particularly around the immediate patient-handling area (such as the surgical table, lights, robots, and trolleys), may have also become contaminated with blood or other tissues and materials during the procedure. In many cases these surfaces may be protected during a procedure with various protective coverings (e.g. operating room light handles and general surface coverings). These coverings should be routinely changed and discarded between patients. It is good practice for general surfaces, in particular those that have not been otherwise covered or may have become soiled, to be wiped down (including cleaning for visual cleanliness) with a disinfectant between patient procedures. It is also common practice for certain procedure areas, including operating rooms and particularly frequently touched surfaces, to be wiped down with an appropriate disinfectant at the end of a working day;

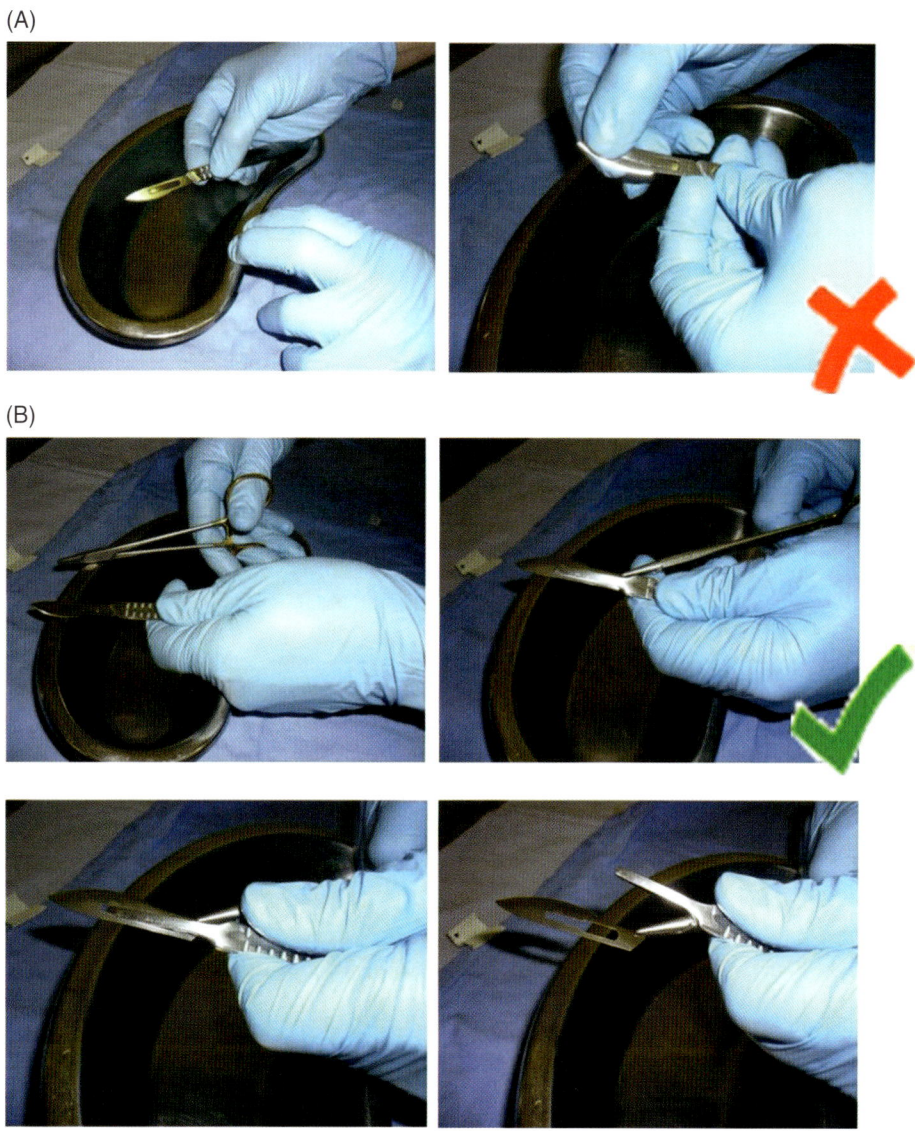

Figure 7.2 Correct disassembly and handling of single-use blades from reusable BP handles. (A) Do not remove the blades by hand. (B) Staff should be trained on the correct removal methods. An example is shown using a needle holder (other devices or tools may also be safely used). Slide the blade up and away from the handle body, allowing it to drop into a container, and discard the blade according to the facility's sharps procedures.

in certain circumstances these areas may also be subjected to "deep" cleaning (including the use of disinfectants and/or fumigants; see Chapter 9 on chemical disinfectants).

Next, devices may be transferred to a separate, distinct site from the procedure area, preferably in an adjacent room, placed back in the tray in which they arrived, and set aside for POU treatment, before being contained, labeled as (bio)hazardous, and transported to the CSSD.

Point-of-use treatment

Traditionally, POU treatment has been thought of as a (pre)-cleaning step. Many people have assumed that it is executed to make the processing staff's work easier. Others have considered it as unnecessary and a waste of operating room staff time. In truth, what is or is not done for POU treatment has a measurable impact and its importance cannot be understated.

Following a procedure, devices and equipment may be contaminated with a variety of materials such as blood, serum, skin, tissue debris, microorganisms, cements, saline, and so on. These materials can pose health and safety risks, such as:
- Risks of infection and cross-contamination.
- Damage to device surfaces (e.g. salts can attack the surface of stainless steel and promote rusting).
- Damage to device operation (e.g. internal lumens or hinge joints may become blocked from soil drying/coagulation).
- Development of biofilm (communities of microorganisms, either single or multiple types, that have developed on or within surfaces and are held together by carbohydrate/protein strands, collectively termed "extracellular polymeric substances" or EPS; see Chapter 5, the section on microbiology and infection prevention/control), whose chemical components are deposited by a range of microorganisms and persist throughout the processing cycle.
- Difficulty in subsequent cleaning if the soil on devices is allowed to dry.
- Soil drying on or in devices significantly increases the cleaning challenge and increases the risk of cleaning endpoints not being achieved, particularly in device areas that have restricted access. In order to minimize these risks, an initial treatment of soiled devices is conducted at the POU. In many cases, device manufacturers specify POU treatment in the instructions for use as an essential step in the overall processing. Contaminated devices should be handled as little as possible at this stage as staff are most at risk of infectious hazards when handling contaminated devices.

Guidelines and standards globally are consistent in the recommendation that POU treatment needs to start as soon as practically possible after or even before the end of the clinical procedure. Devices and equipment are generally kept free of gross soil during a patient procedure to allow for their practical use. During surgery, nursing staff will usually gently wipe down the devices with a sponge or lint-free cloth moistened with sterile water or saline solution to keep them relatively clean. But there are some precautions to the use of liquids at this time. Saline, in particular, is water with added salt and can be very aggressive when used on devices such as those made of metals, causing pitting, rusting (see Chapters 6 and 15), and dulling of sharp edges. Both physical and chemical means are used to loosen and remove gross soil. Generally, soaking devices in the procedure room is not recommended.

If devices cannot be returned to the processing area in a timely manner, it is important that they are at least kept moist using appropriate methods while waiting and/or during transportation. Soil that is allowed to dry on the surface can cause damage to surfaces, both structurally and functionally. These effects can be particularly rapid if devices are left in such a state for extended periods of time. For example, various types of patient soil can include salts that will attack the material surfaces of devices, particularly stainless steel, copper, and brass. These effects can include premature rusting and other types of corrosion that will limit the practical use of the device. These effects may be obvious or hidden, potentially causing a device to fail in operation during a subsequent patient procedure. Physical effects can include clogging of the device at various working parts or internal lumens. Microbial pathogens such as bacteria and fungi are also likely to be protected from these effects and continue to pose an infection or cross-contamination risk to those handling these devices. Further to this consideration, soil that is allowed to dry and/or harden in/on the surface of the device is much more difficult to remove than moist soil. In addition, dry soil can also contribute to biofilm formation, which may well require more aggressive cleaning processes to remove. As discussed in Chapter 5, biofilms are very complex resilient communities and they form rapidly within hours. Once a mature biofilm has developed, it can be more difficult to remove.

Various methods are employed at this stage (Figure 7.3). One common practice, especially in the past, consists of placing the soiled devices into a basin/container and covering them with a clean, non-linting cloth, large enough to cover all devices, moistened with sterile water. This method is inexpensive and simple to perform, but it may be very inconsistent and can allow for the overgrowth of bacteria, so it has tended to be discontinued. In some parts of the world this method is substituted with the use of pre-moistened bags ("humidity packs") that are designed to maintain a safe and sealed humid environment.

Another practice recommends that devices are soaked in a basin/container in water alone or mixed with some type of detergent, examples including enzymatic and non-enzymatic cleaning formulations (see Chapter 6 for the classification of cleaning chemistries). In some countries cleaning chemistries that include some disinfection efficacy are also recommended; these are proposed to be used to reduce microbial contamination (particularly from bacteria and enveloped viruses) and therefore personnel handling risks. With any products that are used, close attention is required to any labeling or other instructions provided with the product to ensure that it is used optimally and safely (e.g. dilution, temperature, time, etc.). It is recommended that cleaning (or indeed any decontamination product) formulations are used that have been designed for use on medical or surgical devices. Hand soaps, or surgical hand scrubs (such as iodine or chlorhexidine-containing products), should not be used because these chemicals may damage devices, are not labeled or designed for such use, or may cause other patient complications. Fresh water alone may be used but should not be reused; consideration should be given to the recommendations on the use of water and requirements for water quality (see Chapter 15 on water quality and purity). A variety of cleaning aids can be used, such as sponges, cloths, and

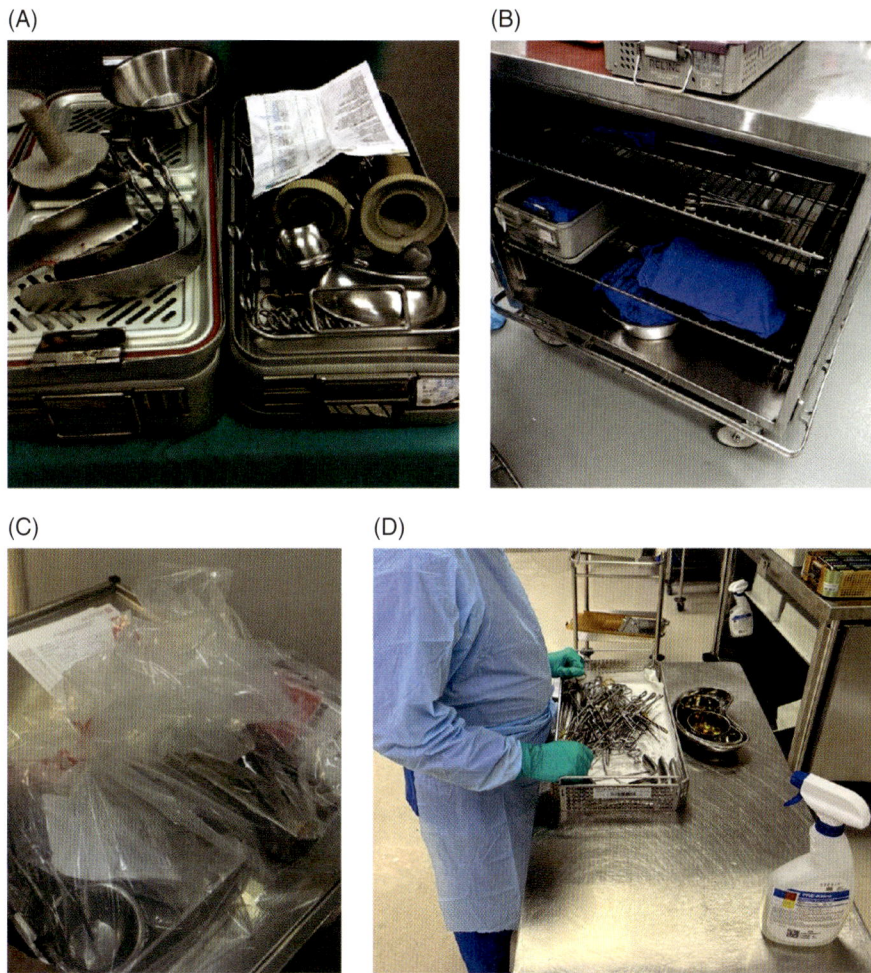

Figure 7.3 Examples of various practices of point-of-use treatment. (A) Devices waiting to be returned in the processing area without any treatment. (B) Several used sets of devices are covered under pre-moistened towels. (C) Soiled devices contained in humidity bags. (D) Devices are placed into the tray and sprayed with a gel ready for transportation.

brushes. It should be noted that abrasive materials and products (e.g. scouring pads) should not be used, as these can damage devices. Depending on the degree of soiling and the type of device, the use of detergent-impregnated wipes may be applicable. There are certain types of soils (e.g. cements) that can be difficult to remove when dried; these should be removed prior to drying (or setting) if at all possible as they can only be subsequently removed by abrasive methods. Soaking methods are helpful to wet all device surfaces, but are also not ideal. Besides the increased costs in time and materials, it poses a safety concern for spills/splashes (by rinsing in water or by cleaning within close proximity to the patient procedure area) and ergonomics, with additional weight during transport to a centralized processing area, likely to result in injury to personnel. When no alternative option is available, it is recommended that the liquid be discarded before transport to minimize the risk of a spill and limit the weight of the container, or else contain the solution to prevent spills and subsequent exposures.

A further method uses specific-purpose products for POU treatment, and these can reduce the risks associated with the other methods discussed. They are available in different types of foam- and gel-based products and are applied quickly by being sprayed over the soiled devices (see Figure 7.4). The optimum product should include the following features:

• Allowing the devices to be directly observed in case any sharps are present. This will reduce any risks to those subsequently handling these devices.
• Preventing the drying of soil on device surfaces; note that any internal device lumens or channels will not readily dry

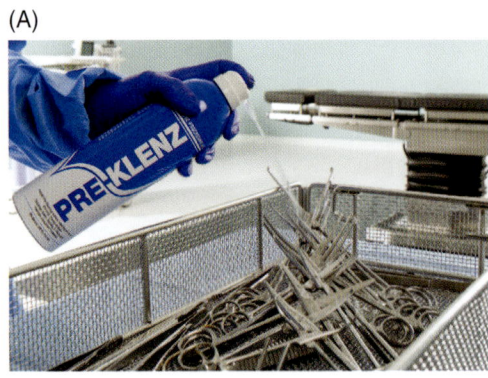 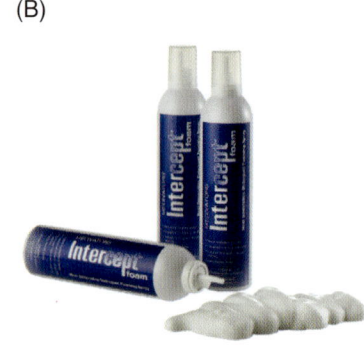

Figure 7.4 Examples of point-of-use treatment with specific-purpose products used on surgical devices. (A) A transparent gel; (B) a foam. Courtesy STERIS Corporation 2024. All rights reserved

out on transport due to the lack of air passage across these internal surfaces, therefore it is not necessary or practical to ensure that such surfaces are fully contacted with applicable products.
- Covering and adhering to device surfaces to maintain moisture in and around the devices.
- Providing bacteriostatic and fungistatic activity (i.e. preventing the growth of bacteria and fungi, respectively), although some products may provide different levels of bactericidal and fungicidal (i.e. killing these respective microorganisms) effects.
- Initiating the cleaning process during transport and preventing drying during elongated storage/transport times.
- Protecting the devices from any damage on elongated storage/transport times.
- Not inhibiting any subsequent processing steps (cleaning, disinfection, and/or sterilization) or causing toxic risks to the following patient.
- Minimizing any potential spillage risks that may present a risk to those handling the devices or others on transport to another processing area.
- Being provided in a manner that will not produce mist, aerosols, or dust.

For certain types of devices, specific instructions for POU treatment are recommended by the device manufacturers. One example is in the use of flexible endoscopes, where a bedside procedure is described. During this procedure gross soil is removed by wiping down the outer surfaces with a moist cloth or sponge that is infused with a cleaning formulation solution and by flushing through the channels of the device (processing of flexible endoscopes is considered in further detail in Chapters 8, 9, and 15). In some cases the distal tip of the endoscope may be encapsulated in a package designed to maintain humid conditions to keep it moist as well as protected during transportation. Another example is in the use of robotic devices that also feature very complex and delicate designs (e.g. small moving components) that are exposed to soils; keeping them moist until the processing starts is essential. Figure 7.5 shows examples of POU treatment of such devices.

Instructions and guidelines can vary in consideration of how much time is allowed between the end of POU treatment and the start of cleaning. Most instructions for use do not provide a specific time limit. Some guidelines state that cleaning should be initiated within one hour or as determined by the facility based on their own documented risk assessment. Overall, the drying of soil prior to cleaning dramatically increases the difficulty of protein/soil removal. The longer the drying time, the harder the cleaning challenge, even after just one hour. Longer drying times, such as over 48–72 hours, are even worse, especially in device areas or features that are considered more difficult to clean due to restricted access (Chapter 8).

Transportation post procedure

Contaminated items should be contained post procedure for transporting to a defined processing area; containment during transport reduces the exposure of staff and others to contaminated materials. The removal of contaminated items from the procedure area should be performed safely and carefully to minimize exposure. It is considered good practice that the next patient procedure should not commence until all contaminated items are safely sorted, removed, or discarded. Materials for transport away from a patient procedure area can include reusable devices, reusable materials (e.g. linens), contaminated items for safe disposal (sharps, single-use devices, etc.), and, potentially, items to be discarded as non-clinical, normal waste. Procedures should be in place for how all these materials are transported. Materials requiring decontamination for reuse are our primary concern in this chapter.

As stated previously, reusable devices should be placed into leak-proof, puncture-resistant containers for transport, and clearly labeled as being biohazardous to allow easy identification that the contents are contaminated (Figure 7.6).

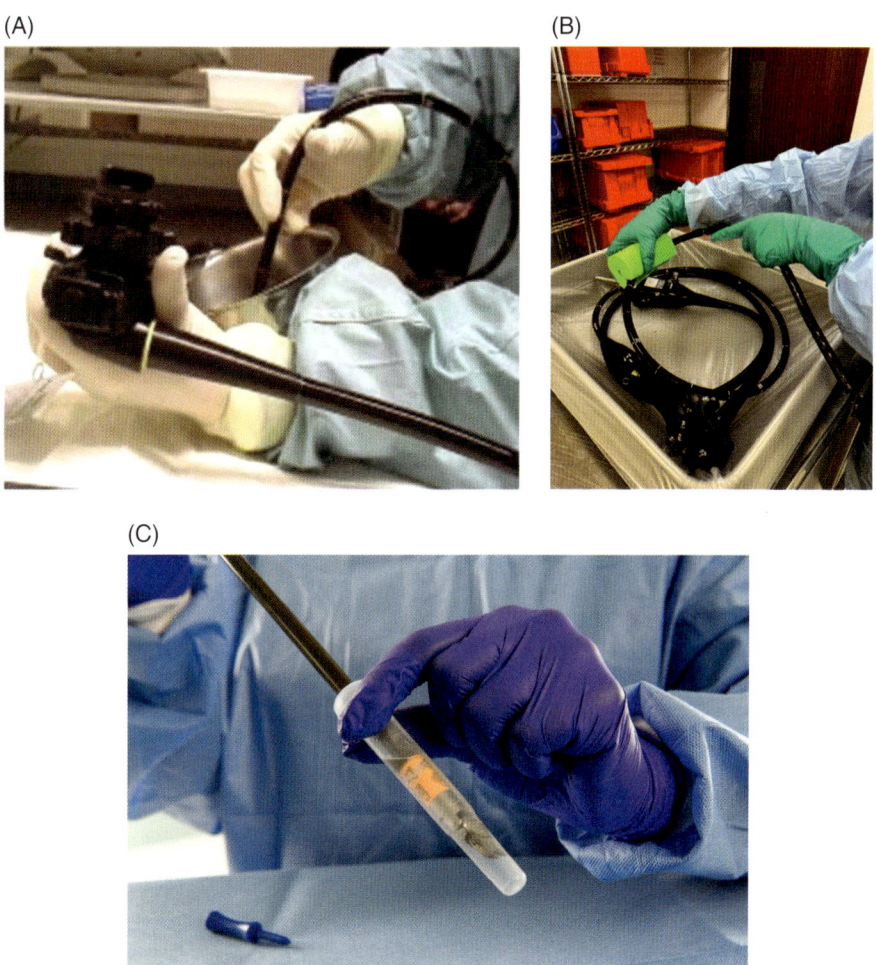

Figure 7.5 Examples of the care of devices with complex features at the point of use. (A) Bedside procedure with a flexible endoscope suctioning a cleaning solution through the internal lumens of the device. (B) Wiping down the insertion tube of a flexible endoscope using a soft single-use sponge. (C) Example of soaking the tip of the robotic forceps, retaining moisture around it and allowing for safe and convenient transportation.

Procedures should be in place to prevent contaminated devices requiring processing from being accidentally mixed with decontaminated and single-use devices being prepared for use in another procedure. Particular attention should be paid to the workflow within these areas, to prevent this from occurring (for discussion on the principles of separating "clean" and "dirty" areas, see Chapter 1, the section on design of a decontamination area).

Contaminated devices can include those that have been used directly with a patient and those that may have been indirectly contaminated during handling, such as carts/trolleys, containers, and so on. It is typical in surgical practices that a set of devices is provided within a tray (in which they have been previously cleaned and sterilized) and the soiled set after a procedure is returned to the same tray. Similarly, transport systems such as trolleys may be used to transport clean devices to a surgical area and then return them to a decontamination area/facility. These transport systems will also require routine processing, either manually or in automated washer-disinfectors (see the section on care of trolleys and containers).

Soiled devices should ideally be transported, in closed trolleys, to a decontamination area for processing as soon as possible after the procedure has been completed. If closed trolleys are not available, open trolleys/carts may be used but should be adequately covered (e.g. using unsoiled towels, wraps, or other materials) to provide a degree of protection. In some cases, where the patient procedure room is in close proximity to

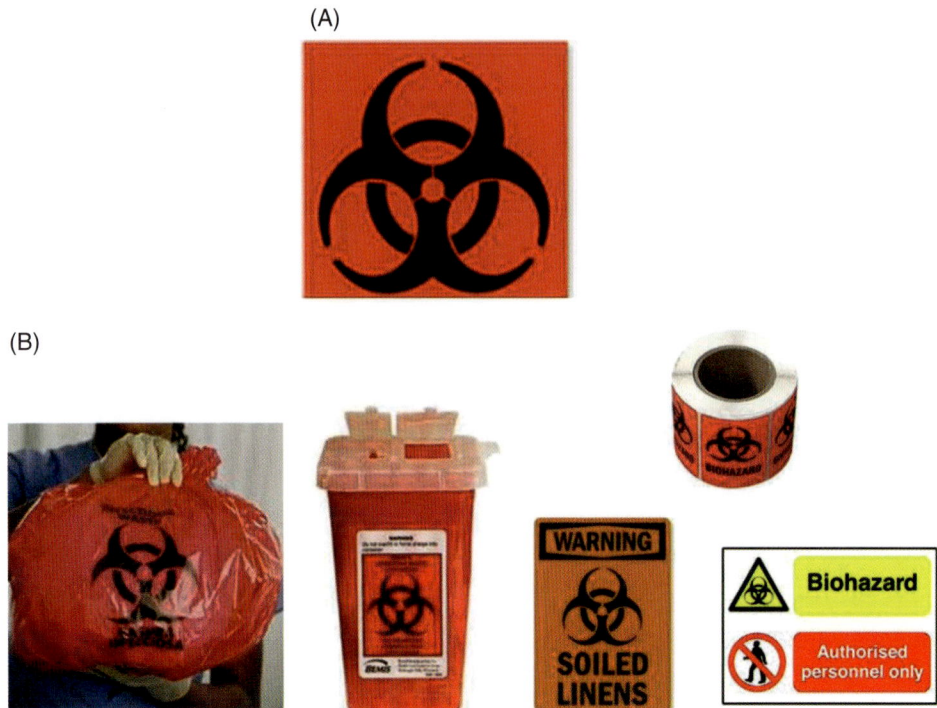

Figure 7.6 (A) The internationally recognized symbol for a biological or biohazard may be presented in different colors, typically orange, red, and yellow. (B) Examples of a clinical waste bag and sharps container, with various examples of biohazard labels.

the decontamination area, devices may be carried directly by hand, keeping trays parallel with the floor (in order to avoid shifting of the devices) and ensuring that soils or soiled materials are not allowed to spill or be dropped on transport. Even in such cases, it is still best practice to place the devices in a leakproof, puncture-resistant, and covered container. Such containers should not be overloaded, to avoid the risk of instrument damage and ensure that they are not too heavy for lifting (leading to risks of lifting/carrying-related strains and accidents).

Similar transport systems and procedures should be in place for any contaminated and reusable linens, as well as for the transport of disposable, contaminated waste (to prevent accidental spillage, etc.).

Transportation systems

A variety of transport systems may be used to transfer contaminated devices and device sets to a processing area (Figure 7.7).

A device set may consist of an individual device needed for a simple or unique task, a tray of devices used for a specific procedure, or a specialty set of multiple trays of devices. A tray of devices can range from a few handheld devices to over a hundred different items. Therefore there are various types of container systems that can be used, based on the facility's needs.

Items may be transported manually by carrying the used device containers directly to a designated area or by using a designated transport system such as a manual or motorized trolley. Trolleys serve an important function in reducing the risk of injury to staff carrying a device tray (some of which can be heavy) from one point to another. Contaminated items should always be completely separated from clean/sterile items during transportation. It is important that a system is put into place to ensure that there is a distinction between soiled and reprocessed (clean/sterile) devices, in order to ensure that soiled devices are not mistakenly used on patients. The concept of clean and dirty separation (see Chapter 1 on design of a decontamination area) does not only apply to the devices themselves but also to the transport aids such as containers and trolleys. Sterile or otherwise decontaminated items, importantly for critical and semi-critical procedures, should be transported in separate closed containers in clean, dry conditions in a way that will not compromise their disinfected/sterilized state and provide mechanical protection to prevent damage to the items or any associated packaging. Sterile packs, for example, should ideally be transported in closed solid-walled containers on covered or enclosed trolleys with solid-bottom shelves.

A two-container or two-trolley clean-and-dirty system is always preferable, but is not essential if effective safeguards are in

Point-of-use treatment and transport

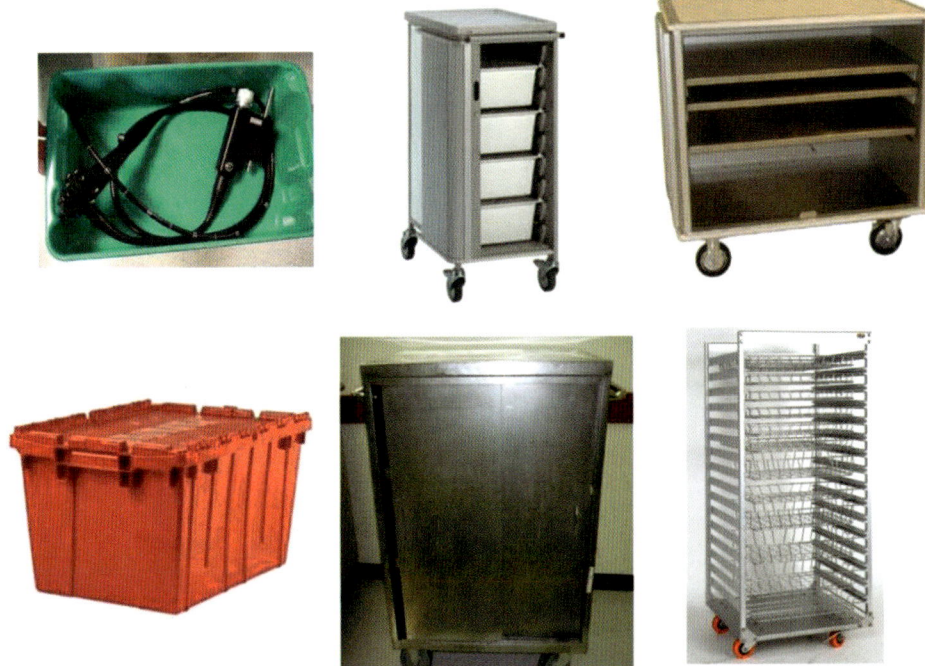

Figure 7.7 Examples of various types of transport systems, including examples of open and closed container systems and trolley systems.

place and monitored to prevent mix-ups. Similarly, "open" trolley systems can be effectively used where systems are in place to prevent mixing of dirty and clean devices/materials, and the risk of public exposure to contaminated items is considered low (e.g. in a staff access only surgical facility with a defined, internal decontamination facility). Closed transport carts/trolleys should always be used for transporting contaminated items between healthcare areas via other departments or for external transport.

Container and containment systems

There are various types of open and closed container systems available, which include trays, trolleys, impermeable bags, lidded bins, and rigid container systems (Figure 7.7). Transport containers should protect both the equipment and the handler from accidental contact during transit. Soiled items should be preferably placed into closed leak/splash-proof and puncture-resistant containers. Remember, all patient soiled items (especially those containing blood or other bodily fluids) should be considered biohazardous and correctly tagged or labeled as such, or according to policy as infectious. The ideal container/containment system should be:

- Easy to clean and disinfect, either manually or in an automated washer-disinfector.
- Specifically designed for transport of contaminated (and also disinfected/sterilized) items where greater protection than normal dust protection is required.
- Stable to prevent spilling or items from falling over or off any cart/trolley during transport.
- Closed to prevent contact with other healthcare personnel and patients in public areas leading to (or away from) any reprocessing area. The practice of locking using a cable tie, tamper-evident seal, or other means to ensure that the container is not opened when transported by a third party such as a courier should be considered.
- Covered, sealed, and leak-proof to minimize contamination and soiling of any transport vehicle/person due to leakage of contaminated fluids.
- Carefully packed with lighter devices on top of heavier devices and to protect sharps and delicate devices from damage.

Specially colored, marked, or labeled containers should be used for transporting soiled items. Red is usually the color of choice as it universally signals danger. Consideration should be given to any national, regional, local, and/or facility regulations regarding the handling and transportation of biohazardous materials. These may be different within and between facilities.

Transport trolleys

In some cases trolleys can be used to help transport devices and materials to a defined processing area. Distances between procedure and processing areas can often be long and over multiple floors within larger institutions, restricting safe and practical transport. A variety of trolley systems can be used to aid in the transport of device sets from one area to another (Figure 7.7). They are generally open or closed in design. They also range from simple push-type trolleys to motorized trolleys and sophisticated, automated transport systems for carrying a variety of supplies/materials around a facility.

Transport trolleys used for distribution of disinfected/sterilized items to users or for returning contaminated items from various sources within a facility to a processing area should be designed for handling and transporting items safely. All transport trolleys (motorized or manual) should be constructed from a material that allows for proper cleaning, which is particularly important if the trolley is transporting alternating decontaminated and contaminated items.

To avoid cross-contamination, contaminated items should, where possible, be transported to a processing area in a covered, enclosed trolley/cart with a solid-bottom shelf to prevent contamination of the floor from the trolley during transport. Items should preferably be transported via a dedicated passage and/or lift that opens directly into or close to the processing area. It is generally recommended that contaminated items are not transported through patient or general public areas; particular care should be taken in these cases to provide container and trolley system procedures that minimize any safety risks.

Only trained personnel wearing personal protective equipment (PPE; see Chapter 13) fit for this purpose, which includes at least protective gloves, should be involved with transporting. If potentially dealing with fluids where splashing could occur, safety goggles/visors and a facemask are also recommended. Care must be taken to prevent accidents while transporting; when either pulling or pushing the trolley, it is important to have a clear path of view in front and on either side of the trolley. For uncovered trolleys, it is better practice to transport by pulling to reduce the risk of contaminant/chemical exposure.

The trolley design should be stable and easy to maneuver with a combination of fixed and swivel wheels and ball bearings to maximize maneuverability. It should ideally have a handle to allow for easier and safer handling in narrow passages. For longer-distance transport between areas, closed, lockable-door trolleys are recommended. The trolley must be large enough for the amount of equipment being transported, but not too large to be difficult to maneuver. Items/containers should be placed securely in a flat position and should not extend beyond the edge of the shelf or outside the trolley in any way. For the greatest flexibility, trolleys with adjustable-height shelves or a number of shelves may be considered. The trolley must at no stage be left unattended in an unsecured location.

External/road transport

When using off-site or outsourced processing facilities, particular care must be taken regarding the containment of contaminated items. Transport vehicles should be completely enclosed and allow for ease of loading and unloading. As in the case of every transport system, soiled items should be adequately separated from disinfected/sterilized items. For example, condensate may occur on plastic or metal surfaces that have been moved from an air-conditioned to a non-conditioned environment. Extremes of temperature and humidity may also be a consideration (e.g. freezing).

As contaminated items are considered to be biohazardous, transport of such materials may be closely regulated by local, regional, and national agencies. At a minimum, such items should be clearly marked as biohazardous and adequately contained (i.e. secure, tamper-proof, leak-proof, sealed, rigid containers, trolleys, or carts). Containers and trolleys/carts should be preferably locked and secured in position to prevent movement during transit. Transport vehicles should be designed to be routinely cleaned/disinfected on a regular basis.

General good practice dictates that personnel dealing with contaminated items are trained on how to handle items safely, including use of PPE and how to handle accidents such as spills (e.g. location and use of a biohazard spill kit).

Care of trolleys and containers

Trolleys and containers are recommended to be routinely decontaminated, preferably after each use. These are considered non-critical items, but as they are potentially contaminated with biohazardous materials, they may need to be subjected to the same essential processes as those used to clean any other contaminated medical devices. This is particularly important to protect staff and to prevent cross-contamination in situations where these same trolleys/containers are used to transport sterile or disinfected goods. This can be achieved manually or in automated cart/container systems (Figure 7.8); recommendations regarding the processing and maintenance of hospital-designed trolleys/containers should be provided by their manufacturers.

In addition to processing instructions, cart/trolley manufacturers' instructions should be provided and consulted regarding maintenance, such as lubrication of any hinge joints and wheel castors. Removal of debris and materials from trolley wheels will prevent jamming and difficulty with maneuvering over time. It is recommended that a maintenance schedule should be in place for washing and maintaining trolleys.

During the design of processing facilities, it is important to consider the use and processing of containers, carts, and trolleys. For example, the parking area may be significant in size. Designated unloading, processing, cart storage, and reloading areas are important to design into the workflow of these areas, not just the medical and surgical devices themselves. It is valuable to consider modeling the throughput of operating hours to determine how much parking space is required for trolleys in the processing department versus how many trolleys are out in the clinical areas.

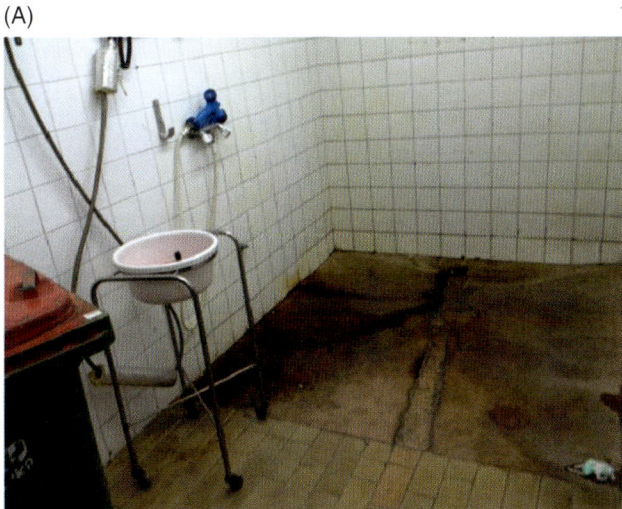
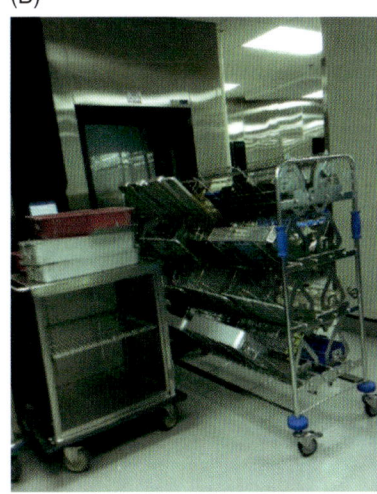

Figure 7.8 Examples of (A) manual and (B) automated systems for processing trolleys and containers. The automated systems shown are commonly referred to as trolley/cart-washer or trolley/cart-washer-disinfectors.

Manual processing of transport systems

At a minimum, containers and various parts of the trolley (particularly shelving) should be wiped down with a hospital-grade disinfectant (to aid in cleaning and low-level disinfection) between each use. Typical disinfectants that can be used include at least low- or intermediate-level disinfectants that are labeled for cleaning and disinfection (Chapter 9). Chlorine (or other halogen) based disinfectants (e.g. "bleach" or sodium hypochlorite solutions) are generally not recommended as they may lead to rusting and damage to carts/trolleys. More detailed and thorough cleaning of the inside and outside of the entire trolley is necessary periodically, as blood and bodily fluids can seep into joints, seams, and under surfaces of shelving and doors. Procedures should be put in place to ensure an appropriate workflow and/or physical separation of dirty and cleaned carts, trolleys, and containers to avoid mix-ups.

To aid with trolley/cart manual cleaning, a wet-working area should be designated within the decontamination area. This can be equipped with a pressure washing system (spray gun) to allow for manual cleaning, for automatic mixing of a cleaning chemistry/detergent with water, and for water rinsing (Figure 7.8). These areas also have both hot and cold water. A typical cycle will include washing (with detergent), rinsing, and drying. Washed carts should be dried (generally manually) with lint-free cloths, which may be aided by the use of 70% alcohol.

Automated processing of transport systems

It is preferable for automated systems to be used for processing of transport systems. These include device washer-disinfectors and specifically dedicated cart washer-disinfectors.

For device washer-disinfectors, specific cycles are usually defined to provide cleaning, rinsing, and low- to intermediate-level disinfection of containers by hot water (thermal disinfection); container systems may also be specifically designed to hold the medical/surgical devices during cleaning–disinfection/sterilization and are therefore reprocessed in the same cycles as those devices. The use of specific, shorter cycles is often preferred to maximize capacity for the use of the washer-disinfectors and the efficiency of the processing area.

Cart-washers (also referred to as cart washer-disinfectors, trolley washers, etc.) are larger washer-disinfectors for the processing of carts and trolleys (Figure 7.8). They can also be used in combination for the processing of containers and other non-critical items at the processing facility (such as footwear, wheelchairs, etc.). A variety of processing cycles can be defined in these washers in order to reduce time, energy, and water consumption. For example, rinse water collected from one stage of a cycle may be collected and reused for a subsequent stage of another cycle. A typical cycle includes pre-cleaning with water (to remove gross soil), cleaning with a detergent formulation, rinsing, disinfection (thermal or chemical), rinsing (if applicable), and drying. Thermal disinfection is the most common method, with a typical recommended cycle at 80°C for one minute or the equivalent (e.g. in accordance with ISO 15883, *Washer-Disinfectors Parts 1 and 6*; see also Chapter 9 on automated cleaning), although chemical disinfection may also be used (in accordance with ISO 15883, *Washer-Disinfectors Parts 1 and 7*). Specific cycles range widely depending on the region or area in use and local requirements.

Tracking and traceability

Tracking and traceability should be considered an integral part of processing. Traceability is the ability to verify the history, location, or application of an item by means of a documented recorded identification system. Traceability can only be achieved if the items are uniquely identified and relevant data about items is captured and recorded. This can be traditionally achieved manually by a paper-based system, but that is increasingly being replaced by computer-based systems, including unique identifying codes provided on individual devices and with sets of devices. Today most individual devices are not provided with unique identification codes and most tracking systems are used to track sets of surgical devices; this will change over time with the greater availability of tracking abilities for individual devices.

A traceability or tracking system should be in place (in particular for medium to larger institutions) that records the progress of individual devices or sets through each stage of the processing cycle (including clinical use and transport) and allows a retrospective reconstruction of the history of that set, including the patients on whom it was used. Tracking records that permit verification that a set or reusable devices have been through an approved processing cycle (cleaning, disinfection, and/or sterilization) should be maintained; these can include details of each set, batch, or load, date, cycle reference numbers, and so on, which in the event of a recall or adverse patient incident would allow the devices to be investigated. The tracking system may also be used to enable identification of patients on whom the device/sets have been used, as it is important that the relevant patients can be identified in the event of exposure to any potential health risk. It may also be used to control inventory, and to understand the availability of devices and device sets for particular (especially surgical and endoscopic) procedures.

For an efficient system, the first requirement is to uniquely identify the items to be tracked by an identification system (manual or automated, e.g. by manually recording a number/code or by bar coding). This can be done by tracking either the individual items or more commonly a set of devices. In computerized systems, such item identification can then be communicated to other members of the processing and supply chain cycle. In some countries it is recommended that devices within a set used in a patient procedure should remain together and be tracked and reprocessed together; individual devices should not in this case be allowed to move from one set to another. In such cases, individual device tracking systems may be necessary. As most devices today are not provided with unique identification codes, facilities often consider and provide onsite marking and identification methods.

Following transport from a site of surgical/medical use to a processing area, it is important that the devices and all associated accessories (particularly parts associated with devices that are reused) have been received and accounted for. If items or parts are missing they will need to be located or replaced.

A more detailed discussion of tracking and traceability in device processing is offered in Chapter 14 in the section on tracking and traceability.

8 Cleaning

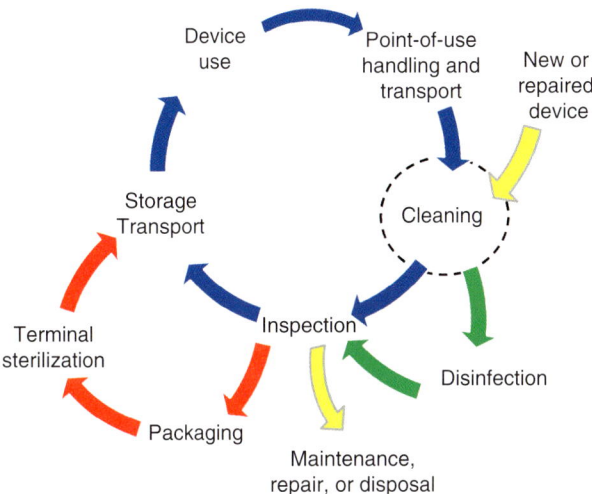

Cleaning is the removal of soil (or contamination) from an item to the extent necessary for its further processing and its intended subsequent use. Soils can be made up of a variety of components, including organic and inorganic materials from the patient or various chemicals used during the medical/surgical procedure (e.g. gels, lubricants, cements, etc.; Table 8.1).

Cleaning may be the only required step in the processing cycle to allow a device to be reused (for example in some cases with non-critical devices; see Chapter 1, the section on goals of decontamination and the Spaulding classification). But for most reusable devices cleaning is an essential step prior to and to ensure effective disinfection and/or sterilization as part of the processing cycle. The presence of soils can interfere with the activity of disinfection or sterilization products or processes against target microorganisms, thereby reducing their effectiveness. The presence of soils can also lead to adverse reactions in patients, such as toxicity and immune reactions, as well as damage to device functioning. Cleaning is therefore an essential step, and often considered the most important step, in the processing cycle.

The cleaning process should produce the result of the devices being clean. This can be defined as their being visually free of soil (visually "clean"), but also can be further scientifically defined as being below specified levels of analytes. Analytes are chemical substances that can be measured to indicate the presence of residual contamination, and these include some of the major chemical contaminants found on reusable devices following patient use, such as proteins, hemoglobin, and levels of organic carbon. Proteins are major components of human, animal, and microbial structures (Chapters 2 and 5) and are therefore an important measure of cleanliness. Carbon is another useful measurement as it will be present in many materials that make up human tissues and microorganisms (e.g. proteins and lipids; Chapters 2 and 5), as well as other materials such as detergents (Chapter 6). The acceptable levels for these analytes to be considered clean will be considered later in this chapter.

In many healthcare situations cleaning may be considered adequate if the surface or all parts of the device are visibly clean. This may appear straightforward on exposed, visual surfaces, but on closer inspection may not be the case. The use of better light or magnification may improve visual inspection, but there is still the difficulty of inspecting a device where all parts cannot be directly seen (e.g. within lumens or requiring device disassembly). The presence of soil in these cases, even at what may appear to be low levels, can pose a patient risk including affecting the outcome of any subsequent disinfection/sterilization step depending on the intended use of the device.

In addition, some bodily fluids may not be visible to the naked eye, including tears, pericardial fluid, synovial fluid, cerebrospinal fluid, and so on. As such, the device may look clean but is not and may still present a patient risk. For these reasons, in addition to detailed visual inspections, other methods may be used to confirm the surfaces/devices are at an acceptable level of cleanliness below what we can see.

Decontamination and Device Processing in Healthcare, Second Edition. Gerald McDonnell and Georgia Alevizopoulou.
© 2025 John Wiley & Sons Ltd. Published 2025 by John Wiley & Sons Ltd.

Table 8.1 Examples of various components of soil found on devices following use on/in patients.

Organic materials	Inorganic materials
Blood, mucus, feces, urine	Salts, such as NaCl
Tissues, such as those in skin, muscles, bone, etc.	Metals, including iron
Proteins, carbohydrates, lipids/fats, lipopolysaccharides[1]	Other elements and molecules, such as calcium and iodine
Microorganisms such as bacteria, viruses and fungi	Cements (used in orthopedic procedures)
Gels and lubricants	Chemicals used on the skin or directly on the device pre-operatively or post-operatively

[1] A lipopolysaccharide is a molecule that includes a lipid ("lipo") and polysaccharide (carbohydrate) part.

These are further considered in Chapter 10 on inspection and later in this chapter.

Cleaning and decontamination practices should be conducted in an environment designed to protect members of staff (or indeed the general public) who may come into contact with contaminated devices (e.g. during transport following patient use or preparing them for further processing steps). It is best practice in healthcare facilities throughout the world that cleaning and decontamination of equipment and instrumentation should occur in designated processing areas or facilities. If this is not possible or practical, standard procedures should be developed to ensure these safety requirements. Note, as discussed in Chapter 7, that point-of-use treatment can often be conducted at the site of device use (e.g. in or in close proximity to a surgical room) or the cleaning process initiated before transport to a processing area. Cleaning can be achieved manually (e.g. in a sink), semi-manually (using a machine to aid in or as part of the cleaning process), and automatically (using a washer-disinfector). In many cases it may include all these steps. A washer-disinfector can be defined as a machine that cleans and disinfects devices; this definition is applicable internationally in the context of medical, dental, pharmaceutical, and veterinary practice. Automated cleaning is often preferred to manual cleaning as it can reduce the risk to staff and can allow for greater consistency in the defined process steps, but this will depend on the design and labeling of the automated system. The specifics of the cleaning process will depend on the instrument or device being processed, ranging from simple to complicated and/or multi-part devices (Chapter 4). It is important to remember that it is the responsibility of the reusable device manufacturer to provide adequate instructions to users on how to safely and effectively process such devices, including cleaning. When such items are sold to a facility, in the absence of detailed instructions, they may be inadequately processed, compromising patient safety and opening the hospital to litigation. Staff who are handling devices in a healthcare facility should have detailed training (and demonstrate competency over time) that will include the safe and proper use as well as the correct processing of a device, to include dismantling, cleaning, inspection/maintenance, reassembly, and subsequent disinfection/sterilization (where applicable). This will include training in the use of all processing equipment.

The key components required for cleaning are:
- A cleaning chemistry ("detergent," cleaning formulation) to break down, loosen, and assist in removing the soil (proteins, lipids, etc.).
- Friction produced by mechanical action (manual or automated) to remove the soil. Examples include flushing, brushing, spraying, ultrasonics, wiping, etc.
- Water to aid in the process of removal and rinsing away soil (including residual detergents).

If all three components are not present or are sub-optimal, effective cleaning cannot take place; this presents a particular challenge in many countries where water and other resources are limited.

Receiving and sorting

The receiving and cleaning (dirty) area should be functionally separated (preferably with physical barriers) from all other areas (e.g. packaging, sterilization, or storage) of the processing facility (Chapter 1). Staff must assume that all items arriving at or returning to any processing facility are contaminated; it is unacceptable to process only those devices that are known or thought to have been in direct patient contact. All reusable instruments and instrument trays opened in the clinical environment should be decontaminated between uses (Figure 8.1). This will include the devices and, in certain situations, the external surfaces of containers that have been touched by staff in the clinical area or have been in contact with bodily fluids. Examples of contact include during surgery with handling by the scrub nurse, surgeon, circulating nurse, or anyone else assisting with a surgical procedure. Remember, soiling and contamination may not always be visible.

Staff working in this area must be fully attired in recommended personal protective equipment (PPE). This is designed to reduce hazards, including microbiological (from patient soil), chemical (e.g. with the cleaning chemistry), and sharps (device) risks. PPE is therefore particularly important and must be mandatory (Figure 8.2). Care should be taken to ensure that staff are comfortable wearing PPE, that they comply with written protocols, and that they are consistent in the way they behave when carrying out this activity. If the PPE is uncomfortable in any way, it is likely that it will not be used efficiently, despite the risks to health. Close collaboration with staff in these areas is important to ensure their safety. There is increasing evidence of the risks associated with aerosolization of contaminants during cleaning processes that can pose a significant risk to staff and visitors. Further, PPE should be inspected to be fit for purpose. An example is with gloves, which should be immediately replaced if torn or otherwise compromised.

Recommended PPE for handling, sorting, and cleaning will include:

- Face protection, which can be a full-face shield or separate eye and mouth protection. The eyes, nasal passages, and mouth are the highest health risk areas. Facemasks can provide a certain level of protection. If mouth/nose masks are used, staff should be trained in the correct method for using these masks (ensuring that the mouth and nose are correctly

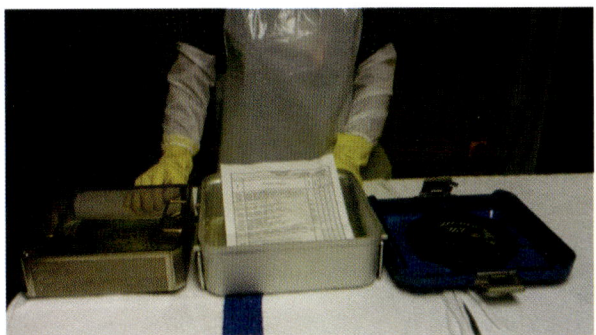

Figure 8.1 An example of a set of instruments, including container and trays, being received into the decontamination area and prepared for sorting. Note: a device set checklist is shown (middle) as part of the facility tracking system (see Chapter 14 on tracking and traceability).

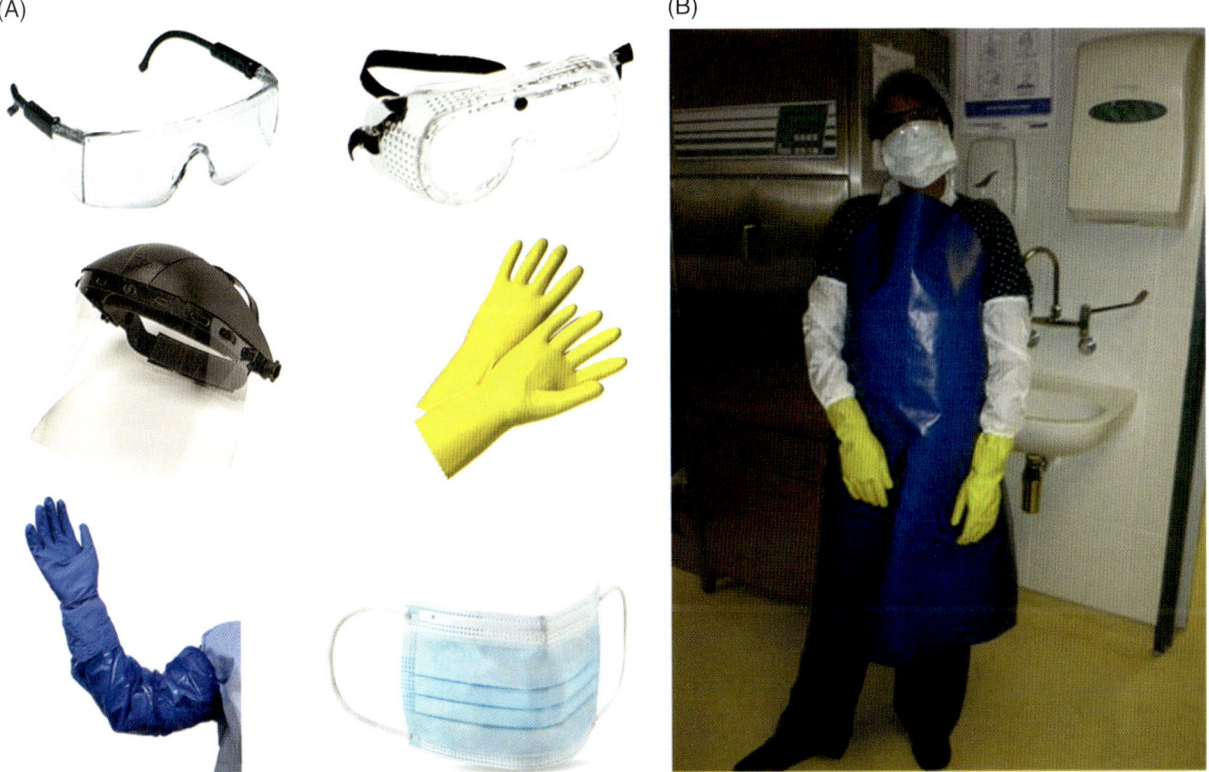

Figure 8.2 An example of typical personal protective equipment (PPE) used during handling, sorting, and cleaning of patient-soiled devices. (A) Safety glasses, face shield, gloves, and a facemask. (B) A typical example of full PPE.

protected). When used, safety glasses should have side shields to prevent splashing from occurring from the sides. It is a useful training exercise to provide a new facemask or safety glasses to a staff member, allow them to do manual cleaning, and then show them what is present on the glasses/facemask over time. This allows for visualization of the risk and increases optimum use.

- Full-length waterproof gown (or in some countries at least a plastic apron), to protect clothing from splashes and spillages. Ideally separate clothing (including shoes) is provided to staff to be worn for sorting and cleaning of soiled devices. This will prevent the accidental contamination of personal clothing and transfer out of the cleaning area. Clothing for use in these areas can remain confined within designated areas and periodically subjected to laundry (Chapter 15). Other considerations can include head/hair protection and liquid-resistant shoes (or shoe covers).
- Heavy-duty gloves (e.g. nitrile gloves). These are usually longer gloves to cover the wrists and lower arm. It is recommended that jewelry and artificial nails are not used, as these can lead to glove damage. Jewelry may also be accidentally damaged during the manual cleaning process. Gloves may also be supported by arm protectors (as shown in Figure 8.2) that go further over the elbows.
- Other PPE should also be considered, such as hair/head protection and liquid-resistant foot protection (e.g. boots and protected footwear, such as steel-toed, to minimize risks from dropping or spillage accidents).

On arrival in the cleaning/decontamination area, any remaining soiled single-use items or miscellaneous materials should be safely discarded. All reusable items should be removed from the transport cart/trolley and containers, sorted, checked, and prepared for cleaning. Due diligence must be always shown when sorting and dealing with contaminated items. If not already conducted at the point of use, all waste materials and single-use devices should be disposed of in accordance with the local waste policy (see Chapter 13 on waste management and Chapter 7 on post-procedure sorting) and any laundry items similarly sorted (see Chapter 15 on laundry). It is best practice that such materials are discarded or separated at the point of use (Chapter 7); when this is not the case, management should work closely with staff in these clinical/surgical areas to ensure safe practices.

Procedures should be in place to ensure that personnel can safely handle reusable devices and minimize any risks of accidental injury. Two important risks are accidental exposure to pathogenic microorganisms (via the hands, eyes, nose, and mouth) and sharps-related injuries. Given the wide range of cutting, dissecting, injecting, and other devices used (particularly surgically), sharps-related injuries are high risk and should be minimized. Not only can they injure the skin, the consequences of cross-infection are high. Examples include safe removal, disposal of single-use blades at the point of use (see Chapter 7 on post-procedure sorting), ensuring technicians can directly see all devices in a set, and using a sorting instrument tool (instead of using the hands directly to remove devices) for sorting (Figure 8.3).

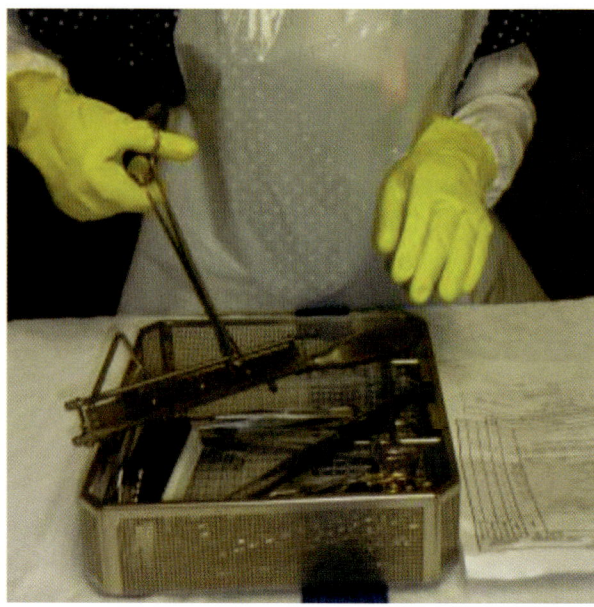

Figure 8.3 Safe sorting of surgical devices using a swab holder. Items are handled and sorted in accordance with any local policy. In this case the instrument being used for handling is dedicated for this purpose and *not* an integral part of the set.

The responsibility for the safe disposal of single-use blades, needles, and other materials should lie with the user designated at the site. If they are discovered in the sorting/cleaning area, this should immediately be reported to the line or facility manager as a failure of the user to comply with operational procedures and thereby putting staff health and safety at risk. In the event of a needlestick or sharps injury, the incident must be reported immediately and any facility policy implemented.

Medical and surgical instruments are often delicate and should be handled accordingly. They should not be dropped, thrown into baskets/sinks, or handled roughly, as this can damage the instrument and affect its functionality. Sets/trays should be carefully checked against any contents list on receipt prior to washing and any missing or damaged items recorded and reported. Remedial action for missing or damaged equipment should be taken in accordance with the department's quality system. It is recommended that where there is more than one tray of devices (e.g. for hysterectomy and some orthopedic sets), such sets are sorted and organized into a limited number of numbered trays required for such procedures.

Certain items may need special attention and should be sorted or handled accordingly. These include:
- Cannulated (lumened) instruments, which may need to be flushed using a high-pressure water system or otherwise cleaned as specified by the manufacturer of the device. Consideration should be given to reducing any risks of staff exposure to aerosols that can be generated during cleaning. As an example, this can be minimized by cleaning the device under water.
- Non-immersible items – devices that cannot be immersed in water, such as types of electrical drills – must be cleaned according to the manufacturer's written instructions and protected from contamination wherever possible during the surgical procedure. Delicate items that have specialized cleaning procedures should be handled and cleaned as recommended by the manufacturer.
- Contaminated reusable devices that are not to be subjected to processing at the site but are to be shipped to another site for processing or further handling. Examples can include devices on loan to be returned to a commercial provider or to be shipped to another site that specializes in processing. In these cases, remember that the devices are considered biohazardous and should be properly contained and labeled in accordance with any local requirement for the transportation of dangerous goods (see Chapter 7 on transportation post procedure). It is overall best practice for devices, including loaned devices/equipment, to be decontaminated (cleaned and disinfected) at the site of use prior to shipping.
- At the time of writing, high-risk devices that may be or are known or have been exposed to prions require separate consideration. Special precautions should be in place (where the device is used and in the decontamination area) in handling these devices, such as separate processing (including chemical and steam sterilization protocols) or incineration (see Chapter 15, the section on devices known or suspected to be contaminated with prion material). In some cases these devices may need to be isolated in accordance with any local policies.

Protocols should be in place that instruct staff members on the minimum requirements for processing of each type of medical/surgical instrument. This is generally based on the Spaulding classification system, which defines critical, semi-critical, and non-critical devices (see Chapter 1 on the goals of decontamination and the Spaulding classification). As an example, dental equipment, such as extraction forceps, scalpel blades, bone chisels, and surgical burs that may have penetrated soft tissue or bone during a procedure, are classified as critical and should be thoroughly cleaned and sterilized after each use. Dental instruments that may accidentally penetrate oral soft tissue or bone (e.g. amalgam condensers, air-water syringes) are generally considered as semi-critical and must also be thoroughly cleaned and at least be high-level disinfected.

Devices can also be classified based on their complexity for cleaning. This can simply be based on the probability of soil retention associated with device features. Minimal-risk devices are those with design features where all surfaces are exposed or visible, therefore they do not require any unique intervention to ensure cleaning. Moderate-risk devices have accessible design features but require some specific intervention to ensure access for cleaning. Examples of such features include lumens (or cannulas) that require flushing or brushing to ensure cleanliness, or mated surfaces (e.g. areas between two contact surfaces such as between the blades of two scissors or the hinge point (or screw) between two blades). In some cases they can be disassembled to allow them to be readily cleaned, but this is not always the case. Therefore disassembly (when described by the manufacturer) or specific intervention into these design features is required to ensure cleanliness. Maximal-risk (or high-risk) designs are complex features that cannot be readily accessed or inspected and require more detailed cleaning steps. These present a high risk of soil accumulation. Care in following cleaning instructions is essential and often includes specific cleaning methods such as the use of ultrasonics or other methods (e.g. using specific accessories provided by the manufacturer) that can better penetrate these areas. It is not unusual to have complex devices that have a mixture of minimal, moderate, and maximal design features. However, it is the features that present the highest probability of soil accumulation that pose the greatest challenge to cleaning.

Consideration should also be given to the handling, processing, and storage of any transport containers and trolleys that are used in this area; this is discussed in more detail in Chapter 7 in the section on transportation post procedure.

Finally, it is best practice during processing that devices and device sets are tracked, using a manual (Figure 8.1) or automated (computerized) system (Figure 8.4; also see Chapter 14 on inventory management). This will allow recording of the presence of devices received for processing, through the processing steps, and for future traceability requirements. Therefore, at this stage there will be a need for devices (and/or sets of device) to be entered into the tracking and traceability system in use by the facility (as discussed in Chapter 7, in the section on tracking and traceability; and in Chapter 14, in the section on materials management). It is possible at this stage for lost or misplaced devices to be identified and potentially located at the previous point of use.

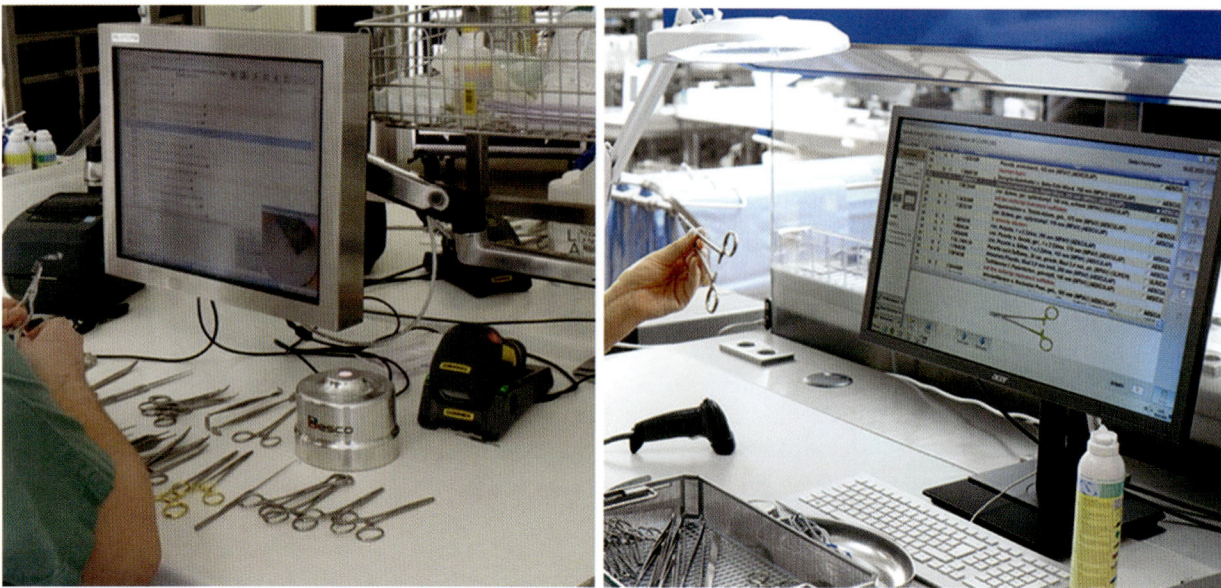

Figure 8.4 Examples of automated/computerized device tracking systems.

Disassembly and preparation for cleaning

If it is safe to do so, devices composed of more than one part or moving pieces should be opened and disassembled to the smallest part in order to expose all surfaces to the cleaning process (Figure 8.5). Before disassembly is considered, always refer to the manufacturer's guidelines for device-specific instructions and follow the recommended procedures. These guidelines should specifically provide any disassembly instructions that are required to ensure adequate cleaning.

As already described, surgical instruments can be divided into three groups based on device complexity and challenge to cleanliness: minimal (or simple challenge), moderate, and maximal (or complex challenge) (Chapter 4). Minimal- and moderate-challenge instruments, such as needle holders, scissors, handheld retractors, hemostats, and so on, have simple moving parts and articulation points (e.g. box locks), hinges, or screw joints. These instruments are typically designed to be hardy and can be processed by a manual and/or automated cleaning and decontamination process. Such instruments can become a greater challenge to clean if gross soil is allowed to remain and dry on the instruments for an extended time (as discussed in Chapter 7 in the section on post-procedure sorting). Complex instruments, with device features that are hard to access, often have multiple moving parts, are powered by electric motors, compressed gas (pneumatic), or batteries, and have long cannula (lumens). They will need special treatment, with close attention to detail provided according to the manufacturer's guidelines.

Maximal-challenge instruments usually require multiple steps to effectively disassemble and clean them. An example of a maximal-challenge device would be a self-retaining retractor that has multiple locking screws and securing ratchets that will need to be opened and retractor blades that will need to be removed to allow proper cleaning. Some of these complex instruments can only be cleaned manually, while others are recommended to be cleaned manually followed by automated cleaning. An example of this is a flexible endoscope, where manual cleaning is recommended alone or in addition to automated cleaning. Endoscopes and other lumened devices provide a notable challenge, as the internal surfaces of such devices cannot be visually inspected (to check for cleaning efficacy) and, in many such cases, the presence, number, and interconnections of lumens in these devices can be difficult to understand. Further, these devices can have an array of moving parts and accessories (including reusable parts such as valves) that are used as part of surgical/medical procedures (see Chapter 4, in the section on endoscopy). Some of these devices can be very heavily soiled due to their clinical use, such as colonoscopes.

Unfortunate mistakes made in the cleaning and processing of these types of devices are well published, in most cases due to device complexity and inadequate understanding of the steps required to safely reprocess. Further examples are delicate microsurgical instruments that normally need to be disassembled and are often recommended to be hand washed and rinsed with water (high-quality water due to the risks associated with these types of devices; see Chapter 15, in the section

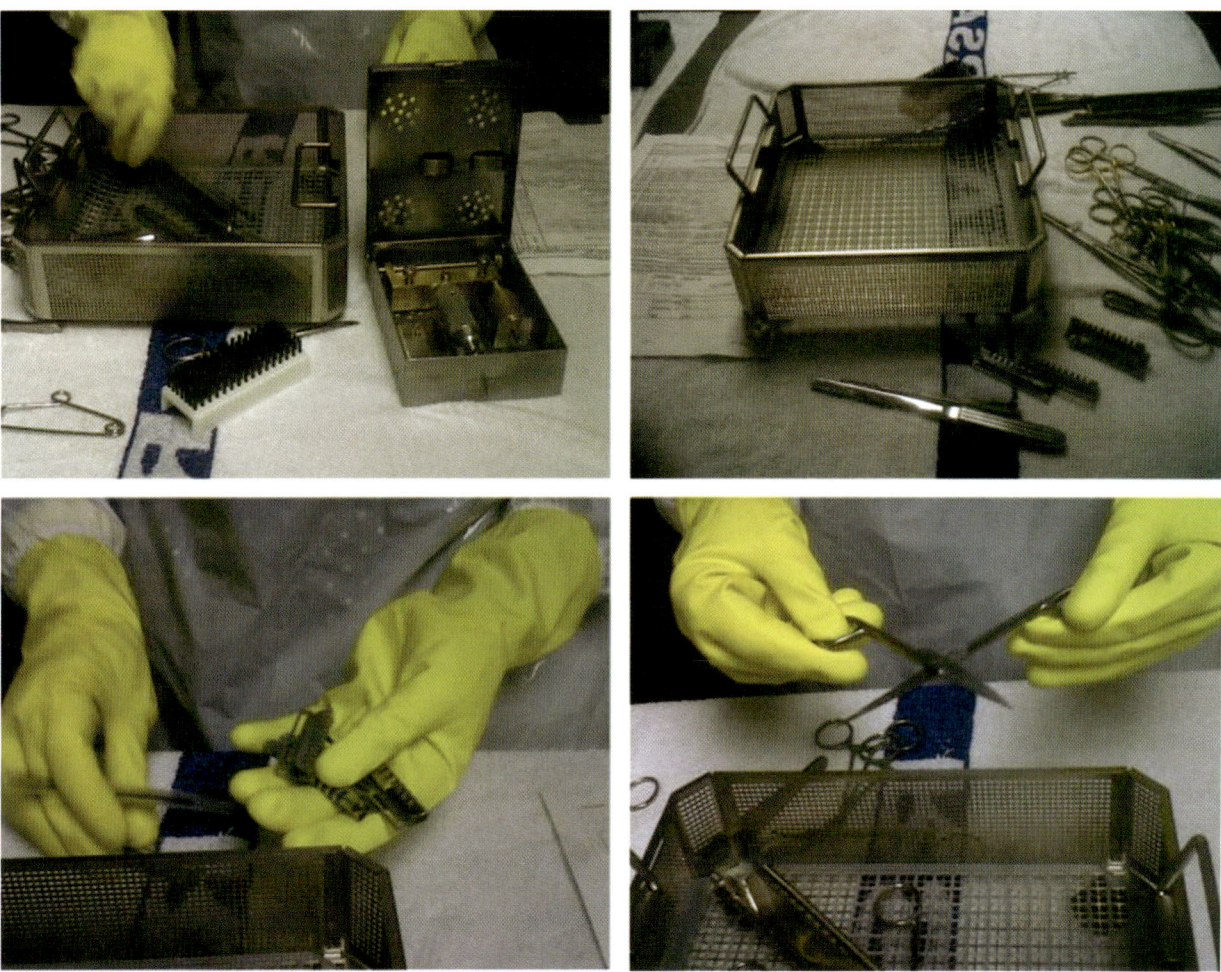

Figure 8.5 Disassembly and preparation for cleaning.

on water quality). Wherever possible these are protected and secured before being passed through an automated cleaning process. Instruments used in orthopedic procedures are examples of the range of device challenges that present significant processing problems for any processing facility (Figure 8.6). Many such instruments require manual and ultrasonic cleaning because bone, tissue, and in some cases cement can become embedded in them (drill bits and guides, cutting blocks, tibial keel punches, and drills are among the instruments that often retain bone and tissue). It is important to note in this case that cement is a particular challenge (if not impossible) to remove from a device surface when it has set; for this reason, it is recommended that cement should be removed at the site of use (e.g. in the surgical theater) prior to its setting (becoming solid) and then needing to be transported (Chapter 7).

Most orthopedic instrument trays contain many devices, being designed with multiple layers and containing large, medium, and very small devices. These are often provided by manufacturers as loan sets that move from hospital to hospital (note: loan sets are further discussed in Chapter 15). Close inspection of such manufacturers' processing instructions is essential. Processing facility staff must understand how these device trays should be handled, disassembled, and processed. For example, they should ensure that tray lids are removed, all instruments may need to be removed (big and small), and some may require disassembly, before the instruments are adequately cleaned. Remember that these sets can contain reusable instruments and single-patient use implants. The instruments are designed to be reusable, but the implants are typically not. In these cases, the implants can be processed, including sterilization, in accordance with the manufacturer's instructions, but not if they have been used in a patient procedure, damaged, or otherwise soiled during handling. They should also not be exposed to certain types of

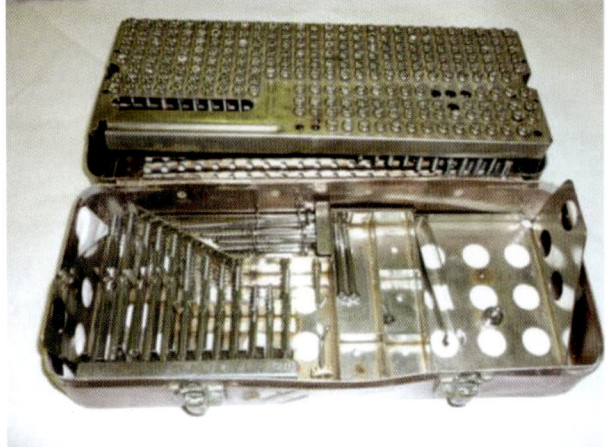 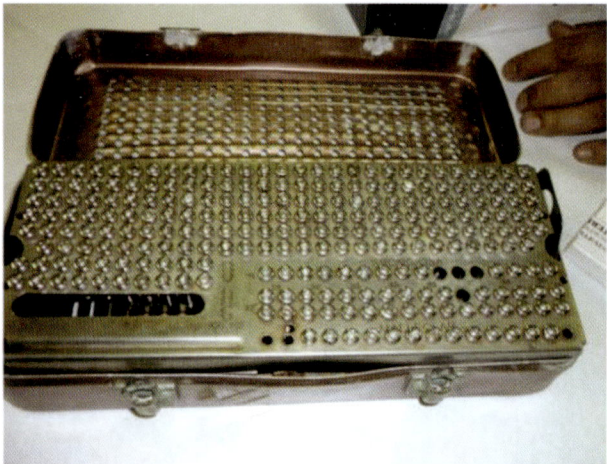
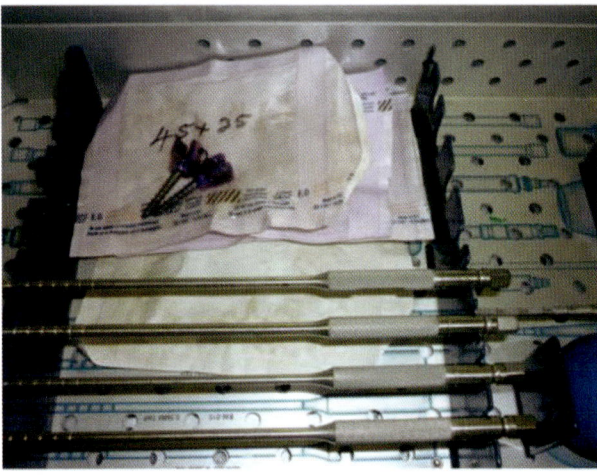 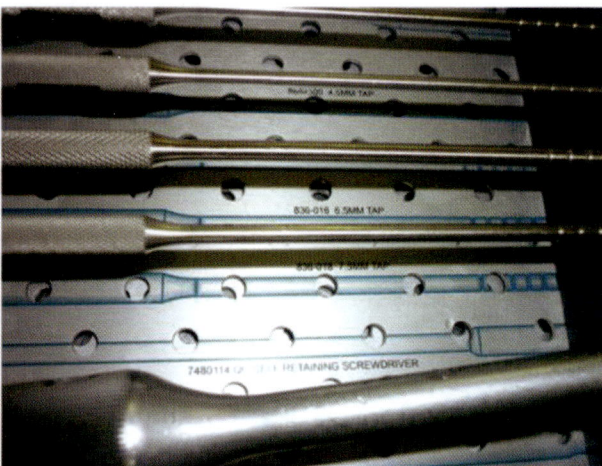

Figure 8.6 Examples of devices used in complex orthopedic sets.

chemicals that can cause damage or leave residuals on them (e.g. with the traditional use of lubricants used automatically in washer-disinfectors). All pins, plates, screws, and other parts (including any implants that are designed to remain in a patient) should be carefully inspected; this may require magnification and particular handling following cleaning and prior to sterilization (Chapter 10). Overall, orthopedic instrument sets provide an example of special challenges because of their size, weight, and number of required trays, multiple layers of instruments, different complexity of design features, as well as the fact that they are usually loan sets that need to be returned following use. It is often advisable to break down multi-layered trays into single-layered trays so that they can be more easily handled and processed safely and effectively. Further consideration to loan devices/sets and implants is given in Chapter 15, in the section on loan devices, sets, and implants.

Basic principles of cleaning

Cleaning is often considered the most important step in the processing cycle. If an item is not cleaned it will be unacceptable to use for medical or surgical purposes for the following reasons:
- Visually, the use of a soiled device is unacceptable to staff and patients. Would you use a device on yourself if it was visually soiled with material from a previous person?
- Foreign materials, particularly if they are left on or injected into a wound during surgery, can lead to the need for further surgery and the patient being exposed to further risks.
- Microbiological and infection risk: microorganisms, particularly pathogens (disease causing), can be present and be transferred to a patient. The presence of soil can compromise the effectiveness of disinfection and sterilization.
- Chemical toxicity risk: residual materials, despite the presence or absence of microorganisms, can lead to toxic reactions

in patients and especially in certain types of surgery such as in ophthalmology. Certain types of "dead" bacteria release toxic substances that can also lead to adverse patient reactions (e.g. endotoxins, see Chapter 5).

• Instrument damage: the presence of soil can damage the device, chemically (e.g. rusting, Chapter 7) and/or physically (e.g. loss of device function/operation). Cleaning can be attained using a variety of methods, including manual and automated cleaning. Right from the start, the appropriate cleaning method for a particular device will depend on its design features, and the manufacturer's instructions should always first be reviewed to determine how a device is properly cleaned.

Consideration has previously been given to the chemical aspects of soils (see Chapter 6 and its introduction to cleaning and accessory chemistries). Soil that remains on device surfaces following their use on a patient can contain a variety of organic and inorganic materials from the patient or items used during the procedure; these could include blood, tissues, surgical preparation chemicals, and microorganisms. The amount and type of soil can vary depending on the medical/surgical procedure the devices have been used for and if any point-of-use treatment has occurred (Chapter 3). Further, the devices may have dried soils present that are an even greater challenge to cleaning. As discussed in the introduction, the minimum expectation is to visually clean each individual device, with particular attention given to those devices or device parts that cannot be directly visually examined (such as lumened devices). Despite this, the required endpoints of cleaning (in order to claim or prove that a device can be called "clean") may require more detailed analysis, such as microbiological (e.g. levels of bacteria), biochemical (e.g. levels of protein), or chemical analysis (e.g. total organic carbon; see the introductory section and the section on trouble-shooting cleaning problems). This detailed analysis is required in the development and validation of the instructions for use by the manufacturer, but verification of some of these endpoints may need to be carried out clinically on a regular basis and periodically reviewed to ensure that any sudden changes are investigated and the cause(s) resolved.

The key components required for cleaning have already been introduced as the cleaning chemistry, a method of friction, and water. The various types of cleaning chemistries have been introduced in Chapter 6. They are classified based on their use and/or type of chemistry: enzymatic (containing enzymes) and non-enzymatic, such as neutral or alkaline detergents. In all cases they are formulations, being a variety of ingredients, including active and inert ingredients, combined into a product for its intended use. In some cases, especially with manual cleaning, cleaning chemistries are often used that have additional, generally low-level, antimicrobial activity. As a note, low-level disinfection during cleaning can be considered helpful to reduce staff handling risks, but is not considered necessary as part of the processing cycle (although it is specifically recommended in certain countries).

Methods of friction include mechanical means to aid in the cleaning process, which can be achieved by manual (e.g. hand washing or using brushes) and automated (e.g. spray, immersion, and ultrasonic) methods. Water plays a particular role in assisting the cleaning process and in rinsing away soil, as well as any cleaning chemistry residues on device surfaces prior to disinfection/sterilization. The combination of these components under the right conditions and time can provide effective cleaning. These essential components are considered in further detail in this chapter.

Cleaning itself is commonly a multi-step process. A typical cleaning process (manual or automated) will include:

• Pre-rinsing or pre-washing (with water and/or with a cleaning chemistry). This is usually conducted at temperatures of less than 45°C (<45°C), in order to remove any gross soil that is present and ensure that soil is not fixed or clumped (which can happen on exposure to higher temperatures). Fixing or clumping of soil components, such as proteins, on devices can leave them even more difficult to clean. Pre-rinsing may be conducted at (or near to) the point of patient use (Chapter 7), manually within a designated processing area, or in an automated washer-disinfector.

• Washing is performed with a cleaning chemistry used at the right concentration (dilution), temperature, and recommended conditions. This is the main stage of cleaning and the optimal conditions for this to occur should be recommended by the manufacturer (of the chemistry and/or the device being cleaned).

• Rinsing is performed with water to remove any residues of soil components and cleaning chemistry to render the device "clean" and ready for subsequent patient use or further reprocessing. This may require single or multiple rinses of water, depending on the chemistry type being used, the device being processed, and the cleaning process being used.

Cleaning can be achieved by manual and/or automated processes. In manual cleaning, devices are generally immersed in a sink or basin containing the cleaning chemistry at the right concentration and temperature. Specific accessories may need to be used and provided by the manufacturer or supplied locally to aid in this process; examples are lumen adapters that allow for a syringe to be attached to a device port and facilitate flushing of internal lumens/surfaces. Care should be taken not to use any accessory (such as hard metal brushes and scouring pads) that could lead to device damage. Metal brushes and scouring pads can significantly damage surfaces such as stainless steel and plastics. In the case of stainless steel, this can lead to loss of the passivation layer and provide opportunities for rust development (see Chapter 10, Figure 10.6). If such an accessory is required to remove stubborn soils (e.g. cements), it is recommended that the soil is removed prior to hardening at the site of use.

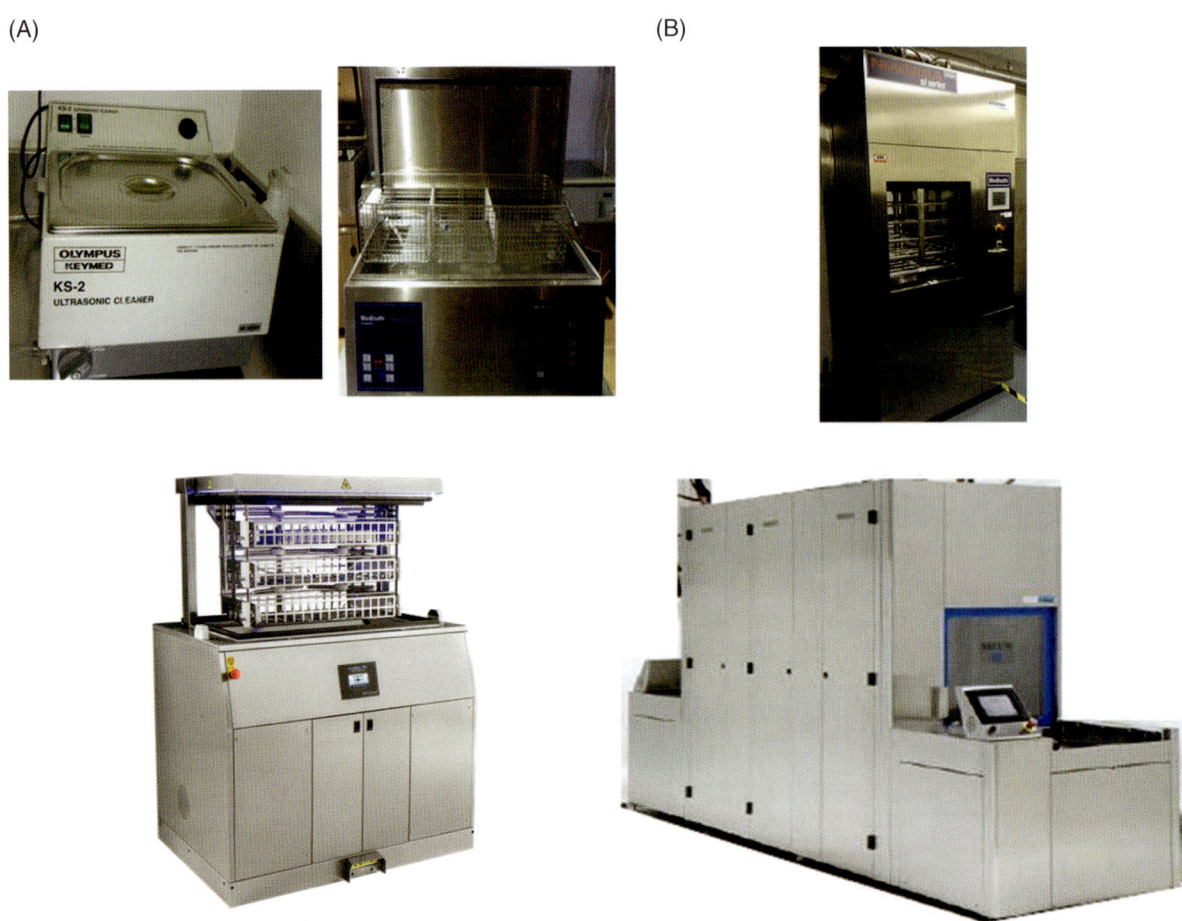

Figure 8.7 (A) Ultrasonic baths of various sizes, used to aid in manual cleaning. Courtesy STERIS Corporation 2024. All rights reserved. (B) Ultrasonics are also used in larger automated washer-disinfectors (single or as part of a multi-chamber washer), for pre-cleaning and/or automated cleaning processes.

A semi-automated cleaning process can include the use of an ultrasonic bath (Figure 8.7). Ultrasonic baths come in a range of sizes, from table-top machines to free-standing baths, to those integrated into washer-disinfectors and as a module in a tunnel or multi-chamber washer-disinfector (see automated cleaning). These allow for devices to be immersed in a cleaning chemistry and cleaning aided by sonication. Sonication is a process using ultrasonic (sound) waves to cause the disruption and removal of soil from surfaces (see the section on immersion including ultrasonic cleaning). In some ultrasonic bath designs, lumen devices can be attached to flow ports designed to allow water and cleaning solutions to flow through the device and aid in the cleaning process. Many ultrasonic baths are just designed for washing and do not provide any rinsing, while others can include a full cleaning process with multiple steps.

Fully automated cleaning processes can be conducted with various designs of washers and washer-disinfectors (see the section on automated cleaning). These allow for the automated programming of standardized cleaning cycles, generally using immersion and more commonly spray systems to clean, rinse, and even dry devices.

The cleaning chemistry is an important part of the cleaning process. As introduced earlier and in Chapter 6 (in the introduction to cleaning and accessory chemistries), cleaning chemistries can be classified on how they are used and the main types of active chemistries that they use for cleaning (such as neutrals, acids, alkalines, and enzymes). Remember that a cleaning chemistry is a formulation or mixture of chemicals for a desired purpose (in this case cleaning). A good cleaning chemistry should:
- Assist in the cleaning process.
- Protect the device from damage (e.g. from water or even the aggressive effects of the cleaning formulation itself).
- Be able to function in the presence of varying qualities of water (e.g. presence of organic and/or inorganic contaminants,

such as microorganisms and various chemicals; see the section on water quality).

Cleaning chemistry formulations can range significantly in their abilities in each of these areas and the benefits/weaknesses of each product type should be closely considered. For example, neutral (~pH 7) formulations are good general cleaners but are generally not as efficient at organic soil removal as alkaline cleaners. Alkaline cleaners range significantly in pH (see Chapter 6 in the section on the pH scale: defining acids and bases), from mild (pH 7–10) to highly alkaline (pH 10–14); higher pH does not necessarily mean better cleaning or indeed that the product is more aggressive on a surface. It will essentially depend on the formulation of the product when prepared in water, where the manufacturer should be readily able to provide evidence to support claims of efficacy and safety. Equally, enzyme-containing formulations can also range significantly, and the presence of enzymes alone should not be considered as being sufficient to remove certain types of soils; enzyme formulations can vary considerably in their activity and formulation composition (e.g. presence of different types of surfactants). Acid cleaners, in contrast, are particularly used in combination cleaning processes as "neutralizers" (following the use of an alkaline cleaner and to ensure that after cleaning the device surfaces are returned to a neutral pH) or specifically for the removal of rust or other inorganic contaminants (e.g. scaling). Overall, care should be taken that the cleaning chemistry being used is fit for purpose (designed and labeled for use for cleaning devices/instruments) and that instructions for use (including any benefits/limitations) provided by the manufacturer are closely reviewed. This may include reading the label (including what is provided on the detergent container or provided separately by the manufacturer), associated documentation, and safety data sheets.

Choosing a cleaning chemistry is only the first step, as any cleaning formulation is only as good as the way it is used. We have already addressed the impact of the cleaning process itself in assisting cleaning (such as manual and automated cleaning methods), but there are a number of key considerations to ensure that a product is used correctly and safely. These include:

- Product design: some products are designed specifically for manual, ultrasonic, or automated cleaning, while others are designed to be used in all three applications. The choice may depend on the features/benefits of the product, as well as its esthetic qualities (e.g. smell is often a concern in manual cleaning, to mask the odor associated with soil but at the same time not be irritating to those using the product).
- Product concentration: this refers to the amount of a chemistry that should be used. Instructions for use should provide details on how the product should be diluted in water (usually within a given range, such as 4–10 mL in 1 L water). For guidance on understanding weights and volumes in measuring, see Chapter 6, in the section on weights, measures and other physical considerations. Overuse of a product can lead to device damage, a requirement for additional rinsing (to remove chemistry residuals), and excessive foaming in manual or automated cleaning (where foam can prevent cleaning from occurring and even cause damage to automated cleaning systems). Foaming may be caused by two major factors: the cleaning chemistry itself and the presence of protein. The cleaning chemistry will contain various types of surfactants to assist cleaning (particularly removal and solubilization of soils) and foaming should therefore be expected. This is not always a negative sign, as in some cases foaming is used to optimize the effect of the product in cleaning, but excessive foaming can prevent the devices from being seen during manual cleaning and can hinder the mechanical actions in ultrasonic and automated (spray-type) washers. It can also be difficult to rinse water from a surface, requiring repeated rinsing. Protein foams when mixed with water; this can be from the cleaning product (e.g. enzymes are proteins) or from patient soil. Excessive foaming can be due to the fact that the instruments being cleaned are particularly heavily soiled. This may be overcome by the cleaning chemistry formulation and by doing pre-washing/rinsing. Under-use of a product can lead to inadequate cleaning and device damage (e.g. if immersed in bad-quality water).
- Washing temperature: temperature plays an important role in the activity of a product, sometimes positive and sometimes negative. All cleaning chemistries should be provided with the recommended temperature conditions. As a general rule, the warmer the water is the more effective the cleaning action; similarly, the higher the water temperature the greater the antimicrobial activity that may occur during cleaning (Chapter 6). However, this is not always the case. One example is that during pre-cleaning if higher temperatures (>45°C) are used then proteins and other soil components can become fixed onto surfaces and make them more difficult to clean. Another is that higher temperatures can cause the inactivation of enzymes present in some chemistries, thereby losing any enzymatic activity as part of the cleaning process. Close attention should be paid to the temperature ranges (upper and lower) recommended with enzymatic chemistries, as their optimal activities are very dependent on having the correct temperature.
- Quality of water: water is one of the most important ingredients for cleaning and is also widely used for disinfection/sterilization in its various forms (see Chapter 15 on water quality). Although it is easy in many parts of the world to take water for granted, in other parts it is a rarer commodity. The chemical quality of water can include various types of dissolved and suspended components that can cause problems during cleaning (introduced in Chapter 6, in the section on mixtures, formulations and solutions, summarized in Table 6.2). These vary depending on the water source (reservoir, lake, water table,

etc.), any purification steps (e.g. to render it safe for drinking), how it is transported to and within a facility, and if any further treatment is performed within the facility. Water quality will also vary over time and between seasons. Common problems include hardness (particularly calcium carbonate, $CaCO_3$), which is dissolved in water but when it is heated becomes insoluble and deposits/sticks on surfaces to form a white or otherwise colored, chalky-type of precipitate/deposit known as "scale" (see Chapter 15, in the section on water quality/purity). Potable (or drinking) tap water usually has various types of chemical added such as chlorine-releasing agents that are used to control microorganisms (Chapter 6), but when heated these can become aggressive on metal surfaces and may cause instrument corrosion. Various other types of chemicals in water can lead to a variety of damage and changes in color. The impact of water quality on the processing of devices is considered in further detail in Chapter 15. Overall, it is recommended that the quality of the water provided to a site of use for cleaning and reprocessing is periodically tested chemically and, if it is found to be unacceptable or at a high risk of causing instrument damage, then pre-treatment is considered.

- Staff training: staff should be trained in using the cleaning chemistry safely and effectively, as well as in the whole cleaning and processing cycle approved by a facility. Staff can lead to the greatest variation in cleaning practices, particularly in manual cleaning. But equally, although automated systems (such as ultrasonic baths and washer-disinfectors) can provide greater consistency, they can only work as well as humans allow them to. It is also important to remember that cleaning chemical formulations are designed to remove and/or break down patient soil components, and will therefore present safety risks to any staff members associated with their use.

An often underestimated principle of correct cleaning is the final step, rinsing. Rinsing should ensure that any cleaning chemicals or residuals remaining on the device surface following washing are safely removed. Cleaning chemistries are designed to remove and break down soil from surfaces, and there is no doubt that patient complications can occur if such chemicals remain on the device through any subsequent processing step (e.g. sterilization) or even direct use on a patient. Such residues may also lead to damage to the device, particularly if it is subsequently treated with another chemistry or with heat. Therefore, rinsing is considered an essential step to ensure that the device can be safely used/further processed. The most effective and widely used method is by using water, with a recommendation that the final rinse water should be of critical quality (see Chapter 15 on water quality/purity). The extent (e.g. number of rinsing cycles and volume of water used) will depend on the cleaning chemistry, and instructions regarding safe rinsing should be provided by the device and cleaning chemistry manufacturer. As pointed out earlier, some high-alkaline cleaning chemistries require neutralization with an acid chemistry (to ensure that the pH on the device surfaces is returned to neutral, around pH 7) and then rinsing to remove the acid cleaner residues. Note that in these cases the amount of acid used to neutralize needs to be carefully controlled, as too much acid can leave the device with a lower (acidic) pH and too little will not adequately neutralize the alkaline, leaving the device with a higher (alkaline/basic) pH.

Following the basic cleaning cycle and depending on any requirement for further processing (disinfection and/or sterilization), the devices may then need to be dried. Drying in this case may be defined as the removal of water or residual moisture. This will be generally true if devices are for immediate patient use and particularly if they are being prepared for steam or gas sterilization. In other cases drying may not be necessary and it may be sufficient to remove excessive water from and, if applicable, within devices prior to further processing or use. Drying may also be conducted manually, within a washer-disinfector or a separate drying cabinet (which uses hot or compressed air and fans to assist drying). In the case of manual drying, care should be taken not to resoil the devices using dirty towels or cloths that are inappropriate at this stage of the process.

Manual cleaning

Manual cleaning may be used as a pre-cleaning step prior to automated cleaning and/or as a full cleaning step when mechanical cleaning facilities are not available or not recommended. For example, many types of delicate or complex instruments that have to be carefully taken apart are often recommended only to be manually cleaned and certain types of devices cannot be submerged in water, such as some electrically operated or air-powered drills or certain parts of complex endoscopes.

When cleaning manually (by hand) caution must be exercised by staff to reduce hazards. These include microbiological (from patient soil), chemical (e.g. with cleaning chemistries) and sharps (device) risks. PPE is therefore particularly important and should be mandatory in manual cleaning (see the section on receiving and sorting and Figure 8.2).

Recommended PPE for manual cleaning (as discussed in the section on receiving and sorting) will include:

- Face protection, which can include a full-face shield or separate eye and mouth protection.
- Waterproof apron, to protect clothing from splashes and spillages.
- Heavy-duty (utility) gloves (e.g. nitrile gloves), which should be longer to cover the wrists and lower arm. Shorter gloves may also be supported by arm guards that go over the elbows.
- Other PPE should also be considered, such as hair/head protection (to protect the operative's hair from aerosols/sprays

that may occur in this area when using sprays or during the action of manual cleaning) and special foot protection (e.g. boots and protected footwear, such as steel-toed, to minimize risks from dropping accidents, which should be enclosed to protect against spillage accidents).

Manual cleaning is only as good as the person performing it and the tools provided to allow it. The most important consideration for cleaning staff is training, to ensure that they are trained on safe and effective cleaning methods for the variety of devices they may encounter. In the cleaning area, lighting should be good so that the person can visualize the devices for cleaning and to prevent injury. A double sink (or two-section sink) set-up is recommended, to allow cleaning in one sink and rinsing in another sink. A triple sink can be even more efficient to allow for pre-cleaning, cleaning, and rinsing in separate sinks (Figure 8.8). In contrast, all steps may be performed with one sink, but particular care should be taken in training on the correct method and quality/quantity of water used for each step, especially for final rinsing to ensure that soil/residual chemistry is adequately removed (see Chapter 15, in the section on water quality/purity). Remember, these sinks should only be used for device cleaning and should not be used for washing of hands or other purposes. A separate, dedicated sink should be provided for hand washing. The volume of the sink should be indicated to allow for consistent and accurate water or cleaning chemistry dilution to be utilized by potentially multiple users. The sinks are generally recommended to be deep, to minimize splashing during cleaning, and should be positioned at the right height for staff to use comfortably. Adequate draining is clearly an important consideration in designing manual cleaning areas. The sink may also be equipped with a spray-hose system, to allow water to be sprayed over devices for pre-cleaning and rinsing; consideration should be given to reducing risks of aerosol generation in such cases. In addition, it is useful to have a manifold system with various tips that are able to accommodate various lumen sizes. Ready access to compressed (instrument-quality) air is also common to allow residual water/chemistry to be flushed from devices (particularly lumened devices).

It is increasingly common to see sinks being equipped or specifically designed with various equipment that allows the manual cleaning process to be better controlled. Examples include temperature probes (to ensure the optimal use of the cleaning chemistry), dosing systems (which automatically dose in a controlled volume of chemistry, to minimize waste and over/under-dosing), and level indicators/sensors (which ensure that the quantity of water used is effective). Sinks are also being designed to allow for adjustable height settings, to improve their safe (ergonomic) use by multiple users.

When not in use, sinks should be cleaned, disinfected, and dried. Specific cleaning accessories are designed for certain types of devices, such as endoscopes to allow for leak testing and cleaning (flow) of internal channels.

As highlighted earlier in the chapter, a variety of manual aids are often provided to aid in the cleaning process. Examples include various types of soft or specifically designed brushes, syringes (for lumen cleaning/flushing), and sponges. Such cleaning accessories are readily available in most countries. Care should be taken in using them, in particular sponges, which should be replaced on a frequent basis (at least daily if not more), as if they are left wet, bacteria and fungi can multiply in and on them, providing an additional risk. It is preferable that such accessories are single-use, disposable items, but if this is not economically viable, reusable

(A)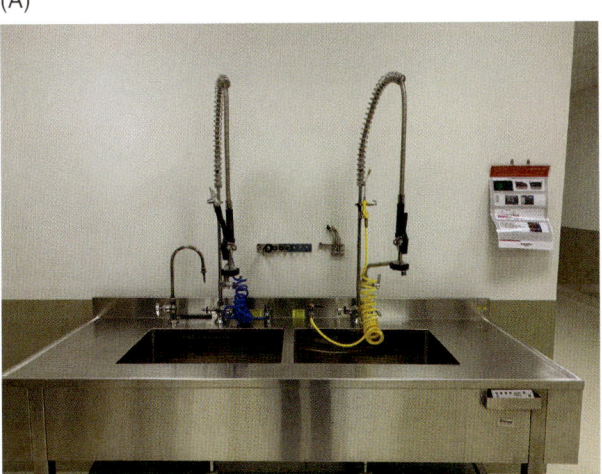

(B)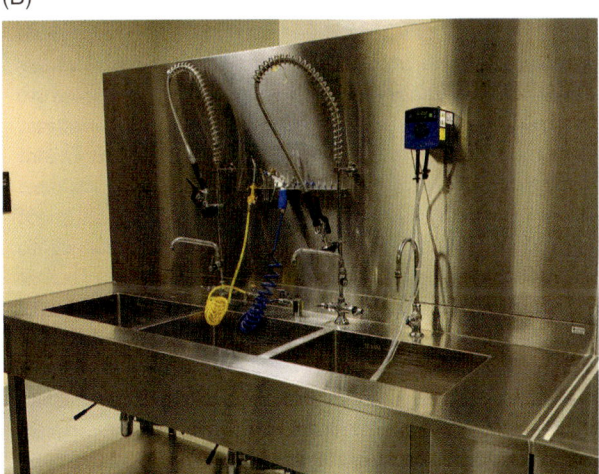

Figure 8.8 (A) A typical double-bay and (B) a triple-bay sink system used for manual cleaning.

accessories are recommended to be frequently decontaminated (rinsed, heat-disinfected, and kept dry when not in use). Accessories such as scouring pad should not be used, as they can damage device surfaces. If specific types of accessories are required by a device manufacturer to allow cleaning, such as specialty brushes, information regarding brush specifications and how these can be obtained should be provided.

Some cleaning chemistries have been specifically designed and labeled for manual cleaning (others can be used for both manual and automated cleaning). Any cleaning chemistry can be used for manual cleaning if instructions are provided by the manufacturer for that purpose. Choose a good-quality product with the applicable labeling, being careful to review the labeling and instructions for use carefully. Cleaning chemistries should be used that have been designed for medical/surgical device use. All cleaning chemistries have health risks, but some (such as high-alkaline or low-acidic chemistries) are often considered of greater risk to staff. For this reason, neutral or mild alkaline chemistries are widely recommended for routine cleaning, which may or may not include enzymes. All chemistries should be handled as if they are potentially damaging to health and particular care given to reviewing the safety data sheets provided with them. It is also recommended to make provisions for potential large spills of these chemicals, such as having designated spill kits.

Whatever cleaning chemistry is used, the chemistry supplied should be prepared and used according to the manufacturer's instructions. Pay particular attention to the concentration, temperature, and recommended exposure times, as well as any requirements for rinsing. Rinsing instructions can range from one to multiple steps (including exposure times and water volumes). Training on the correct use of the cleaning chemistry is essential to prevent the over- or under-use of the chemicals.

During manual cleaning, minimize any splashing or aerosolization. It is recommended that devices should be cleaned under water (immersion method) and particularly when using brushes or when flushing lumened devices. All surfaces of the instrument/device must be cleaned. To do this, some disassembly may be required (see the section on disassembly and preparation for cleaning). Remember that inaccessible areas will be difficult, if not impossible, to manually clean and this should be considered in the device instructions. Items that cannot be immersed should be cleaned in a manner that will minimize the production of aerosols/sprays and with particular attention to the instructions provided by the device manufacturer.

Manual friction is the basis of manual cleaning, with the cleaning chemistry aiding in the removal and breakdown of soil from surfaces. The following guidelines are given:
- Appropriate PPE should be worn at all times. Strong gauntlet gloves, a plastic apron, eye protection, and a facemask are recommended to protect staff and reduce the risk of splashes and cuts from sharp items.
- A double (or double-section) sink method is recommended to be used with a dedicated washing sink and a separate rinsing sink.
- Fill the clean sink with the appropriate measured amount of water and detergent, according to the detergent manufacturer's instructions. The ideal water temperature and concentration should be specified. Water at a temperature of <45°C is preferable for any pre-cleaning (to remove gross soil), as hotter water may coagulate protein materials (found in blood, sputum, etc.) making them very difficult to remove. Water temperatures of greater than >55°C will be too hot for comfortable manual cleaning by staff.
- Medical-grade cleaning chemistries that are specific to the type of soil on the instruments/equipment should be used. In most cases these will be neutral or alkaline-based detergents, with or without enzymes; inorganic soil contaminants (such as rust and scale) can be removed using acid-based chemistries (see later discussion). Do not use household or hand soaps as they are not labeled for such use, can be highly foaming, make rinsing difficult, and can leave unwanted residues (e.g. fatty acids in the household soap may react with hard water to form a soap "scum" on the instruments).
- Dismantle/disassemble/open all instruments before cleaning, paying special attention to joints, serrations, tips, or crevices. A clean, soft brush or soft cloth/sponge may be used to clean the surfaces. Do not use abrasive or metal brushes as these will damage the instruments. It is recommended that the number of devices placed and washed in the sink at any time is limited (e.g. no more than six devices). Wash the device using manual friction (e.g. using a brush) below the surface of the water, in order to avoid aerosols and minimize splashing. Pay special attention to grooves, teeth, and device joints when brushing to remove any soil. The brush should be cleaned and rinsed before use and after each use; any cleaning accessories should be left dried when not in use (or otherwise discarded). Lumened items should be washed externally, but particularly all lumens brushed according to manufacturer's instructions using appropriately designed brushes. Some lumens may require irrigating with a high-pressure water-jet spray gun; this should be done below the water surface to prevent aerosolization. Note: manual lumen cleaning is required for two reasons: to remove patient soil and to ensure that lumens are free-flowing (not blocked). Blocked lumens will prevent subsequent disinfection/sterilization and may render the device inoperable. Automated systems (e.g. specifically designed ultrasonic washers, irrigator systems, and washer-disinfectors) may be used to replace manual cleaning, but in these cases the system manufacturer's instructions and written claims should be closely inspected and followed to ensure they allow the flow and detect the potential blockage of the range of lumen sizes

that can be present in any lumened device (flexible or rigid; see Chapter 10, in the section on rigid endoscopy, flexible endoscopy).

• While cleaning, visually inspect the item to ensure that all parts are clean. If an instrument is broken, attempt to locate any missing pieces and follow the broken/missing instrument procedure (generally to discard and replace the device).

• Replace cleaning and/or rinsing water after each set of devices or when the water is obviously soiled/contaminated.

• When rinsing, fully immerse or rinse cleaned items in a separate sink with clean water in order to rinse off all soil and detergent residues. The number of rinses required may vary depending on the number of devices being cleaned, types of devices, and any manufacturer's instructions. Data from the cleaning chemistry manufacturer should be available to support the rinsing requirements (e.g. lack of toxicity after the stated number of rinses). Any chemistry or soil left on the items can reduce the effectiveness of further processing and can lead to other patient complications. The chemical quality of the water will need to be controlled, especially for rinsing, and if the water quality being provided to a processing area is not considered safe for such purpose it must be further treated (for further guidance see Chapter 15 on water quality/purity).

• If required, instruments should be manually dried before patient use or further processing (e.g. when devices are being prepared for packaging and steam or gas sterilization). At a minimum, any large amounts of water remaining on or within a device should be removed, and devices should be dry before gas sterilization.

• Complete any relevant documentation associated with the facility quality and/or tracking/traceability system.

Note that for both manual and automated treatments, brown staining is often observed on device surfaces during cleaning and on inspection. This can be due to rusting (Figure 8.9), dried patient soil, or residual iodine (which is sometimes used as a surgical scrub and pre-operative preparation and can accidentally contaminate device surfaces). It can often be hard to differentiate these, but in general patient soil and iodine will be easily removed during the cleaning process, rusting will not. Rusting can be removed by spot treatment with an acid-based, rust-removing cleaning chemistry that is used to dissolve inorganic contaminants such as rust.

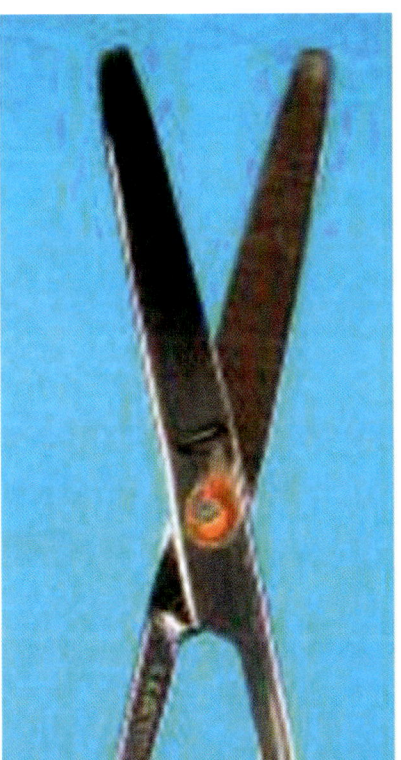 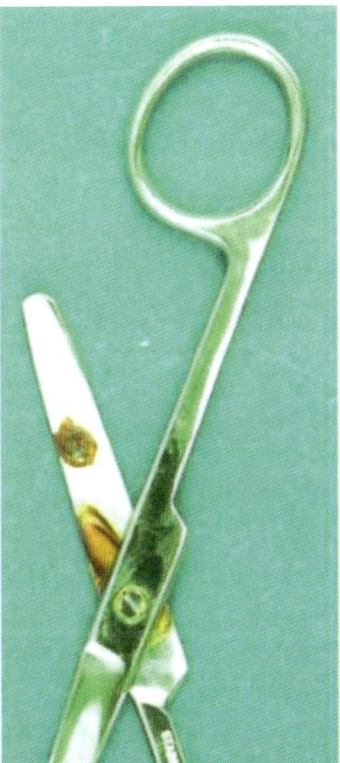 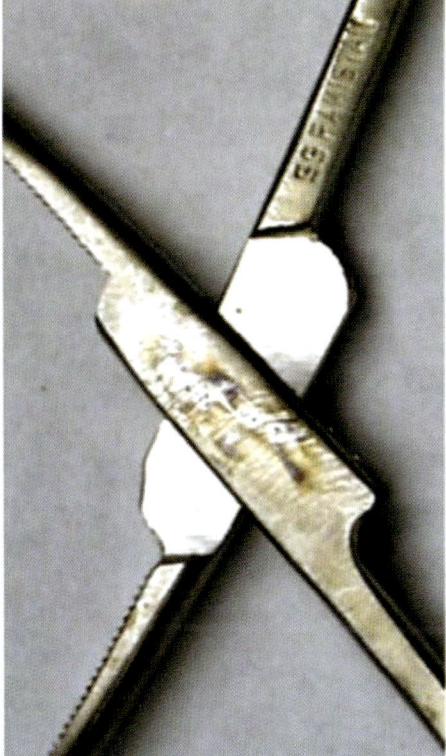

Figure 8.9 Rusting present on a device. Rusting is a sign of damage on a device surface, in particular on stainless steel devices where two metal surfaces interact (e.g. the hinge joints of forceps). Rust (chemically known as ferric oxide) builds up on the surface when it becomes visible as a brown stain or deposit.

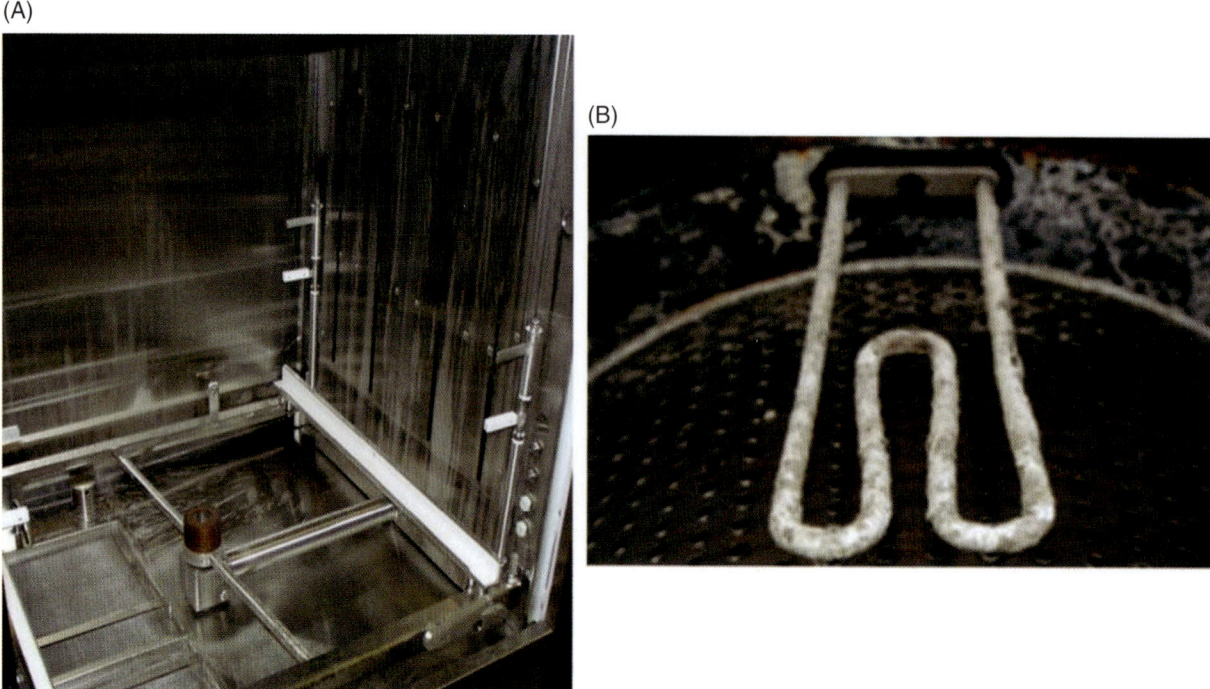

Figure 8.10 An example of "scaling" due to water hardness (A) in a washer-disinfector and (B) on a water heater. Note the white precipitate.

Remember that the brown staining of rust is a sign of underlying surface damage; you can remove the rust, but the damage remains present, particularly under microscopic examination. A further use of such acidic chemistries is for the routine removal of hardness or "scale" deposits on a surface (generally seen as a white chalky precipitate; Figure 8.10). Excessive use of acid-based cleaners can itself actually promote surface damage and rusting, so care should be taken in reading the instructions supplied with such chemistries and in their use. In the case of scale deposits, this clearly indicates poor water quality; correct control of the water chemical quality is important to consider in order to prevent device and equipment damage over time.

Automated cleaning

Most modern device processing facilities in developed countries use an automated cleaning system that results in minimal handling of contaminated equipment by staff, enabling process standardization and a larger handling capacity of device sets through the processing cycle. Unfortunately, this is not always the case in developing countries, which exposes staff and patients to increased safety risks. At the same time, mechanical washers and washer-disinfectors, like any other tool, will only be effective if designed and used correctly.

In comparison to manual cleaning of devices, mechanical cleaning is the method of choice as it can remove soil and microorganisms, with minimal risk to staff, through a consistent, repeatable automated cleaning and rinsing process, provides higher standards of cleanliness, and can be validated (Table 8.2).

Most, but not all, modern instrument washers also incorporate a thermal or chemical disinfection cycle capable of destroying various numbers and types of microorganisms; these are officially known as washer-disinfectors but may also be referred to as "washers," "washer-pasteurizers," and other similar terms (see Figure 8.11). A washer-disinfector is defined as a machine that cleans and disinfects medical devices and other articles used in the context of medical and dental settings (but is equally applicable to other areas such as veterinary and research settings); "clean" in this context is defined as being visually free of soil and quantified as being below specified levels of analytes. Remember that soil refers to any unwanted contaminant(s), including patient materials, and process/procedural residues. Also, analytes include any chemical substance that is the subject of chemical analysis (e.g. protein and residual detergents). The design and performance requirements for a washer-disinfector, according to international standard requirements, are defined in the ISO 15883 (*Washer-disinfectors*) series of standards (see the section on cleaning guidelines, standards, and testing). Essentially, all the

Table 8.2 Manual versus automated cleaning.

Manual cleaning	Automated cleaning
Advantages	**Advantages**
Often recommended for handling delicate, complex devices	Fully automated programmable cycle, including cleaning, rinsing, and (in most cases) disinfection
Required for non-immersible devices	Automated cycles that should expose the device to the same conditions for each cycle, record cycle parameters, and can be validated
Often considered cheap	Minimizes instrument handling and safety considerations
Direct and visual inspection during cleaning	Performance can be more easily monitored and documented
Disadvantages	**Disadvantages**
Difficult to ensure reproducibility and to validate that a process is consistent	Often unsuitable for certain types of items, such as non-immersible devices
Cleaning depends on individual performance	Equipment and maintenance can be more expensive
Safety issues	Cleaning outcome is design specific, where inadequate designs can lead to problems when not considered carefully
Labor intensive and time consuming	

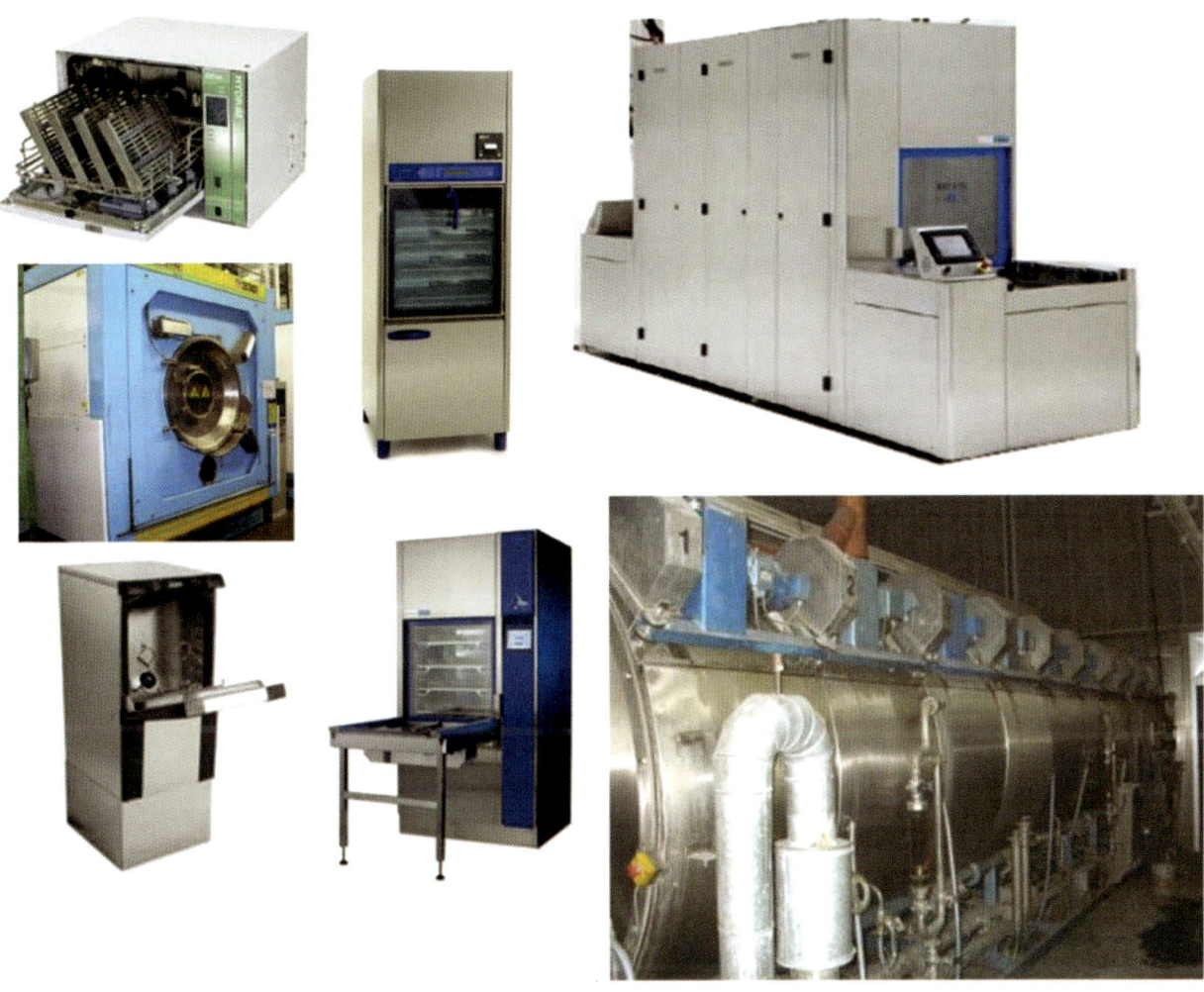

Figure 8.11 Various types of automated washers and washer-disinfectors. These may be used for washing alone (with or without rinsing) or with a chemical or thermal disinfection cycle. They come in different sizes, specifications, types, and with additional accessories.

cleaning principles described in the section on the basic principles of cleaning are equally applicable to automated cleaning, but in this case the cleaning process is done by a machine rather than a person. This provides many advantages, but it should always be remembered that the machine (and the processes it is programmed to control) will only be as good (safe and effective) as it is designed to be if used by staff as intended by the manufacturers and maintained in accordance with recommendations.

Washers vary considerably in their design, varying from those that are only designed to assist in part of a manual cleaning process to those that provide a fully automated cleaning, and optionally disinfection and drying, process. The same three components for the cleaning process (as outlined in the section on the basic principles of cleaning) are still required: water, cleaning chemistry, and a method of friction. In the case of automated washers, the methods of friction include ultrasonics, flow systems (e.g. those that flow water through devices lumens), immersion, and spray-type mechanisms. One or a number of these mechanisms may be employed within the same washer. As examples, an ultrasonic bath includes immersion and ultrasonics, but may also be equipped with a dedicated flow system; tunnel (or multi-chamber) washers can include immersion/ultrasonics in one chamber and a spray-type system in another. In considering the installation and use of an automated washer, important factors will include the size and shape of the washer, required water volumes (and in some cases temperature ranges recommended), water quality/purity requirements, electrical and draining specifications, and even the types of cleaning (or other accessory) chemistries that may or may not be used. All of these requirements, in addition to recommended process cycles, maintenance schedules, and instructions for use, should be provided by the washer manufacturer. A common example is the choice and use of cleaning chemistries. As for manual cleaning, certain types of cleaning chemistries are specifically designed for automated cleaning and should be labeled as such. A common concern is the production of excessive foam during the cleaning process (Figure 8.12); foaming is not a bad attribute (in many cases it can be a benefit), but excessive foaming can lead to inadequate cleaning/rinsing as well as damage to the machine's pumping systems, potentially leading to pump cavitation, where the presence of air (in the foam) reduces the efficiency of the pump and significantly impacts the water pressure being employed for flow or spraying.

Although it will depend on the washer design, the washer should always be capable of providing a consistent process that can include pre-washing, washing, and rinsing. Some washers will only be designed for one, two, or all of these stages, with most being capable of being specifically programmed to run one or a number of washing cycles to meet the needs of a facility. In all cases, care should be taken to ensure that the cycle settings (which have been designed and tested to meet the facility requirements) are fixed; the ability to change cycle

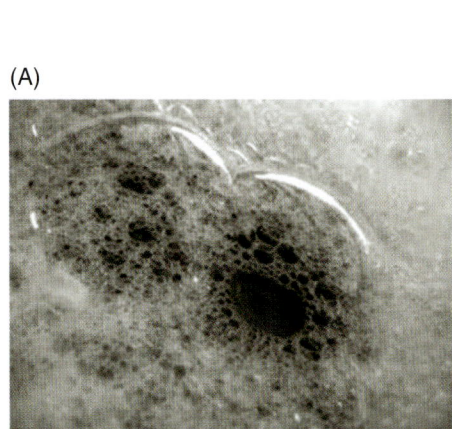

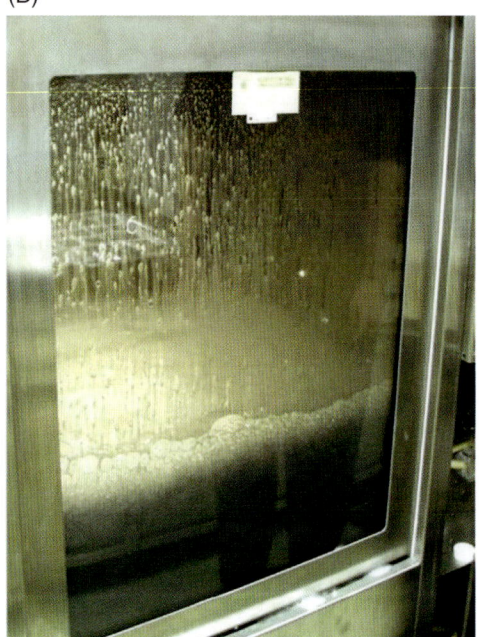

Figure 8.12 (A) Foaming and (B) an example of excessive foaming in a washer-disinfector.

parameters (including chemistry dosing volumes, cycle times, etc.) should only be possessed by staff members authorized to do so and who understand the risks and requirements when such parameters are changed. When defined machine cycles are fixed, staff should be trained on the correct use of the machine, including cycle choice, loading/unloading of devices into the washer, and alarm resolution.

The main benefits of automated washers should be to reduce handling risks and to provide a consistent, more efficient cleaning process. This, however, may not always be the case, and inappropriate washer design, maintenance, or use can lead to problems. Consider some of the following examples that have been reported:

• Open sonication baths can cause aerosolization of microorganisms and chemicals into the processing area and can affect the health of those working in this area.
• Washing processes may appear to and have been recorded (documented) as being successfully completed, but in fact have not been (e.g. no cleaning chemistry was dosed into the machine or spray arms/flow ports were blocked, thereby not allowing flow for cleaning).
• National and/or international safety designs have not been adequately considered, despite the obvious risks of mixing electrical components, mechanical parts, and water/chemistry within the same machine.
• Devices have not been loaded into the washer correctly, thereby not allowing the process to have full contact with the various internal or external parts or not allowing for adequate draining/rinsing.
• Machine alarms being ignored or even turned off by facility staff, due to lack of servicing/maintenance.

For these reasons, greater attention has been paid in recent years to the adoption and use of washer-disinfector standards (the ISO 15883 series, as international examples) to reduce these risks.

The correct use of the washer will also depend on various accessories that are provided to be used with it, such as loading tray, racks, and flow connectors (Figure 8.13). Many types of

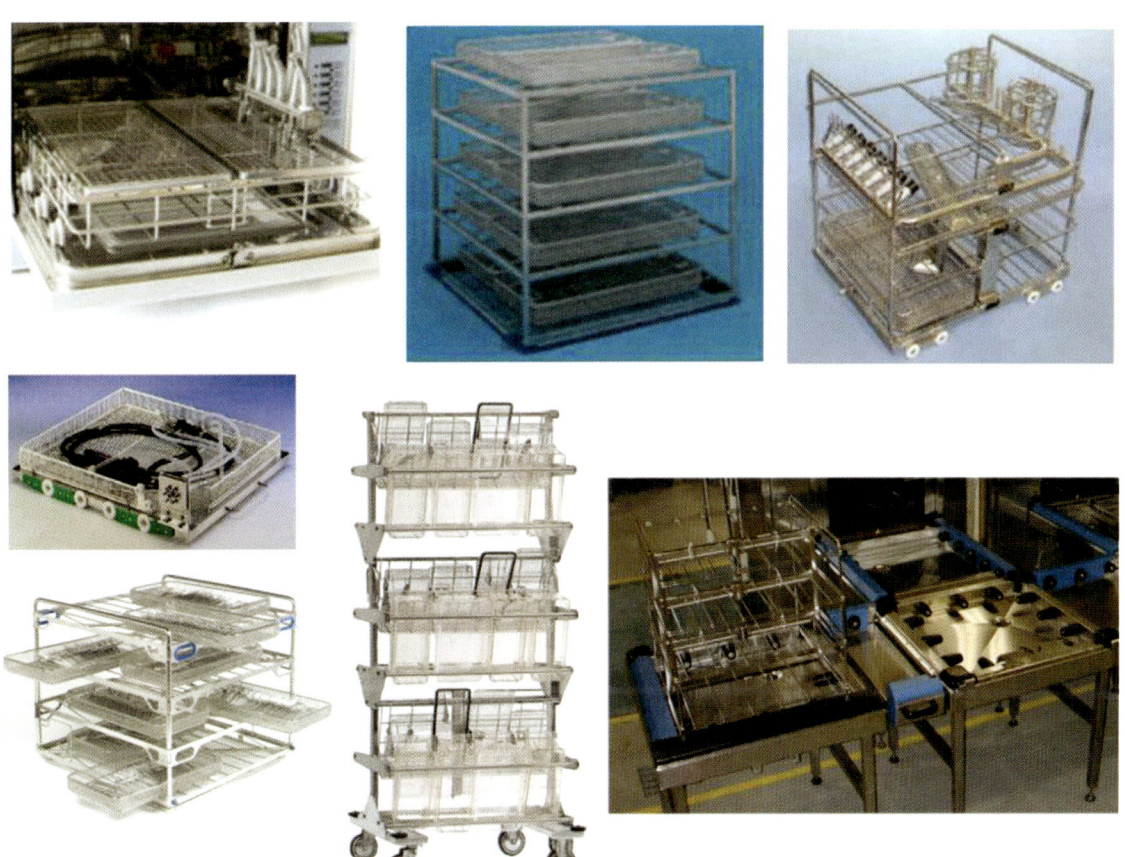

Figure 8.13 Various types of accessories (racks and trays) used with automated washers.

accessories can be specifically designed for the processing of unique device designs, to include the correct positioning of devices in the washing process and connectors for lumened devices to allow for flow (which may or may not include designs that allow for flow not only through lumens but around the connection sites to the device). Instructions on the correct use and maintenance of all accessories should be provided by the washer manufacturer.

Overall, despite the obvious benefits of automated cleaning, the washing process is always dependent on those using the machine. Therefore, training is important and should, at a minimum, involve the following:

• Safe and correct use of chemicals (e.g. when changing the chemical provided to the machine or during accidental spillages). In some cases the same cleaning chemistry can be used for manual, ultrasonic/immersion, and automated cleaning, thereby minimizing mix-ups and simplifying staff training. In such cases, the cleaning chemistry should be labeled for each specific application.

• Preparation of devices for loading into the washer. Particular attention should be paid to device disassembly (when required), ensuring that hinged instruments are open and that device trays are not overloaded (Figure 8.14).

• Loading and unloading of devices in trays/racks into the washer. This can be manual or assisted by an automated loading/unloading design within the facility. Particular attention should be given to any safety risks in using automated loading/unloading systems as they include automated moving parts that can cause accidental injury. Manual or automated loading/unloading systems are generally designed to improve ergonomics (preventing or minimizing lifting/pushing/pulling) and to maximize throughput of the available washing machines.

• Correct cycle selection. Washers are often set up with different cycles to be able to handle different types of loads.

• Handling and reporting of any alarms. Alarms can be visual, audible and/or otherwise recorded. For example, most modern washers have independent process monitoring installed (see the section on cleaning guidelines, standards, and testing) and inspection of computer-generated reports or data records may be required to ensure the correct process has been attained. Some washers may sound an alarm but once a cycle is complete or the alarm has been turned off there is no record, while others will sound an alarm and prevent further use of the machine until the problem is rectified.

• Any subsequent processing steps. For example, ultrasonic and immersion baths may only wash the devices and require subsequent manual or automated rinsing. Similarly, devices may require drying following the cleaning/disinfection cycle.

• Routine maintenance is required for all machines and recommendations should be provided by the manufacturer. Failure to follow these guidelines can lead to damage or failure of the washer. Typical examples of recommended maintenance include inspection of drains (not clogged and free-flowing), that spray arms are freely moving (not stuck) and spray jets are not blocked, and regular draining and disinfection of immersion baths.

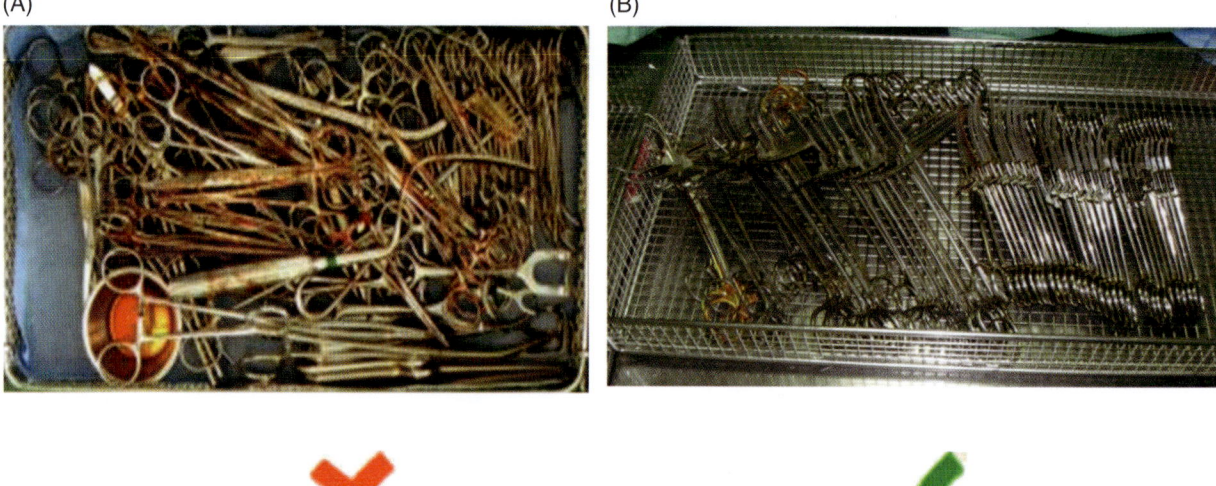

Figure 8.14 (A) Overloading and improper assembly of a device tray. (B) A better assembled tray. Note the opened hinged devices to allow access to the cleaning process.

Figure 8.15 Examples of acceptable personal protective equipment (PPE) being used in an automated cleaning area. By all accounts the recommended PPE is similar, if not identical, to that described for manual cleaning (Figure 8.2). In general, similar to manual cleaning, a full water-resistant gown with sleeves is preferred and is mandatory in some countries.

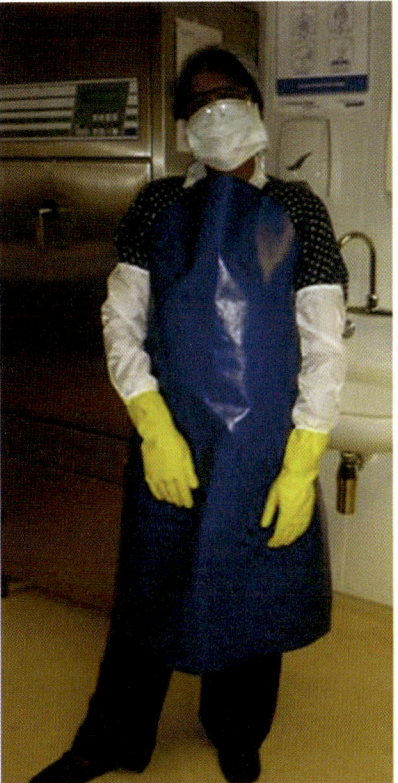
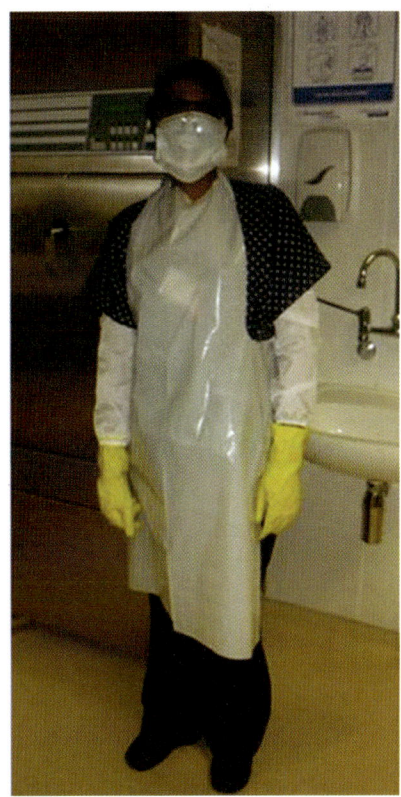

- Routine testing. As mentioned previously, there are international standards now in place (e.g. the ISO 15883 series) and users should follow the advice given and carry out the recommended periodic testing. The results of all tests should be logged for each individual machine and retained for future inspection.

As a final note, despite the use of an automated washer, PPE requirements will be similar to those specified for sorting (see the section on receiving and sorting) and manual cleaning (see the section on the basic principles of cleaning). Although the risks associated with splashing, aerosolization, and sharp instruments may be less, it is not unusual for staff involved with automated cleaning to be also conducting sorting, disassembly, pre-cleaning, and manual cleaning in the same area; therefore PPE consistent with requirements within the area should be considered (Figure 8.15). Devices that are only subjected to washing alone (e.g. with some ultrasonic bath designs) are still potentially contaminated with microorganisms that could pose a staff safety risk and should be handled with this in mind. Consideration should also be given to rinsing and drying of these devices prior to their inspection and preparation for sterilization. Others that have been subjected to a full washer-disinfector process may be considered safe for handling, but may require further processing (such as packaging and sterilization) to ensure they are ready for safe patient use.

Immersion, including ultrasonic baths

Various types of immersion baths can be used for cleaning and can provide the benefit of controlling various cleaning variables such as temperature and friction mechanisms. The most commonly used are ultrasonic baths (Figure 8.16).

Sound (or "sonics"), including the sensation of hearing, is based on a mechanical vibration (or pressure variation); sound, as we perceive it, is essentially a vibration within a certain range (known as a frequency range). "Ultrasonic" or "ultrasound" refers to sound that is at a higher range than that perceived by the ear (generally >20 kHz). These mechanical vibrations (at high frequencies) can be used for a variety of medical applications including medical imaging (where very high frequencies are used to visualize various internal organs and structures, such as during pregnancy, known as an "ultrasound" or sonography) and treatments (e.g. high frequencies used to fragment kidney or gall stones into smaller pieces, in a process known as lithotripsy). Lower frequency levels, but still at or higher than those that we perceive as sound, are used for cleaning purposes, such as in dental practices (teeth cleaning) and with surgical/medical devices. Cleaning in these cases is assisted by the production of ultrasonics in water/cleaning chemistry.

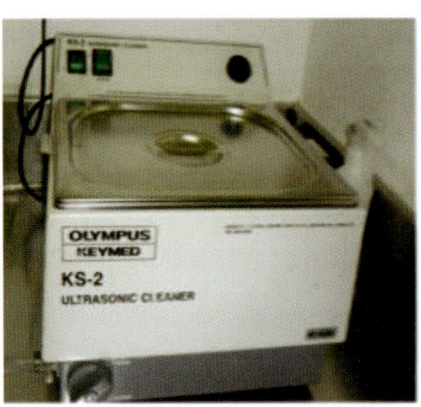
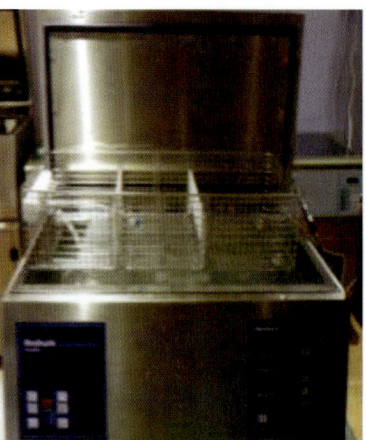

Figure 8.16 Ultrasonic baths.

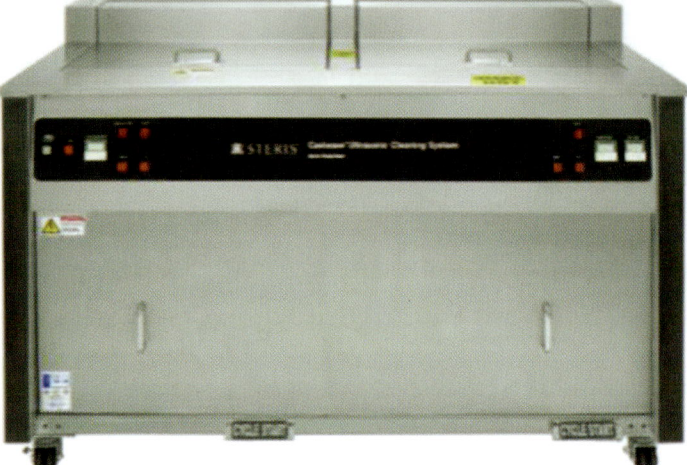

An ultrasonic cleaning process is assisted by an effect known as cavitation, where ultrasound production within a liquid causes the production and collapse of small bubbles along the surface of the device that causes soil disruption/removal. A cleaning chemistry should always be present, which also assists in the removal of soil and in preventing soil from reattaching to the device surface when the ultrasonics are turned off. The cleaning chemistry should be designed for ultrasonic use, or at a minimum not cause any negative effect on ultrasonic production or cleaning. Some ultrasonic bath designs allow lumened devices to be attached to a flow system provided in the bath that circulates cleaning chemistry through the device to aid in cleaning.

An ultrasonic washer (also known as a "sonicator" or "sonication bath") can be particularly effective in the presence of a cleaning chemistry to remove soil and hardened debris from instruments, including contact areas or those that are harder to reach manually. They may be used for pre-cleaning purposes or as part of an automated cleaning process (including cleaning and rinsing). Highly contaminated and difficult-to-clean instruments (such as those containing tight hinge joints; see Chapter 4 on basic everyday instruments) are often recommended to be pre-cleaned in an ultrasonic bath. For pre-cleaning purposes the use of an ultrasonic bath is preferred to manual immersion cleaning, as it reduces direct contact with contaminated items, decreases the risk of cuts/puncture wounds to staff, and can be an effective cleaning step. It is important to note that some device manufacturers may recommend the use of ultrasonics for cleaning, while others will not (or even recommend against the use of ultrasonics, due to the risks of damage to the device); such recommendations or limitations should be clearly stated in their instructions for processing.

Staff are recommended to always wear PPE, including heavy-duty gloves, fluid-resistant masks, protective eyewear, and a gown, when handling contaminated instruments and working with ultrasonic baths. Protective headwear should also be considered. The following are general instructions

for using ultrasonic baths, but can vary depending on the ultrasonic bath type and manufacturer:
- Fill the tank with water (typically potable or drinking water) to the manufacturer's designated level (defined volume).
- De-gas the water as recommended by the machine manufacturer. This sonicates the water to remove dissolved gases (see Chapter 6, the section on mixtures, formulations and solutions) that could interfere with the cleaning process.
- Add the cleaning chemistry to the defined concentration, ensuring the manufacturer's recommendations (for the chemistry and/or ultrasonic bath) are followed. It is advisable to use a suitable neutral or mild alkaline detergent (with or without enzymes) that is effective at lower temperatures (as for manual cleaning).
- If the tank has a heater, set the temperature control to the set point as defined by the ultrasonic manufacturer and/or as defined by the cleaning chemistry manufacturer's recommendations.
- When the specified temperature has been reached, place the opened/dismantled instruments either directly into the ultrasonic tank or into an accessory basket. Place the basket of instruments into the tank, ensuring that the devices are completely immersed in the diluted cleaning chemistry. Never put instruments directly onto the base of an ultrasonic washer as this can short-circuit the ultrasonic transducers and damage the washer.
- In some designs, lumen devices can be connected directly to flow ports and connectors provided within the washer; ensure that these devices are connected correctly (and do not become disconnected during washing) and that they are completely immersed. The contact parts at the connectors/device ports may need to be manually cleaned prior to attachment and/or checked for debris following cleaning. If the sonicator does not contain flush ports, lumens must be flushed with solution before submersion. For sonication to be effective, fluid has to be present in all features of the device.
- Set the timer control to the time specified by the machine or device manufacturer, or initiate the pre-programmed cleaning cycle.
- After the washing cycle has been completed, remove the basket (or individual devices) from the tank and rinse the items with clean water – unless the machine has an automatic rinse stage, or the load is to be transferred directly into a washer-disinfector for further processing. As for manual cleaning, the quality of water used for rinsing may need to be controlled; potable water may not be sufficient (see Chapter 15 on water quality/purity). Cleaned devices may be further processed, dried, and/or used clinically (depending on the Spaulding classification recommendations; see Chapter 1 on goals of decontamination and the Spaulding classification).
- Completely drain the bath chamber. If the ultrasonic bath is to be used again, it is to be refilled with fresh water and the previous steps repeated. If it is not being used again (e.g. over two to three hours), the chamber can be dried (using a non-linted cloth) and stored dry.
- Record the instrument(s) that has/have been processed according to facility requirements (such as the method and solutions used and details of the staff member who completed the procedure).

Similar procedures are recommended for other types of immersion (including irrigation) baths.

Automated washers/washer-disinfectors

Most automated washer-disinfectors today are designed for cleaning, disinfection, and drying. These processes are introduced here with an emphasis on the automated cleaning phases of the cycle; disinfection specifically is discussed in further detail in Chapter 9. The cleaning and disinfection process is intended to make the items clean but also safe (microbiologically) for staff to handle (as a prerequisite for packaging and sterilization), reducing the load of microorganisms on device surfaces, and also often for direct/indirect use with a patient (in particular for non- and semi-critical devices; see Chapter 1 on the goals of decontamination and the Spaulding classification). Examples of devices that typically go through a cleaning-disinfection process prior to direct patient use include flexible endoscopes (used for semi-critical procedures, as is generally the case with investigational colonoscopy and gastroscopy; see Chapter 15 on endoscopes and other lumened devices) and miscellaneous non-invasive devices such as trays/carts, wash bowls, and reusable footwear. Most surgical devices are typically (although not always) passed through a cleaning and/or disinfection process, packaged, and then subjected to a sterilization process.

A typical cleaning-disinfection process consists of a number of separate phases, which include:
- Cleaning, usually including a prewash with water (<45°C), a washing phase, and rinsing; the number of prewashes, washing steps (including type(s) of chemistry used), and rinsing steps can vary depending on the cleaning process.
- Disinfection, using hot water (for devices that are thermo-resistant) or various chemical disinfectants (for thermosensitive devices). In most cases where chemical disinfection is used, the disinfectant is required to be rinsed away at the end of the disinfection phase. Thermal (hot water) disinfection (also known as pasteurization) is achieved by the action of moist heat maintained on the surface to be disinfected at a particular temperature for a particular time. In accordance with international standards for washer-disinfectors, this time–temperature relationship can vary depending on the types of devices being processed (e.g. non-critical or critical devices) and the design of the washer-disinfector, which is further discussed in

Chapter 9 in the section on physical disinfection. Lubricants (as accessory chemicals) can be added automatically to device surfaces during the disinfection phase (to ensure that devices, in particular hinged devices, are operating optimally), but it is more common for lubricants to be applied manually to individual devices that require lubrication in accordance with manufacturer's instructions following cleaning and disinfection.

- Drying, if and when applicable. Drying is performed using the circulation of dry/heated air within the washer and can be assisted using a chemistry (rinse aid). The rinse aid assists in dispersion of water droplets, making them easier to evaporate (from liquid to gas) and be removed by the drying system. Note: any chemical rinse aid used should be non-toxic, including testing to show that it does not become toxic to patients both directly (in the case of non-critical devices) and following sterilization (e.g. by steam) that can change the chemicals.

There are many different sizes and types of washers (Figure 8.10). They may be single- or multi-chamber, single (one) or double (two) door, and varying in size/design. In single-door designs, the devices or materials (referred to as the "load") are introduced and removed from the same door, while double-door designs allow for introduction and removal through separate doors (pass-through design). Pass-through door washers are preferable as contaminated items can be loaded in the "dirty" area and removed in the "clean." The disadvantage of a single-door washer is that the contaminated and clean items are loaded and unloaded through the same door from the "dirty" side.

The major components of a washer-disinfector will include:
- Washing chamber and draining system, to hold, circulate and remove water/chemistry during the cleaning process.
- Water-pumping system, including pipework, pump(s), and spray/flow systems.
- Dosing system, for the delivery of any chemistries used during the process. Chemistries are normally dosed as liquids using designated pumps and the number of individual dosing pumps can typically vary from one to four. Solid dosing systems are also used, being integrated into the water-pumping system directly or indirectly. Manual dosing systems are rarely used.
- Air-handling system, for use during drying but also during rinsing phases to remove larger volumes of water/chemistry from the devices and minimizing the use of water.
- Computerized control system allowing the cleaning-disinfection process to be automatically controlled, according to defined programmed process conditions; these include process phases (cleaning, rinsing, disinfection, drying), dosing of any associated chemistries, temperature, pressure (used for the control of the flow of water through the system), exposure times, and other parameters required for the specific washer design. The control system is therefore linked to sensors that monitor the performance of the process (such as temperature sensors). It is typical for the control to include a recording system (either printed out on paper and/or collected by a computer system) to allow for a record of the cleaning–disinfection process to be confirmed/archived.

In addition to the main control system, most modern washer-disinfectors are equipped with an independent monitoring system (as defined in the ISO 15883 series on washer-disinfectors). This system is often separate from the main computer control system and its associated sensors (e.g. temperature, pressure, etc.), where independent sensors are used to verify that the controlling sensors are operating correctly. As an example, if a dosing system for cleaning chemistry has malfunctioned or the chemistry container is empty (and is now dosing air), the main control system may record that chemistry was delivered to the washer at the right volume/concentration even though it was not. The independent monitoring/sensor can be used to detect that this had occurred. Similar types of systems are often found in modern sterilizers (see Chapter 11 on steam sterilizer design). In some cases the independent monitoring system is integrated into the control system to immediately alarm and inform staff of the problem, preventing the washer-disinfector cycle from proceeding until the problem is fixed; in other cases the data collected from an independent monitoring system needs to be manually checked by staff to ensure that all the cycle variables were within a given specification (range). Overall, care should be taken to ensure that staff understand how the independent monitoring system operates to ensure its correct use. These systems are designed to reduce the risk of an automated process failing, not to remove the risk.

Washers are also designed to accept single or various types of loading racks that allow devices (directly or within trays) to be placed and introduced into the washer (Figure 8.12). These are designed to be used as part of the washing process; a common example is that the rack is designed with spray arms that connect directly with the water flow systems within the washer chamber and allow water to be sprayed over and/or under the devices for cleaning–disinfection. Typical surgical instrument racks are multi-layered, designed to accommodate a number of wire mesh baskets full of instruments, or can be more widely spaced to accept and correctly position large bowls, instrument trays, reusable rigid containers, and similar items. Specific types of racks commonly used include those to accommodate anesthetic equipment and accessories, as well as racks to assist in the washing of minimally invasive surgical (MIS) and endoscopic (rigid and flexible) devices. These will often include different types of irrigation systems to accommodate the inclusion of device lumens in the washing–disinfection process.

Loading/unloading of automated washers

As already discussed, devices are usually introduced into the washer using a system of baskets and racks. For example, commonly used terms in the capacity of a washer are "DIN" or

"ISO" tray/baskets, which refer to the number of standard-sized trays into which devices/device sets are placed in the washer chamber. Typical examples widely used in Europe include 10 and 15 DIN tray racks and washer designs.

Despite the design of the washer and rack system, automated washing will only be effective if the devices/trays are loaded correctly according to the manufacturer's instructions and the cleaning process can contact the various parts of the device. The following is a guide to device loading:

- Do not overload trays or racks (Figure 8.14); if the washer is overloaded, then not all devices may be cleaned effectively, increasing the rejection rate (the number of devices that are rejected on visual inspection as not being adequately cleaned and requiring recleaning, manual or automated).
- When loading, make sure all items are placed into a basket in a manner that will enable them to have direct exposure to the water/detergent (e.g. the spray system). For example, hinged instruments should be placed in the open position.
- Ensure that the correct racks are used for loading the various types of instruments in the load; different types of racks are often designed for specific types of loads/devices.
- Separate multi-level sets of devices and remove lids to ensure access to devices.
- Certain types of accessories such as silicone mats may need to be removed.
- Do not place hollow or larger materials (such as bowls/basins) over other instruments as this can cause "shadowing," where the instruments are blocked from contact with the cleaning process. Hollow items must be turned upside down, otherwise water/cleaning chemistries will collect in them during the process.
- Ensure that spray arms are freely moving within the washer and are not blocked or obstructed from circulating by the load (particularly those integrated into the rack design). Inspect any spray jets or connectors within the washer or rack/tray designs to ensure they are not blocked or damaged. Racks should be correctly positioned within the washer chamber to ensure contact with the washer pipework/pumping system (according to the washer manufacturer's instructions).
- Devices and loads should not be left for extended periods of time in the washer, especially if it is only used for cleaning and not disinfection/drying. Residual moisture can lead to corrosion on some instruments over time.

Smaller washer-disinfector designs will obviously have smaller loading racks and device capacity; devices are usually manually loaded in and out of the washer. Similarly, larger washer-disinfectors (e.g. for carts, beds, and wheelchairs) are most often manually loaded, but automated loading–unloading systems are also available. For larger-capacity devices and other material washers (e.g. laundry, see the section on surgical and medical laundry), the load can be very heavy and difficult to handle for staff without the high risk of back/arm/hand injuries. Ergonomics refers to the design of procedures and equipment to reduce operator fatigue, discomfort, and injury. In this case, automated loading–unloading systems are used to minimize the risks of carrying/pushing/pulling and also to improve the operational capacity of the available washers within a department. Automated loading–unloading systems can range from semi-manual types to fully automated systems (Figure 8.17).

In a typical example, the empty racks are placed on a conveyor belt that is under the control of a computer/sensor system. The device-containing trays are then individually loaded onto the rack shelves and once ready can be advanced to an available washer-disinfector. Various levels of complexity and automation design can go into such systems. For example, the conveyor system may assist in moving the rack to and into the washer under control by a person, followed by manual selection and initiation of a washing cycle. In contrast, the loaded racks can be automatically moved along floor-, ceiling-, or wall-mounted conveyor systems and when a washer is detected as being free (or available to take a load), the system automatically moves the rack to the washer, detects the type of devices associated with that rack (e.g. surgical instruments), and instructs the washer to automatically open, receive the load, close the door, and initiate the defined cycle. Equally, in a typical double-door washer design, similar unloading systems are used on the clean side of the washer to remove the load, which can be manually or automatically moved to an area for packaging and sterilization. Overall, safety considerations are important in the design and use of automated systems, to reduce any risks of accidents.

Tunnel (or continuous process) washers

A tunnel washer consists of a series of interconnected, open chambers (essentially a tunnel) through which devices are passed through in a continuous process (Figure 8.18); these should not be confused with multi-chamber washer-disinfectors (see the section on automated washers/washer-disinfectors), which consist of separate, distinct chambers with doors separating the chambers from each other. Tunnel washers were popular in the past, but they were not generally designed for cleaning complex or cannulated instruments. These washers typically featured two to five interconnected open chambers, each with a specific processing task. The instruments move through the prerinse, washing (spray, immersion, and/or ultrasonic) rinse, and drying cycles on a conveyor belt. Water can typically be sprayed from the top, bottom, and sides. For device cleaning, the tunnel washers have largely been replaced by multi-chamber washers, but tunnel washers are still used for certain types of devices and laundry applications.

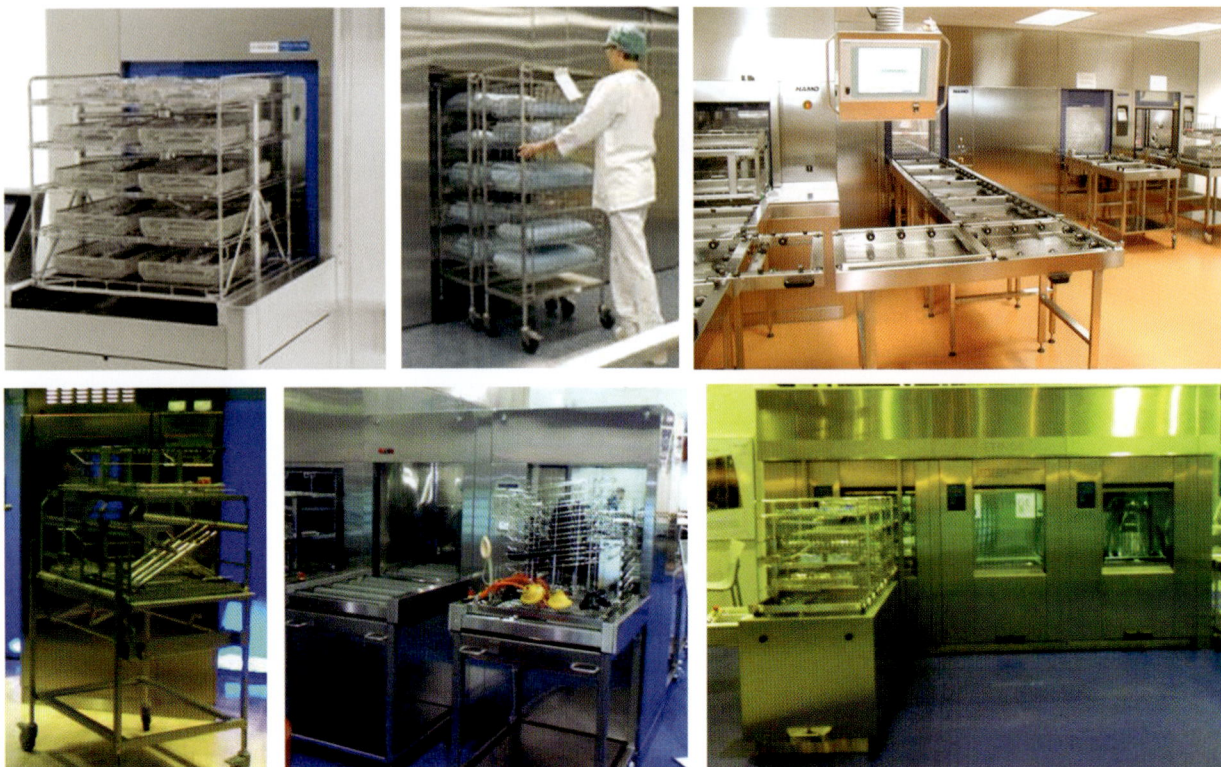

Figure 8.17 Examples of various types of loading/unloading systems. They range from manual to semi-manual and fully automated (with fully automated examples shown on the right).

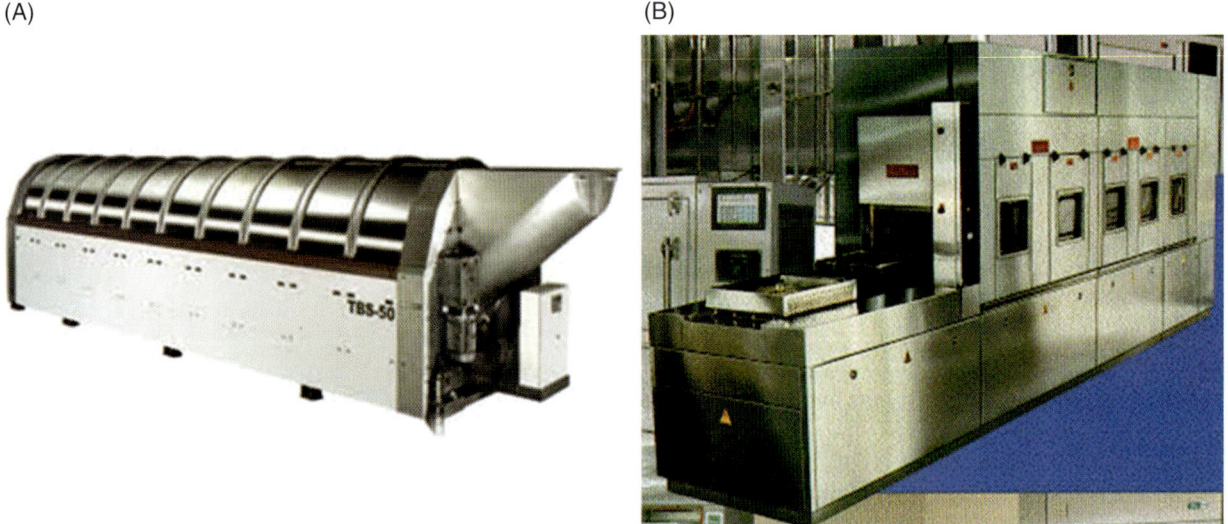

Figure 8.18 Examples of tunnel washers. (A) A laundry washer and (B) an instrument washer.

Multi-chamber washers

A multi-chamber washer is similar to the tunnel washer in that it has two or more (typically up to four) chambers, but the similarity ends there; these machines have separate chambers with doors at either end and at intermediate positions between chambers (Figure 8.19).

Instead of an open chamber each chamber is separated by an interlocking door and each chamber has a specific, distinct process associated with its design. During the process, the devices are passed through each chamber sequentially. Only the entry or exit door on each chamber can be open at any given time to prevent cross-contamination between the clean and dirty areas or recontamination of a chamber containing a processed load. By placing chambers and processes one behind the other, loads can be prepared and passed in sequence through the cleaning–disinfection–drying process (depending on the washer design).

Multi-chamber machines have more than one chamber, with separate stages of the processing cycle being performed in each chamber. The typical phases are cleaning (including a

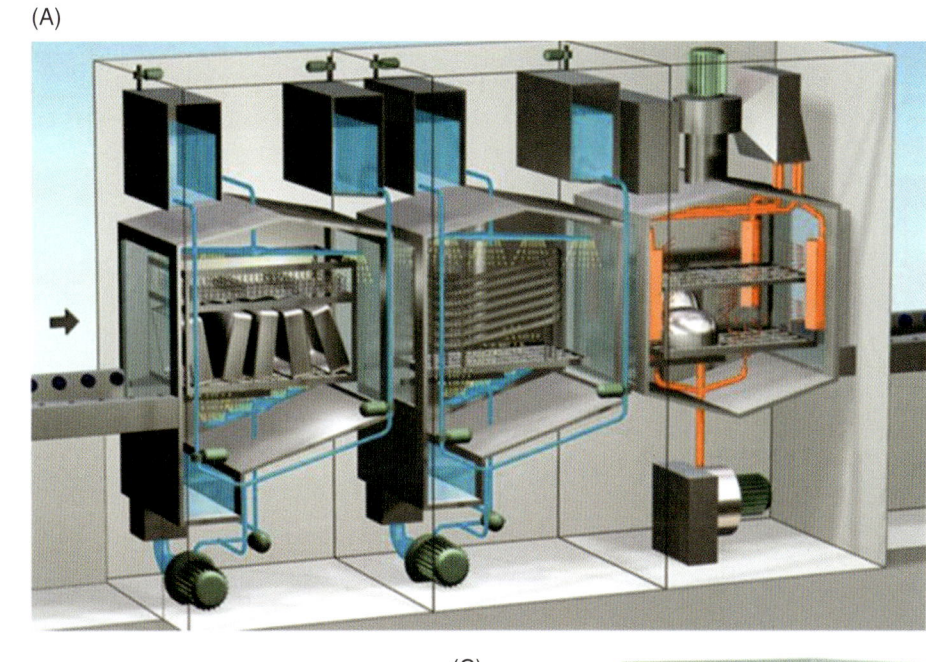

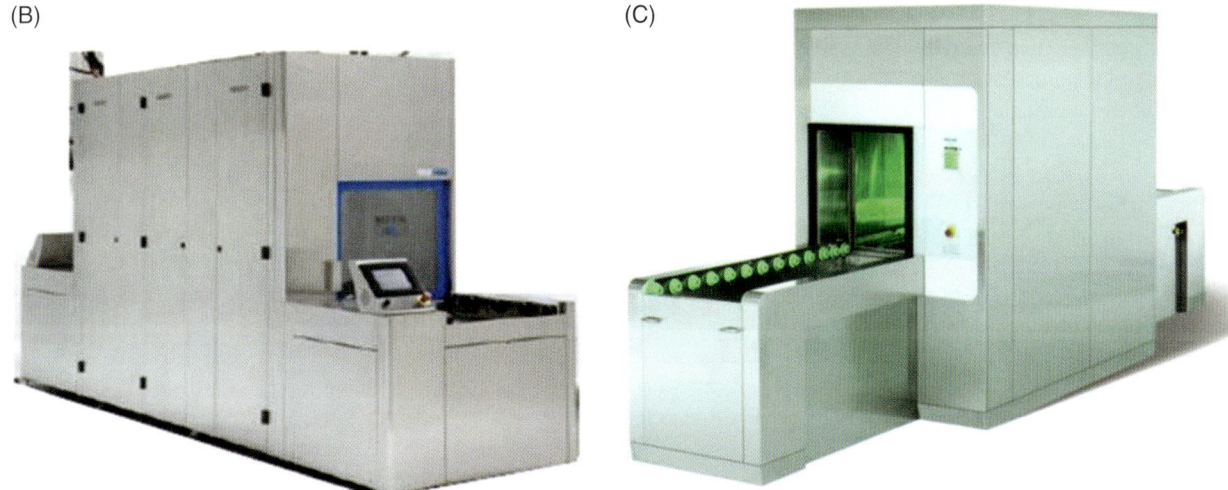

Figure 8.19 Multi-chamber washer-disinfectors. (A) A representation showing three chambers each with a separate process ongoing (cleaning, disinfection, and drying). (B) A three-chamber and (C) a two-chamber washer-disinfector.

pre-wash for gross debris, cleaning chemistry wash, and rinsing), disinfection, and generally drying. Additional chambers can include separate pre-cleaning or cleaning chambers (e.g. an ultrasonic bath into which the device rack is lowered for cleaning). Since the load is moved through the machine and separated from phase to phase, it is possible to get physical separation between dirty and clean loads. The full range of process stages is only completed when the load is delivered from the final chamber. Typically, individual chambers will be dedicated to cleaning, disinfecting, and drying. Compared with single-chamber machines (where the full washer-disinfector process is included in one chamber), multi-chamber washers have a higher continuous throughput of devices/loads for a similar process, but have a larger footprint requirement (being longer in design they take up greater space within a facility). Although they can provide efficient throughput of devices over time, if these systems require maintenance or malfunction the overall ability of the processing facility can be significantly impacted if workflow alternatives are not available.

Single-chamber washers

Single-chamber washers are widely used for processing a variety of devices and other materials. They range in size from smaller table-top washers to large-load (such as cart) washers; they may also be single-door or double-door designs. Over time, they have replaced manual cleaning due to their ability to provide a consistent and documented process, to minimize handling risks, and to free up staff time from manual cleaning. The entire wash cycle is in one chamber; that is, prewash, main wash, rinsing, and typically disinfection and drying (if applicable). Since all stages of the cycle take place in the same chamber, it is not possible to get physical separation between the dirty and clean stages of the cycle within the washer. Assurance that the load will not be recontaminated is dependent on the efficacy of the cleaning and disinfecting stages in decontaminating the interior of the washer as well as the load. Physical separation within the processing area between a "dirty" and a "clean" area is possible with double-door designs, with soiled devices being passed into the washer on one side and removed from the other, typically into a "clean" area (e.g. packaging room). Depending on the design and use of the washer, the machine can include a variety of dosing pumps (with chemistry being applied from outside or inside the washing chamber), pumping/spraying/flowing/immersion systems, and an air-handling system (particularly when drying is performed).

Three examples of single-chamber washers are:
- Endoscope washer-disinfectors (Figure 8.20). These are specifically designed for the reprocessing of rigid and/or flexible endoscopes. They are generally smaller sized (including table-top or under-counter washers), but can also be larger, single or double-door design. In some examples, the washer may be used for a variety of different device cleaning processes, where specific racks are provided for the handling of basic devices or rigid or flexible devices and associated accessories. Racks can be designed to allow for the support and specific flow of water/cleaning chemistry through the internal device lumens. These are widely used with minimally invasive devices (including rigid endoscopes) and are often referred to as MIS racks. MIS instruments are also automatically washed in some types of immersion/ultrasonic baths that control the various phases of the cleaning cycle (but most ultrasonic baths are semi-manual, see the section on immersion, including ultrasonic baths). In another example, the washer is only designed for use with specific devices, which is typical with flexible endoscope washer-disinfectors. These can include immersion or spray-flow type systems, which allow for cleaning and chemical disinfection outside and within (lumens) of the device. Flexible endoscope washer-disinfectors can be simple or complicated in design; these can be simply immersion baths with or without specific flow connectors for attachment/flow of lumens, or more complicated systems that are designed to ensure that the correct number of lumens are connected and flow connectors are checked to ensure that they are not blocked/occluded before, during, or after the cycle. They can include a leak-test phase that ensures that the flexible endoscope can be safely immersed in water, specifically that no holes are present on/in the device that would allow water to leak into the internal (fiberoptic) parts of the device. Cleaning and disinfection chemistries can be provided in a variety of ways, and provisions should be made for the correct quality of water (generally, bacteriologically free water) to be used for rinsing of the chemistry following disinfection. Cleaning is historically conducted with neutral, enzymatic cleaning chemistries, but any neutral or mild-alkaline chemistry may be used if labeled as compatible with flexible endoscopes.
- Surgical (including dental) device washer-disinfectors. These can be bench-top, under-counter, or larger-chamber washer-disinfectors. They can also be single or double door in design (Figure 8.21). They are used for processing the variety of surgical/medical instruments, sometimes with multiple, programmed cycles to include critical or non-critical device loads. They commonly have specified cleaning, disinfection, and drying phases of processing cycles, where a higher quality of water may be required for use in the final rinsing (following cleaning), and thermal disinfection of instruments and potable (acceptable for drinking) water is used for cleaning. Such washers most commonly use thermal disinfection. Many larger processing facilities will employ the use of automated material handling systems with multiple single-chamber washers. Such systems position multiple single-chamber washers side by side to reduce the floor space required within a department. The machines are then connected by a loading

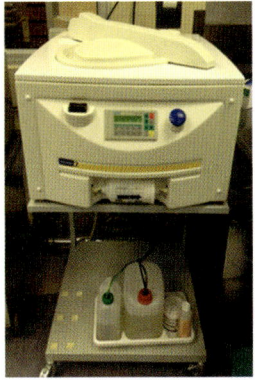 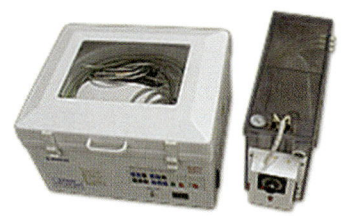 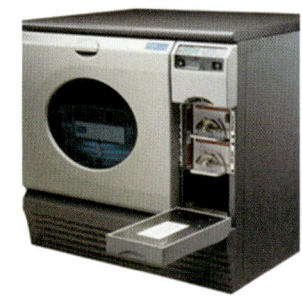

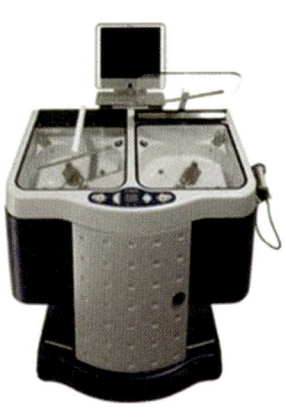 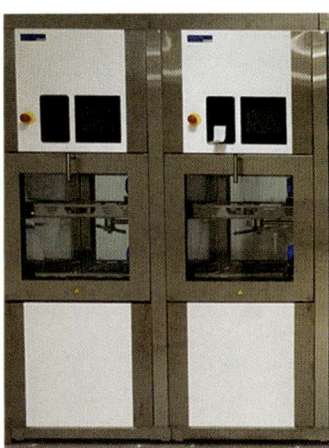 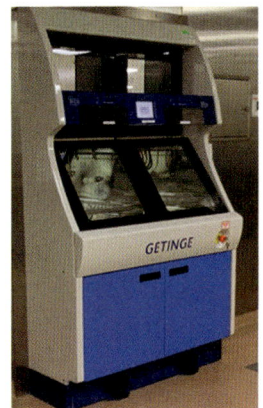 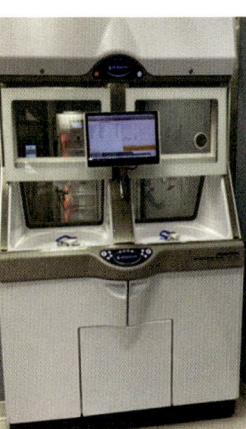

Figure 8.20 Endoscope washer-disinfectors.

(and unloading, on the clean side) conveyor belt positioned at a right angle to the line of washers, with docking stations at each washer. These can be fully or semi-automated and assist the staff in handling and loading of devices for reprocessing (Figure 8.17).

- "Cart" washers: these are commonly referred to as cart or large-chamber washers, but are used for the processing of a variety of non-critical materials such as carts, trays, trolleys, bed-pans, and wheelchairs (Figure 8.22). They may also be used for processing instrument trays and, if labeled and validated for use, for processing instrument sets (in compliance with manufacturer's instructions). Larger devices are placed in the washer in a tilted position to enable water to drain out and prevent restriction of any moving parts within the washer. Due to the volume of water used in such designs and for non-critical items, it is now common for water used for various phases to be collected and reused between cycles; for example, rinse water may be reused but should be monitored to ensure that any soil or chemical load within the rinse water does not accumulate over a safe level that could cause problems. If designed, installed, and programmed for such purpose, cart washers can also be used as larger washers for critical surgical/medical devices. In these cases, it is typical for a higher level of disinfection to be programmed. Although chemical disinfection can be used in such washers, they more commonly employ thermal disinfection.

Special cleaning considerations

This section discusses the cleaning challenges with specific types of devices due to their design. It is important to remember, as highlighted throughout this chapter, that every device requiring processing may or may not require specific handling procedures during cleaning. This can include disassembly, limitations on types of cleaning method or chemistries that can be used, and adequate rinsing. Processing instructions should be provided by the device

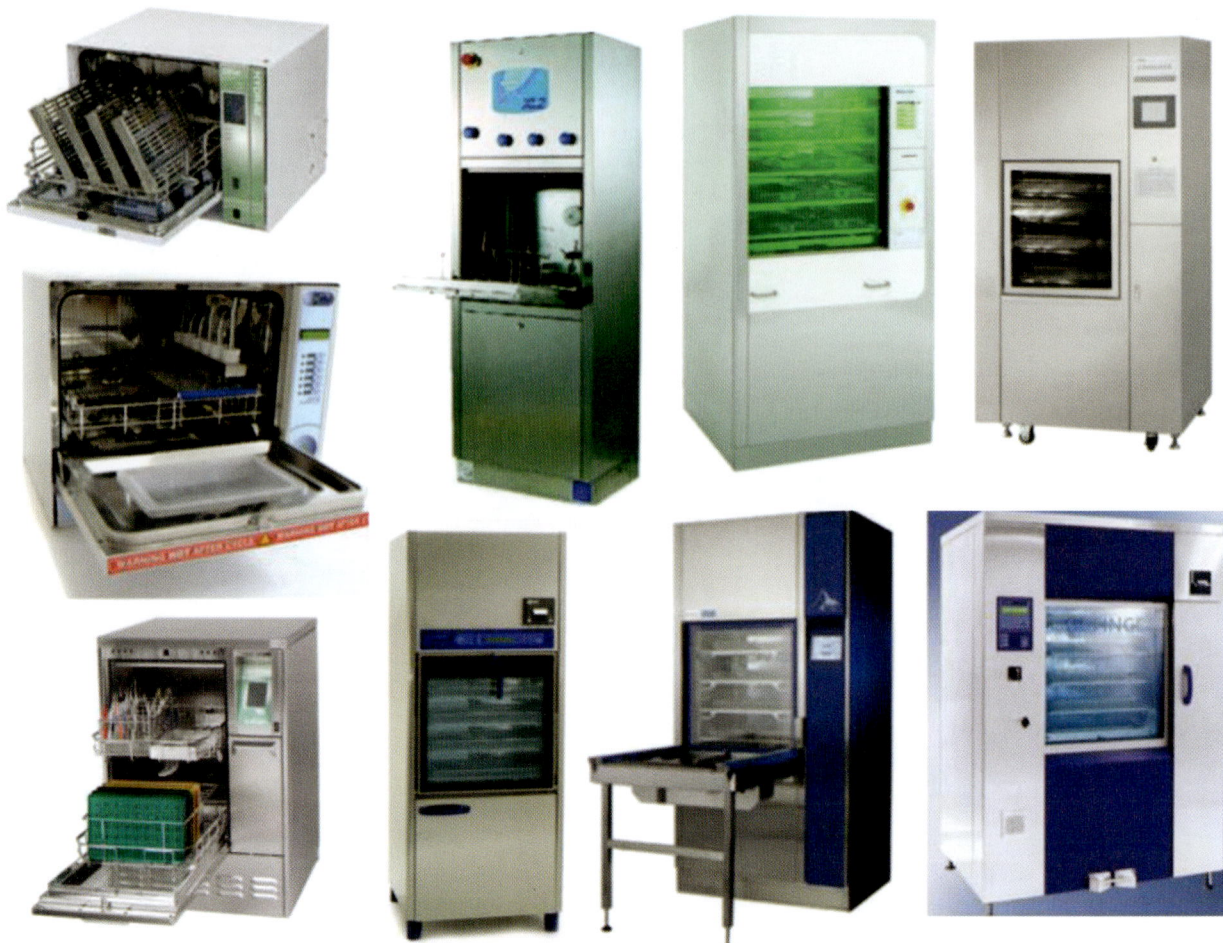

Figure 8.21 Single-chamber surgical and dental device washer-disinfectors.

manufacturer, in accordance with international guidelines and standards (in particular ISO 17664-1 *Processing of health care products – Information to be provided by the medical device manufacturer for the processing of medical devices – Part 1: Critical and semi-critical medical devices*, and ISO 17664-2 *Processing of health care products – Information to be provided by the medical device manufacturer for the processing of medical devices – Part 2: Non-critical medical devices*). This section only considers some of these devices as examples, so it is important to remember that many devices may appear to be simple but may need special considerations.

Microsurgical, including ophthalmological devices

Microsurgical devices are generally small and delicate, and are often used for surgical procedures using a microscope for magnification. They are used for a wide range of surgical procedures, including those on the eye (ophthalmology surgery). Processing such instruments can be a challenge as they are easily damaged during handling or in contact with different types of cleaning methods (including chemistries). Cleaning is a challenge due to the size of the devices and difficulty in inspecting such small parts for soil residuals. As highlighted in the section on the basic principles of cleaning, various types of soils or chemicals (from the cleaning process or even from the water used for rinsing) that remain on instrument surfaces can lead to toxicity risks in patients; this is particularly true with microsurgery and can be highlighted with toxicity concerns following ophthalmology procedures. Toxic anterior segment syndrome (TASS) is a rare and potentially devastating complication of routine intraocular surgery due to a non-infectious toxic agent entering the anterior (front) segment of the eye during the procedure, causing an inflammatory reaction and patient

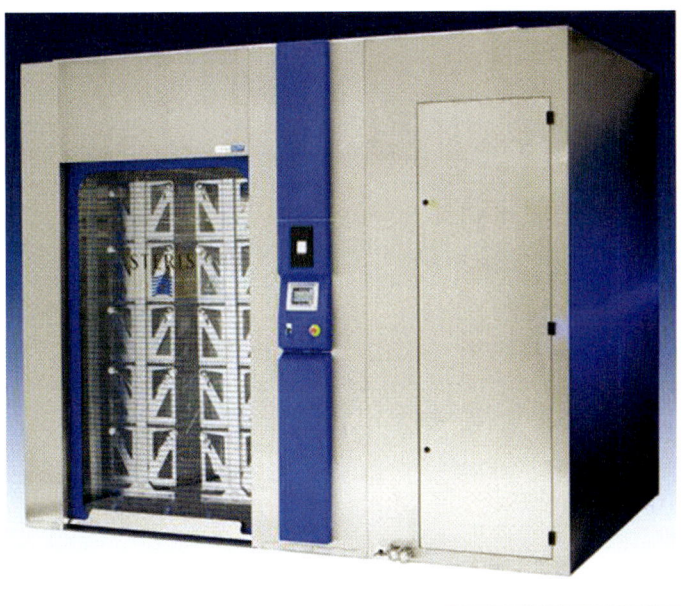
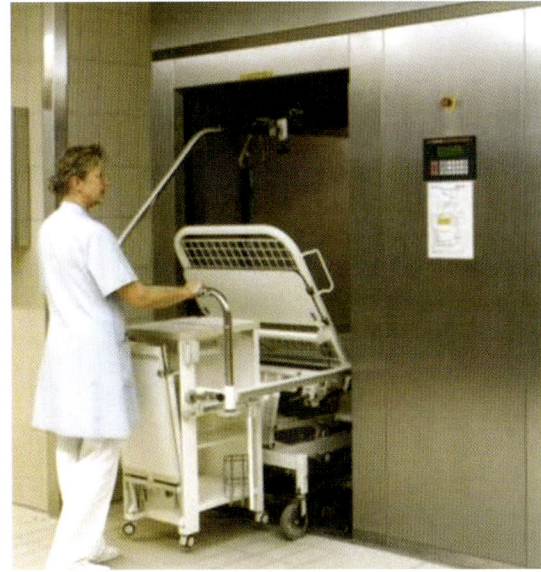
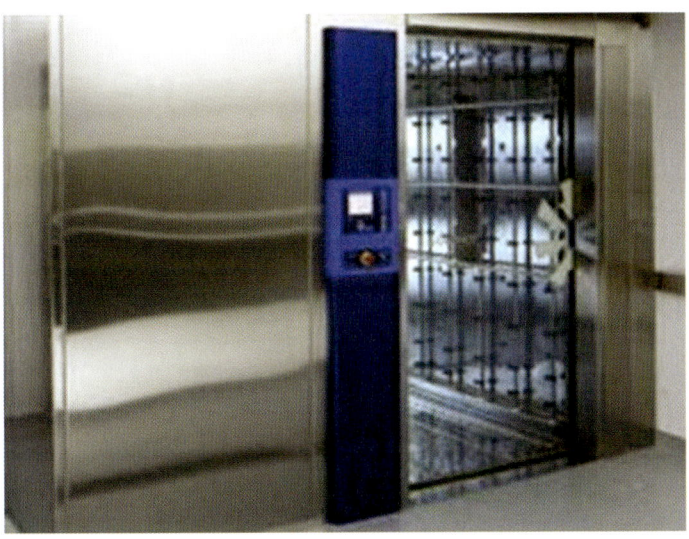
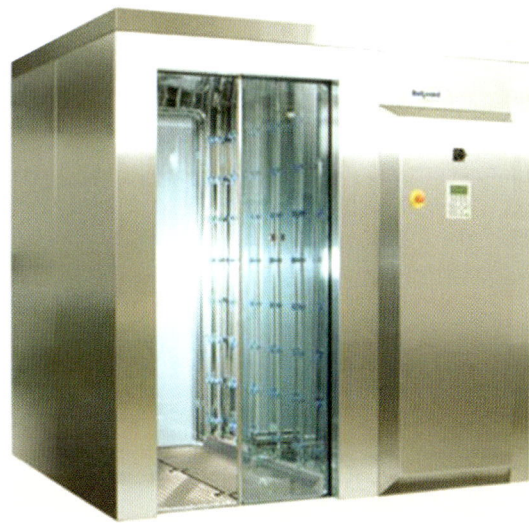

Figure 8.22 Cart or large-chamber washers.

complications. TASS has been repeatedly reported following cataract surgery and lens implantation, with complications ranging from partial to complete loss of the eye. The main suspected causes of TASS related to device use include cleaning chemistry residuals, remaining soil (inadequate cleaning), materials (such as toxins, particularly endotoxins; see Chapter 5 on bacteria) present in water used for processing, poor steam purity, and rusting or other chemicals or chemical/physical damage. Equally, TASS may also be caused by particulate contamination, possibly by other materials used during the procedure, such as talc from gloves, topical ophthalmic ointments, lint (from materials), and so on. Although not well described, other toxic effects may also be expected from the improper processing and use of other microsurgical devices. To reduce these risks the following guidelines are given:

- Follow the device manufacturer's guidelines regarding handling and processing.
- Ensure cleaning chemistries are correctly prepared and used according to the manufacturer's guidelines. This requires accurate measuring and dilution of the chemistry; do not overdose the chemistry, as it can lead to unexpected problems with rinsing. Some guidelines have recommended not using certain types of cleaning chemistries due to frequent non-compliance

with cleaning and rinsing instructions (particularly with enzyme-containing chemistries).
- Check if automated washer-disinfectors can be used to process devices. If an ultrasonic system is used, it is recommended to empty, clean–disinfect, rinse, and then dry devices after use or at least daily.
- Pay close attention to the quality of water used to rinse the devices post cleaning (and during any subsequent disinfection and sterilization processes; remember that chemical impurities, sometimes at high levels, can be transferred in steam onto a device surface). In some countries it is recommended that high-purity water (e.g. distilled or reverse osmosis water) is used for rinsing and subsequent reprocessing following cleaning (see Chapter 15 on water quality/purity).
- Closely inspect the devices following cleaning (and disinfection, if applicable; see Chapter 10 on inspection).
- Ensure that lint-free drying, inspection, and packaging materials are used following cleaning. An example is the use of powder-free gloves during inspection and packaging after cleaning.

Loan devices and device sets (including orthopedic sets)

In many situations the devices and equipment used by a healthcare unit will not belong to the facility, but are borrowed from or on loan from the manufacturer, supplier, or another facility. Examples include orthopedic device sets, when specific devices are needed for patient implantation (e.g. screws/pins that are selected during the surgical procedure based on the immediate need of the surgeon; Figure 8.23), the use of experimental devices/equipment, or when the required equipment is not routinely available at that facility. These are commonly referred to as "loan" devices or sets. There should be a detailed contract with the owners of the loaned sets on how they are to be handled at the facility, to include financial arrangements, receipt, storage, return procedures, and requirement for processing.

Loaned device sets often include reusable devices (or instruments) that are designed to be repeatedly used and processed multiple times, as well as single patient use implantable devices. Close attention to the labeling and processing instructions is important. While the instruments are expected to be used and soiled during the patient procedure, the implants are generally not unless they are used and remain in the patient. Implants that have been used, damaged, or soiled but have not remained in the patient are typically required to be discarded. As single patient use implants, they can be processed and resterilized when not used/soiled, and may also be subject to limitations in the number of processing cycles that can be conducted over time.

Facilities can have many different types of arrangements in place with suppliers, so it is important to understand these as they can vary. In some cases the devices or equipment may be

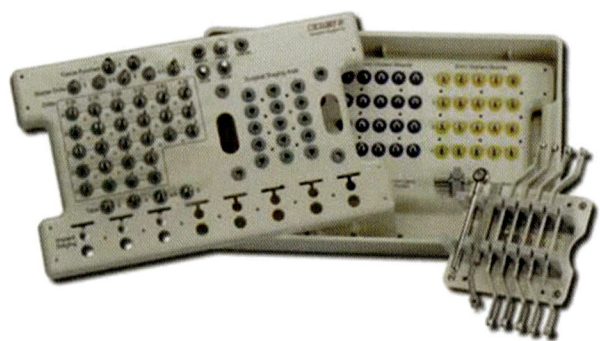

Figure 8.23 An example of an orthopedic loan set. Sets can include reusable instruments for use during the procedure and implantable devices. Note in this case a series of small orthopedic screws/pins that are designed for selection and implantation during a surgical procedure. The instruments are designed to be used (therefore soiled) and then reused, following processing. The implants are different as they are typically labeled as single patient use devices. Once they are implanted into a patient, damaged, or used/soiled during surgery they should not be reprocessed; but implants that have remained intact can be resterilized in accordance with manufacturer's instructions for the next procedure.

used and returned soiled to a manufacturer or third-party processing facility; the risks of exposure to blood-borne pathogens are important in these cases as multiple handlers are at risk during transportation. In other cases the devices are processed within the same facility and provided for a further procedure (at the same or a different hospital). For surgical devices, this can include only cleaning and disinfection (to render them safe for handling/shipping) or the full processing cycle (e.g. to include inspection, packaging, and sterilization). With the range of contract situations that may be in place, the risks associated with such sets/devices should be closely controlled. Written instructions and procedures for staff are essential.

The following guidelines are given when handling/processing loaned instruments:
- A written procedure should be in place at the healthcare facility receiving loaned devices/sets, describing how they need to be handled and processed (before and after surgical use, as applicable). Staff should be trained on the procedure, particularly in any disassembly, cleaning, rinsing, and inspection instructions. This should be considered in advance of receipt of the instrument(s).
- Carefully follow the manufacturer's processing instructions. Many loaned sets may provide various types of implantable and non-implantable patient devices, small and large. Processing procedures and particularly cleaning processes should ensure the adequate cleaning, rinsing, and subsequent processing of each device. In some cases the complete set may need to be disassembled from the set tray(s) or multiple trays removed from set containers to ensure adequate cleaning/rinsing.

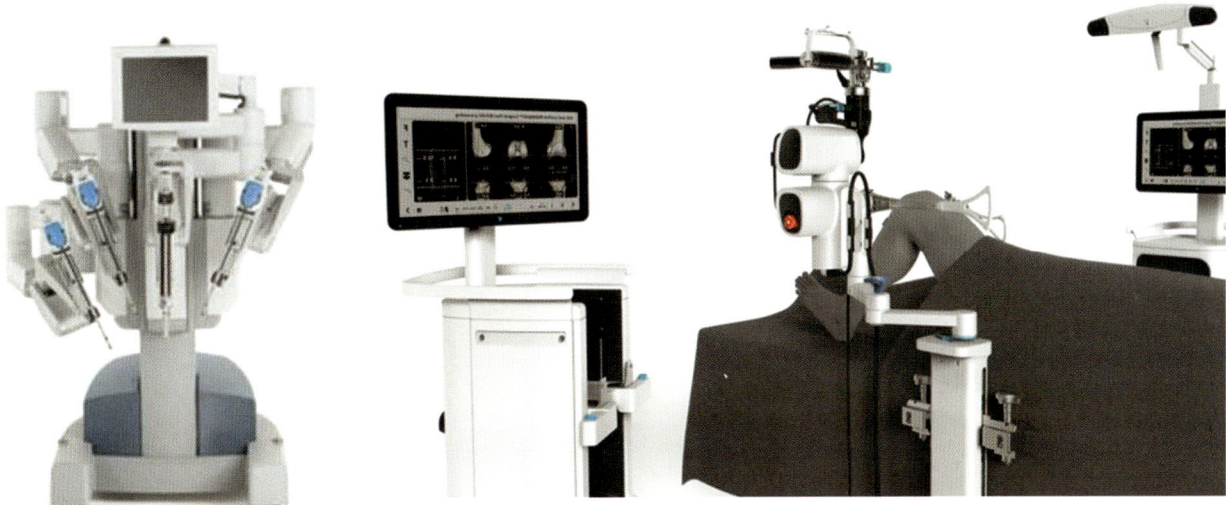

Figure 8.24 Examples of robotic systems that can include attachments of a variety of device types that may or may not contact the patient during surgical procedures.

Safe practice dictates that all items entering the processing facility are treated as contaminated, whether open or unopened and whether they appear to be used or not. Loan surgical sets should always be opened, cleaned, inspected, and sterilized before they are issued to an operating room, unless a quality assurance certificate has been received from the previous processor/device manufacturer. Such devices/sets that are not packaged (or if packaging has been compromised) should be considered contaminated and be processed according to documented policies and procedures.

- Inspection during processing can include detailed examination for cleanliness, damage, maintenance requirements, and, when applicable, dryness. Detailed examination of single patient use devices (screws, pins, etc.) is particularly important and may be challenging.
- Many loaned sets of devices, particularly orthopedic sets, can be large, complex, and often heavy. Care should be taken in lifting and moving sets to prevent injury. In addition, because of the weight and complexity of many of these sets, they should be carefully inspected for dryness following cleaning–disinfection and sterilization, as longer dry times may be necessary (in accordance with manufacturer's instructions and the capabilities of the equipment used during processing).

Electrical and robotic systems

Many devices contain various internal electrical components (Chapter 4) and can often be very sensitive to damage. Care should be taken in the handling but also in the cleaning of such devices. For example, it is not usual (although sometimes surprising to find) that a particular device or part of the device cannot be immersed in water. In such cases, close attention should be paid to the manufacturer's instructions. An example is a part of a device that is inserted into a patient for a particular procedure, while another attached part never touches the patient and is connected to an electrical source; this occurs with various types of flexible endoscopes, which are further discussed in the next section. In this case the patient-contacting part of the device may be manually cleaned in a sink, while the other parts of the device are cleaned with a wetted cloth. Protecting this kind of device from patient contamination will assist with the decontamination and can limit the extent of soiling. Manufacturer's instructions will provide specific guidance on handling and processing requirements in these cases.

Robotic-assisted surgery is a growing area of patient care and can include a variety of associated devices such as flexible/rigid endoscopes, light guide cables, light guide cable adaptors, camera arm sterile adaptors, camera sterile adaptors, instrument sterile adaptors, graspers, scissors, large and small needle drivers, blade instrument arm cannulas (sheath), cannula adaptors, obturators, and reducers. All or most of these can contain electronics and microprocessors built into them, and it may not always be possible to submerge them in water, which presents a challenge when cleaning. A further consideration is the various parts of the robot itself (examples are given in Figure 8.24) that may require routine cleaning/disinfection (typically considered as non-critical equipment but within the surgical area around the patient). In some cases various part of the robotic equipment may be covered in single-use sterile drapes or other barriers to reduce risks and prevent contamination during surgery. But it is considered best practice to clean and disinfect such equipment between patient uses, unless otherwise defined by the manufacturer or facility-specific requirements.

Cleaning instructions can vary depending on the specific device/component, to include the cleaning process and type of chemistry that can be used. These can include a manual cleaning and disinfection wipe, immersion in a sink, or the use of ultrasonic, automated cleaning. In all cases manufacturer's instructions should be closely reviewed.

Endoscopy

Endoscopes are complex viewing instruments (see Chapter 4) and are generally classified as rigid or flexible in design. They are delicate devices (particularly due to their internal structure, containing lenses and fiberoptics) and are composed of a variety of parts that are assembled together. They can range in materials from stainless steel (particularly rigid endoscopes) to plastics, elastomers (flexible endoscopes), and glass. In addition, many of these designs include internal channels (or "lumens"), ranging from one to seven lumens that can often be interconnected, as well as a variety of complex features that can be challenging to clean (see Chapter 4, Figures 4.57 and 4.58). The endoscope can also have a number of reusable accessories (see Chapter 4, Figure 4.60, and Chapter 15) that will also need to be considered for cleaning and subsequent disinfection/sterilization. Overall, care needs to be taken in the processing of these devices and particularly during cleaning to prevent damage; damage may occur during their handling and from the various types of chemicals, processes, and accessories used for cleaning. Flexible endoscopes are particularly sensitive due to their complex internal structures and the various types of soft plastics used in their construction. Depending on their use, the levels of soil (including microorganisms) can be very low, but in contrast they can also be very high; consider, for example, the use of a colonoscope for the inspection of and often receiving a sample from the colon (part of the lower intestines).

Endoscopic systems may or may not consist of many parts, such as the endoscope itself (the part that contacts the patient) and a remote power source to which the endoscope is connected (either directly or indirectly; Figure 8.25). The power source can enable the device to provide light, to view and capture internal pictures of structures within the body (on a video screen), but also to provide a source of water (from a designated water bottle), air (or another gas), and suction that are also used during the procedure. The emphasis for cleaning will be on the endoscope itself (as a critical or semi-critical device, depending on its use), although periodic cleaning (and disinfection) may also be required for the power source. Maintenance may also be required for any utilities (water, gas, etc.) that are provided as part of this equipment.

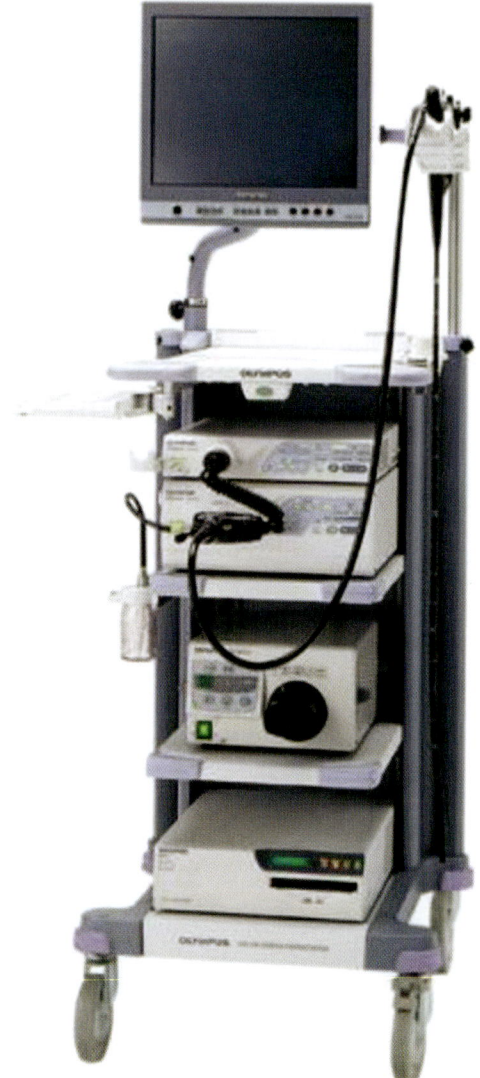

Figure 8.25 An example of an endoscopic system. This is a typical flexible endoscopic system including the endoscope (hanging on the right and connected to the control system), the control system (center), video screen (top), and water source (middle left).

The following recommendations are given for endoscope cleaning:
- Ensure that staff have been correctly trained on the handling and cleaning of endoscopes and any associated endoscopic equipment. Written procedures should be required and considered for individual devices, in particular for flexible endoscopes that contain multiple internal lumens or complex features (see Chapter 4, Figures 4.57 and 4.60). Remember that following patient use all lumens will be contaminated, not just the main working channels. One of the most common mistakes

made during endoscope processing is not understanding the device design, in particular how many lumens are present, and neglecting to clean all the lumens. Other problems occur with complex device features, such as moving parts and the elevator mechanism at the distal tip of duodenoscopes (see Chapter 4, Figure 4.57).

- Care should be taken in the handling of endoscopes to ensure they are not physically damaged during cleaning. Flexible endoscopes, for example, have a minimum bend radius (how tightly they can be coiled) defined by the manufacturer and sinks or cleaning containers should be provided into which the device can be safely accommodated and cleaned with adequate room for the process.
- Immediately following a patient procedure with a flexible endoscope, it is the normal process for the major working lumens of the device to be flushed with water and/or a cleaning chemistry and for the outside of the scope to be wiped down with a cloth. This is the recommended point-of-use treatment, often referred to as the "bedside process" as it is usually conducted in the patient room before the endoscope is disconnected from the control system (Figure 8.26; see Chapter 7 on point-of-use treatment). This serves to remove gross soil from the device lumens and surfaces prior to transport for processing. It may also be possible to flush other lumens at this time, which is important as they can become soiled during use in/on the patient.
- Endoscopes should be processed as soon as possible following use in a patient procedure. Guidance in different countries can include recommendations of no longer than one hour post procedure.
- Endoscopes may need to be prepared for immersion in water prior to cleaning. For example, flexible endoscopes are provided with water-resistant "soaking" caps that are placed over the exposed electrical components on their light guide connector ends (Figure 8.27). Newer generations of flexible endoscopes are completely waterproof and the soaking cap is no longer required.
- Before cleaning, the device should be inspected for any signs of damage that may restrict if and/or how the device should be cleaned. An example is with flexible endoscopes, where the device is recommended to be leak tested before being immersed in water. The internal compartments of the flexible endoscope contain various electrical and fiberoptic components that are not designed to contact patient materials or water; however, in some cases the internal lumens or external parts of the device may become compromised (e.g. through a tear or puncture on the various surfaces) and allow materials to enter these compartments. It is therefore important to make sure that these parts do not further contact water during cleaning/disinfection. During a leak test the internal compartment of the endoscope is pressurized with air using a leak tester (Figure 8.28) specifically designed for this purpose and the endoscope design. The leak tester usually connects to a specific port on the light guide end of the endoscope. The leak test can be performed manually (with a handheld or electrical leak tester)

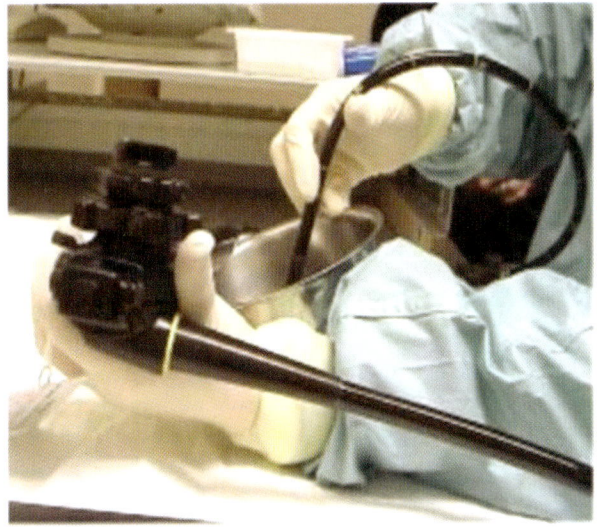

Figure 8.26 Bedside procedure with a flexible endoscope showing the device lumens being flushed with water/cleaning chemistry (by suctioning) prior to transport for processing.

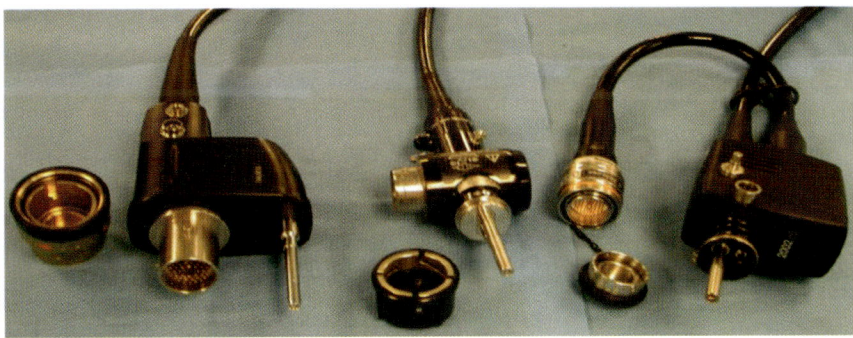

Figure 8.27 Flexible endoscope soaking caps (three different designs shown).

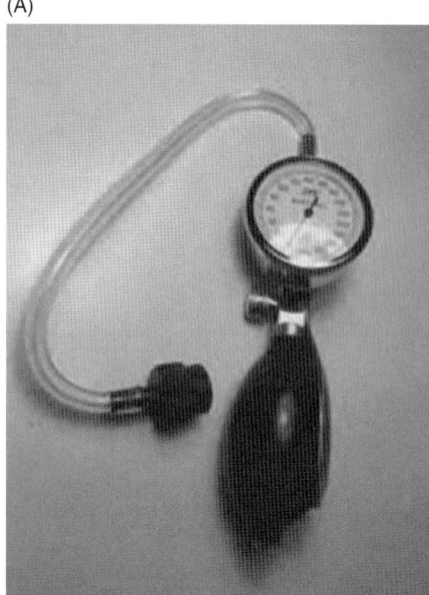 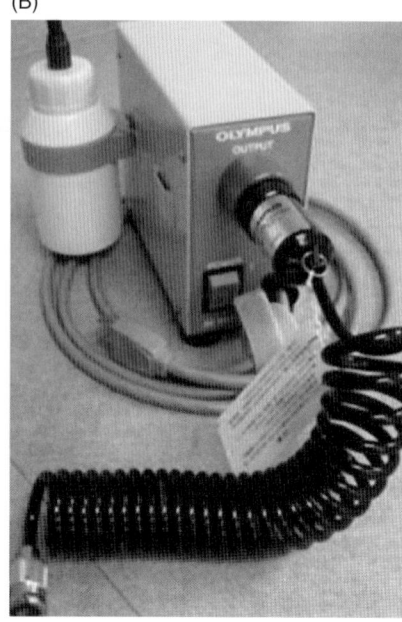

Figure 8.28 Flexible endoscope leak tester. (A) Manual and (B) electrical examples. They should periodically undergo verification testing and applicable maintenance, based on manufacturer's instructions.

and/or in an automated system. During manual dry leak testing, if a large leak is present a rapid pressure drop will be observed by the pressure monitoring gauge/system; the test should be repeated and if a leak is confirmed the device should not be immersed in water. In a wet leak test, the endoscope can be completely immersed in clear water to detect a continuous stream of small bubbles emerging from it on inflation. It is important to check for any leaks around all areas, including the tip, the knobs, and the bending rubber of the device. It is also important to consider that the devices should not be overpressurized as this can also lead to damage. Devices that have failed leak tests or are otherwise damaged should be sent for repair in accordance with facility requirements and manufacturer's instructions.

- Ensure that the device is disassembled and each reusable part is cleaned according to instructions. Some parts or accessories may or may not be immersed in water. Other accessories (such as valves or "buttons" used with flexible endoscopes) require special cleaning to ensure that all parts are adequately cleaned (e.g. by actuating, essentially repeatedly opening and closing, valves in the cleaning solution to ensure cleaning of all contact surfaces).
- Recommended cleaning chemistries can vary depending on the device or chemistry manufacturer. This can include neutral to mild alkaline cleaning chemistries. Neutral chemistries (with or without enzymes) are most commonly used. It is recommended that a fresh solution of cleaner/water is prepared, used for manual cleaning, and discarded after each use.
- Manual cleaning is often described by the manufacturer, with or without any subsequent automated cleaning. During manual cleaning, the device should be cleaned on the outside as well as any internal lumens (Figure 8.29). Manual cleaning of internal lumens is performed for two particular reasons: for cleaning purposes (to remove soil) and to ensure that the lumens are free flowing (not blocked or occluded). Internal lumens can be cleaned by flushing with water and cleaning chemistry and/or the use of specifically designed brushes/sponges (Figure 8.30). This should always be done under water to minimize the risk of aerosol formation during cleaning that could pose a safety risk to staff. Care should be taken to only use the correct brushes/sponges for the size of the lumen; when too small they will not be able to clean the lumen and when too big they can damage the internal structure. Older brushes/sponges should not be used, as parts could fall off and get stuck within or otherwise damage the lumen.
- Semi-automated irrigation systems may be used to assist in the cleaning process. It is important to ensure that any lumens are correctly attached to such systems to ensure irrigation (flow of cleaning chemistry/water) through the lumens. Some systems may be capable of detecting a blocked or occluded lumen while others may not. It is important to understand the specifications and limitations with such systems, including those within washer-disinfector or automated endoscope (re) processing (AERs) systems. Ultrasonic baths with appropriate cleaning chemistries are often used for cleaning of endoscopic accessories, but it is important to check with the device manufacturer's instructions if the device is compatible or not with ultrasonics. Not all ultrasonic systems are the same (e.g. different ultrasonic power, recommended exposure times,

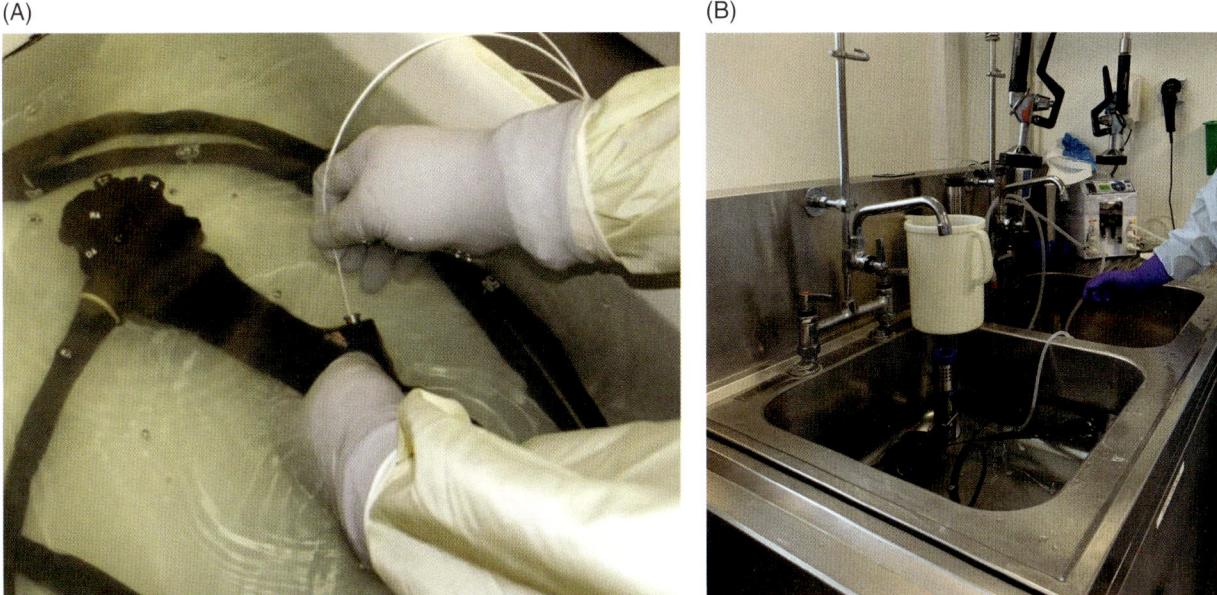

Figure 8.29 Manual cleaning (brushing) of a flexible endoscope. (A) The brush is shown being passed through the biopsy port of the device and then down the patient end of the endoscope (suction/biopsy channel). Note that the device is brushed while under water to prevent aerosolization. (B) The endoscope is soaked in detergent solution and channels irrigated with the aid of a semi-automated irrigation system.

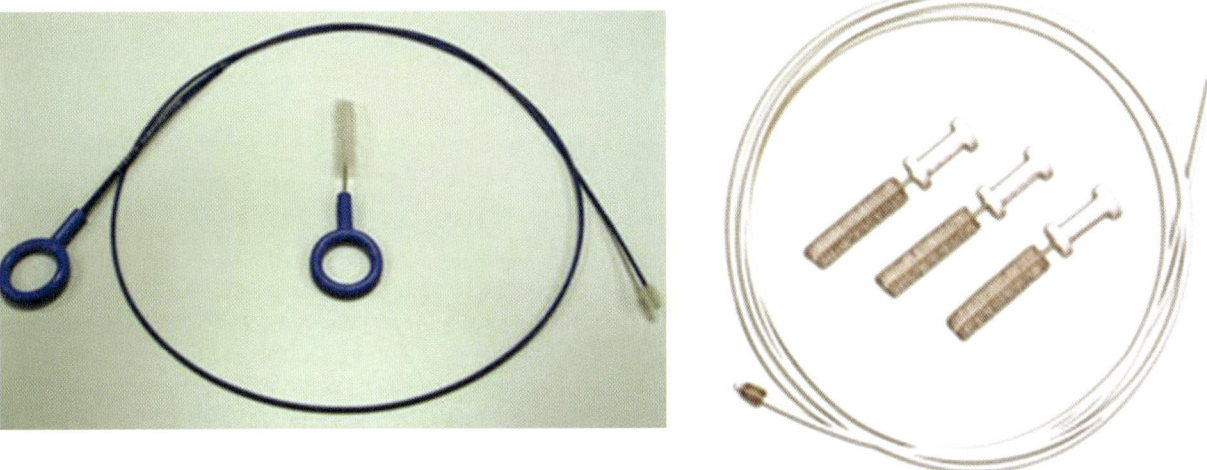

Figure 8.30 Examples of specially designed brushes and sponges used for cleaning of endoscope lumens.

temperature control, etc.) and some devices may be damaged under certain exposure conditions/limits.

- Ensure that correct rinsing is performed on all external and internal structures. The temperature and number of rinsing cycles with fresh water will vary depending on the cleaning agent used. Correct rinsing to the manufacturer's requirements is important to ensure that residual enzymes (which are proteins) or other chemicals do not remain on the device prior to disinfection/sterilization.
- There are many different designs of endoscope washer-disinfectors or AERs that can be used for automated cleaning (see the section on automated washer/washer-disinfectors and Figure 8.9). They range in complexity, including immersion and/or spray systems for cleaning the outside of the

endoscope and general irrigation systems for lumen cleaning. Some washers use specifically designed connectors that attach to the endoscope and irrigation/flow system of the machine, while others use a pressurized system at the control head of the scope to provide flow (connector-less washers). They may or may not provide a variety of features such as a leak test, lumen blockage test, irrigation control, detection of connector attachment/detachment, cleaning process parameter control, rinse-water quality control, and so on. Information should be provided by the washer manufacturer regarding the testing and validation of cleaning efficacy, preferably in compliance with local national or international standards/guidelines (see the section on cleaning guidelines, standards, and testing). At a minimum, the washer should be provided with at least one cleaning process that has been shown to be effective for the claimed endoscope types compatible with the system.

Devices known or suspected to be contaminated with prion material

Prions are unusual infectious agents (see Chapter 5, in the section on prions and other infectious proteins). They are considered infectious proteins and are implicated in causing a group of rare diseases known as transmissible spongiform encephalopathies (TSEs), with the most common example being Creutzfeldt-Jakob disease (CJD). They are known to be transmissible through contaminated tissues (particularly brain and other nervous tissues/organs) on items such as reusable devices, and are considered to have a higher resistance to decontamination methods. In most countries in the world (including recommendations by the World Health Organization published in 1999), additional precautions and handling procedures are recommended in known or suspected cases of prion disease. These are considered in further detail in Chapter 15, in the section on devices known or suspected to be contaminated with prion material.

There have been multiple investigations on the effectiveness of cleaning to reduce the risks of surface prion contamination, and the following conclusions have been drawn to date:
- As prions are proteins, and cleaning is designed to remove protein, cleaning is considered one of the most important steps in processing device surfaces known to be or considered at high risk of being contaminated with prion materials.
- Prions are hydrophobic (water-hating) proteins and therefore have a high affinity to attach to device surfaces, making them harder to remove, especially with water. The use of surfactants and other cleaning mechanisms can assist in the removal process.
- The highest risk of prion contamination is a device in direct contact with brain and spinal cord tissue. This is not to say that other tissues do not pose a risk, but the risk with these tissues is much less. In some cases, with a specific form of the disease known as variant CJD (vCJD), other tissues may provide a higher risk, such as lymph nodes and in certain types of eye procedures (e.g. that contact the optic nerve). Despite this, standard precautions against prions should be considered if there is a high risk of them being present (e.g. patients with known or highly suspected TSEs and contact with brain tissue during the surgical procedure).
- Drying of prion-contaminated material (similar to any soil present on a device after surgical or medical use) on a surface has been shown to increase the difficulty of its removal or inactivation during subsequent processing. Soil should not be allowed to dry on device surfaces prior to decontamination. Cleaning alone can significantly reduce the risk of prion surface contamination by physical removal and even (depending on the cleaning chemistry and process) degrade the prion material. This is, however, not always the case. In some cases cleaning chemistries have been shown to *increase* the resistance of prion material; in others they *decrease* the risk. This appears to be specific to the cleaning chemistry formulation. Therefore, in high-risk cases it is recommended that cleaning chemistries should be used only if they are supported by data that demonstrates directly that the individual cleaning chemistry has been tested and shown to safely reduce the risk of surface prion contamination. It is not sufficient to claim a product to be effective because it is of a certain type (e.g. alkaline or enzymatic). As an example, proteins are generally broken down by enzymes called proteases (see Chapter 6, Table 6.2), but prion proteins are known to be extremely resistant to the effects of most proteases.
- Most cleaning processes alone will not be effective in completely removing the risks associated with prion or indeed microbial contamination. Therefore, cleaning should always be followed by routine or prion-specific inactivation protocols (see Chapter 8, the section on devices known or suspected of being infected with prion material).

The following cleaning guidelines are given when handling known or potentially prion-contaminated reusable devices. These can be considered in consultation with regional or country-specific guidance, which can vary and is periodically updated:
- Ensure that a written facility policy is in place regarding the safe handling and processing of reusable devises. In many cases, device processing is not recommended and the device may need to be destroyed or otherwise taken out of use.
- Reduce any risk of devices drying following surgical or medical use and prior to pre-cleaning/cleaning.
- Cleaning chemistries used should be supported with data that shows that such products have been demonstrated to reduce the

risks of prion contamination. Cleaning conditions (product concentration, temperature, and contact time) should be closely followed, in addition to the normal cleaning guidelines (e.g. manufacturer's instructions regarding disassembly).
• Ensure that devices are correctly rinsed and prepared for subsequent disinfection/sterilization and/or specific prion decontamination recommendations.

Textiles and laundry

Laundering of reusable surgical/medical linens and textiles should follow the same basic processing steps as other surgical/medical devices. This should include the following:
• Post-procedure sorting and separation of waste from materials to be processed (see Chapter 7, in the section on post-procedure sorting).
• Safe transport to a processing site (see Chapter 7, in the section on transportation post procedure).
• Cleaning.
• Disinfection (Chapter 9) and/or sterilization (Chapter 11) as required (e.g. if used directly or contacting critical devices used directly for patient procedures).
• Drying, ensuring laundered items are stored dry and in a manner to prevent cross-contamination.

Laundry items (linens, textiles, drapes, etc.) can be considered as devices in their own right, and in some parts of the world may be described as such from a regulatory and legal point of view. They can be provided and labeled as single use or reusable. Similar to devices, reusable items may be considered critical (therefore needing to be provided clean and sterile) or non-critical (clean and disinfected, often referred to as "low bioburden").

All reusable, soiled textiles should be washed and disinfected/sterilized. Depending on where they are used, some textiles such as gowns and drapes may seem to play a negligible role as sources of infection, but they can act as carriers of infectious microorganisms and allow these to be released into the environment. Examples can include cross-contamination of items used in a dirty area of a processing department (which should not be worn outside of these controlled areas) or the use of sterile gowns within a surgical suite so as not to cross-contaminate the sterile core environment (see Chapter 3 on principles of aseptic (or "sterile") technique). Bacterial and fungal contamination can also accumulate in textiles (e.g. when used multiple times or stored wet) that can offer an even greater risk.

Conventional surgical gowns and drapes were typically made of cotton; however, cotton materials are not considered a safe barrier against fluids and microorganisms in high-risk environments and may also release lint (fluff or fragment) particles that can cause patient complications. Lint can be released into the environment during patient procedures and, if introduced into the patient (particularly during surgery), the body will recognize it as a foreign body and cause patient complications (e.g. impaired wound healing). Low-linting fabrics with more effective barrier properties are therefore recommended in higher-risk areas.

The laundry process should begin at the point where the items are used (e.g. in the operating theater) with the proper collection and sorting of textiles into specially provided containers (see Chapter 7 on post-procedure sorting). All items should be correctly sorted to include single-use, disposable items (textiles and devices) for waste disposal and multiple-use, reusable textiles and devices. Devices should be separated from textiles. A common hazard posed by contaminated linen is negligent waste disposal by staff at the point of use, where instruments such as sharps (needles, razor blades) and surgical instruments are accidentally mixed with textiles. It is for this reason that contaminated textiles are often defined as "laundry that has been soiled with bodily fluids or other potentially infectious material or may contain sharps." The risk to users in these cases is clear. Textiles may also be heavily soiled, posing a contamination/infection risk to staff. Therefore, the same protection methods (PPE, see the section on receiving and sorting) should be used in handling soiled linens as described for instruments. Any textiles that may have been exposed to patients, whether used or not, are assumed to be contaminated. Standard or universal precautions are always recommended when handling such items.

The processing process with textiles needs to consider safety (to staff and patients), ensuring that cleaning is adequate to remove visible soiling and staining, disinfection/sterilization requirements, and that the textiles are of acceptable quality to ensure patient comfort and textile durability. Surgical laundry, such as gowns, drapes, and surgical towels, may have to be kept separated from general hospital or heavily contaminated waste. If textiles are heavily contaminated, as much organic material as possible must be rinsed off before placing them into the machine with other washing. Remember that aerosolization is an important staff risk in these cases when manual cleaning. The type and cause of stains will affect the acceptance or rejection of laundered items. For example, linen with stains from substances, such as lubricants, blood, or bodily fluids, that cannot be removed is unacceptable. The lack of cleanliness may affect the disinfection or sterilization process and the textiles should be rejected. Chemical stains, such as those from dyes including methylene blue, may appear unsightly but will not necessarily affect the functioning of the textile. A stain protocol should be in place establishing stain acceptance and rejection criteria.

Cleaning and disinfection of textiles (laundering) are usually conducted in specialized washer-disinfectors that can be single-chamber, multi-chamber, or, commonly, tunnel washer-disinfectors (Figure 8.31). A typical cycle will include cold water pre-cleaning, cleaning, rinsing, disinfection, and

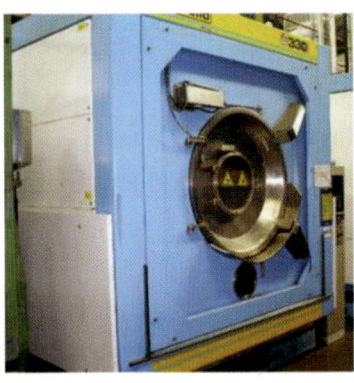 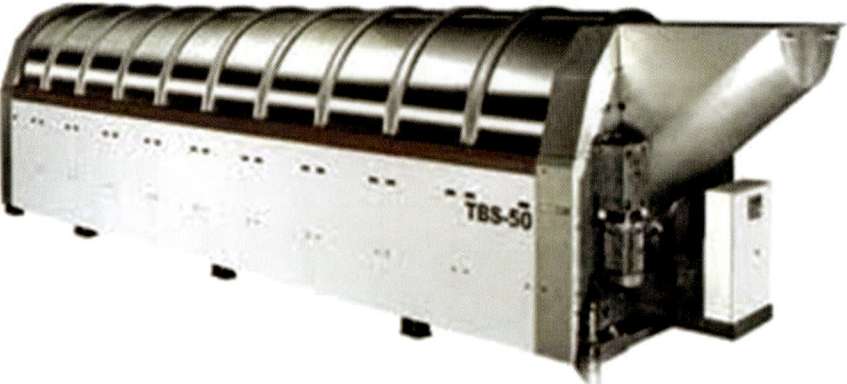

Figure 8.31 Examples of single-chamber and tunnel washer-disinfectors used for textiles.

removal of water/drying. Drying may be in the same machine or in a separate system. Depending on the institution the laundry may be an in-house department (separate to or part of a central reprocessing area) or an off-site facility, which often combines general-use and surgical textiles laundry. The textiles may also be owned by either the laundry (therefore on loan) or the medical facility. A variety of cleaning chemistries may be used, similar to those described in the section on basic principles of cleaning, including neutral, alkaline, and enzymatic-based chemical disinfection (see Chapter 9 on chemistries). Alkaline and enzymatic chemistries are typically used. Adequate rinsing (and in the case of some alkaline chemistries, correct neutralization with an acid) is important to reduce risks of skin irritation on clinical use. Accessory chemicals may be used for conditioning the textile load (to improve softness). Disinfection is performed by thermal (>65°C) and/or chemical means (<60°C, e.g. using ozone, peracetic acid, or chlorine-releasing solutions under controlled temperature conditions; see Chapter 9, in the section on chemical disinfection).

The following guidelines are given regarding the processing, including cleaning, of linens and textiles:
- Similar to other devices, textile items can be provided as single use or multiple use. "Textiles" are often used to described reusable items, while "non-wovens" refer to single use. Single-use items are designed to be discarded when used/soiled and are not recommended to be reprocessed.
- Facility staff (including those using, transporting, and reprocessing textiles) should work closely together to set standards and allocate responsibilities. A facility has a health and safety responsibility to ensure that there are clear separation and handling procedures for soiled/used materials and clean materials ready for patient use. Decisions should be made regarding what type of laundry equipment and how many systems will be needed to process the anticipated volume, who will be responsible for transporting both soiled and unsoiled items and how they will be transported, who has the responsibility for inspecting textiles, who will assemble packs, and whether the laundry or the healthcare facility will store new or uncirculated textiles.
- Reusable textiles should be separated from instruments and single-use items at the point of use. Particular care should be taken to remove any sharp devices, which will be a risk to laundry staff. All temporary labels, tape, and so on should also be removed from the textiles prior to returning them to the laundry. Standard/universal safety precautions should be followed when handling contaminated textiles, including the use of PPE. Hand-washing facilities, including a hygienic sink, soap dispensers, and paper towels, must be provided in the laundry area. The laundry facility should be designed to have a barrier or functional separation between areas in which soiled textiles are received/processed and areas in which cleaned textiles are handled, stored, and/or sterilized for distribution to the facility.
- Soiled textiles should be sorted and checked before being loaded into the washer, to prevent damage to machines from other materials (such as paper, sharps, and instruments). Some textiles that are heavily soiled may require pre-washing, pre-wetting, or the use of a pre-soak chemical to reduce staining.
- Laundry washer-disinfectors are currently excluded from the scope of the international standard for washer disinfectors (ISO 15883), but many of the requirements included in these standards are equally applicable to laundry applications. These include verifying the correct dosing of chemicals (including cleaning chemistries), verification of temperature control/distribution, correct rinsing, and disinfection requirements.
- As in cleaning of instruments, the way the washers (and dryers) are loaded is also important; if they are not loaded correctly, are overloaded, or sometimes underloaded, it may affect the process. An example is the exposure of all surfaces to the

cleaning chemistry: if a washer is overloaded there may be insufficient water/chemistry to be effective or lack of sufficient contact for cleaning; and if under loaded, in washers that are calibrated with a given level of chemistry to handle a given load, there may be overuse of chemistry and inadequate rinsing.
- Drying is an important consideration, as the presence of moisture will allow for the growth of microorganisms (bacteria and fungi) when textiles are stored, particularly if these materials are not packaged and sterilized for use. This may be assisted by hot-air drying in dedicated machines and ironing.
- Inspection of laundered materials should include inspection for cleaning and particularly staining. Textiles can be visually inspected, with the assistance of a light table, for stains, physical defects, foreign debris, and labels/tape, against a written quality procedure/standard. Although stained, processed materials may be safe for use, they may be unacceptable to patients/staff. If applicable, the critical zones of gowns, drapes, table covers, and sterilization wraps should be particularly inspected. Stains must be removed/remediated and then processed if possible, holes must be repaired with heat patches, foreign debris (hair, lint) must be removed, labels and so on removed, and tapes on gowns repaired.
- In some cases materials are separated and packaged for sterilization; these processes should follow the same guidelines as for instruments (Chapters 10 and 11).
- Cleaned/disinfected textiles must be protected from contaminants in the environment, including during transportation and storage, to avoid recontamination. Unwrapped textiles should be placed into transport carts or hampers and covered for transport to a designated area for storage. If the transport cart does not have a solid bottom, it should be lined with heavy plastic before placing clean textiles inside. Protective packaging may also be used to prevent accidental soiling of materials during transport and/or storage.
- During storage, unwrapped textiles should be handled as little as possible and be placed preferably in a dry, positive-pressure, temperature-controlled (68–98°F), properly ventilated area with limited access in order to prevent accumulation of dust and lint. Shelves for clean textiles should be typically 2.5–5 cm (~1–2 in.) from the wall, 15–20 cm (~6–8 in.) from the floor; and 30–46 cm (~12–18 in.) below the ceiling; textiles should never be stored on the floor.

Cleaning guidelines, standards, and testing

There are a variety of cleaning guidelines and standards that are used in specific countries and internationally; a number of these are summarized in Table 8.3. Staff and managers should be familiar with any local, area, or country guidelines and standards that apply to their facility; in the absence of specific guidelines, consider the use of international standards and guidance.

The ISO 15883 series of standards apply internationally to washer-disinfectors. They define the minimum design, performance, and testing requirements for washer-disinfectors. At the time of writing the series includes seven parts:
- Part 1: General requirements, definitions, and tests. This standard is applicable to all washer-disinfectors and should be used in conjunction with Part 5 (defining cleaning requirements) and the applicable other standards for the specific type of washer.
- Part 2: Requirements and tests for washer-disinfectors employing thermal disinfection for surgical instruments, anesthetic equipment, hollow articles, utensils, glassware, etc.
- Part 3: Requirements and tests for washer-disinfectors employing thermal disinfection for human waste containers. Examples include bed-pan washers.
- Part 4: Requirements and tests for washer-disinfectors employing chemical disinfection for thermo-labile endoscopes. This part considers the processing of flexible endoscopes (which use chemical disinfection).
- Part 5: Requirements and test method criteria for demonstrating cleaning efficacy. This part was initially published as technical specification (or guidance) that summarized various methods used around the world to test cleaning efficacy. This was subsequently modified to harmonize requirements for cleaning, and is used together with Part 1 of the series for all washer-disinfectors.
- Part 6: Requirements and tests for washer-disinfectors employing thermal disinfection for non-invasive, non-critical medical devices and healthcare equipment. An example would be a cart-washer.
- Part 7: Similar to part 6, but for washers employing chemical disinfection for non-invasive, non-critical items.

Each standard describes the necessary requirements for the design, performance, and validation of the washer-disinfector, including cleaning. Design requirements include the mechanical, electrical, safety, and control components. Performance requirements include how the washer should perform for cleaning, as well as for disinfection, rinsing, and drying (if appropriate). These requirements are tested by the manufacturer and also confirmed (validated) by testing a washer-disinfector when installed in a facility. The minimum requirement for cleaning efficacy is visible cleanliness, being dependent on detailed inspection following cleaning. Additional requirements are also defined for semi-critical and critical items, based on the chemical evaluation of the presence of residuals below what can be observed by the eye. These include defined levels of analytes (or chemical substances) that are typically found on reusable devices such as protein and organic carbon. The levels of analytes defined in the standard are given in Table 8.4. The presence of soil components below the alert levels is considered acceptable (clean) and above the action levels is a fail (dirty). Analyte concentrations between

Table 8.3 Various internationally used cleaning guidelines and standards. This list is only an example of some of the most widely used documents. It should also be noted that these standards/guidance are periodically updated/revised.

Guideline/standard	Title	Description
ISO 15883 series	*Washer-disinfectors*	A series of standards describing the design, performance, and testing of washer-disinfectors, including cleaning requirements. The essential requirements are provided in Part 1 (*General requirements, terms and definitions and tests*), which describes the requirements for all washer-disinfectors and is used together with Part 5 (*Performance requirements and test method criteria for demonstrating cleaning efficacy*) for cleaning requirements. Subsequent standard parts provide more details on specific types of washers (e.g. those used for the processing of surgical instruments or flexible endoscopes).
ISO 17664-1	*Processing of health care products – Information to be provided by the medical device manufacturer for the processing of medical devices – Part 1: Critical and semi-critical medical devices*	Information to be provided by the device manufacturer on the processing of reusable critical and semi-critical medical devices, including preparation at the point of use, preparation, and cleaning
ISO 17664-2	*Processing of health care products – Information to be provided by the medical device manufacturer for the processing of medical devices – Part 2: Non-critical medical devices*	Information to be provided by the device manufacturer on the processing of non-critical medical devices, including cleaning-disinfection instructions.
ISO 9398 series	*Specifications for industrial laundry machines*	Series of standards on laundry machines, including definitions, testing of capacity, and consumption characteristics. For example, Part 3 considers washing tunnels and Part 4 washer-extractors.
ANSI/AAMI ST65	*Processing of re-usable surgical textiles for use in healthcare facilities*	US standard for the proper handling, processing, and preparation of reusable surgical textiles, including cleaning. Addresses on-site and off-site recommendations.
AS/NZS 4187	*Reprocessing of reusable medical devices in health service organisations*	Australia/New Zealand recommendations on the processing of devices, including sorting, cleaning, and safety aspects. Note: replaced by AS 5369 in 2023 (*Reprocessing of reusable medical devices and other devices in health and non-health related facilities*)
AS/NZS 4815	*Office-based health care facilities – Reprocessing of reusable medical and surgical instruments and equipment, and maintenance of the associated environment*	Similar to AZ/NZS 4187 but with an emphasis on office-based (including outpatient) facilities. Includes recommendations on cleaning and associated facilities.
ANSI/AAMI ST98	*Cleaning validation of health care products – Requirements for development and validation of a cleaning process for medical devices*	US standard on requirements for cleaning validations, including process definitions, test soils, test methods, and endpoints.
AAMI TIR 30	*A compendium of processes, materials, test methods, and acceptance criteria for cleaning re-usable medical devices*	US guideline regarding test protocols, test soils, and acceptance criteria to validate cleaning processes for reusable devices (replaced by AAMI ST98).
AAMI TIR 12	*Designing, testing and labeling re-usable medical devices for reprocessing in healthcare facilities: a guide for medical device manufacturers*	Like ISO 17664-1, this US guidance provides information to device manufacturers on developing and testing cleaning processes, including requirements at the point of use, preparation, and cleaning.
AORN	*Instrument cleaning*	US recommended practices for point of care, transportation, cleaning, and general care of surgical instruments.
SGNA (USA)	*Standards for infection prevention in reprocessing of flexible gastrointestinal endoscopes*	US recommendations and guidelines on the care, handling, and cleaning of flexible endoscopes.

Table 8.3 (cont'd).

Guideline/standard	Title	Description
ANSI/AAMI ST79	*Comprehensive guide to steam sterilization and sterility assurance in health care facilities*	US standard for device processing, including requirements for cleaning and cleaning verification
WHO	*Decontamination and reprocessing*	General guidance on device processing, including cleaning requirements
HSPA	*Sterile processing technical manual*	US learning resource for the processing of reusable devices, including preparation and cleaning/cleaning processes.
CAN/CSA-Z314 (Canada)	*Decontamination of re-usable medical devices*	Canadian standard describing safe handling, transportation, and biological decontamination of contaminated reusable devices. Biological decontamination includes thorough cleaning and disinfection.
ESGE	*Guidelines on cleaning and disinfection in gastrointestinal endoscopy*	European recommendations and guidelines on the care, handling, and cleaning of flexible endoscopes.
HTM 01-01	*Decontamination of surgical instruments*	UK guidance on device decontamination in various parts. Cleaning requirements are included in Parts A (management and provision) and D (washer-disinfectors).
HTM 01-05	*Decontamination in primary care dental practices*	UK guidance for processing, including cleaning, in dental practices.

Table 8.4 Acceptance criteria for cleaning efficacy for semi-critical and critical devices. The levels of analytes are given as the total concentration per surface area of the device ($\mu g/cm^2$) or the whole device (in the case of endotoxins). Note: non-critical devices are required only to be visibly clean on inspection.

Test or analyte	Alert level	Action level
Visual examination	No visible soil	Visible soil
Protein	$\geq 3\,\mu g/cm^2$	$\geq 6.4\,\mu g/cm^2$
Total organic carbon	$\geq 6\,\mu g/cm^2$	$\geq 12\,\mu g/cm^2$
Carbohydrate	$\geq 0.9\,\mu g/cm^2$	$\geq 1.8\,\mu g/cm^2$
Hemoglobin	$\geq 1\,\mu g/cm^2$	$\geq 2.2\,\mu g/cm^2$
ATP	≥ 10 femtomoles ATP/cm^2	≥ 22 femtomoles ATP/cm^2
Endotoxin	≥ 2.2 EU/device	≥ 20 EU/device

ATP, adenosine triphosphate.

the two require further investigation as they may indicate a concern over time (e.g. a device feature that is difficult to clean and may build up soil over time). Other tests included in the standard are used to detect the presence of other process residuals on device surfaces such as those from cleaning chemistries.

In addition to the testing done by the manufacturer to demonstrate compliance with the standard, testing is also recommended to be performed routinely or periodically, to ensure that the washer is operating correctly. Various checks and tests should be determined with the washer manufacturer, but the following are given as a guide:

- Daily tests:
  ○ Check that devices are visually clean. In some countries more sensitive tests are recommended for periodic verification of cleanliness levels below visual detection. These can include, as examples, swab-based protein or adenosine triphosphate (ATP) detection methods or direct detection of protein on device surfaces.
  ○ Check that any nozzles, flow attachments, filters, and rotating spray arms (in the machine and on racks) are clean/free flowing.
  ○ Inspect door seals.

- Confirm that the correct type and volume of chemistry are available for the day.
- Manually clean around the areas, including any carts/conveyors/loading areas so that they are not left soiled.
- Check printouts (including paper where available) and/or that associated computers collecting cycle data are working (where relevant).
• Routine tests (these may be quarterly, six monthly, and/or yearly):
  - Calibration of various washer instruments, such as thermometers, pressure sensors, dosing systems, etc.
  - Washing tests, including chemistry dosing and cleaning studies.
  - Thermometric test for thermal disinfection.
  - Water quality tests (note, washers can use up to three different sources of water: cold, hot, and treated, e.g. deionized or reverse osmosis water).
  - Check for wear and tear on various washer parts (including seals, pumps, racks, and other accessories).
  - Verify security and settings of door safety switches and interlocks.

While such testing is often carried out with washers, little to no testing is conducted with manual cleaning, which can often lead to concerns about the safety of such processes. It is recommended to minimize any risks with manual cleaning by ensuring that written procedures are given, staff are periodically trained, tools are provided to minimize any variables (such as PPE, automated chemistry dosing, and sinks with indicated water volume levels), and regular auditing of manual cleaning practices is conducted.

Manual cleaning variables can be routinely verified, including volume of water used for cleaning (e.g. indicated in the sink), dosing of cleaning chemistry (dilution amount in water), temperature, and compressed air pressure/quality. Some types of modern sinks can have such monitoring or control systems integrated into their design, and often have further benefits such as adjustable height levels to accommodate different operators (see Chapter 13 on ergonomic safety).

The minimum requirement after cleaning is visible inspection of devices for any signs of soil (visual inspection); this can be enhanced using correct lighting and a lighted magnifying glass (Figure 8.32). Rigorous inspection of devices is recommended at a minimum to ensure devices are correctly cleaned and fit for further processing or patient use.

Ensuring a consistent cleaning process provides a further level of security that sufficient cleaning has been performed. For manual cleaning, this can be encouraged by having written protocols, well-trained staff, and periodic audit. Greater assurance can be provided with washers and washer-disinfectors by monitoring various process parameters (including temperature, pressure, chemical dosing, etc.); however, these do not replace the need for correct staff training, audits, and device inspections.

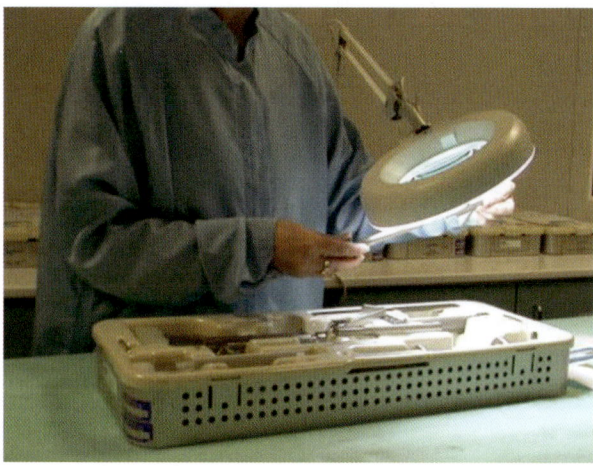

Figure 8.32 Visual inspection of a device set following a cleaning process.

As mentioned earlier in this chapter, visual cleanliness is a minimum requirement following cleaning. Other endpoints of cleaning (for semi-critical and critical devices) are now in widespread use and include biochemical and chemical tests (Table 8.4). It should be noted that most of these methods of assessing the efficacy of cleaning are laboratory based and are generally not considered to be routinely used in healthcare facilities. Examples include the detection of protein or total organic carbon on surfaces following a cleaning process. These are primarily used by manufacturers (of devices, materials, washers, and cleaning chemistries) to assess cleaning in or with their various products. Despite this, some tools and methods are being recommended and used to assess cleaning methods or cleaning endpoints in healthcare facilities. These include:

• Laboratory-prepared cleaning soils that are used to soil devices and then tested for being clean after a cleaning process. ISO15883-5 describes the test requirement for such soils to be considered effective and provides examples of soil types. Examples include coagulated blood, defibrinated blood soil, and biofilm test soils (Table 8.5). Most of these are made in a laboratory setting from given recipes, but a few are available commercially (Figure 8.33).

• Detection kits that are used for the specific identification of certain components of soils, such as protein, blood, and ATP (a molecule found in most living cell-based materials). These include the use of chemicals that react with these soil components, in accordance with manufacturer's instructions, to give a reaction (e.g. a color change) that is indicative of the concentration of analyte present. In many cases they are swab-based tests that require the use of use the swab provided to sample the device surface for detection. In others chemicals are provided to the device surface to allow for direct detection on the

Table 8.5 Various types of test soils used for testing cleaning efficacy.

Test soil	Components	Uses
Coagulated blood	Commercially available heparinized or citrated blood, activated chemically to coagulate immediately prior to use[1]	General surgical instruments, endoscopes, and anesthesia equipment
Edinburgh test soil	Egg yolk, defibrinated blood, hog mucin. Includes an original and a preferred modified form (also known as defibrinated blood soil or DBLSO)	Surgical instruments, surgical instrument trays, bowls, and dishes
Two-component blood test soil	High-protein and hemoglobin-based soil prepared in two components in salt solutions and mixed together prior to use	General surgical instruments
Artificial test soil (ATS)	Blood- and serum-based soil containing various chemicals	Gastrointestinal endoscopes
Biofilm	Bacterial (*Pseudomonas aeruginosa*) biofilm developed on the inner surfaces of lumens	Flexible endoscopes

[1] Note that the coagulation of blood can change its affinity to and difficulty in removal from surfaces. This also simulates exposure to blood in surgical or medical use.

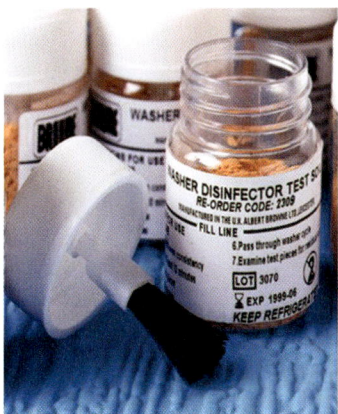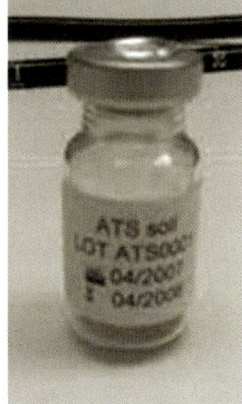

Figure 8.33 Two types of commercially available test soils.

device using equipment provided. These often offer soil detection at lower levels than are visually observed (Figure 8.34).
- Washer indicators (Figure 8.35) that are defined surfaces (e.g. stainless steel or plastics) that have a known amount of soil applied and dried. They are used to test the efficacy of cycle process performance in washer or washer-disinfector.

These are all useful to test washer performance, but, as for all types of indicators and tests, they can be used to ensure that a cleaning process has taken place but cannot ensure that the devices in the process are clean. Examples include the difficulty of using swabs to sample areas of a device that are difficult to access (and often to clean), and an indicator used in a washer-disinfector that shows a clean result, but the devices have not been loaded correctly into the washer to ensure they are contacted at all internal and external surfaces.

Troubleshooting cleaning problems

Inadequate cleaning is a common problem in the processing of devices/materials. This can be observed directly by the presence of visual soil or by using other more sensitive soil-detection methods (e.g. protein detection). This should be detected during inspection following cleaning, but unfortunately may not be observed until the point of patient use. In both cases the device or devices should be rejected and returned for further cleaning and processing (note: it is not best practice to perform "spot" cleaning in these situations). It is useful for the processing facility to monitor these occurrences, such as by reporting a rejection rate (the number of devices rejected compared to the number processed). Rejection rates should be absolutely minimized and rejected items investigated for potential causes. Any rejected devices will need to be recleaned and subjected to further processing before clinical use, which in some cases can lead to patient procedure delays and even cancelations. Examples of the most common causes of inadequate cleaning, including with automated washers, are:

- Staff not being familiar with the details of instructions of use. Devices may often have exposed or hidden device features that present a challenge to cleaning. Unfortunately, in the past device processing instructions have been reported to be inadequate in the level of detail required to ensure cleanliness.
- Devices not disassembled according to instructions or not placed in the optimum position for cleaning. A typical example is with hinged instruments that are not opened prior to washing, thereby not allowing cleaning to occur within the joint. If certain hinged instrument designs are constantly being rejected, despite being placed in the open position, these devices may require specific manual pre-cleaning or disassembly.

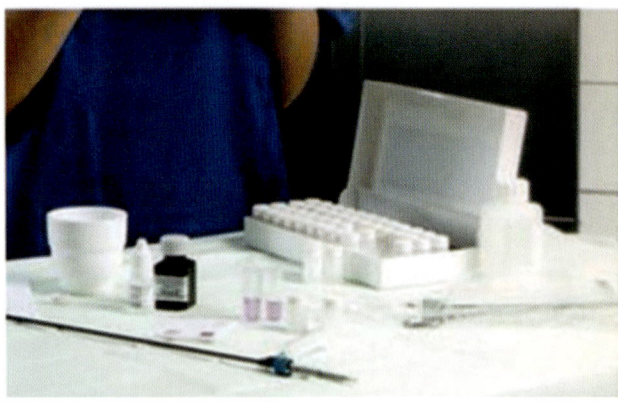
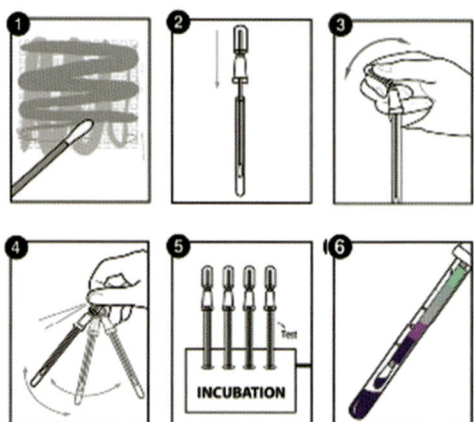
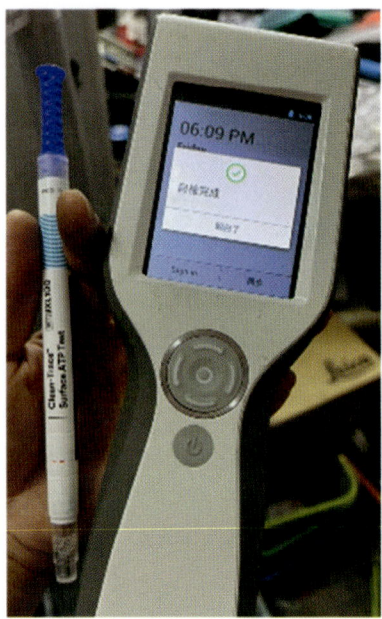
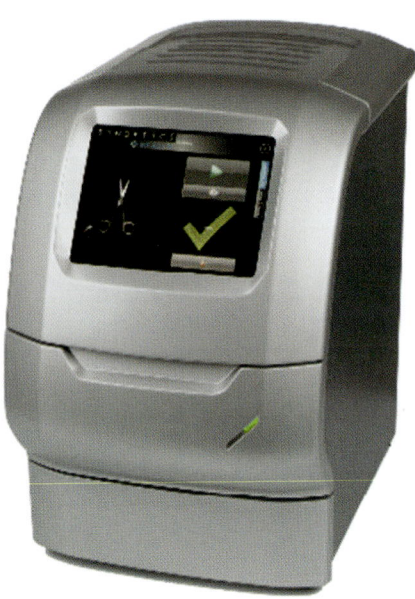

Figure 8.34 Various types of soil-detection kits.

- Inappropriate use or malfunction of cleaning equipment, detergents, or water. Examples include not using detergents in accordance with manufacturer's instructions, poor water quality, poor maintenance of equipment, or even inoperable automated systems.
- Overloaded baskets/trays in automated systems allowing some items to shadow others from spray jets (e.g. a bowl placed over instruments) or cleaning processes.
- Inadequate maintenance of immersion/ultrasonic bath, including build-up of soil in the bath that is carried over on the device to a subsequent processing stage.
- Blocked spray jets and/or spray arms that are not free to rotate or apply their cleaning impact. These should be periodically checked. A common problem is that the washer racks are not correctly aligned/attached to the water flow system within the washer.
- No cleaning chemistry used (e.g. dosing system is broken or chemistry has run out in automated systems). This may or may not be detected by the washer-disinfector design.
- Blocked strainer in the washer-disinfector chamber base, leading to inadequate draining from the chamber and spray patterns for cleaning.

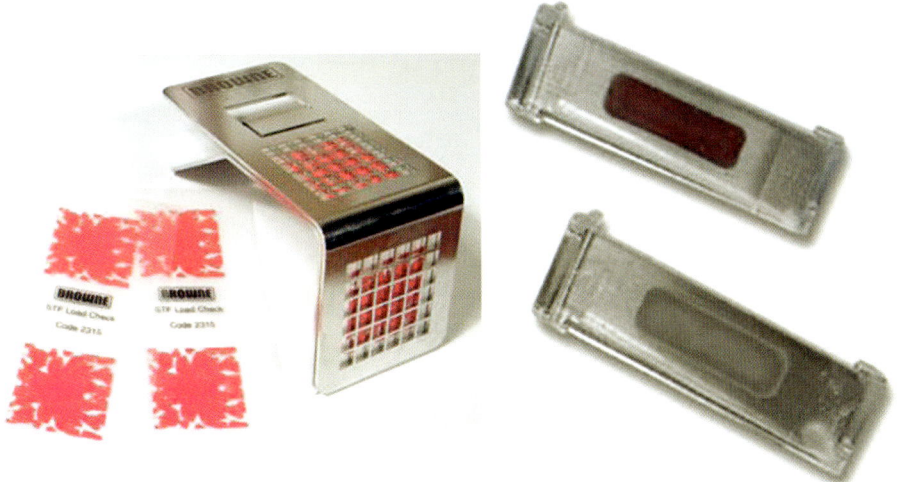

Figure 8.35 Various types of washer indicators used to test cleaning process performance.

- Soiled instruments that have been stored for prolonged periods with no pre-cleaning or pre-treatment. Blood, protein, and other materials can become fixed and coagulated when dried, making soil difficult to remove. A difficult example is orthopedic cements that dry hard and insoluble onto device surfaces.
- Inadequate cleaning process designs: this can include many variables such as pre-cleaning, subjecting devices to high temperatures (45°C) prior to cleaning (allowing soil to be fixed onto the device), cleaning chemistry (type, concentration, temperature, and exposure time), and inadequate rinsing.
- The water quality being used (for cleaning and rinsing): the formulation of the cleaning chemistry should be able to work under good or poorer water qualities, but this is formulation specific and even then has limitations. Water hardness (scale) is a particular concern and is often detected by the presence of "spotting" or a white, grainy deposit on device surfaces. It is insoluble in water and can only be removed by treatment with an acid or acidic-based chemistry (see Chapter 6 on non-enzyme-based cleaners). Repeated observation of this is a strong indicator of poor water quality that needs to be addressed with facility management staff.

In addition to these common problems, the type of soil observed may also be a challenge based on its source. Soils can be from the patient, various chemicals used during or following the procedure on the device, or even from the processing cycle itself. Care should be taken to inspect for the presence of patient soil compared to other materials that may be present. The methods used to remove the problem can be different. In the case of patient soil or chemicals such as iodine (due to inappropriate use in surgical or other medical procedures), these should be removed by repeating the normal cleaning process. Other types of soils will not be removed by repeating the normal cleaning process, with examples being the development of rust, water hardness, and the presence of cement. The first two are generally water quality concerns, although rusting can be promoted by aggressive cleaning or other chemicals used on the device (in particular low-quality stainless steel devices). Rusting may often be mistaken for dried blood, as they can have the same brown appearance; a simple test for rusting (and hardness deposits) is to place a small amount of an acid cleaner onto the material and it should quickly dissolve, while patient soil will not. Both can be removed using an acid-based chemistry, but this only hides the problem, which will persist unless the water quality is improved and/or better cleaning chemistries are used. Cement is a particular concern with orthopedic devices, as when it dries it becomes very hard on a surface; it is recommended that cement deposits should be removed at the point of a patient procedure, as when cement sets it may only be removed by chipping off the surface (also assisted by an acid cleaner), which may damage the device.

Overall, in many cases inadequate cleaning rates can be reduced by staff training for both manual and automated cleaning procedures. This may include the correct handling and inspection of not only the device but also any of the tools used for cleaning (chemistries, machines, loading systems, etc.). Other problems, such as persistently high rejection rates, appearance of chemical deposits, and device damage, may require more detailed analysis of the cleaning process in place and the variables associated with that process. Note that many of these problems will be seen following cleaning, disinfection, and/or sterilization. A simple process of elimination can be used to investigate such problems. For example, if rusting is not observed following cleaning and disinfection (on inspection prior to packaging) but appears to be present on a device presented to a theater, this potentially highlights a problem with the steam sterilization and/or drying/storage process. Another example is the sudden occurrence of a problem when the cleaning and other processing steps have remained unchanged; this often highlights a problem with variable water quality that can change from season to season within a facility (Figure 8.36). These surface changes include:

- White to gray, grainy deposits or films. This is typically an indication of high hardness levels in water being used for cleaning or rinsing. Hardness (or scale) refers to the concentration of calcium and magnesium ions in water, measured chemically as parts per million (ppm) or milligrams per liter (mg/L) $CaCO_3$. Water can have high concentrations of hardness (e.g. over 400 ppm) without its being seen, but such high concentrations will precipitate out when heated. The precipitate may also be colored, appearing as more green or brown for example, due to the presence of other metals such as copper in the water that precipitate with the hardness. At lower concentrations, hardness may appear as "spotting" or brown rings on a dried device surface. To reduce these effects, hardness levels in water of ≤ 150 mg/L $CaCO_3$ are recommended for cleaning. In some countries ≤ 10 mg/L is recommended for water used for disinfection/final rinsing.

- Reddish brown, partial discolorations or crater-shaped or pinhole-type impressions on the device surrounded by brown or multi-colored edges. These are the hallmarks of corrosion or rusting; rusting is a visual sign of surface damage, particularly on stainless steel devices. The main cause of rusting is chlorine (but also other halogens such as iodine and bromine) that can be present in patient soil (e.g. in blood), water, and other solutions (such as iodophors used in theaters and physiological saline, which is sodium chloride, NaCl). High levels of chloride in water are a common concern, particularly when heated. Typical recommended chloride levels for cleaning should be ≤ 250 mg/L. Chloride concentrations greater than 250 mg/l chlorine can be very damaging to stainless steel and plastic surfaces, with higher temperatures being more aggressive at even lower concentrations (in the 10–120 mg/L range). Other causes can be

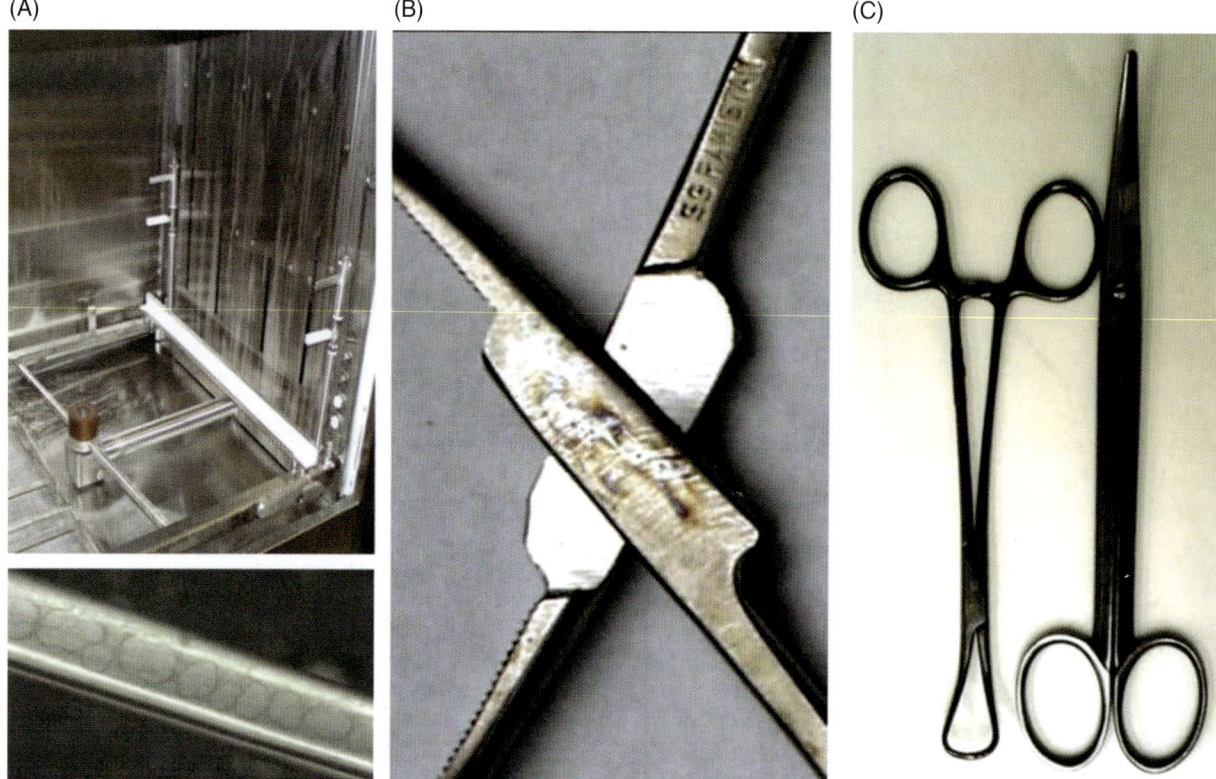

Figure 8.36 Examples of various types of surface changes commonly observed following cleaning, disinfection, and sterilization processes. They include (A) water hardness deposition (seen as white precipitate in a washer-disinfector and "spotting" on a device surface), (B) rusting, and (C) staining (black staining on stainless steel devices).

due to wear and tear (e.g. in hinge mechanisms) and aggressive cleaning chemistries (especially acid chemistries). Significant damage or rusting on a device is a common indicator of the end of life of a reusable device, where the device may need to be repaired or discarded.

- Multi-colored stain (often seen as a rainbow or other colored effects including yellow, brownish, blue, and violet) covering large areas or drop-shaped or irregular, insular shapes. These are usually due to increased content of silicates in water, particularly the final rinse water. They can also be seen on stainless steel devices on exposure to excessive (often dry) heat.
- Whitish gray corrosion or deposits on surface of carbon steel and naturally anodized aluminum. This is usually due to incorrect chemicals (e.g. strong acid or alkaline chemistries) being used that are incompatible with such metals. In these cases, cleaning products that are labeled as being "aluminum safe" should be used, such as neutral and mild alkaline cleaners (depending on the formulation and specific manufacturer's claims).
- Orange-brown staining. This is often due to high levels of phosphates in the water or is even sometimes associated with the cleaning chemistry.
- Black staining. This is typically due to levels of acid remaining on device surfaces (e.g. when used for neutralization of an alkaline cleaner or for removal of rust in manual cleaning).
- Other types of deposits, including white or otherwise colored grainy films observed on drying. These may be simply due to residual chemistries remaining on the device because of inadequate rinsing; when dried the chemistry remains. Close attention should be paid to rinsing post cleaning. In contrast to hardness deposits, these should be more easily dissolved/removed with water alone. In some cases white spots can be due to high levels of silicates or sulfites in water used for processing.

Although these are the most common problems associated with cleaning, other stains can be observed after steam sterilization, such as any of those listed associated with water (used to make steam) or purple/black stains (due to overdosing of amines often used to prevent corrosion of steam lines) and gold tinting (from chlorine and other chemicals present in water treatment systems).

As many of these problems are associated with water, the quality of water used for the various stages of processing is an important consideration and is further discussed in Chapter 15, in the section on water quality/purity.

9 Disinfection

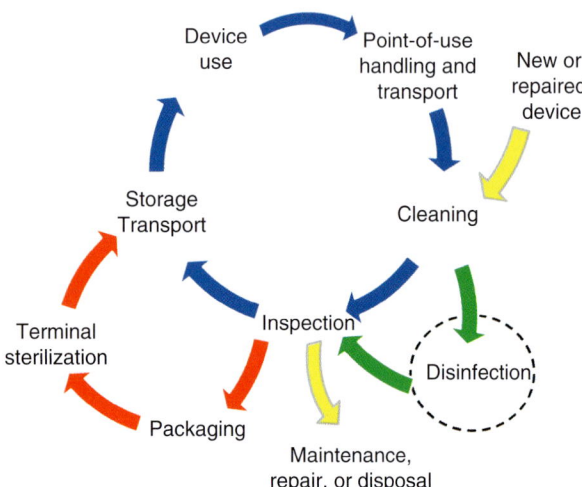

Disinfection is defined as a process to inactivate viable microorganisms to a level previously specified as being appropriate for a defined purpose, to include further handling or use. A disinfectant is a chemical and/or physical agent used for disinfection. This chapter addresses the disinfection of reusable devices. During the decontamination cycle devices may be subjected to cleaning, disinfection, and/or sterilization prior to patient use, depending on their classification (see Chapter 1 on the decontamination process). Some consideration is also given to the various types of disinfectants used for other, general-surface applications. Microorganisms present on reusable devices can be transferred to those handling the devices or to patients, and are therefore sources of infection. Antimicrobial products and/or processes such as disinfection are designed to reduce these risks when using devices or materials with patients, as well as to protect staff handling these devices. As introduced in Chapter 1, reusable devices can provide different levels of risks to a patient and therefore various levels of disinfection or even sterilization are recommended to reduce these risks (as summarized in Table 9.1).

In device processing cycles, disinfection should follow cleaning (see Chapter 8). Cleaning itself can significantly reduce the number of microorganisms on a reusable device, and may be considered as the only step required for processing of non-critical devices (those that may contact intact skin). But even in these cases, low- or intermediate-level disinfectants are also often used to inactivate microorganisms, either as part of or as a separate step to cleaning. A "high-level" disinfection process is the recommended minimum requirement for semi-critical devices that can directly contact patients' mucous membranes. The different levels of disinfection are considered further later in the chapter. Disinfection is also used as an interim step in the processing of critical devices, such as in a washer-disinfector process with surgical devices to render the devices safe for handling during subsequent inspection and packaging for sterilization. Other terms such as pasteurization (use of moist heat disinfection) and antisepsis are forms of disinfection; other definitions such as sanitization may have local, specific definitions and care should be taken to understand the data provided to support any disinfectant product claims and local requirements (for further discussion see Chapter 6 on disinfectants, including preservatives).

As introduced in Chapter 5, microorganisms consist of a wide range of viruses, bacteria, fungi, protozoa, and helminths. They range in their resistance levels to disinfection, as summarized in Figure 9.1 (also introduced in Chapters 1 and 6, in the section on disinfectants, including preservatives). Different levels of disinfection are traditionally defined based on their ability to inactivate such microorganisms. A common classification includes the designation of high-, medium-, or low-level disinfection, which are dependent on the types of microorganisms that it kills. Specific definitions of disinfection levels can vary from country to country, with a widely used example given in Figure 9.2.

Sterilization is the highest level of microbial inactivation and is the recommended minimum practice during the processing of critical (and in many cases semi-critical) devices. Sterilization is more than the demonstration of a product's or

Decontamination and Device Processing in Healthcare, Second Edition. Gerald McDonnell and Georgia Alevizopoulou.
© 2025 John Wiley & Sons Ltd. Published 2025 by John Wiley & Sons Ltd.

Table 9.1 A summary of the Spaulding classification system, recommending various levels of disinfection or sterilization for the reprocessing of devices based on their potential risk to patients.

Patient contact	Examples	Device classification	Minimum inactivation level
Intact skin		Non-critical	Cleaning and/or low/intermediate-level disinfection
Mucous membranes or non-intact skin		Semi-critical	High-level disinfection
Sterile areas of the body, including blood contact		Critical	Sterilization

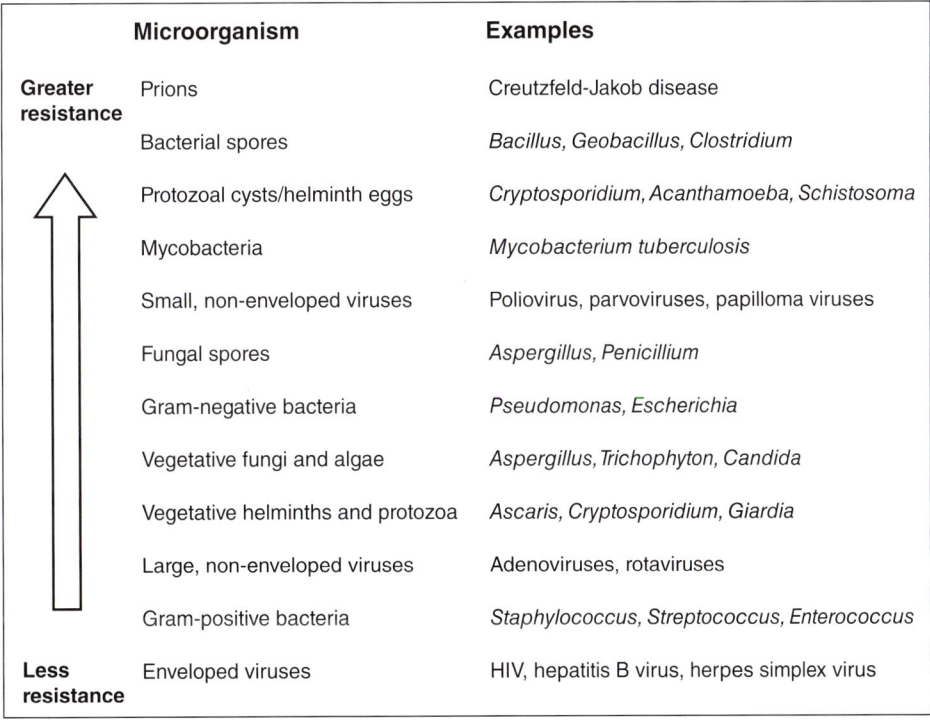

Figure 9.1 The resistance of microorganisms to inactivation. Microorganisms are listed as being of lower (bottom) to higher (top) resistance to inactivation. This list is given as a guide only, as the actual level of resistance can vary depending on the disinfection/sterilization method used. For example, the designation of prions as showing the highest resistance is generally accepted but is not always the case. Also, bacterial spores are often considered the most resistant to disinfection/sterilization, but in some special cases other types of microorganisms are equally or even more resistant. Certain types of microorganisms are not as well studied from a disinfection or sterilization point of view, but this list gives an estimate of what is known.

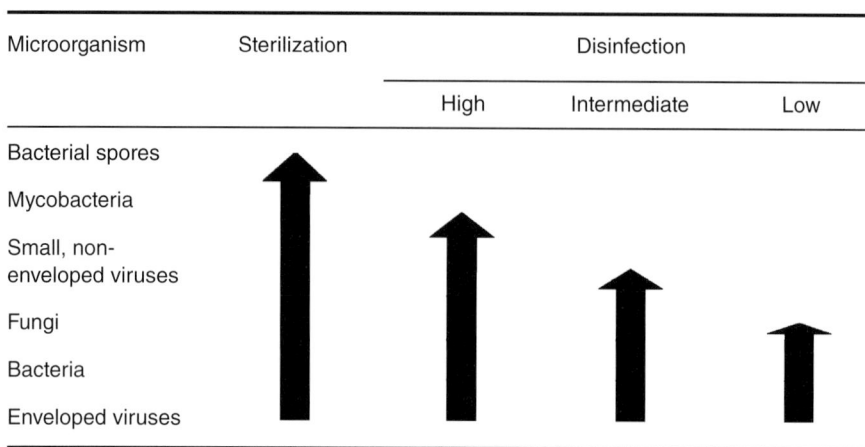

Figure 9.2 A commonly used classification system for disinfectants, describing their different levels of efficacy against various forms of microorganisms. The definition of the specific disinfection levels and their requirements for efficacy can vary from country to country.

process's effectiveness at killing all types of microorganisms. The various thermal/chemical methods used in healthcare facilities are described in further detail in Chapter 11. According to the classification scheme we are using here, high-level disinfection is considered effective against a range of microorganisms, including mycobacteria, and even has some activity against bacterial spores. Examples include disinfectants based on aldehydes or oxidizing agents (e.g. peracetic acid), as well as moist heat processes at greater than or equal to ($\geq$) 90°C for one minute. Another term that is widely used is "chemical sterilant," describing a high-level disinfectant that is effective against bacterial spores but might require extended contact time for such activity. This can only be effective as a sterilant under the specific conditions that are recommended by the manufacturer. Intermediate-level disinfection includes activity against enveloped viruses, most fungi and non-enveloped viruses, and bacteria, but not necessarily mycobacteria. Due to their unusual structure, mycobacteria are highly resistant to disinfection in comparison to other types of bacteria (see Chapter 5). Finally, low-level disinfection is also considered effective against enveloped viruses and most bacteria, but might only be practically active against some types of fungi and not more highly resistant forms such as non-enveloped viruses and mycobacteria.

These defined levels of microbial inactivation and the types of microorganisms that a disinfectant is effective against are (or should be) confirmed by standard test methods, such as those defined by the Association of Analytical Communities (AOAC), ASTM, the European Committee for Standardization (CEN), and the Organisation for Economic Co-operation and Development (OECD). In many countries such disinfectant claims are regulated by national agencies such as the Food and Drug Administration (FDA; for medical devices) and Environmental Protection Agency (EPA; for environmental surfaces) in the United States and the Therapeutic Goods Administration (TGA) in Australia; this is, however, not always the case. As different countries or regions can have different requirements, care should be taken to ensure that any disinfection or sterilization claims are substantiated and, if necessary, approved for use in your particular area. In addition to statements of effectiveness against specific microorganisms (e.g. "effective against HIV") or levels of disinfection, other commonly used terms with disinfectants include the following:

- The suffix -static, implying the ability of a product to inhibit the growth of a specific microorganism, for example bacteriostatic, sporistatic, or fungistatic.
- The suffix -cidal, implying the ability to kill a specific microorganism, for example bactericidal.
- Bactericidal, the ability to kill bacteria. This may be misleading. It is clearly not possible to test all types of bacteria and so surrogates are generally selected. In the United States, a bactericidal claim is based on testing against three types of bacteria: *Staphylococcus aureus*, *Pseudomonas aeruginosa*, and *Salmonella enterica*. This is also specifically referred to as a "germicidal" claim. It does not, however, include mycobacteria.
- Mycobactericidal, the ability to inactivate mycobacteria. In some regions this is different to a specific tuberculocidal claim, referring specifically to a test method to confirm activity against *Mycobacterium tuberculosis*.
- Sporicidal, activity against bacterial spores. As bacterial spores (or more correctly "endospores") are generally considered as some of the more resistant microorganisms, this will typically imply activity against other dormant forms in particular fungal spores. The test methods to verify sporicidal activity can range considerably from region to region.

- Virucidal, the ability to inactivate viruses. There are two major types of viruses based on their resistance to disinfection (see the section on viruses in Chapter 5): enveloped (being relatively sensitive) and non-enveloped (demonstrating higher resistance). Non-enveloped viruses can be further sub-classified into large and small forms based on their resistance profiles (see Chapter 5, Figure 5.2). Therefore, specific virucidal claims can vary, ranging from an individual virus tested (which may be enveloped but demonstrating low resistance) to a range of viruses (e.g. one test virus from each type/group).
- Fungicidal, the ability to kill fungi.
- Other, less used terms may include cysticidal (effective against specific types of protozoan cysts) and priocidal (referring to reducing the risk of prion contamination).

Disinfection can be considered as physical or chemical in nature, though both can be employed together. The main mechanisms of antimicrobial activity are summarized with examples in Table 9.2. The most common physical methods are various forms of heat, including the use of hot water (also known as pasteurization). Other physical methods can include radioactive or light sources (e.g. ultraviolet or UV light); these are considered only briefly here as they are rarely (if at all) used for the processing of reusable devices, but have become more widely used for environmental disinfection (e.g. in patient rooms). Chemicals (chemical disinfectants) are widely used for environmental surface (including many non-critical device surfaces) and device disinfection; they are also used as part of controlled processes for sterilization (see Chapter 11). Chemical disinfectants are designed for use under specific conditions, which may include the correct control of various physical factors (such as temperature; the combination of a chemical/thermal process can be referred to as "chemothermal" or thermo-chemical).

Disinfectants and disinfection products are provided or conducted in a variety of forms, such as:
- Boiling water baths.
- Washer-disinfectors, where disinfection can be achieved by chemical, thermal, or thermo-chemical methods.
- Disinfectant concentrates, which require dilution and/or suspension in water prior to use.
- Ready-to-use products, which require no dilution prior to use.
- Wipe or cloth or disinfectant-impregnated wipe/cloth.
- Two (or more) component or activated disinfectants, requiring two or more parts to be mixed together to prepare the disinfectant (some products will require a certain "activation" time to allow the disinfectant chemistry to be generated prior to use).
- Electrochemically generated systems, which generate the disinfectant from water/chemical mixtures.

In addition, as is typical with many high- to low-level disinfectants, they can be designed for single or multiple use, depending on the product design and labeling. These terms differentiate utilization of a single-use disinfectant for a particular application once and then discarding it, while multiple-use disinfectants are prepared (if applicable) and used for many applications, even over multiple days.

Basic principles of disinfection

Disinfection products and processes are designed to reduce the level of microbial contamination on surfaces (but also in the air or water). Device disinfection is used to prepare a device for direct patient use or staff handling, and also as an intermediate step in the processing cycle (e.g. prior to packaging and sterilization). This can range from the use of a low- or intermediate-level disinfectants to wipe down various types of

Table 9.2 Examples of disinfection and sterilization methods. These are given as examples only. Note that the formulation and use of a chemical disinfectant can have a dramatic effect on the activity of an antimicrobial chemical (biocide). Exposure time is also a critical variable and the manufacturer's written instructions (see product labels) must be followed.

Inactivation method	Examples
Sterilization	*Physical*: Steam (e.g. at 121°C for 15 minutes or 134°C for 3 minutes)
	Chemical: Ethylene oxide or hydrogen peroxide gas
High-level disinfection	*Physical*: Moist/wet heat (e.g. hot water at 90°C for 1 minute), ultraviolet (UV) light
	Chemical: Glutaraldehyde, peracetic acid, ortho-phthalaldehyde (OPA), sodium hypochlorite (chlorine), hydrogen peroxide
Intermediate-level disinfection	*Physical*: Moist/wet heat (e.g. hot water at 80°C for 1 minute), UV light
	Chemical: Phenolics, sodium hypochlorite (bleach) (chlorine), iodophor, alcohols
Low-level disinfection	*Chemical*: Quaternary ammonium compounds (QACs/QUATs), alcohols

equipment used medically with the patient such as blood pressure machines or monitors, to high-level disinfectants and high-temperature processes used to treat more critical devices. The choice of disinfectant will depend on two major considerations:

- Efficacy or how effective the product is. As described in the introduction to this chapter (Figure 9.2), this depends on the designation of the device as critical, semi-critical, or non-critical, and the ability of the disinfectant to inactivate various types of microorganisms. While low-level disinfectants have limited effectiveness to include enveloped viruses and most bacteria, high-level disinfectants or processes are expected to practically inactivate all forms of microorganisms with the exceptions of high numbers of bacterial spores (and unconventional agents such as prions).
- Safety, including primarily the safety of the patient and protection of the functionality of the device. An example of a patient safety consideration is the use of a chemical disinfectant, where residuals of the chemical or its by-products remain on or within the device; these can lead to toxic problems in patients. Similar safety risks will apply to members of staff who use the disinfectant or could be exposed to the device following disinfection. Device safety will also include compatibility, the ability of a disinfectant to be used on the device without damaging it. Compatibility (or indeed incompatibility) can be obvious following treatment or may only be observed over time. For this reason, it is highly recommended that any disinfectant being used on a device, particularly a semi-critical or critical device, is labeled as safe for use on that device. A typical example is the description of a device as "thermo-sensitive" or "thermo-resistant"; thermo-sensitive devices are designed with components/materials that cannot tolerate high temperatures (generally >60°C) that are required for thermal disinfection/sterilization. Such devices can only be processed in low-temperature disinfection or sterilization processes; flexible endoscopes are a common example, see Chapter 15). Thermo-resistant devices are less restrictive, in particular in their ability to withstand higher temperatures. Equally, many devices cannot tolerate certain types of chemicals or formulations due to negative effects on their construction materials; examples include the chemical compatibility of various types of adhesives (glues) that are used to bond materials together. Other safety considerations include any risks to those using the disinfectant, with close attention needing to be given to the safety data sheet (SDS) that should always be provided with the disinfectant) and any environmental concerns (which is an important issue in many parts of the world, restricting the use or disposal of certain disinfectants).

Efficacy and safety are the major considerations, but there are others:

- Product design and practical considerations. Formulation plays a major role in the efficacy of a chemical disinfectant (see Chapter 6 on mixtures, formulations, and solutions). Therefore, close attention should be paid to the product labeling (including any associated documentation provided by the manufacturer) to ensure that the product can be safely used for a given application. First, is the product designed for this particular application? Many disinfectants are to be used only on general, environmental surfaces and are not designed for device use. Second, how is the product to be used? Is it to be diluted, used directly, or activated prior to use? What is the required exposure time? The product might be effective against a particular organism but may take an impractically long time to be effective. The concentration of the active chemicals (or biocide) in the product is important to ensure efficacy and safety, but so are other variables such as recommended exposure times, concentrations, temperatures, and so on. Close attention should be given to the types of test methods that have been used to prove that the disinfectant is effective against various types of microorganisms; in some countries these claims are tightly controlled while in others they are not. Instructions on how the product is used are important; these should be provided by the manufacturer and closely followed by the user. Some products may only be designed for manual use, while others are for automated disinfection. In manual-type applications care should be taken to ensure that all surfaces of the devices (particularly internal surfaces) are fully exposed to the disinfectant for the required exposure time/conditions. Many disinfectants or device instructions may have the requirement that devices are rinsed with water after use of the disinfectant (and often multiple rinses) to remove harmful residuals. As with other chemistries, the choice of a disinfectant or process may also depend on its esthetic qualities (e.g. smell and low foaming are common concerns in manual disinfection).
- Regulatory approval. Is the product/process approved for use in a general country/region? Note: the fact that a product is available for sale does not mean that it meets the legal requirements of the country/area.
- Product efficacy variables. These include the concentration, temperature, mode of preparation/use, exposure time, and so on, which can all significantly influence disinfectant effectiveness. Low temperatures can decrease a product's efficacy, depending on its design; temperature control is essential in the case of thermal washer-disinfectors, for instance. Equally, low concentrations of chemical disinfectants can be ineffective but may also allow bacteria/fungi to grow within the formulation; this can be a particular concern in multiple-use disinfectants, where in many semi-critical applications chemical indicators (CIs) are available to check that the product is capable of disinfection (see Chapter 14).
- Water quality. Some chemical disinfectants can essentially lose their activity if the water quality is inadequate; this should

always be clearly stated in the instructions for use/labeling of a disinfectant. Thermo-chemical disinfection can also cause some concerns, for example the presence of high levels of chlorine when heated can cause significant damage (pitting/corrosion) to stainless steel surfaces and damage other types of materials. The impact of water quality is considered in further detail in Chapter 15.

- Staff training and competency. Disinfectants, physical and chemical, are designed to kill microorganisms and these effects can also have immediate or even long-term effects on staff after constant or accidental exposure. Essentially there is no such thing as a "safe" disinfectant and all disinfection products/processes should be treated with caution. Staff should be trained in using the disinfectant safely and effectively. This will include, where applicable, the preparation, handling, use (or reuse), rinsing, checking, and disposal of the product. Care should be taken to ensure that the correct personal protective equipment (PPE) and environment are provided to ensure staff safety; examples include ventilation, safety cabinets, accidental spill procedures, access to water, and so on. This is particularly important in manual disinfection. As highlighted previously, automated processes can provide greater assurance, but staff need to be trained on their use and equipment needs to be maintained and serviced according to manufacturer's guidelines.

It should be noted that all of these considerations not only apply to disinfection but are also important for cleaning or sterilization processes. It is clear that close attention should be paid to reading and understanding the instructions for use, labeling, and associated materials provided with a product and/or process used for disinfection.

Disinfectants can be classified in many ways, with the most common including:

- Type of antimicrobial agent, usually classified as physical or chemical. This classification is considered in further detail in the rest of this chapter.
- Sterilization or various levels of disinfection for critical, semi-critical, and non-critical devices; the use of a disinfectant/sterilant for these applications was considered in the introduction to this chapter. Note: the use of a disinfectant for these applications will depend on its associated labeling; if the product is not described for use for a particular medical application then it should not be used for that purpose. A common example is antiseptics (disinfectants designed for use on the skin/mucous membranes) being mistakenly used to disinfect devices used on patients because they are considered medical grade. If the product is not labeled for purpose it is not fit for purpose!
- Manual or automated disinfection. Examples of manual disinfection include the use of disinfectant-impregnated wipes and soaks, while automated disinfection is most commonly by means of a washer-disinfector.

Physical disinfection

Physical methods of disinfection include heat (thermal disinfection), radiation, and filtration. Heat can include dry (hot air) heating and moist/wet heat (essentially hot water). Wet heat methods are the most commonly used and reliable methods of disinfection, for instance in thermal washer-disinfectors or boiling water baths. All other physical methods including dry heat, radiation methods, and filtration are less often used for device disinfection but may be used as part of another process; these are discussed later in this section.

Moist/wet heat disinfection

Hot water is a very effective and simple disinfection method. Most microorganisms, with the exclusion of heat-resistant bacterial spores, are inactivated at temperatures in excess of 65°C; however, the intrinsic resistance of various types of microorganisms can vary depending on the temperature. Most bacteria and fungi, in their vegetative form, are unable to grow at temperatures greater than 45°C (113°F) and are inactivated at ~60–65°C (140–149°F). This is essentially the basis of pasteurization methods that are widely used to treat liquid foods, including milk (e.g. 65°C for 30 minutes). Most viruses are inactivated at this range but some have been shown to be more resistant, for example requiring 70–80°C (158–176°F) to be inactivated. These direct high-temperature effects cause the coagulation and loss of structure/function of the various parts that make up a microorganism (see Chapter 5).

It is widely accepted that heat disinfection is based on a time–temperature relationship: essentially as the temperature increases, less time is required for disinfection. Therefore, examples of thermal disinfection conditions used for the processing of surgical devices will include:

- 80°C (176°F) for 10 minutes.
- 90°C (194°F) for 1 minute.
- 100°C (212°F) for 0.1 minute.

Such time–temperature relationships are used to define the disinfection conditions for immersion disinfection and washer-disinfectors. An example is the A_0 concept described in the ISO 15883 series of standards for washer-disinfectors. A_0 is defined as the equivalent time (in seconds) at a temperature of 80°C (176°F) for disinfection; this definition is with reference to microorganisms with a z-value of 10°C (the z-value is a concept further discussed in steam sterilization, which is also based on time–temperature relationships; see Chapter 11 on steam (moist heat) sterilization). It is mathematically given as:

$$A_0 = \sum 10^{[(T-80)/z]} \times \Delta t$$

A minimum temperature of 65°C (149°F) is required. From this concept, recommended levels of disinfection are given in various parts of ISO 15883 and times/temperatures can then be applied in order to provide these levels (Table 9.3). Essentially, as the exposure temperature increases, the time for disinfection decreases. It should be noted that temperatures over 65°C within such disinfection processes to reach the defined minimum temperature and also cooling down below 65°C after the defined exposure time will also contribute to the overall disinfection efficacy (a summary of this is shown in graph form in Figure 9.3).

In defining such a disinfection process, it is important to consider that the water temperature alone is not sufficient to confirm thermal disinfection; the temperature distribution in the exposure chamber and particularly the load to be disinfected need to be within the required temperature ranges during disinfection.

Thermal disinfection of devices is usually conducted by a water immersion or spray method (Figure 9.4). Water immersion, where devices are immersed in hot water for a given period of time, used to be a common method but is less used today. It is still effective, but care should be taken to ensure that the water temperature and exposure time are controlled and that air bubbles do not collect at the device surface. The safe handling of devices during or following disinfection is important, to ensure that staff are not burned during the process of placing devices in the bath and then removing them, and also that devices are not recontaminated following

Table 9.3 Examples of A_0 values and their practical application in disinfection processes.

Device types	Disinfection level	A_0[1]	Examples
Non-critical, e.g. bed-pans, wash bowls, carts	Low or intermediate	60	80°C (176°F) × 1 minute 90°C (194°F) × 6 seconds
Semi-critical or critical, e.g. surgical instruments	High	600	80°C (176°F) × 10 minutes 90°C (194°F) × 1 minute 100°C (212°F) × 6 seconds

[1] The minimum recommended A_0 is accordance with ISO 15883.

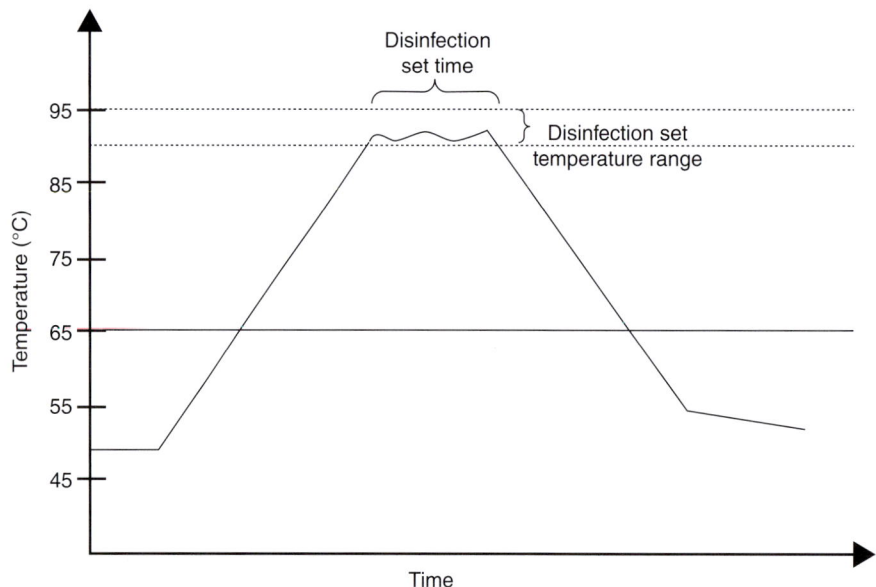

Figure 9.3 An example of a thermal disinfection process in a washer-disinfector. Thermal disinfection is based on a time–temperature relationship; the graph shows this relationship with time on the X (horizontal) axis and temperature on the Y (vertical) axis. The temperature over time is plotted during the disinfection cycle. In this example, a minimum disinfection time and temperature are set (the temperature at 90°C, but in a range of 90–95°C; dotted lines). Under these conditions, the minimal A_0 is based on the time at the set temperature of 90°C but the actual A_0 can be determined based on the amount of time at each temperature above 65°C (solid line across the graph).

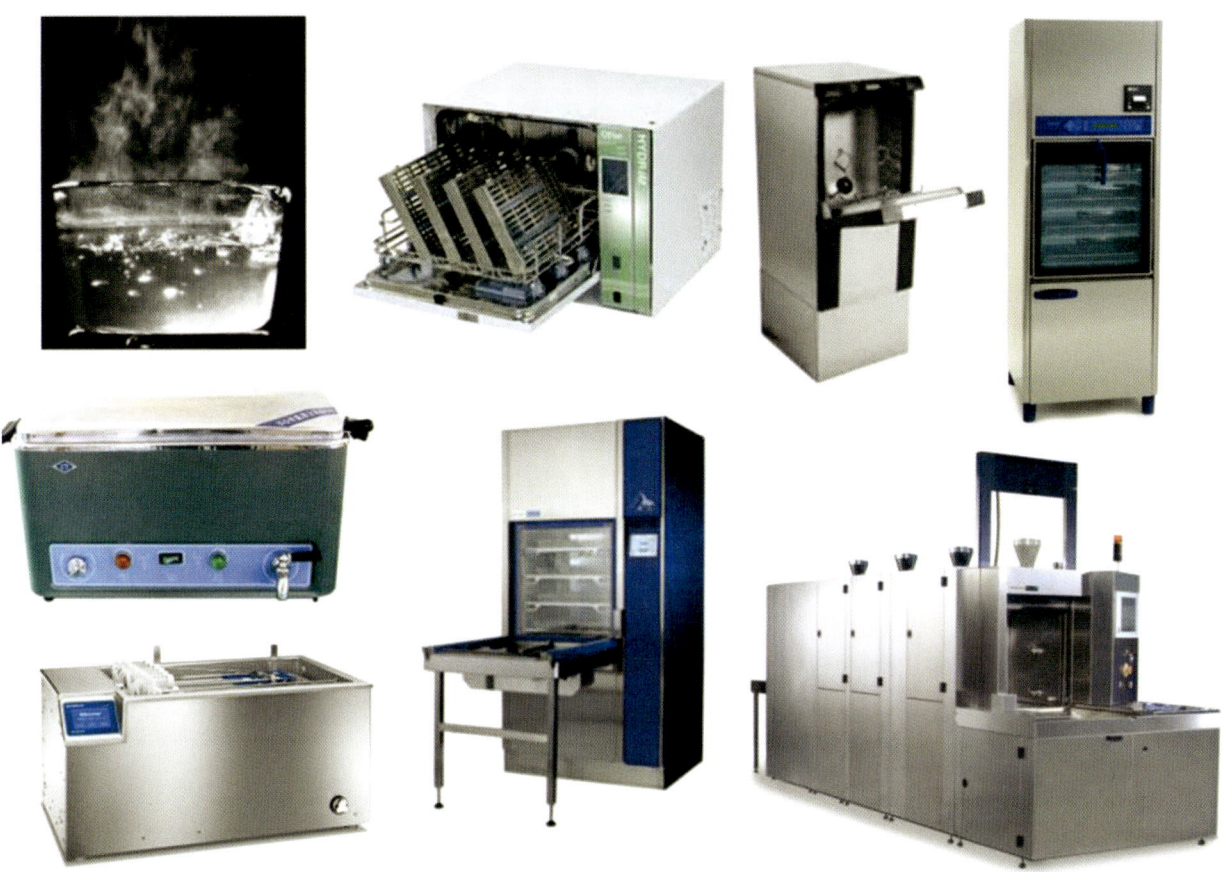

Figure 9.4 Examples of thermal disinfection methods. On the far left are various types of immersion methods, including a simple pan of boiling water (top) and specially designed immersion disinfectors. On the right are various types of washer-disinfectors using thermal disinfection, including bench-top, single-chamber, and multi-chamber washer-disinfector. The design of various types of washer-disinfectors is discussed in further detail in Chapter 8.

the process (particularly if being prepared directly for patient use). Spray-type methods are used in many types of washer-disinfectors for thermal disinfection (Figure 9.4). Washer-disinfectors are defined as machines intended to clean and disinfect devices and other articles. They are widely used in medical, dental, pharmaceutical, and veterinary practice. They have already been introduced and discussed in detail in Chapter 8 for automated cleaning. They are provided in a variety of sizes and designs, ranging from smaller bench-top or under-counter disinfectors to larger free-standing machines (Figure 9.4). With the emphasis on thermal disinfection in washer-disinfectors, water is generally introduced into the load chamber, circulated by a pump system including a spray system, and heated to the programmed disinfection temperature. The load is then held at a given range of temperatures (e.g. between 0 and +5°C of a set temperature, which at 90°C is 90–95°C) for the required disinfection time and then drained. This is commonly achieved by spraying the load using the same mechanism as during the cleaning cycle (see Chapter 8). The load may then be cooled (with or without drying) prior to removing it from the chamber (to reduce any risks of burns). Different types of chemicals can be applied during the disinfection phase to include lubricants and drying/rinsing aids (see Chapter 6 on the classification of cleaning chemistries). Lubricants are applied mechanically as an alternative to manual application to ensure that devices, in particular hinged devices, are in good working order. Rinse aids assist in water droplet dispersion, making them easier to remove during drying. In both cases, these chemicals should be proven to be non-toxic to patients, either on their own or if to be subsequently sterilized.

In addition to direct heating of volumes of water for thermal disinfection (in immersion or spray-type systems), steam-exposure chambers may also be used, where steam is provided or generated within a chamber under atmospheric pressure and allowed to contact the device load for the desired temperature/time. Although the mechanism of heating is different, these types of disinfectors follow the same principles of time/temperature as immersion/spray-based disinfectors; in all cases, the distribution of the correct temperature within the load is important to ensure the correct disinfection process.

Dry heat

Dry heat disinfection follows the same principle as wet/moist heat but in the absence of moisture/water. Many types of bacteria, enveloped viruses, and vegetative fungi are inactivated by drying alone and this can be enhanced at higher temperatures; however, it is important to note that the mechanisms of action and efficacy of dry heat are different to those of wet/moist heat. For sporicidal activity in particular, much higher temperatures and exposure times are required for dry heat to be effective than for moist heat, and for these reasons dry heat methods have not been as widely used for disinfection historically. Dry heat disinfection/sterilization can be achieved in specific machines, also referred to as ovens or convection ovens (Figure 9.5). Convection refers to the method of heat transfer through a liquid (water) or gas (air), in this case through hot air; conduction is another term that refers to a method of heat transfer from one surface or material to another. Dry heat disinfection is effective by the transfer of heat by conduction and convection. Note that if a device is placed wet into a dry heat disinfection process, the water will be heated and the presence of this moisture actually increases the effectiveness of the process by moist heat mechanisms.

Dry heat may be considered a reasonable method for low- or intermediate-level disinfection, even at temperatures of 70–80°C (158–176°F) over time to ensure that treated surfaces are dried; higher temperatures may be used to achieve higher levels of disinfection, such as up to 140°C (284°F) for one hour. Even higher temperatures and extended exposure times (over many hours) are used for some sterilization methods to accommodate efficacy against bacterial spores and validation requirements (see Chapter 11). Types of devices/materials that are disinfected with dry heat have included oils/powders, needles, glass syringes, and some clothing; many devices are restricted from dry heat disinfection due to risks of damage at higher temperatures.

Radiation

Radiation and various forms of light (high-energy sources such as X-rays and γ radiation) can have disinfection and sterilization properties; they are, however, not widely used for reusable device processing and are not covered in detail here. The various different forms of radiation were identified in Chapter 6 (in the section on light, radiation, and the electromagnetic spectrum). High-energy radiation sources and generators are more widely used by device and materials manufacturers for the disinfection and sterilization of single-use materials/devices within healthcare facilities such as bandages and types of single-use devices. There are three forms that are

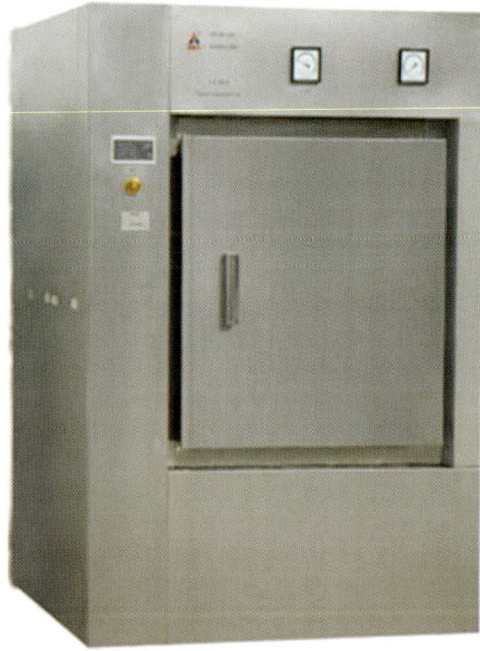
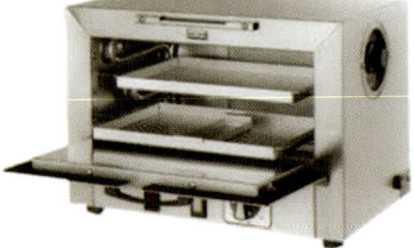
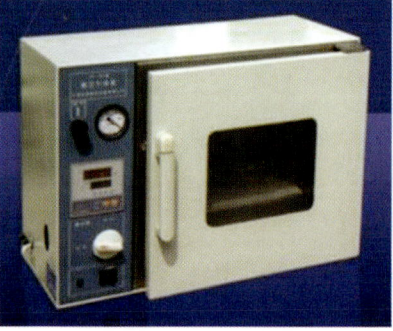

Figure 9.5 Dry heat disinfection ovens.

utilized in healthcare facilities, either on their own right or as part of a particular system. These are:

- UV light. Light is much greater than what we see, which is known as "visible" or white light. In technical terms, light refers to the electromagnetic spectrum (see Chapter 6, Figure 6.9). UV light refers to wavelengths of light that have a higher energy level just above visible light (specifically in the 10–400 nm wavelength range). UV light is generated from specifically designed types of lamps; the most effective range of UV against microorganisms is in the 200–280 nm wavelength range. UV light is primarily used for exposure to general environmental surfaces (including various types of equipment/devices that may be present in a given area), the air, and liquids (e.g. in water treatment). UV light is not very penetrating and therefore will only be effective on those surfaces or liquids that directly make contact with the light. It is used for both preservation and disinfection, but rarely for direct disinfection of devices. The specific efficacy of different types of UV disinfection systems can range considerably, therefore close attention should be paid to the claims and support evidence provided by suppliers.

- Infra-red (IR) light. Both IR light and microwaves are on the opposite end of the visible light wavelength range to UV light, being lower in energy (longer in wavelength). IR light is in the 0.7–1000 μm wavelength range; at this range it is considered to have low to no direct antimicrobial properties, but is used as a method of applying dry heat (see the section on dry heat).
- Microwaves. Microwaves are commonly used for heating purposes (for foods/liquids); they have an even lower energy level than IR and, similarly, have little to no direct antimicrobial activity. Microwaves are used as a heating mechanism for water or materials, thereby acting as an indirect moist heat disinfection method (see the later section on physical disinfection).

Filtration

Filtration is commonly used as a physical mechanism of disinfection (and even sterilization), especially with air, gases, and liquids (including water). It is distinct from the other methods of disinfection discussed in this chapter in that it is primarily by physical removal of microorganisms rather than their inactivation. The theory of filtration is presented in Figure 9.6.

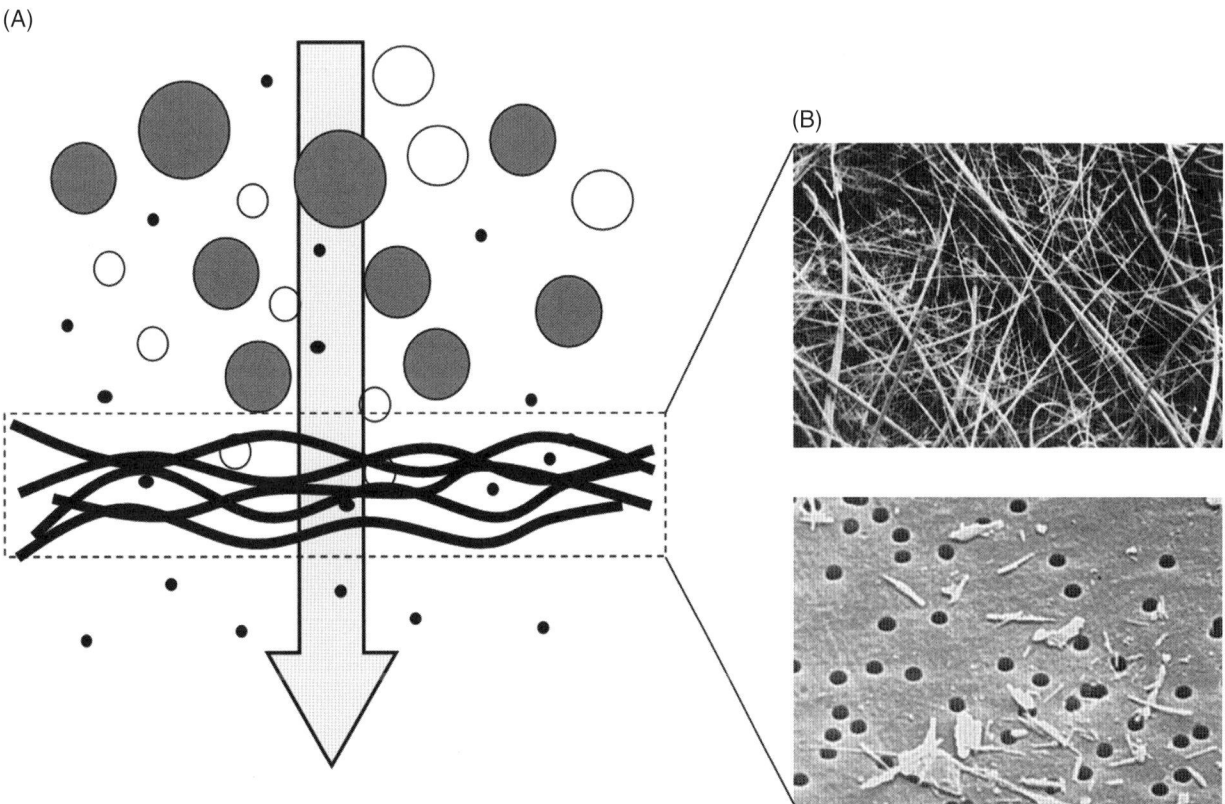

Figure 9.6 Mechanisms of physical removal of microorganisms by filtration. (A) An example of a liquid/gas containing particles at various sizes being passed through a filter (center); only the smallest particles will pass through the filter (this is often called the "filtrate") while the others are retained on the dirty side of the filter. (B) Examples of the microscopic structure of the two types of filters.

Filters are used to remove various microorganisms by size. The filter itself (also known as a membrane) is essentially a mesh of fibrous material, or contains holes of specific sizes as defined by the manufacturer. If the microorganism, chemical, or any other substance is too large it will be trapped on one side of the filter, while those that are smaller can pass through.

Filters can be designed out of a variety of types of materials and in a variety of forms, depending on their application. Typical examples include high-efficiency particulate air (HEPA) filters used for filtering air in controlled-environment (e.g. packaging) rooms and water filters (Figure 9.7). Some types of filters are used to remove different types of chemicals from water, liquids, or gases (including air), with examples being carbon filters or reverse osmosis (RO) membranes used in water treatment (see Chapter 15).

Microbiological filters are generally classified based on their size exclusion characteristics (or the size of particles or microorganisms whose passage they can prevent). Examples of various types of filters and their size exclusion capabilities are shown in Figure 9.8.

In addition to being designed for size exclusion, some filters are made to specifically remove various contaminants by attachment to the filter material; examples include carbon filters and HEPA filters. Carbon (also known as charcoal or granular activated carbon) filters are composed of activated (positively charged) carbon and are used for water treatment; they can, depending on their design, remove particles down to ~1 µm (therefore including some bacteria), but actively bind chlorine that can be present in the water. They are often used for pre-treatment of water prior to further purification (e.g. by RO).

HEPA filters are used to filter air, but are designed to have a variety of retentive abilities (often designated by letters/numbers such as E10, H13, and U17). These filters can have the capacity to retain particles down to a 0.3–1 µm range (thereby removing most bacteria), but this will depend on their specific design. They can also cause the removal of smaller

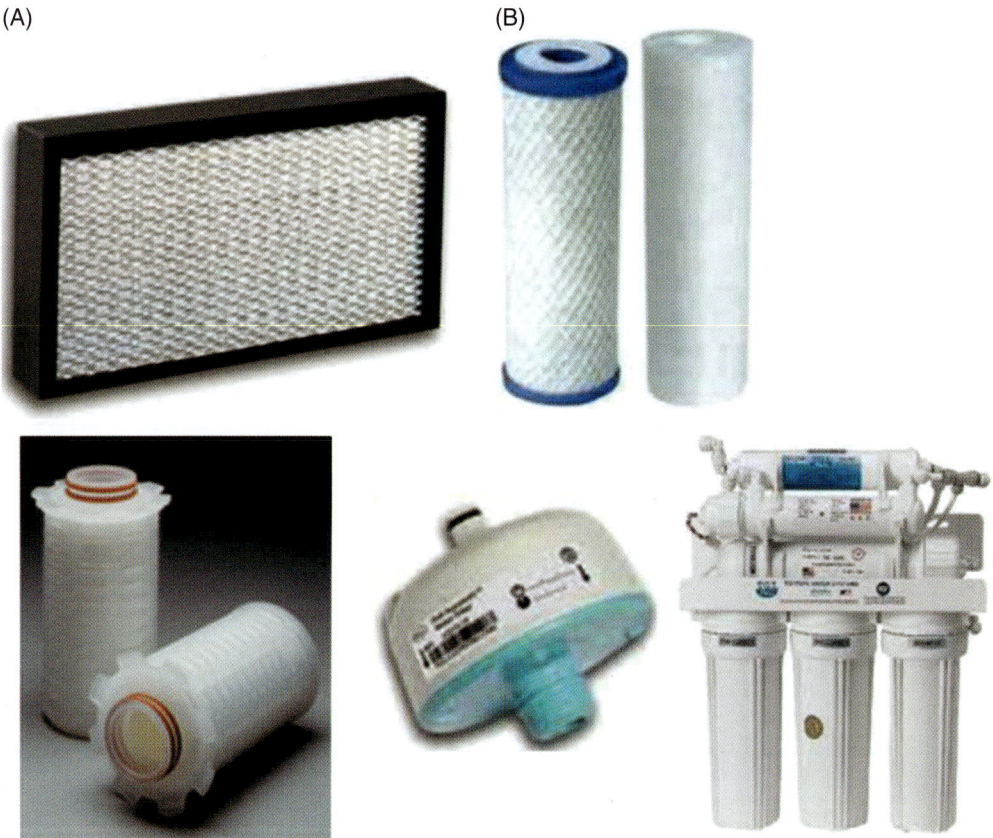

Figure 9.7 Examples of types of filters. (A) Air filters, with a high-efficiency particulate air (HEPA) filter (top) and sterile air filters (bottom). (B) Water filters of various types (top), a tap filter (lower left) and an under-counter reverse osmosis filter system (lower right).

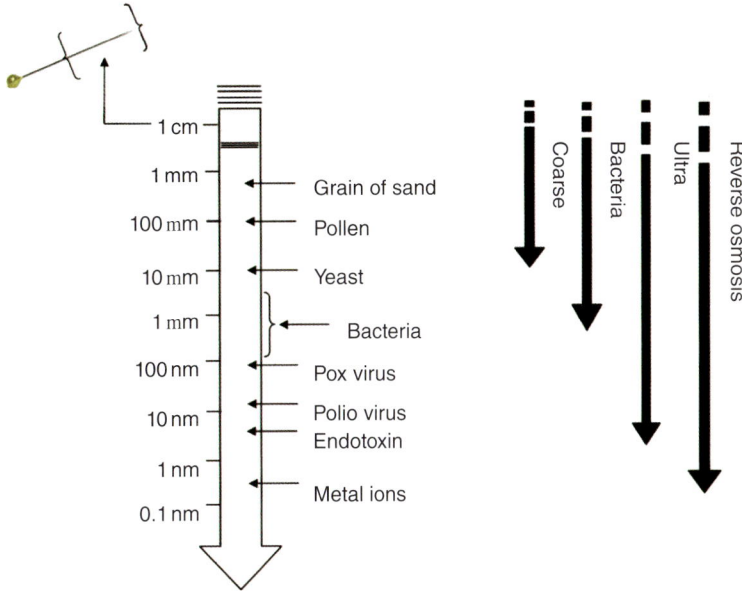

Figure 9.8 The various sizes of microorganisms, particles, and chemicals and types of filtration methods. The head of a pin is shown for perspective (note: there are 10 mm in 1 cm). Filters can therefore be referred to as coarse (or gross), bacterial-retentive, ultrafilters, etc. The specific retentive abilities of an individual filter will depend on its size and can vary considerably, even within these estimated ranges.

materials due to attachment to the filter. HEPA filters are used for treating air in a defined clean area (such as in surgical theaters and in some "clean" packaging areas of decontamination facilities), as well as treating air that is used in various washer-disinfectors (for drying) or sterilizers (for releasing vacuums during sterilization cycles).

RO filters, known as semi-permeable membrane, are specifically designed for generating purified water in that they can remove most microorganisms and chemicals. The RO process is not just the use of the membranes but includes a designed pressurized system and constant water flow/movement; the water moves along the surface of the membrane and contaminants are continually swept away while the pure water passes across the membrane.

It is important to note that while the various types of filters can theoretically exclude or remove various sizes of materials, the successful use of filtration is dependent on how the filters are used. An example is that mechanical or chemical damage to the filter may not be detected and can compromise it, allowing contaminants to pass through. If filter-based systems are not designed and maintained correctly, they can easily become compromised. There are test systems available to ensure the correct installation and maintenance of filters; these include filter integrity (air or water) and leak tests. Filters can also become blocked, thereby not allowing air/water to pass through; in the case of water, this is typically detected by reduced flow over time. Another example is that while most bacteria are retained by a 0.2 μm micro-filter, some bacteria can "grow through" the filter over time and contaminate the clean side of it. Overall, as with any disinfectant, filters should be used and maintained according to manufacturer's instructions to ensure their correct use.

Chemical disinfection

There are many types of chemicals and chemical processes used for disinfection (Figure 9.9). These were introduced briefly in Chapter 6 (in the section on disinfectants, including preservatives) and are discussed in further detail here. In many publications and guidelines, the different types of biocides used for disinfection are classified as capable of killing certain types of microorganisms and therefore capable of low-, intermediate-, or high-level disinfection (Figure 9.2 and Table 9.2). For example, non-critical devices/surfaces may be treated with a wide range of disinfectants, including those based on surfactants, oxidizers, alcohols, phenols, and aldehydes. A much more limited selection of biocides are used for semi-critical/critical applications, such as the peroxygens and aldehydes. This approach can be useful (as shown in Table 9.1) but is often misleading. The ability of a disinfectant or chemical disinfection process to be effective can vary significantly depending on how the biocide is formulated and how it is used (see Chapter 6 on mixtures, formulations, and solutions). Here we discuss some of the major types of biocides and give some general guidance on their advantages and disadvantages. It should, however, be remembered that specific efficacy claims, methods of preparation/use, and any safety considerations

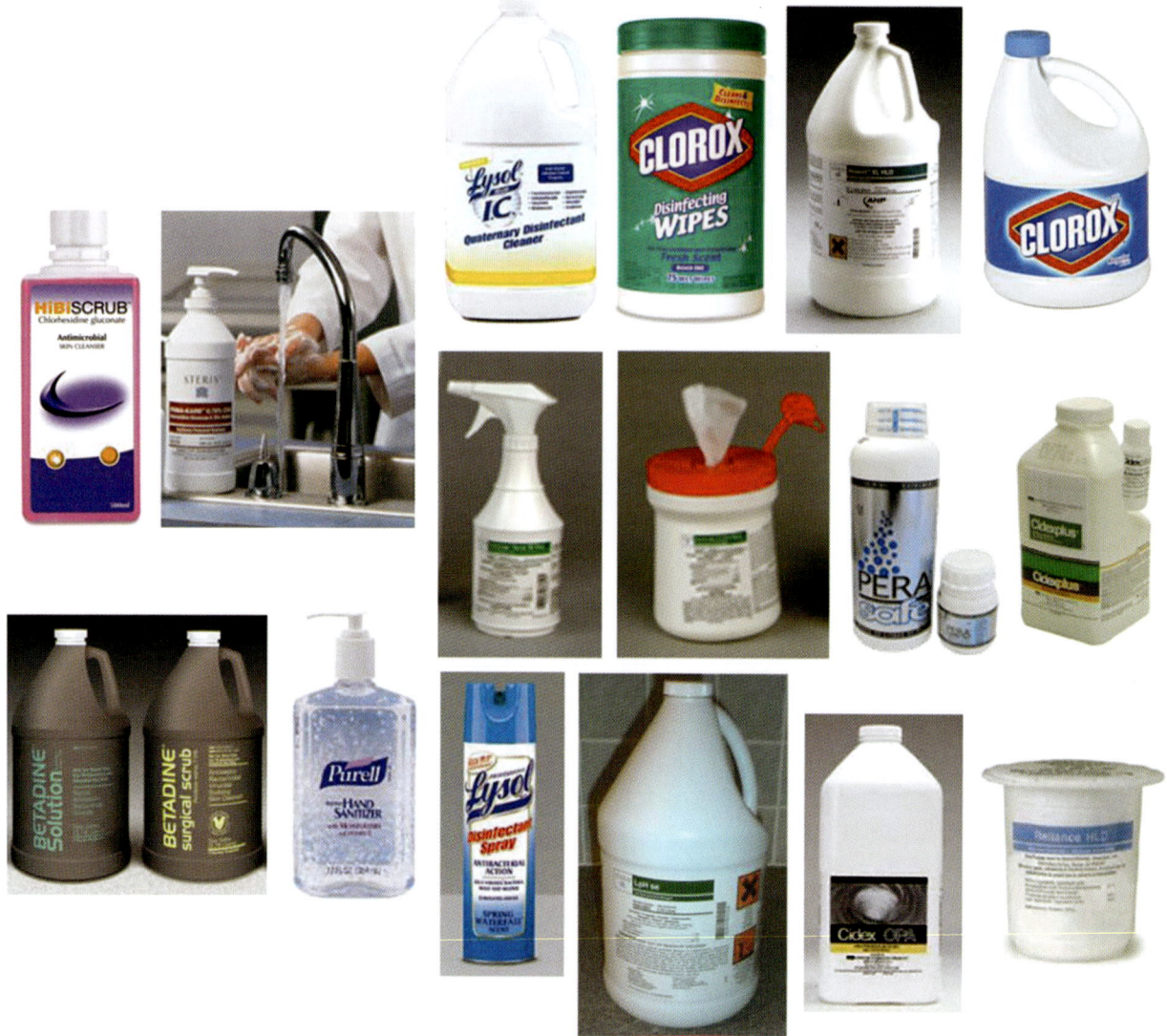

Figure 9.9 Various types of disinfectants, from antiseptics (used on the skin; left) to low-, intermediate-, and high-level disinfectants (from left to right). They include concentrates, ready-to-use, and wipe-type products, as well as one- and two-component chemistries.

should be provided by the disinfectant manufacturer and should always be closely reviewed, included associated instructions and labeling.

Alcohols

There are three types of alcohol used as disinfectants: ethanol ("alcohol" or the major component in methylated spirits), isopropanol (also known as "rubbing" or isopropyl alcohol), and n-propanol. Alcohol solutions are used directly at specified dilutions in water or as formulated products, typically within the optimal 60–80% range (note that although higher concentrations are available they are often *less* effective). Alcohols are widely used as antiseptics, known as hand rubs or hand disinfectants; they have been particularly highlighted for routine use in hospitals and healthcare facilities due to their ease of use (convenience), good antimicrobial activity on the skin, and the fact that they do not require rinsing in water. The formulation of the alcohol can be important to maximize its efficacy, particularly on the skin, but also to ensure that it does not irritate the skin. An example is the use of lower concentrations of alcohol (in the 60–65% range) with other chemical ingredients that help to prevent drying effects on the skin; these extend the contact time of the alcohol on the skin and can leave the skin feeling smooth after use. Some alcohol-based disinfectants can contain other biocides, in particular chlorhexidine (see the section on other biocides), which remain on the skin following use to continue to provide antimicrobial activity (this is known as residual activity or persistence). Alcohols are not generally used as device disinfectants, but can be used to wipe down various environmental surfaces or for device cables during decontamination. They have the benefit of evaporating (drying) very quickly and are therefore often used to aid in the drying of devices, in particular lumened devices such as flexible endoscopes. Remember that alcohol preparations usually contain water (e.g. 70% alcohol, 30% water) and, while alcohol can be used to remove residual water from device lumens, water and alcohol can still remain and require the consistent passage of air through the device lumens to ensure drying. This can often take a significantly long time.

Alcohols are generally considered as intermediate- to high-level disinfectants. They have rapid bactericidal activity (including against mycobacteria), are somewhat slower but effective against fungi and viruses (with the exception of most non-enveloped viruses), and have little to no activity against bacterial spores. This is a good example of how the resistance profile of microorganisms can sometimes vary depending on the biocide type and use (Figure 9.1).

Alcohols have the advantages of being easy and rapid to use as disinfectants, with little odor, few residues (depending on the product/preparation), and low toxicity. Disadvantages include no sporicidal activity (and limited activity against some non-enveloped viruses), their flammability risk (at high concentrations), and the fact that they can damage/irritate surfaces, including skin, by drying.

Aldehydes

The main types of aldehydes used as disinfectants are glutaraldehyde, orthophthalaldehyde (OPA), and formaldehyde.

Glutaraldehyde and OPA are widely used as high-level disinfectants for temperature-sensitive devices, in particular flexible endoscopes and other semi-critical devices that may not tolerate sterilization processes. They are available as single- or multi-use types of disinfectants. They can also be used for low/intermediate-level disinfection for non-critical types of devices, and rarely in the case of some glutaraldehyde-containing products for environmental surfaces in some jurisdictions.

Glutaraldehyde has been traditionally used as a high-level disinfectant for over 60 years, but its use has been decreasing over recent years due to safety and efficacy concerns. It is typically used for disinfection in the 1.5–3% range and is supplied as one- or two-component chemistries. The one-component (usually stabilized acidic formulated) chemistries do not require any pre-activation and can be used immediately (either directly or by dilution in water); two-component formulations require

activation (mixing and contact time) before they are used for disinfection. They are generally provided in two parts: an acidic solution containing the aldehyde to which a smaller activator is added to make the solution neutral or alkaline for use. Once prepared the product is ready for use, within the defined shelf-life of the activated solution (e.g. 14 days or as defined by the manufacturer). Remember, in these cases the product is not effective as a disinfectant unless it is activated correctly. As with any activated and/or multiple-use formulation, care should be taken to follow the manufacturer's instructions and in particular regarding any means provided to ensure the disinfectant can be safely used; an example is the use of a CI provided by the manufacturer that is specifically developed for use with the disinfectant to show that it is correctly activated/fit for use (Figure 9.10). Glutaraldehyde-containing formulations may also include high concentrations of other antimicrobials that work together with the aldehyde to provide the disinfection efficacy; examples include various types of surfactants, acids, alcohols, and phenols (Table 9.4).

OPA formulations are normally provided as concentrates or ready-for-use solutions (not requiring activation), and are typically used at the ~0.4–0.6% range for disinfection at room temperature (18–25°C). With both OPA and glutaraldehyde, the efficacy of disinfection increases at higher temperatures (e.g. within a heated bath or washer-disinfector); in these conditions low concentrations may be used (by dilution in water) in accordance with any label claims (Table 9.4).

As high-level disinfectants, the biocidal properties of glutaraldehyde and OPA have been well described, being effective against most bacteria (including mycobacteria), viruses, and fungi. Glutaraldehyde is also effective, in particular over

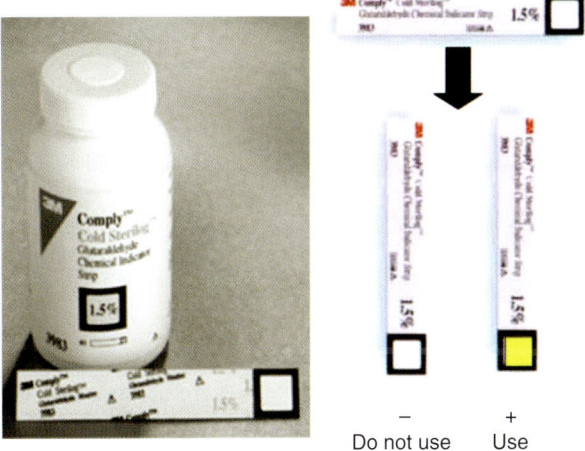

Figure 9.10 A glutaraldehyde-based disinfectant chemical indicator, used to confirm that the disinfectant is activated/safe to use. In this case, a white to yellow color change indicates that active glutaraldehyde is present.

Table 9.4 Examples of label claims on glutaraldehyde and ortho-phthalaldehyde (OPA)-based high-level disinfectants. Note: due to country- or region-specific regulatory requirements, the recommended disinfection time may vary on the same product. These are typical claims on US Food and Drug Administration registered products.

High-level disinfectant	Recommended exposure conditions
2.5% glutaraldehyde with surfactants	35°C for 5 minutes; 28-day reuse One component
3.4% glutaraldehyde with 26% isopropanol	20°C for 10 minutes; 14-day reuse Two component (activated)
1.12% glutaraldehyde with 1.93% phenol	25°C for 20 minutes; 14-day reuse Two component (activated)
2.5% glutaraldehyde with surfactants	25°C for 90 minutes; 28-day reuse Two component (activated)
2.4% glutaraldehyde	25°C for 45 minutes; 14-day reuse Two component (activated)
0.55% OPA	20°C for 12 minutes; 14-day reuse 25°C for 5 minutes; 14-day reuse One component

extended exposure times (e.g. as a chemical sterilant in the United States), against bacterial spores; OPA is considerably less effective against spores, although this activity may be enhanced at increased temperatures. Both aldehydes are considered effective against protozoal vegetative forms, but not always the dormant (encysted) forms, in particular *Cryptosporidium* oocysts and *Acanthamoeba* cysts. Some types of mycobacteria, other bacteria, and fungi have demonstrated the ability to develop high-level resistance to aldehydes (in particular with glutaraldehyde).

Both glutaraldehyde and OPA are well recognized as high-level disinfectants for flexible endoscope and other device (e.g. dialysis machine) disinfection. Formulations generally show good material compatibility and are often provided at lower costs. OPA is considered less irritating than glutaraldehyde, due to its lower vapor pressure (essentially it evaporates into the air less), but can cause staining of materials in the presence of protein (often indicating poor cleaning processes prior to disinfection). Aldehydes are cross-linking agents, therefore (as is the case for all disinfectants) devices should be well cleaned prior to aldehyde disinfection, as any remaining materials can become fixed onto device surfaces and can lead to complications over time.

Care should be taken to follow the manufacturer's instructions regarding activation (for two-component disinfectants), handling, use (in particular reuse to ensure the disinfectant remains active), and disposal of aldehyde-based disinfectants. An example of bad practice often observed in the use of aldehyde disinfectants is referred to as "topping up." This is where the reusable disinfectant is used for a certain time and then a smaller amount of a freshly prepared solution is added to the disinfectant so that it can be used for longer. Such practices are not safe and are unlikely to be recommended by the disinfectant manufacturer (if they are this should be verified in writing).

Glutaraldehyde and OPA can be irritating to the skin, mucous membranes, and respiratory tract; in addition to short-term effects, long-term exposure to either biocide can have other consequences. Glutaraldehyde has been reported to lead to dermatitis and asthma, with some debate regarding its being classified as a carcinogen (an agent that can cause cancer). OPA is also known to be a potent sensitizer, but overall is less studied than glutaraldehyde. In both cases, risks can be reduced with the proper design of the facility using the biocides for disinfection; this particularly includes the use of closed baths (preferably enclosed washer-disinfectors) and correct ventilation (e.g. 10–15 air changes/hour in the room or the use of a chemical fume hood). Some facilities recommend the use of respirators for all staff handling or using aldehyde-containing baths. The use of adequate PPE is important, to include safety glasses, face shields, and nitrile/rubber gloves when handling solutions. In certain countries, staff's levels of glutaraldehyde exposure are recommended to be closely monitored, with a typical "safe" level being considered to be at or below 0.05 ppm; at the time of writing no such level has been set for OPA. Glutaraldehyde monitors including personal or area monitors and periodic or constant sensors are available for such purposes. High levels of glutaraldehyde and OPA remaining on device surfaces following disinfection are also a concern, in particular after reports of colitis (irritation of the colon) and complications following eye surgery. Care should be taken to ensure that any high-level disinfected devices are correctly rinsed, according to manufacturer's instructions, prior to patient use; this may include up to 4–6 individual fresh water rinses, ensuring that all surfaces (internal and external) are correctly immersed in water for each rinse. Finally, specific instructions are usually provided on the safe disposal of aldehyde disinfectants due to environmental concerns; in certain regions/countries there is a requirement for the neutralization of glutaraldehyde-based disinfectants (e.g. by mixing with other chemistries such as glycine or sodium bisulfite) prior to disposal down a public drain. Such instructions will be provided by the manufacturer or by local agencies.

Formaldehyde is considered separately, as today it is not widely used for disinfection in healthcare facilities. It is, however, more widely used for gas sterilization applications and this is considered further in Chapter 11 (in the section on formaldehyde gas). It includes humidified formaldehyde gas and chemical vapor (formaldehyde with alcohol) sterilizers used in certain parts of the world. Formaldehyde is particularly used in pathology laboratories as a disinfectant/preservative for tissue; it is primarily used as "formalin," a 37% solution of formaldehyde in water/methanol. Older liquid disinfection applications used dilutions at 4–8% in water and/or alcohol, but these are no longer recommended due to material compatibility and toxicity concerns. Such formulations were considered to provide intermediate- to high-level disinfection but at recommended long contact times (e.g. 4% formaldehyde at 24 hours); although liquid formaldehyde is effective against most bacteria, viruses, and fungi, efficacy concerns were observed with some types of bacteria (with resistance mechanisms), non-enveloped viruses, and bacterial spores requiring higher concentrations and/or extended contact times. Of particular concern are the safety aspects of using formaldehyde, as it is associated with irritating fumes; it is a known carcinogen, but also with known short- and long-term toxic effects (such as dermatitis and asthma-like complications). The recommended safety level is in the range of 0.75 ppm.

In addition to liquid use, gas-based formaldehyde was traditionally used for laboratory and even hospital area disinfection (also known as fumigation). In these processes, the gas is produced by heating paraformaldehyde (a dry form of formaldehyde) or formalin solutions in the presence of high humidity (>80%) and holding this in a room/area for many hours (e.g. 7 hours); the room is then aerated (typically over 12–24 hours) to remove the gas. Overall, long cycle times and safety concerns have limited the use of liquid or gas formaldehyde for healthcare disinfection applications.

Halogens

"Halogens" describe a group of similar chemicals (see Chapter 6), some of which are widely used as disinfectants, particularly chlorine and iodine. Both have been used as disinfectants for many years and in a variety of applications.

Iodine (specifically in water, the biocidal molecules I_2 and HOI) is used for both antiseptic and general surface disinfectant (low, intermediate, or high) applications; it is not generally recommended for reusable medical device reprocessing. Iodine is traditionally provided in two forms: tinctures (for use on skin/wounds, e.g. iodine dissolved in ethanol) or iodophors (iodine-releasing agents, e.g. povidine–iodine or PVPI). A common example is the Betadine® range of iodophor-containing hand washes and surgical scrubs (see Chapter 6 on antiseptics). Iodine, depending on the biocidal concentration and contact time, can provide high-level disinfection including bactericidal, fungicidal, virucidal, and even sporicidal activity. Antiseptic products are generally used at lower biocidal concentrations to minimize damage to the skin and at higher, sporicidal concentrations for general surface disinfection. Note: these products should not be used for device disinfection unless labeled for such use. At higher concentrations iodine can be staining (browning), irritating, and damaging to some surfaces, but the alternative use of iodophors has reduced these negative effects.

It is hard not to come across the use of chlorine on a daily basis, as it is one of the most widely used chemicals for disinfection. Chlorine is widely used as a general surface, water, and in some cases device/equipment disinfectant. When chlorine is dissolved in water, the main active molecules are Cl_2, HOCl, and OCl^-; they are provided by directly dissolving chlorine or chlorine-containing chemicals, with common examples being sodium hypochlorite (NaOCl; typical household "bleach" solutions contain 5% NaOCl in water but this can vary depending on the product), calcium hypochlorite (solids or tablets), and chloramines (e.g. monochloramine or T-chloramine). Chlorine should not be confused with chlorine dioxide (ClO_2), which is a peroxygen-based chemistry and is considered separately for its associated safety and efficacy in the section on peroxygens. Similar to iodine, the antimicrobial activity of chlorine is dependent on its available active concentration over time; it is widely studied and tested as being effective against all microorganisms, with higher concentrations or contact times being required for dormant forms (spores and cysts); high concentrations/exposure times (e.g. 2.5% sodium hypochlorite for one hour) have also been particularly shown to be effective in degrading prions (see Chapter 15). Note that many chlorine-containing products do not have associated disinfectant claims, such as household bleach, while others are registered disinfectants with specific recommended dilutions/preparation methods and claims; despite this, chlorine solutions such as those based on household bleach are widely used for environmental disinfection applications. For example, many guidelines recommend the use of a 10% household bleach solution, which can be misleading. Inspection of household bleach products will show that they range in concentration; typical concentrations are in the 5–6% range of sodium hypochlorite and other ingredients may also be present (e.g. surfactants). The 5–6% sodium hypochlorite is approximately equal to 50,000–60,000 ppm of available chlorine (depending on the product formulation and its age/storage conditions). As a guideline, freshly prepared bleach dilutions at ~500 ppm available chlorine (a 1:100 dilution of a 5% sodium hypochlorite solution in water) are considered effective low-level disinfectants at contact times of ~1–2 minutes. However, bleach solutions are readily neutralized by many materials and the "10% household bleach solution" or about 5000 ppm available chlorine is more reliable as an intermediate- to high-level disinfectant; mycobacteria might be inactivated in ~5 minutes whereas 10 minutes or more might be needed for many types of bacterial/fungal spores. Further important variables include the quality of water that chlorine-based products are diluted into, which may also affect the actual available activated chlorine concentration, and the types of surfaces on which it will be used. The presence of soil, as for most disinfectants, can dramatically affect the antimicrobial activity, as available chlorine reacts with the soil and may therefore not be available for inactivation of the microorganisms that are present.

For device or equipment disinfection applications, staff should ensure that chlorine will not damage the surfaces (referring to manufacturer's instructions); one of the leading causes of rusting on stainless steel devices is chlorine (particularly in water when heated as part of cleaning, disinfection, or sterilization applications). Other material compatibility concerns will include the "bleaching" (loss) of colored materials, hardening of plastic surfaces, degradation of some types of rubber materials such as O-rings used in many types of device designs, premature wearing of devices/general surfaces, and degradation of anodized aluminum.

Chlorine is widely used as a water disinfectant, where a low level of chlorine is often present to continue to maintain the microbial content in the water to a low and safe level for drinking. Levels of chlorine can range from season to season and even from day to day. In addition, chlorine is often used at high levels as a disinfection method for equipment and facility pipework/water-handling systems. An example in hospitals is the treatment of a facility's water pipework to reduce the levels of certain infectious microorganisms such as *Legionella* (the causative bacteria in Legionnaires' disease). As already highlighted, chlorine can be a leading cause of device damage (e.g. rusting) when present in water used for processing and particularly when heated (e.g. during thermal disinfection or sterilization). Therefore, it is important to monitor and potentially control the levels of chlorine in water used for processing of devices (see Chapter 15 on water quality/purity). The typical recommended level of chlorine in water used for cleaning and disinfection is less than 120 mg/L available chlorine, with even lower levels being recommended when heated to a higher temperature (such as for steam sterilization, where it is <10–120 mg/L; note in this case that chemically 1 mg/L is ~1 ppm).

Chlorine-based products are widely used and inexpensive disinfectants, with good broad-spectrum antimicrobial efficacy (depending on the available chlorine concentration and including sporicidal activity), are fast acting, and have generally low associated toxicity. The "chlorine" smell is commonly associated with cleaning/disinfection. Higher concentrations of chlorine can be irritating and sensitizing, depending on the concentration and the individual. Chlorine can also damage surfaces (metals and plastics), ranging from loss of color (bleaching) to more serious damage such as pitting and rusting. Chlorine products should never be mixed with acid chemistries (e.g. descalers), as the reaction can lead to the release of chlorine gas that is poisonous. Chlorine chemistry is very pH dependent; when stored as an alkaline solution (household bleach) it is quite stable, but on dilution with water the pH drops and the solution is more rapidly active but less stable. Diluted chlorine-based products can be unstable (in particular in the presence of poor-quality water and soil), therefore they are not recommended to be stored for extended periods of time and should be prepared fresh for use (unless otherwise described by the product manufacturer).

Chlorine-generation systems are also used (although rarely) for device, general surface, and even wound disinfection applications. These are referred to as "activated," "electrolyzed," or "super-oxidized" water applications (Figure 9.11). Most of these systems work on a process known as electrolysis, where an electrical current (or other form or energy) is applied to water with a low concentration of salt (typically NaCl, sodium chloride). The salt solution has little to no antimicrobial activity, but when the electrical current is applied active chlorine species (primarily HOCl but also Cl_2 and OCl^-) are formed and can be concentrated in the design of the generator. Other antimicrobial molecules can also be formed during this process that add to the disinfection activity (such as ozone). These preparations have powerful antimicrobial activity (based on their oxidation potential) for use when diluted into water for device disinfection (e.g. with flexible endoscopes and other semi-critical devices) and water disinfection (including low concentrations added into water to be used for disinfectant rinsing). The preparations are, however, not stable, therefore activated water is not stored but is freshly made at or close to the time of use (although this may vary depending on the exact generator type, e.g. stored for up to 24 hours). The concentrated antimicrobial solution prepared is at a very low pH and this may be modified by the generator (in concentration and pH) for different applications depending on the specific antimicrobial process designed and tested. Overall, depending on the concentration and pH used, it can provide low- to high-level disinfection (and has even been used as a sterilant, due to powerful sporicidal activity). Its antimicrobial activity is generally very rapid, with typical intermediate- to high-level disinfection (at 100–250 mg/L available chlorine) for 2 minutes and 5–10 minutes for sporicidal efficacy. Similar to chlorine solutions (discussed earlier), the quality of water used and the presence of soil (in the water or on the device/surface being disinfected) can affect the antimicrobial activity (depending on the dose). In addition to providing powerful antimicrobial

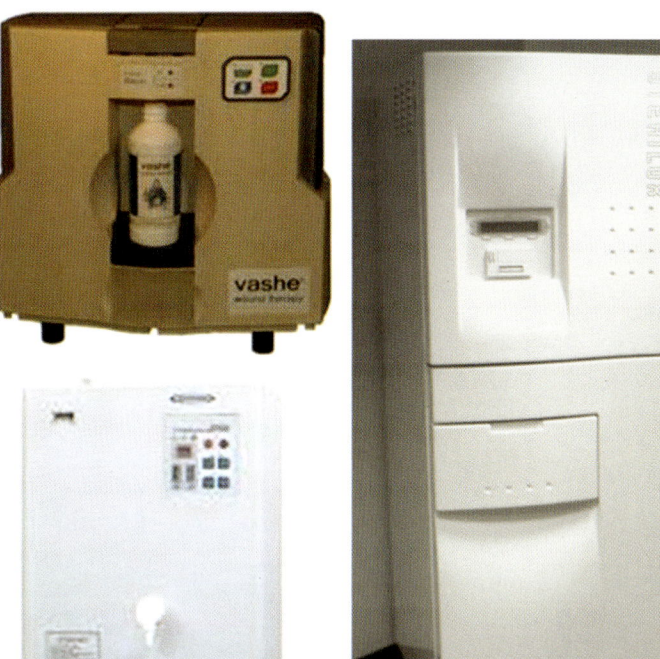

Figure 9.11 Examples of super-oxidized or activated water generators.

activity, these systems are easy and generally safe to use. Activated water does not have the strong odor/irritation associated with high-level hypochlorite solutions and, after the initial purchase of the generator, the overall running costs are considered low. Disadvantages have been reported to include device damage (e.g. with flexible endoscopes protective coatings are often recommended to be applied prior to use to prevent damage to the external surfaces of these devices) and the importance of controlling the quality of the water used for generation (poor-quality water can lead to other negative effects in the generator and surfaces treated with the activated water produced, such as strong odor and device damage).

Peroxygens

Peroxygens are a group of chemicals widely used for disinfection; they include hydrogen peroxide (H_2O_2), peracetic acid (CH_3COOOH, often called PAA), and chlorine dioxide (ClO_2). In addition, ozone (O_3) is also considered in this section. Depending on how they are used, all are potentially effective disinfectants and sterilants (including sterilization applications that are further discussed in Chapter 11).

Hydrogen peroxide is widely used in liquid and gas forms. Simple liquid solutions of peroxide in water (such as 3–6%) have been traditionally used on wounds or in laboratories for wiping surfaces, being considered low- to high-level disinfectants depending on the concentration and exposure time. However, these have now been largely replaced by hydrogen peroxide–containing formulations that have been developed to enhance the antimicrobial activity of peroxide and minimize the negative effects on device compatibility, thus allowing the use of lower concentrations of peroxide to achieve the same effects that would not be possible with the unformulated chemical alone. These formulations are specifically developed for certain applications (environmental surface or device disinfection) and may or may not contain other biocides (e.g. PAA-containing products always contain a certain low concentration of hydrogen peroxide, and some products that are primarily hydrogen peroxide might contain some additional peroxygen compounds, including PAA). Peroxygen concentrations used in formulation range from <1% to 10%. An example is a series of "accelerated" peroxide formulations used for low- to high-level disinfection within 5–10 minutes; at higher concentrations, this includes high-level disinfection of reusable devices. The material compatibility of these peroxide-containing preparations can vary significantly, therefore care should be taken to examine any evidence provided of compatibility with metals and other materials sensitive to oxidation damage. The antimicrobial activity also depends on the specific formulation, but these typically provide high-level disinfection with some activity against bacterial spores.

Other liquid formulations mix 6–8% peroxide with silver (as an antimicrobial metal), claiming a combined benefit in antimicrobial activity; these are used for environmental surface applications and in particular in the generation of peroxide/silver-containing droplets/gas mixtures that are released into the air for the purpose of air/surface disinfection within a room/area. Hydrogen peroxide gas is also a very powerful antimicrobial, being much more effective than liquid preparations at lower concentrations (e.g. 0.00001–0.001% in gas form is typically used). Depending on the concentration and contact time, peroxide gas is a rapid bactericide (including against mycobacteria), fungicide, cysticide, virucide, and sporicide; it has also been shown to be effective under certain conditions against prions and to penetrate over time through organic soils (including blood) that may be associated with microbial contamination. The gas is easy to make (usually from liquid preparations ranging from 6% to 55% peroxide in water) by heating/aerosolization and can also degrade naturally into water and oxygen, therefore it has a good safety (including environmental) profile. In addition to being an effective antimicrobial the gas, when correctly controlled, is safe for use on most materials, including electricals and electronics. For these reasons, peroxide gas in used for a variety of disinfection and sterilization applications. For disinfection, its major use is for room/area and equipment fumigation; fumigation refers to the use of disinfectant indirectly within an area (as opposed to manually applying a liquid disinfectant). These include routine or high-risk (e.g. isolation wards) areas within a facility. With the use of gaseous peroxide, equipment may also remain in or be specifically taken into an area during the fumigation process as a method of disinfection (such as hospital beds, stands, and other non-critical items). A variety of peroxide gas generators are used for this purpose and vary in their application methods, generation methods, and safety/efficacy claims (Figure 9.12). Some systems are used to generate gas-phase (also known as vapor-phase) peroxide only while others make a mixture of gas and liquid peroxide or even just liquid alone. They can vary in the type and concentration of peroxide used as part of the process. Some generators are designed to make peroxide gas and then safely remove it (to allow staff to re-enter the room) and others just generate a peroxide liquid aerosol, leaving it in the room to naturally degrade. Peroxide gas can be noxious at low concentrations (e.g. 5–10 ppm) and a recommended safety level within an area is typically defined at 1 ppm. Overall, the safety and efficacy data associated with any system should be closely inspected prior to use as they can vary significantly. Sterilization applications with peroxide gas are considered in Chapter 1.

Thus hydrogen peroxide in liquid or gas form can be a powerful disinfectant; liquid products can vary depending on their formulation and gas/aerosol products depending on their concentration and process control. Gaseous peroxide is a particularly effective antimicrobial, including sporicidal activity, but its use is constrained to areas not under active occupation. Peroxide has a relatively good safety profile and has become a popular alternative to other biocides with greater safety (staff, patient, or environmental). Although liquid concentrations at 3–6% can be safely handled, even at these lower concentrations they should be respected as potent chemicals (use of PPE, including gloves and safety glasses); higher concentrations (e.g. 35% solutions used to generate gas peroxide) can have serious effects, such as skin burns, on contact. Low concentrations of the gas can be irritating (especially to the eyes) and at higher concentrations (e.g. at 75 ppm) can do

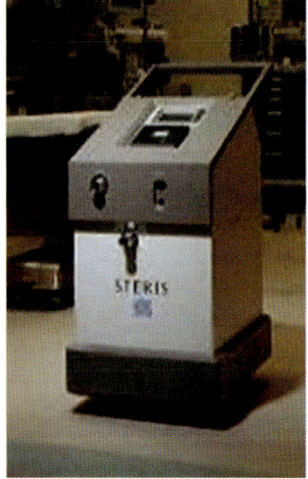 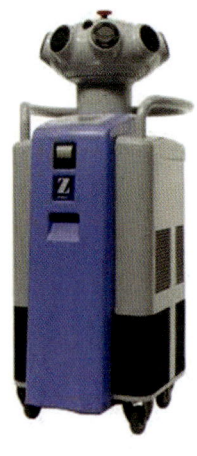 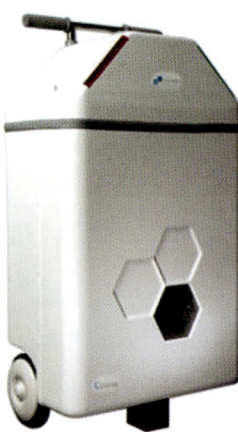

Figure 9.12 Various types of hydrogen peroxide gas- or aerosol-generating systems used for disinfection applications.

significant damage to various tissues, including the lungs, with potentially serious complications. Depending on the application/product, peroxide can lead to loss of color (bleaching). It also degrades on contacting certain types of materials (e.g. paper, wood, and brass/copper, thereby losing disinfectant activity) and can damage some surfaces. These side effects can vary significantly depending on the formulation and/or process used for disinfection.

PAA is primarily used in liquid form for disinfection; it has not been widely used to date in gaseous form in healthcare applications. Solutions of PAA always contain a certain level of hydrogen peroxide and acetic acid, with the acetic acid being responsible for the typical pungent odor associated with such products. It is also widely used as a general surface disinfectant in industry, but in healthcare facilities its most important function is as a high-level disinfectant/sterilant for semi-critical and critical devices. Sterilization applications with PAA are considered in Chapter 11 in the section on chemical sterilization. PAA is also used for equipment disinfection, in particular of water-handling equipment (e.g. RO water generation and storage systems). PAA is provided for disinfection applications in many ways (Figure 9.13): as single components (ready for use or diluted in water), two components (requiring mixing to provide the disinfectant or allowing the component to generate PAA), and activated or not. Dry (solid) or liquid formulations are also available as single- or multi-use products for manual application/immersion or as part of a defined washer-disinfector or disinfector/sterilizer processor.

PAA disinfectants can be used in open trays for manual immersion, but the strong odors associated with such applications may be undesirable and can be minimized by the use of chemical hoods or appropriate ventilation (frequent air exchanges) within the processing area. PAA is also used as a common disinfectant in many types of washer-disinfectors for flexible endoscope disinfection (Figure 9.11). These systems not only control exposure to the disinfectant (such as for disinfectant delivery through device lumens and under controlled temperature conditions) but minimize any handling (staff safety) risks and should also ensure that disinfectant residuals are adequately removed prior to patient use.

PAA-containing formulations are very effective high-level disinfectants/sterilants with effectiveness against all types of microorganisms including bacterial spores; relatively low concentrations (e.g. 0.1–0.2%) are required for such activity and can be particularly enhanced by controlling the temperature of the disinfection process (if labeled for such applications). Temperature-controlled processes have been shown to have cysticidal activity, but this can be product specific. Some formulations will also have cleaning and biofilm removal effects, but this strictly depends on the product formulation. PAA is considered an effective biocide at low concentrations even in the presence of organic/inorganic soils. Similar to other peroxygens, it also degrades naturally into safe, non-toxic by-products such as water and a low concentration of acetic acid. There are, however, some disadvantages. Some formulations can have strong, irritating odors that are undesirable when being used or stored. PAA can cause skin burns at low concentrations, with the eyes being particularly at risk from accidental splashing. Material and device compatibility is a frequent complaint with PAA formulations, and this can vary significantly from product to product; as for any disinfectant, compatibility claims should be supported by documentation from the manufacturer and the product should not be counter-indicated by the device manufacturer.

Chlorine dioxide–based disinfectants are popular in many parts of the world for both non-critical device/general surface disinfection and for high-level device disinfection applications. Similar to PAA, chloride dioxide is also used for equipment disinfection, such as water-handling systems, and for water disinfection itself (as an alternative to chlorine). Chlorine dioxide should not be confused with chlorine (see the section on halogens), as they are separate and distinct biocides. Its primary use to date is as a liquid-based disinfectant and it is rarely, if ever, used at this time in gas phase. As it is a very unstable biocide, it is always provided as a one- or two-component generating system where the chlorine dioxide is generated by mixing two components together or by dissolving similar components in dry tablet form into water. A variety of delivery systems have been developed to accommodate the biocide generation. These include two-component liquid systems (to generate a concentrated chlorine dioxide solution that is then diluted in water at the indicated concentration), ready-to-use pump systems (two components are mixed on spraying out onto a surface), tablets (which activate when mixed with water), and wipe systems that are activated prior to use using the indicated mixing method and time. These are used for manual application/device immersion or in automated washer-disinfector systems.

The antimicrobial effects of chlorine dioxide depend on its concentration, formulation, and contact time/temperature; with these considerations it can be similar if not superior to chlorine formulations. Typical bactericidal/virucidal concentrations have been reported in the 0.2–1 mg/L range, with high-level disinfection requiring higher concentrations (1–2 mg/L), at which it is also effective against spores and some types of cysts. It also maintains efficacy in the presence of soil, but this is concentration dependent. Unlike chlorine, chlorine dioxide disinfectants are not associated with strong odors (although they may have a slight "chlorine" odor) or other negative effects observed with chlorine. It is considered non-toxic and safe for the environment, as it degrades naturally. Since such disinfectants require generation, care should be taken to ensure that they are activated correctly according to the manufacturer's instructions at the time of use and this

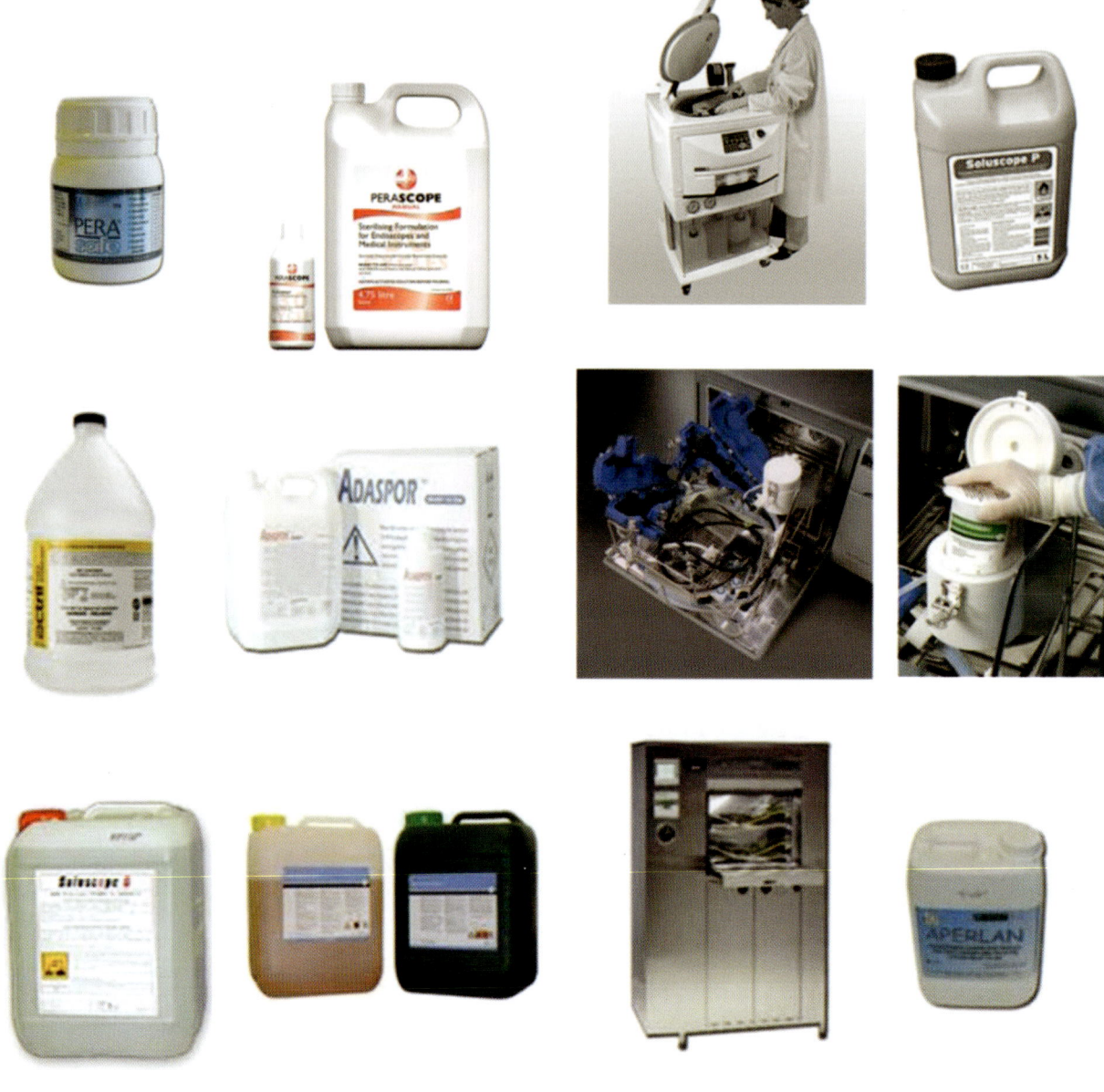

Figure 9.13 Various types of peracetic acid (PAA)-containing disinfectants and disinfection/sterilization systems. (A) One- and two-component formulations (far upper left is an example of a solid product that is diluted in water to generate PAA). (B) Endoscope washer-disinfectors and their associated PAA-containing disinfectants for flexible endoscopes; some designs are restricted to one type of disinfectant and others are not.

should preferably be confirmed using a type of CI specific for chlorine dioxide. High, generally sporicidal concentrations are often considered damaging to certain types of materials (including stainless steel and plastics) but these effects are formulation specific; loss of color is frequently observed over time. Release of chlorine dioxide gas from disinfectants can be a safety concern, with relatively low levels (over 0.1 ppm) considered to be toxic.

Ozone is not widely used for disinfection purposes in healthcare facilities today and is only briefly described here; specific sterilization processes using ozone are considered in more detail in Chapter 11. The main applications for ozone include laundry, for water or waste disinfection, and less commonly for area (environmental) and air disinfection. It is generated in air or water from available oxygen (including water, H_2O, as a source of oxygen) at the point of use (e.g. from an ozone generator or within a washer-disinfector). In a typical ozone-water system, the ozone is generated from air (or from an oxygen gas source) by application of an electrical charge and then, as a gas, bubbled into the water (e.g. using an injector/mixing system; Figure 9.14); the ozonated water is then used in a disinfection process. Ozone has become a popular low-temperature chemical alternative for healthcare laundry applications (typically at 30–35°C), in that it can provide an intermediate to high level of disinfection but also is a deodorizer and degrades naturally to give safe by-products (oxygen), therefore minimizing water consumption. As a gas, it is generated and used directly in the air (for air and surface disinfection) but requires high humidity levels (75–95%) for optimal activity.

Ozone is a particularly powerful biocide and, like other peroxygen biocides, its disinfectant activity will depend on the ozone concentration and process control. For example, in air disinfection and device sterilization applications (see Chapter 11), in addition to ozone concentration the temperature, contact time, and humidity control are important; humidity (usually over 80%) is particularly important to ensure that ozone can be effective and at higher temperatures there can be a benefit of increased activity but a negative effect that degrades the available ozone concentration. Its disinfectant activity can therefore range from low to high level, and it can even be used for sterilization purposes as part of a controlled process. As a highly reactive disinfectant, it reacts with all microorganisms and, with sufficient activity, will render them non-viable. Typical conditions of bactericidal and viricidal activity are in the 0.2–0.5 mg/L range, with higher concentrations generally required to inactivate fungal and bacterial spores, as well as protozoal cysts.

Overall, the advantages of ozone are its wide antimicrobial activity, ease of generation, and being environmentally friendly. Ozone is also used to neutralize various types of chemicals that are associated with foul odors (such as aldehydes and some phenols) and other unwanted molecules. Disadvantages are its rapid neutralization by surface and soil contact, that it can be toxic at low levels (with a typical safety limit being 0.1 ppm), and that it may damage surfaces (including stainless steel and plastics, depending on the concentration and disinfection process).

Phenols

A phenol is a specific type of chemical and is actually not routinely used as a disinfectant; "phenols" or "phenolics" refer to biocides used for disinfection that are based on derivatives of phenol or have a similar chemical structure. Examples include cresols, 2-phenylphenol, chlorocresol, chloroxylenol (commonly known as PCMX), and triclosan. They are used as low- to intermediate-level disinfectants for environmental surfaces, but are generally not considered safe and effective for device processing. They are available as concentrated or ready-to-use disinfectants for general housekeeping (floors, walls, general contact surfaces, etc.), but are often not recommended in certain applications (e.g. in nurseries and particularly incubators) due to strong odors or toxicity (in some cases). Depending on the formulation (including types of specific phenols), concentration, and application time, phenols can provide rapid bactericidal, fungicidal, and virucidal (enveloped) activity, with some formulations having practical activity also against mycobacteria and some non-enveloped viruses. Phenols have little to no activity against bacterial spores. Overall, phenolic disinfectants retain good activity in the presence of soils (used for cleaning/disinfectant activity), are often associated with the "hospital" smell (a sweet, aromatic odor), and some are readily biodegradable (while others may not be). The formulation plays an important role in their activity and, as with many other disinfectants, they are usually combined with surfactants to aid in cleaning–disinfection

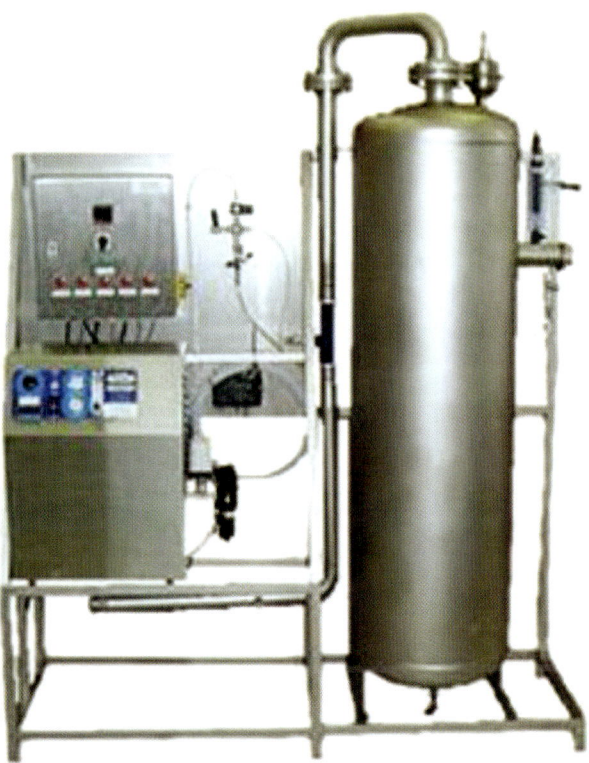

Figure 9.14 An ozonated water–generating system. In this system the ozone is generated as a gas from the oxygen in air by application of an electrical current and then added into the water by bubbling. The ozonated water is then used for disinfection applications.

applications. They are, however, often associated with a strong odor (particularly when used at high concentrations), should not be used in applications where toxic residues could be a concern (e.g. neonatal and food contact surfaces), and (again depending on the formulation) can damage certain types of plastics and rubbers.

Two specific phenolic chemicals, triclosan and PCMX (or chloroxylenol), have been widely used as antiseptics, including for routine (antiseptic) hand washing and surgical scrubbing (see Chapter 6). Other examples of phenol-derived antiseptic-type biocides are hexachlorophene and salicylic acid. These are all considered separate from the hard-surface disinfectants and are distinct in safety and efficacy considerations. Triclosan was one of the most widely used biocides in antiseptics and is often integrated into surfaces that have antimicrobial claims. In antiseptic formulation concentrations typically range from 0.1% to 2%. Its antimicrobial activity is very good against Gram-positive bacteria but poorer against Gram-negative bacteria; the correct formulation is essential to optimize the activity of triclosan for use in antiseptics against a wider range of bacteria. These antiseptics are considered low-level disinfectants and for use only for hand washing (or in combination with alcohol, for hand rubbing) or other specific applications. The widespread use of triclosan in liquid antiseptics and disinfectants has been discouraged due to potential health concerns over time. Chloroxylenol (in the 0.5–4% range) has become more widely used in recent years for antiseptic and disinfectant use. Antiseptics using this biocide often claim activity against fungi (yeast and molds) and enveloped viruses. Both triclosan and chloroxylenol can remain on the skin following washing to give a sustained (persistent, bacteriostatic) antimicrobial activity. Both have been popular in antiseptics due to their low irritation profiles and mildness to the skin, but they have limited antimicrobial (low-level) activity and are often a concern due to their persistence in the environment.

Quaternary ammonium compounds

Quaternary ammonium compounds belong to a group of chemicals called surfactants (or "surface-active agents"). These are unique chemicals that can hold dirt (including fats and oils) in water; for this reason, they are widely used in cleaning and disinfection chemistries (see Chapter 6). Many types of surfactants also have antimicrobial activity, particularly the quaternary ammonium compounds (QACs or QUATs for short). These are usually associated with rather long chemical names such as hexadecylpyridinium chloride and hexadecyltrimethylammonium bromide (commonly known as "cetrimide"). Other types of surfactants used for their disinfection activity are known as the "amphoteric" surfactants (e.g. alkyl dimethyl oxide). QACs are used in disinfectants, particularly low level, for combined cleaning and disinfection. They are also widely used with surfactants in a range of other cleaning and disinfectant formulations due to their soil-removing and capturing activity. They can be particularly effective at inactivating microorganisms (within their spectrum of activity or label claims) but also in the physical removal of microorganisms from surfaces.

QACs are typically provided as concentrates and as ready-to-use and impregnated-wipe disinfectant products for general environmental and non-critical device applications. They are known to have a pleasant, clean odor than can also be used for deodorization in general ward use. Similar to the phenols (see the earlier section on phenols), the QACs range dramatically in activity depending on the particular chemicals (they are often used in mixtures of two or three QAC types) and their formulation. In general, QAC-based products provide good bactericidal and viricidal (enveloped) activity, but can range in activity to include fungi and even (rarely) mycobacteria and therefore might have claims as intermediate-level disinfectants. They have important advantages in being used as both cleaning and disinfectant agents, and are considered non-corrosive and safe for use. They are limited in antimicrobial activity and can be irritating or damaging to some surface materials (e.g. on copper) depending on their formulation.

Other biocides

There are many other types of biocides that can be used for disinfection purposes, in addition to the main types already discussed. It is difficult to consider all of these in detail and, even then, individual products and applications can range considerably. In all cases of existing and new biocides, consideration should be given the claims made with the product, with particular emphasis on safety and efficacy (see the section on the basic principles of disinfection). A few additional biocide types are discussed briefly here.

Glucoprotamine (or glucoprotamin) is used for low- to high-level disinfection of environmental surfaces and device processing (including semi-critical devices, depending on the disinfection product). Formulations can have claimed bactericidal (including mycobactericidal activity at defined contact times/conditions), fungicidal, and viricidal (enveloped viruses) activity. There is little to no activity with certain types of non-enveloped viruses and bacterial spores. Typical concentrations used are in the 0.25–0.5% range in formulation; formulation effects include optimizing antimicrobial activity and surfactants to aid in cleaning activity. Such disinfectants are generally considered to have good material compatibility, but have been reported to be irritating to the skin/mucous membranes.

Strong acids and bases (low or high pH, respectively; see the section on the pH scale: defining acids and bases in Chapter 6) are sometimes used for their antimicrobial activity, especially in product formulations. Examples may include low pH (acidic) and high pH (alkaline) based formulations that may also have some antimicrobial claims (used for cleaning and low-level disinfection), with particular emphasis on bactericidal and viricidal (enveloped) activity. Strong alkaline solutions have been recommended to be effective against prions (such as 1–2 N sodium hydroxide for one hour on surgical devices), but these are not generally recommended for routine use for device reprocessing. Although they may provide some antimicrobial activity, care should be taken in their use from a personal safety and device compatibility point of view (in particular as strong acids and bases can be damaging to device materials). pH also plays an important role in the activity of other chemical disinfectants (as discussed earlier) and is a valuable part of a disinfectant formulation strategy to optimize activity and label claims (see the section on mixtures, formulations, and solutions in Chapter 6).

Chlorhexidine (commonly known as CHG for "chlorhexidine gluconate") is a widely used biocide in antiseptics (hand washes and hand rubs), for general hand washing, preoperative patient bathing, preoperative skin preparation, and as a surgical scrub. It is an example of a group of biocides known as "biguanides." Other examples, although much less used in this group, are alexidine and octenidine in antiseptics and the polyhexamethylene biguanides (PHMBs) for general surface/water disinfection. Chlorhexidine-based antiseptics generally provide bactericidal and virucidal (enveloped) activity, with some activity against fungi (depending on the product). Some products provided a combined effect of chlorhexidine and alcohol (in hand rubs) as well as other formulation effects to increase the overall antimicrobial activity of the product. Typical concentrations range from 0.5% to 4%, but overall activity is based on specific formulation effects. As antiseptics they are considered gentle on the hands but effective against many of the transient bacteria/viruses found on the skin; in addition to its immediate activity during the wash/application, chlorhexidine can remain bound to the skin and provide a persistent antimicrobial activity over time. This is often a benefit during long surgical procedures to prevent the growth of bacteria (in particular under gloves). Despite these benefits, the overall antimicrobial activity is limited (low-level disinfection) and some formulations can be irritating to those using them; residual activity can be neutralized by certain types of skin creams and hand washes (e.g. those containing non-ionic surfactants). The PHMBs are not widely used as disinfectants and then only for general, environmental surfaces as low-level disinfectants (with specific claims dependent on the disinfectant formulation).

Certain types of metals are used for disinfection purposes in healthcare; these particularly include silver and copper. Copper has become more widely used as a naturally occurring antimicrobial integrated into surfaces; these surfaces usually consist of a certain amount of copper mixed with other metals (these are known as "alloys," for example brass is an alloy of copper and zinc). Copper-containing surfaces are used to provide low-level (specifically bactericidal or bacteriostatic) disinfection on surfaces if contacted. Typical applications include light switches, tray tables, and so on. Silver is also used for antimicrobial purposes but rarely for surface/device disinfection and more commonly for certain antiseptic-type applications (e.g. wound dressings). Copper–silver ionization systems (where an electric current is provided to copper/silver plates to release a low level of both biocides into water) are used for water treatment (e.g. to reduce levels of certain types of bacteria such as *Legionella* that can be a concern in water-handling systems). The activity of these types of antimicrobial metals can range considerably and close attention should be given to any label claims, which can include bactericidal/bacteriostatic or fungicidal/fungistatic activity over time. Like all metals, they can be toxic to humans if exposed as higher concentrations.

Disinfection guidelines and standards

As highlighted earlier in this chapter, disinfection claims may or may not be regulated in different countries/regions, with some countries closely controlling the use of disinfectants and others not. Examples include:

- United States: The FDA's Center for Devices and Radiological Health (CDRH) regulates the disinfection and sterilization of devices, including thermal and chemical processes, as well as antiseptics (as they contact the skin/mucous membranes). The EPA regulates the use of chemical disinfectants for general environmental surfaces. Products are registered and approved for use based on scientific evidence of safety and efficacy. Some states may also have specific requirements regarding the use of disinfectants, including restrictions on disposal of chemicals through public drains.
- European Union: In Europe, if a disinfectant or disinfection process is used for processing a device for patient use it is also considered a "device" and is therefore regulated under the Medical Devices Regulations (2017/745). There are various classes of devices depending on the risk to the patient, ranging from the lowest risk (class I) to the highest risk (class III). Device disinfectants and disinfection processes are currently considered as class IIa or IIb devices depending on their labeling. The general (essential) safety requirements for these products are described in the regulation itself and specific requirements are also outlined in applicable European (EN) and/or International Organization for Standardization (ISO) standards. Note: under the Vienna Agreement 1991, there is technical cooperation between ISO and the European Committee for Standardization (CEN) to make such standards compatible or even identical. An example is for washer-disinfectors as defined in the EN ISO 15883 (washer-disinfector)

series of standards. Further considerations for washer-disinfectors and disinfection machines include the Machinery Directive (2006/42/EC, if moving parts are used as part of the process) and electrical safety requirements. There is also a series of EN standards under development regarding demonstration of the antimicrobial activities of antiseptics and disinfectants. These range from simple suspension tests (phase 1) to laboratory antimicrobial tests that simulate the practical use of the disinfectant (e.g. on the hands or a hard surface; phase 2) and "field" tests where the disinfectant is tested as used in practice (phase 3). In addition to these tests, other country-specific tests or requirements may be specified in certain countries, such as tests from the French standardization authority (Association française de normalisation or AFNOR), the British Standards Institution (BSI), and the German Institute for Standardization (Deutsches Institut für Normung or DIN). Chemical disinfectants used for other purposes (environmental or water disinfection) are also affected by other European Directives. These include the Biocidal Products Directive (BPD, 98/8/EC) that regulates chemicals used for antimicrobial purposes, with a particular emphasis on environmental concerns. Others with a similar scope that affect disinfectants (or the use of other chemicals in disinfectant formulations) include EC Detergent Regulation (648/2004) and the REACH Regulation (Registration Evaluation, Authorisation and Restriction of Chemicals, EC 1907/2006). A further exception is that antiseptics are regulated as medicines under the EU Medicinal Products Directives 2001/83/EC and subsequent amendments such as 2004/27/EC.

- Australia: Disinfectants are regulated by the TGA under the Therapeutic Goods Order (TGO) No. 54. This applies to antiseptics and disinfectants. A range of international and national standards and test methods are recognized to establish disinfection efficacy.
- Canada: Disinfectants, including antiseptics, are regulated under Health Canada's Therapeutic Products Directorate (TPD). Products are registered and approved for use based on scientific evidence of safety and efficacy. Antimicrobial hand soaps must also have a Drug Identification Number (DIN) that is displayed on the product label.
- Brazil: Disinfectants to be registered with the National Health Surveillance Agency (ANVISA), including evidence of safety and efficacy (with standard test methods).
- Korea: Disinfectants are registered with the Korean Food and Drug Administration (KFDA), including evidence of safety and efficacy (with standard test methods).
- International: Example of international requirements include the ISO standards (e.g. EN ISO 15883 for washer-disinfectors) and antimicrobial test methods described by the OECD. In the case of ISO standards, although these are internationally harmonized, many countries may specifically decide to modify the text for publication as a local standard and others will adopt them without modification.

In addition to these country-specific requirements, a variety of country- or organization-specific guidelines have been developed and are frequently updated. They generally provide guidance regarding antisepsis and disinfection, including types of disinfectants and local or device-specific considerations regarding safe and effective use. Guidelines are not a replacement for country/region-specific regulations, but they are often used together to establish best practices in facilities. A summary of some types of guidance on disinfection is given in Table 9.5.

Some consideration has already been given to the various parts of the ISO washer-disinfector standards, the ISO 15883 series (see Chapter 8, in the section on cleaning guidelines, standards, and testing). Thermal disinfection is specified as the minimum temperature and contact time necessary to provide an A_0 applicable to the type of washer-disinfector; for example, surgical devices are required, in compliance with ISO 15883 Parts 1 and 2, to be disinfected at a minimum A_0 of 600 (e.g. 90°C (194°F) for one minute). The temperature distribution within the washer-disinfector is verified using temperature sensors (e.g. thermocouples) and associated recording systems (Figure 9.15); these are placed at various locations within the chamber, load, and load carrier (rack, tray, etc.). The measurement system should have specified accuracy, precision, and so on and be periodically calibrated to ensure that it is functioning correctly. For ISO 15883 compliance, the disinfection temperature should be between −0°C and +5°C (32–41°F) of the set temperature; an upper limit is also set to prevent the washer-disinfector from accidentally overheating the load, which could lead to damage.

Testing and confirming temperature distribution may be conducted during the design and installation, and periodically (e.g. yearly) during clinical use. The A_0 concept is now widely accepted internationally as acceptable alone to make a thermal disinfection claim and only in rare cases do thermal disinfection cycles require further verification by antimicrobial test methods (discussed further in this section and summarized in Table 9.6). These test methods and pass/fail criteria will be defined by government regulatory agencies. Although there are tight controls and testing requirements defined in ISO 15883 for automated washer-disinfectors, there are few such controls on manual thermal disinfection; despite this the same concepts can be applied. The temperature of the water used for disinfection should be verified, exposure conditions should ensure that the device is fully immersed for disinfection, and the contact time should be controlled.

Chemical disinfection can be achieved by a chemical disinfectant alone (usually at room temperature, either manually or in a machine) or by a chemical-thermal process (where the temperature and other variables can be controlled during the disinfection process). A wide range of test methods may be used to show that a product is effective as a disinfectant and/or

Table 9.5 Examples of disinfection guidance documents.

Publisher	Title	Description
US Centers for Disease Control (CDC) Healthcare Infection Control Practices Advisory Committee (HICPAC)	Guideline for disinfection and sterilization in healthcare facilities	Recommendations on methods for cleaning, disinfection, and sterilization of patient-care devices and the healthcare environment
Canadian General Standards Board (CGSB)	CAN/CGSB-2.161-97 Assessment of efficacy of antimicrobial agents for use on environmental surfaces and medical devices	Guidance on the registration of disinfectants, including safety and efficacy requirements
British Society of Gastroenterology (BSG)	BSG Guidelines for decontamination of equipment for gastrointestinal endoscopy	Guidelines on cleaning and disinfection of flexible endoscopes
World Gastroenterology Organisation (WGO)	WGO/OMED Practice guideline endoscope disinfection	Guidelines on cleaning and disinfection of flexible endoscopes
Association for the Advancement of Medical Instrumentation (AAMI)	AAMI/ANSI ST58 Chemical sterilization and high-level disinfection in health care facilities	Guidelines for the selection and use of high level disinfectants (and chemical sterilants) approved in the United States
Society of Gastroenterology Nurses and Associates (SGNA)	Guideline for use of high-level disinfectants & sterilants for reprocessing flexible gastrointestinal endoscopes	Guide to the types and use of disinfectants/ sterilants for endoscope reprocessing
American Professionals in Infection Control (APIC)	Guideline for hand washing and hand antisepsis in health care settings	Guidelines on the type and use of various antiseptics in healthcare applications
China	Regulation on the safety evaluation report of disinfecting products WS 628, Technical requirements for the hygiene and safety evaluation of disinfectant products	Required tests to complete a disinfectant safety evaluation report, based on five categories of disinfection products
World Health Organization (WHO)	Infection control guidelines for transmissible spongiform encephalopathies Decontamination and reprocessing of medical devices for health-care facilities	Guidelines for infection control practices against prion diseases, including decontamination[1] Guidelines on device processing including chemical disinfection/disinfectants

[1] These were initially published in 1999 and are now considered outdated.

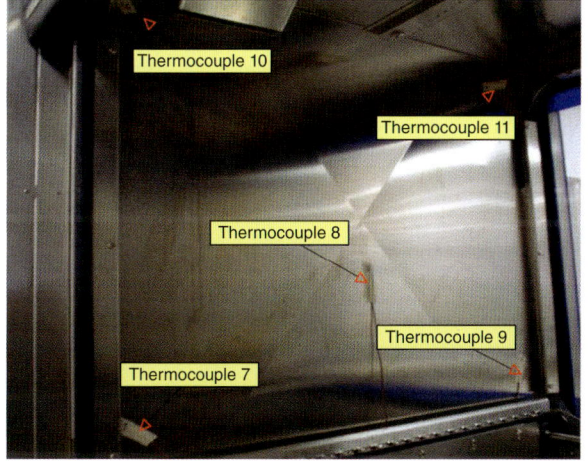
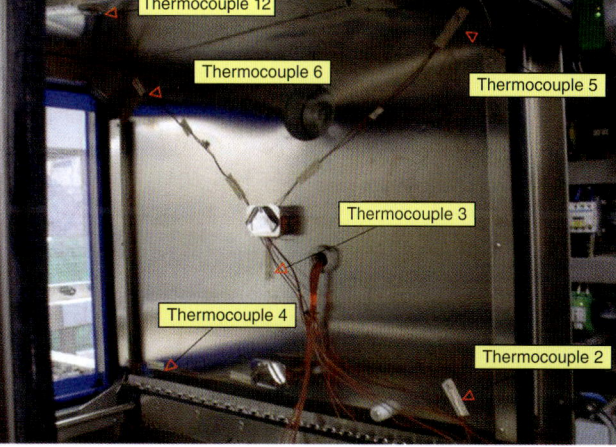

Figure 9.15 Temperature distribution testing within a washer-disinfector chamber. Note the use of various temperature sensors (thermocouples) located at various places in the chamber.

Table 9.6 Examples of published and widely used disinfection test methods.

Test method	Title	Description
EN 1500	Hygienic handrub – Test method and requirements (phase 2/step 2)	Volunteer hands are artificially contaminated with a controlled number of test organisms. The number of test organisms before and after application of the hand rub is tested
EN 14347	Basic sporicidal activity. Test method and requirements (phase 1)	Bacterial spore (*Bacillus* species) suspensions added directly to the disinfectant to test sporicidal ability
EN 13727	Quantitative suspension test for the evaluation of bacterial activity of chemical disinfectants for instruments used in the medical area. Test method and requirements (phase 2, step 1)	Vegetative bacteria (Gram-positive and -negative) suspensions added directly to the disinfectant in the presence of interfering substances
AOAC	965.12 Tuberculocidal activity of disinfectants	*Mycobacterium bovis* (or test modified using *M. terrae*) inoculated onto small cylinders, dried, and exposed to the disinfectant
AOAC	966.04 Sporicidal activity of disinfectants	Two types of spore-forming bacteria (*Bacillus* and *Clostridium*) in the presence of soil inoculated onto two types of carriers, dried, and exposed to the disinfectant
ISO 15883:1	Washer-disinfectors – Part 1: General requirements, terms and definitions and tests	Describes the A_0 concept for thermal disinfection and testing of temperature distribution in a washer-disinfector
ISO 15883:4	Washer-disinfectors – Part 4: Requirements and tests for washer-disinfectors employing chemical disinfection for thermolabile endoscopes	Microbiological testing of a range of microorganisms (including bacteria, viruses, fungi, and spores) inoculated into surrogate lumen devices and tested for microbial inactivation (log reductions) following the disinfection process
ISO 15883:6	Washer-disinfectors – Part 6: Requirements and tests for washer-disinfectors employing thermal disinfection for non-invasive, non-critical medical devices and healthcare equipment	Defines an A_0 requirement of 60 for thermal disinfection and testing of temperature distribution in a washer-disinfector
ISO 15883:7	Washer-disinfectors – Part 7: Requirements and tests for washer-disinfectors employing chemical disinfection for non-invasive, non-critical thermolabile medical devices and healthcare equipment	Microbiological testing requirements for the disinfectant, disinfection cycle, and rinsing requirements for chemical disinfection. Includes antimicrobial activity against bacteria, yeasts, and enveloped viruses
Organisation for Economic Co-operation and Development (OECD)	Guidance document on quantitative methods for evaluating the activity of microbicides used on hard non-porous surfaces	Guidance document describing chemical disinfectant quantitative test methods to verify bactericidal, mycobactericidal, fungicidal, and virucidal activity on hard non-porous surfaces. This is the basis for the ASTM E2197 test methods
ASTM E1174	Standard test method for evaluation of healthcare personnel handwash formulations	Activity of an antiseptic on the hands using an artificial inoculum of *Serratia marcescens*
ASTM E1838	Standard test method for determining the virus-eliminating effectiveness of hygienic handwash and handrub agents using the fingerpads of adults	Activity of an antiseptic on finger pads contaminated with different viruses
ASTM E2197	Standard quantitative disk carrier test method for determining the bactericidal, virucidal, fungicidal, mycobactericidal, and sporicidal activities of liquid chemical germicides	Tests the ability of disinfectants to inactivate microorganisms in the presence of a soil load on disk carriers, representing environmental surfaces and devices
ASTM E2111	Standard quantitative carrier test method to evaluate the bactericidal, fungicidal, mycobactericidal and sporicidal potencies of liquid chemical germicides	Known quantity of microorganisms inoculated onto carriers and exposed to a disinfectant to determine a given reduction

antiseptic. Examples of such tests are given in Table 9.6. It is important to note that these tests are designed to show that a product is effective when tested in a laboratory under a particular set of conditions and that the disinfectant can be effective when used in accordance with labeled directions.

Some of these tests are specifically defined to demonstrate the effectiveness of a chemical disinfection process in a washer-disinfector; examples are ISO 15883 Parts 4 and 7, describing tests for washer-disinfectors employing chemical disinfection. In ISO 15883 Part 4, recommended testing includes a range of microorganisms (bacteria, mycobacteria, viruses, fungi, and bacterial spores). Preparations of each are inoculated into plastic (specifically polytetrafluoroethylene or PFTE) tubes of 2 mm or 1 mm diameter × 150 mm in length and placed at various positions along an overall length of tubing at 1.5 m; two of the 2 mm sizes and one of the 1 mm sizes are then used for testing in the washer-disinfector (during the disinfection process; Figure 9.16). Bacterial spores are used to test for physical removal during the process and the other microorganisms to demonstrate antimicrobial efficacy, where a given level of microbial reduction is expected to be demonstrated. Such tests can demonstrate a combination of physical removal and disinfection.

Other test methods, given in Table 9.6, are used to show that the chemical disinfectant is effective under laboratory conditions and/or within a washer-disinfector. They are used to establish and achieve regulatory approval of a chemical disinfectant as being effective; in certain countries specific test methods are defined and reviewed, while in others they are not. A further series of tests may be required for a chemical washer-disinfector regarding "self-disinfection." A self-disinfection cycle is described as a programmed cycle for use without any load in the washer-disinfector that is used to periodically disinfect all liquid transport systems including piping, chamber(s), tanks, and all other components that may come into contact with the water and/or solutions used for cleaning, disinfecting, and rinsing the load. This is a periodic disinfection cycle designed to reduce the risk of the development of biofilm formation (see Chapter 5, in the section on bacteria), where a different type of chemical or preferably thermal disinfection process is provided within the disinfector to reduce biofilm. This is particularly important in the water-rinsing or storage system provided within the washer-disinfector that may or may not be routinely disinfected.

A further consideration for chemical disinfectants is the use of CIs. Chemical indicators are defined as test systems (usually in the form of test strips) that reveal a change in one or more pre-defined process variables based on a chemical and/or physical change resulting from exposure to a process. They are generally provided as color-change indicators (Figure 9.17) that are used to verify that a chemical or physical disinfectant or disinfection process (or indeed cleaning or sterilization process) is fit for use or has been conducted. CIs are often used with reusable disinfectants (in particular high-level disinfectants), where the disinfectant is verified to be under the right conditions (e.g. presence of sufficient biocide) to be effective according to the manufacturer's claims. In the case of reusable disinfectants, this is important as the antimicrobial activity may become watered down with use over time, be incorrectly prepared/maintained, or be used in a manner that may have exhausted the presence of the biocide. A typical term used is the minimum effective concentration (MEC), where the indicator is designed to show that a minimum amount of the disinfectant is present. CIs are also used for single-use disinfectants/sterilants, for example to ensure that they have been delivered correctly at the right concentration or generated/mixed

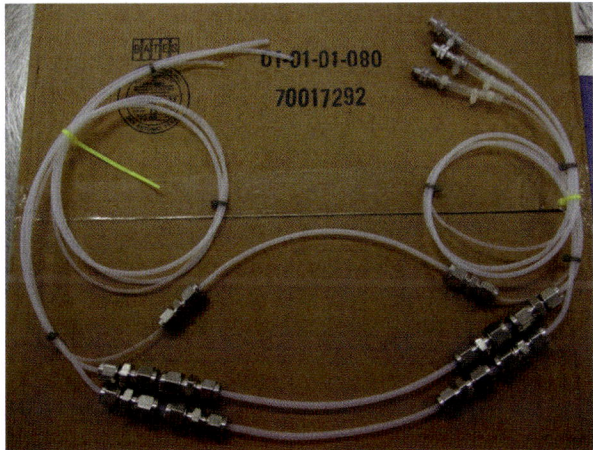

Figure 9.16 Example of a surrogate test device for demonstration of disinfection efficacy in a washer-disinfector.

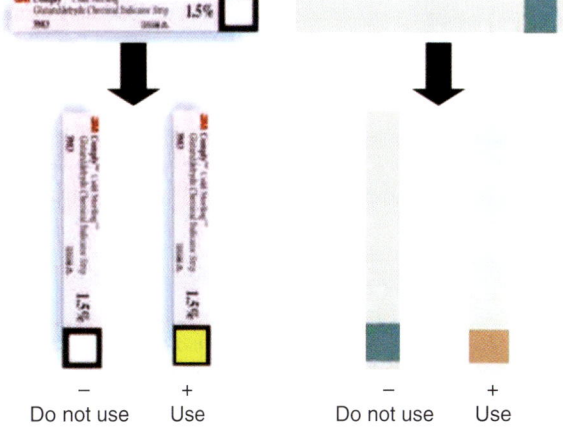

Figure 9.17 Examples of two different types of chemical indicators and their typical color change on exposure to a chemical disinfectant.

Table 9.7 The classification of chemical indicators.[1]

Type	Indicator type	Description
Type 1	Process indicator	Simple indicators to demonstrate exposure to a process and also to distinguish between processed/unprocessed units A pass result may not mean the process has been achieved
Type 2	Indicators for use in specific tests	Used to indicate a specific type of test, generally established in another standard
Type 3	Single variable indicators	Designed to respond to only one critical process variable (e.g. concentration of a biocide)
Type 4	Multi-variable indicators	Designed to respond to two or more of the critical variables (e.g. temperature, time, and concentration of a biocide)
Type 5	Integrating indicators	Designed to respond to all critical variables of the process, in particular to be equivalent to a biological indicator (e.g. indicators containing bacterial spores used to test sterilization processes); see Chapter 11
Type 6	Emulating or cycle verification indicators	Designed to react to all critical variables for a full specified cycle (which may be over and above that matching a biological indicator)

[1] Defined based on ISO 11140 *Sterilization of health care products – Chemical indicators*. Other regulatory agencies may use similar terms and require clearance of their local requirements for testing/labeling for use (e.g. the US Food and Drug Administration or the Chinese GB 18282.1 requirements for chemical indicators).

correctly (in cases where the biocide is made or activated by mixing two chemicals together). In addition to chemical disinfection, they are also widely used to verify thermal and chemical sterilization processes (see Chapter 11).

According to the ISO 11140 series of standards titled *Sterilization of health care products –Chemical indicators*, CIs are defined in six different types depending on their monitoring abilities and the information they may (or may not) provide about the process being monitored (Table 9.7); although this series of standards relates to sterilization process, it is introduced at this stage in reference to the use of CIs for disinfection. At the time of writing there are no standards defining the requirement for CIs used for disinfection, but overall most indicators used with chemical disinfectants are generally similar to 1, 3, or 4 types.

As the various regulatory requirements can change periodically, it is important to understand any local requirements and to review any disinfectant product claims closely. This is particularly important in countries where no specific product registration (including technical review) is required or independently reviewed. Do not hesitate to get an expert microbiological review of any test data to ensure that the disinfectant or disinfection process is fit for purpose.

Special considerations

Many of the special considerations outlined in Chapter 8 on cleaning of various device types apply equally to disinfection. These include close attention to any manufacturer's guidelines on disinfection practices (e.g. restrictions on temperature, preparation, chemical compatibility, etc.) and/or local guidelines, requirements, or legal rules. For example, many biocides or chemicals used in disinfectant preparations may or may not be used in certain geographic regions or will require local registration with an authorized regulatory authority prior to use in healthcare facilities. These may include various efficacy and safety requirements (e.g. environmental safety is a growing concern worldwide). Care should therefore be taken to understand any local requirements and to ensure that any changes or updates are considered in the use of chemical or even thermal disinfection products/processes. The concerns related to microsurgical devices, ophthalmological instruments, loan devices/sets, devices with integrated electrical components, robotics, endoscopes, and textiles should be considered as outlined in Chapter 8 in the section on special cleaning considerations.

Thermal and chemical disinfection will be affected by the quality of the water provided. In some cases chemical contaminants such as high chlorine and water hardness levels can lead to device damage (rusting) or the deposition of chemical deposits (scaling) on surfaces. In both cases these can lead to patient complications. Further, the chemical quality of water can affect the ability of a chemical disinfectant to be effective (such as the presence of water hardness and even heavy metals that can significantly affect the disinfection activity of these products, depending on their formulation). The microbial water quality can also be important. High levels of microorganisms in water used as part of a chemical disinfection process may affect the overall efficacy of the product. This is a further concern in water used to rinse a device following disinfection, where the disinfection may be successful but then the water used for rinsing can recontaminate the device and lead to patient infections; this has been highlighted, for example, in the inadequate processing of flexible endoscopes following high-level disinfection and the inadequate design or maintenance of washer-disinfectors (or automated endoscope-reprocessing machines) used to process such devices. In addition to the microbial risks of infection in these cases, high levels of certain types of bacteria (Gram-negative bacteria) may be present, can be inactivated, but then release toxins (with Gram-negative bacteria endotoxins; see Chapter 5 on bacteria) that can lead to toxic complications in patients. Note that endotoxins are known to be resistant to thermal disinfection and even sterilization process conditions and may not be inactivated by these processes.

Flexible endoscopes

Special considerations in the cleaning and processing of flexible endoscopes have been outlined in Chapter 8 in the section on endoscopy. These apply equally to disinfection. Remember that a flexible endoscope can involve various components, including the endoscope itself used on the patient, its accessories, and the control system (with its own accessories such as to provide water and air during the procedure). The control system is a non-critical device but will require routine cleaning/disinfection of various surfaces using low- to intermediate-level disinfectants (e.g. daily or after each use). Various parts may become soiled or otherwise contaminated during procedures (in particular due to staff handling). Some systems provide a source of water and associated pipework for delivery to the endoscope during the procedure (e.g. for cleaning lenses at the distal tip of the endoscope or for irrigation of internal tissues during the procedure). These water bottles should be provided with sterile water, but also should be routinely cleaned and disinfected/sterilized, or be disposable. This is a good example of how mistakes can happen in processing, where the device is clean and disinfected and the water used for the procedure is labeled as sterile, but the water bottle in the system is contaminated. In this case, the water bottle also requires periodic processing in accordance with the manufacturer's instructions. A typical example is to rinse the water bottle with fresh water, assist drying with 70% alcohol, and steam sterilize. Specific device manufacturer's instructions should be considered regarding the disinfection of the control system, associated water bottles, and other accessories.

Flexible endoscopes are generally temperature sensitive, being restricted to cleaning and disinfection processes below 60°C, and are therefore commonly processed using low-temperature (chemical) disinfectants and sterilization processes. These can be conducted under manual immersion methods or as part of disinfection (washer-disinfection) processes (Figure 9.18).

It is important to make sure that all parts of the device are adequately immersed in the disinfectant to ensure antimicrobial activity, which includes that all internal surfaces of device lumens are contacted (and air removed from them) during manual immersion (e.g. by immersion and flushing of the lumens under the disinfectant) and by correct attachment of all lumens to an automated irrigation system. Further, it is important to consider any accessories that are used as part of the device or during the device procedure (see Chapter 15, Figure 15.3). This will include the control valves ("buttons") used with the device, which are commonly overlooked. Remember that these valves may be single use or reusable and be required to be cleaned and disinfected/sterilized as an important component of the device. Due to their design, they may require to be correctly opened (or actuated, by opening and closing) to ensure that all parts of the valve are correctly exposed.

The various steps in processing of a flexible endoscope include:
- Point-of-use treatment (bedside procedure).
- Manual and/or automated cleaning and rinsing.
- Manual or automated disinfection (or sterilization, if available).
- Rinsing (if applicable). Note that in rare cases rinsing may not be required in certain types of washer-disinfectors; if this is claimed by the manufacturer, it should be verified and documented by the facility.
- Drying, if applicable.

Further consideration is given next to the disinfection and drying stages.

The most widely used disinfectants used for flexible endoscopes include aldehydes (glutaraldehyde and OPA), oxidizing agents (PAA and hydrogen peroxide, as well as chlorine dioxide and super-oxidized water methods), and other miscellaneous biocides or mixtures of biocides such as QACs and glucoprotamine. All of these are used in formulation and individual formulations will vary depending on the required exposure conditions and antimicrobial claims; it is not sufficient to consider the concentration of the biocide (or antimicrobial) alone as this can be misleading. Remember that each formulation will vary depending on safety, efficacy, device compatibility, preparation method, shelf-life (when being used or stored), temperature, monitoring systems (e.g. use of chemical indicators to confirm the MEC; see the section on disinfection guidelines and standards), number and method of rinses, and so on. In all cases, care should be taken to read and understand the label claims and instructions provided with the disinfectant.

In some countries, specific soaking times may be recommended in independent guidelines that are different to product

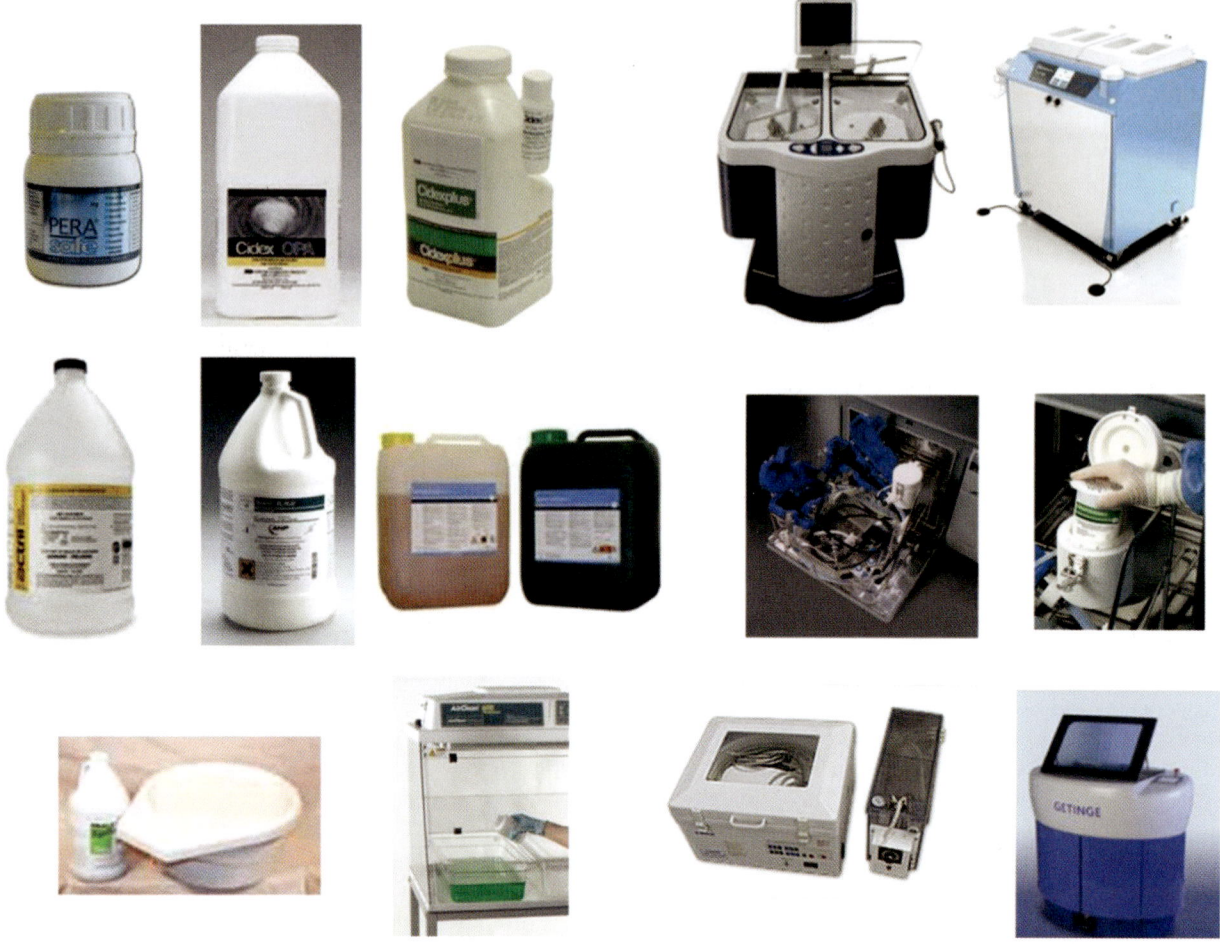

Figure 9.18 Various types of manual and automated flexible endoscope disinfection products/disinfectors. Various types of disinfectants (single- and two-component; upper left), manual immersion baths (lower left) and automated disinfectors (right). Images with permission of Sword Medical Ltd., Johnson & Johnson, and Medivators Inc.

label claims; in these cases this is a facility decision, and should be specified and approved in a written protocol to prevent staff confusion. Due to differences in country/region testing and registration requirements, it is not unusual for the same disinfectant to have different label claims in different countries. It is therefore important to understand any local requirements or restrictions in the use of disinfectants (e.g. certain biocides may not be recommended for use in each region or may have specific handling/disposal requirements).

Some formulations are only designed for use in automated systems under temperature control, while others are designed for manual and/or automated processing. In manual immersion systems, care should be taken to ensure that all surfaces of the device are adequately immersed/covered in the disinfectant, including the internal lumens. The presence of air bubbles, for example, on immersed surfaces can limit contact by the disinfectant with all surfaces. Automated systems generally provide various types of irrigation or flow-type systems that are designed to flow the chemistry through the internal channels; they may also use spray- and/or immersion-type methods to disinfect the outside surfaces of the endoscope.

In addition to ensuring disinfectant/disinfection efficacy, consideration should be given to the safe handling of the chemical disinfectant. Safety considerations include risks to staff, devices, patients, and the environment. All disinfectants are potentially hazardous to health, therefore contact with them should be minimized. This can be done manually using a well-ventilated area, chemical extraction hoods (Figure 9.19), and by covering open disinfection baths. Automated systems are often preferred as they should limit access/exposure to the disinfectant. Safety has been highlighted with the use of aldehyde-based disinfectants due to occupational hazardous

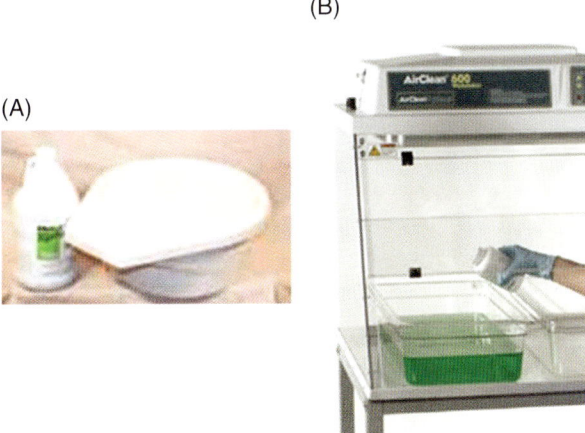

Figure 9.19 Manual immersion safety, showing (A) a covered soaking bath and (B) use of the disinfectant in a chemical safety cabinet.

that were often overlooked (e.g. irritation to the skin, mucous membranes, and respiratory tract; see the section on aldehydes) but may be equally true in the handling of other types of disinfectants. Exposure risks should be specified in the SDSs provided with the disinfectant; if these are not provided the disinfectant should not be used.

Information regarding compatibility with the device and device materials should be provided by the disinfectant manufacturer. It is preferable that a disinfectant is approved for use by the device manufacturer, but failing this a written statement of compatibility should be provided by the disinfectant manufacturer. In general, aldehyde-based disinfectants are widely compatible with flexible endoscopes, while oxidizing agent and other biocide disinfectants can vary considerably.

Rinsing is an important consideration following chemical disinfection, to minimize any patient safety risks. The endoscope should be rinsed, manually or in a programmed/validated automated system according to the disinfectant manufacturer's instructions, to ensure that no chemical toxic residual remains on the device. In some cases, up to five or six rinses in fresh water may be required to ensure that all external and internal surface residuals are correctly removed prior to patient use. Disinfectant residuals have been frequently reported to lead to significant patient complications. A typical example is with the use of glutaraldehyde and OPA; both types of disinfectants can be difficult to rinse away from surfaces and have been associated with complications such as colitis (irritation of the colon) following colonoscopy procedures. Toxicity may be related not only to the biocide but also to the other components of the disinfectant formulation.

There is a further consideration with rinsing: contamination of the rinse water being used. Water can include a variety of chemical and microbial contaminants, even if it has been previously treated to reduce such risks (see Chapter 15, in the section on water quality). Therefore, the control of water quality is an important consideration to ensure that the device is not recontaminated prior to patient use. National and regional guidelines can vary considerably on this point to include:

- Rinsing with tap water, followed by flushing internal lumens with alcohol to aid in (but not as a replacement for) drying.
- Rinsing with filtered water (generally using a "sterile" or bacterial retentive filter).
- Rinsing with water previously sterilized by steam or provided sterile.
- Rinsing with highly purified water, such as deionized, distilled, or RO water of the correct chemical and microbial quality.

All of these methods may be considered safe depending on the quality (chemical and microbial) of the water being used and the subsequent use of the endoscope. For example, the quality of tap water can vary widely, even from day to day, including microbial and chemical contamination. But equally, treated water (by filtration or purification) can become recontaminated on storage or transfer to the point of use for rinsing. For low-risk endoscopy procedures (e.g. an investigational colonoscopy), processing of the endoscope followed by a rinse with tap water can be used to remove disinfectant residuals and bacterial contaminants present in the tap water can be reduced by alcohol flushing and drying; however, tap water and even 70% alcohol can often be contaminated (remembering that alcohol is not an effective disinfectant for certain types of microorganisms, particularly bacterial spores). Therefore, it is always optimal for the microbial quality of the water to be maintained at a low or essentially no contamination level. For microbial contamination, an guideline that is used in the routine monitoring of bacterial contamination is:

- <1 cfu/mL: satisfactory.
- <1–9 cfu/mL on a regular basis: acceptable, indicates that bacterial numbers are under reasonable control.
- 10–100 cfu/mL: unsatisfactory, investigate the potential problem and/or repeat testing.
- >100 cfu/mL: unacceptable, out of service until quality is improved.

These levels may or may not be acceptable depending on the use of the endoscope (procedure, blood contact, etc.). Any system providing, treating, or holding water for rinsing should be correctly maintained to ensure that it does not itself become contaminated; for example, biofilms (e.g. with bacteria such as *Pseudomonas* and *Mycobacterium* species) can easily form within these systems leading to cross-contamination of endoscopes during rinsing. Maintenance may include routine disinfection (by heat and/or chemical) of water storage/handling lines or self-disinfection cycles of the washer-disinfector/separate water-treatment equipment. Equally, certain types of chemical contaminants may cause problems, such as high levels of chlorine leading to device damage over time (see the later section on troubleshooting disinfection). Overall, local guidelines should be considered and regularly monitored in providing staff with facility-approved instructions. In some cases these are required to be validated by the washer-disinfector manufacturer and be routinely monitored by the facility.

Drying of the endoscope is a further consideration, particularly when the device has been disinfected and is to be stored for some time. Drying will prevent the growth of bacteria/fungi in the device lumens during storage. Guidelines are equally variable on this topic and include:
- Purging of water from the device lumens using air and wiping down the external surfaces with a clean cloth.
- Use of alcohol (typically 70%) to assist in lumen drying, following and during air purging as already described.
- Purging of any large volumes of water from internal lumens and placing the device into a specifically designed flexible endoscope storage cabinet that allows HEPA-filtered air to pass through the lumens to dry and/or maintain dryness during storage (an example is shown in Figure 9.18).

Remember that purging is used to remove gross volumes of water but does not ensure that the device (and internal lumens) are dry and could still promote bacterial growth.

Drying may therefore be done as a manual or automated method. Some washer-disinfectors use air to purge the majority of water from the lumens (or external device surfaces) and/or provide a 70% alcohol rinse. Drying with the use of 70% alcohol is sometimes recommended after each and every processing cycle, particularly where tap water is used for rinsing, or more commonly at the end of the day/patient list prior to device storage. Equally, the use of 70% alcohol may not be required or may even be recommended against. At a minimum, flexible endoscopes that have been high-level disinfected and not in use should be stored under dry conditions (including the lumens) in a dedicated area/cabinet to prevent damage (Figure 9.20). It is recommended that they are hung vertically, not over-coiled, and protected from accidental breakage. Specially designed storage cabinets are used for this purpose that provide HEPA-filtered air to pass through the device lumens (when correctly connected) to assist in drying. In most cases, it is recommended that the device is re-disinfected

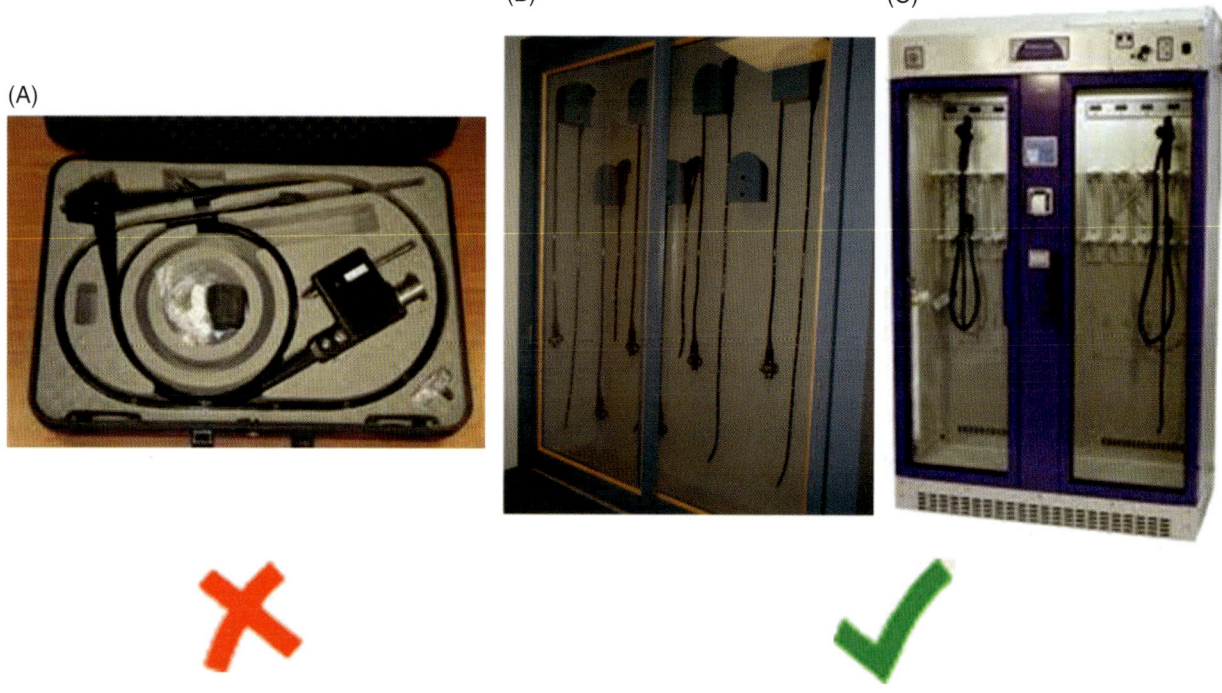

Figure 9.20 Flexible endoscope storage. (A) When not in use, flexible endoscopes should *not* be stored inappropriately, such as in their transport cases. They should be correctly stored in dedicated storage cabinets. (B) Cabinets may simply allow the devices to be safely stored by hanging or (C) for the device lumens to be connected to a high-efficiency particulate air (HEPA)-filtered air source to allow for and/or maintain drying.

immediately prior to patient use following storage; however, if the device has been correctly dried and maintained dry during storage (e.g. according to instructions provided by storage cabinet manufacturers) this may not be necessary. Local guidelines should be reviewed in considering safe and acceptable practices for a facility.

Following disinfection (and drying, if applicable), chemicals may be used for the maintenance of some devices or device components (such as lubricants). These should be used safely under the guidance given by the manufacturer.

A variety of automated systems may be used for the processing of flexible endoscopes, such as disinfectors or washer-disinfectors (Figure 9.16). These can vary in complexity and include immersion and/or spray systems for disinfecting the outside of the scope and irrigation (flow) systems for lumen cleaning. Some washers use specifically designed connectors that attach to the endoscope and irrigation/flow system of the machine, while others use a pressurized system at the control head of the scope to provide flow (connector-less washers). They may or may not provide a variety of features such as lumen blockage testing, irrigation control, detection of connector attachment/detachment, disinfection process parameter control, rinse-water quality control, or fault alarm systems.

Remember that a machine is only as good as it is designed, used, and maintained. A common problem is that a lumen connector has not been attached (or is not attached correctly) or has become detached during the cycle. A further issue is in the maintenance of the system, where bacteria biofilms may develop (particularly in the rinse water system/lines) and can cause recontamination of the device during the automated process. The disinfector manufacturer should provide an assurance that these risks are minimized in the machine's design and associated instructions for use. Information should also be provided by the manufacturer regarding the testing and validation of disinfection efficacy, preferably in compliance with local national or international standards/guidelines. At a minimum, the disinfector should be provided with at least one disinfection process that has been shown to be effective for endoscope disinfection/rinsing. The disinfector may be designed for use with one or many types of disinfectants. Useful standards to consider are ISO 15883 Parts 1 and 4, with Part 4 being specific to flexible endoscope washer-disinfectors.

One of the prevalent causes of failure in flexible endoscope processing is human error. Examples include:
- Failure to clean/disinfect the whole device, including the accessories.
- Failure to ensure that all lumens are cleaned/disinfected and detect if they are not.
- Failure to use the disinfectant or disinfection machine according to manufacturer's instructions.
- Recontamination due to inadequate water quality.
- Inadequate endoscope storage.

These risks should be minimized by correct and frequent training (and competency assessment) of staff; this is particularly important where a department has a high turnover of staff. Flexible endoscope processing can be a difficult task and is often performed in departments that have little time to ensure it is performed correctly. Training should highlight the structure and safe handling of flexible endoscopes, separation of dirty/clean areas within a dedicated processing area, manual cleaning, how to use and troubleshoot automated processing systems, manual or automated washing-disinfection, rinsing requirements (manual or automated), maintenance of the endoscopes and processing equipment, and safety. Health risks should be specifically highlighted, including the risks associated with manual cleaning (including brush), use/disposal of chemicals, and requirements for PPE.

All facilities should have a written policy on the safe processing of flexible endoscopes. Various international and regional endoscopy organizations provide and periodically update guidelines on safe practices. Due to differences from country to country, these may vary and even unfortunately contradict each other, therefore it is important to ensure that the correct local requirements are considered in establishing and maintaining written facility instructions. Some of these organizations are listed in Table 9.8.

Table 9.8 International and regional endoscopy organizations.

North America
AAMI: Association for the Advancement of Medical Instrumentation
AORN: Association of periOperative Registered Nurses
APIC: Association of Professionals in Infection Control and Epidemiology
ASGE: American Society for Gastrointestinal Endoscopy
CSA: Canadian Standards Association
CSGNA: Canadian Society of Gastroenterology Nurses and Associates
SGNA: Society of Gastroenterology Nurses and Associates
Europe
BSG: British Society of Gastroenterology
ESGE: European Society of Gastrointestinal Endoscopy
ESGENA: European Society of Gastroenterology and Endoscopy Nurses and Associates
RKI: Robert Koch Institute and the Federal Institute for Drugs and Medical Devices (BfArM)
Australia
GENCA: Gastroenterological Nurses College of Australia
GESA: Gastroenterological Society of Australia
International
WGO: World Gastroenterology Organisation
WHO: World Health Organization

Laundry

Textile processing (preparation, cleaning, disinfection, and drying) has already been considered in some detail in Chapter 8, in the section on textiles and laundry. Textiles may often become heavily contaminated (soils, such as blood and feces, and microorganisms) and present a risk of transmission to staff/patients, therefore they require safe handling and processing. Standard safety precautions (including PPE) should be taken in handling contaminated or patient-used materials. Disinfection of textiles provides some unique challenges given the types of materials being treated. Healthcare laundry disinfection is usually conducted in a washer-disinfector design (see Chapter 8, in the section on textiles and laundry) and some materials may also require further packaging and sterilization. Disinfection is performed by thermal (>65°C) and/or chemical means (<65°C, e.g. using chlorine, ozone, or PAA under controlled temperature conditions). The cleaning and disinfection process may be conducted as part of the same stage or separate stages of the processing cycle. Other chemicals are used as part of the process, including for cleaning, specific stain removal, and load conditioning.

Thermal disinfection is conducted in the same manner as for instrument disinfection, in a time- and temperature-dependent manner. A typical recommended condition is a minimum temperature of 71°C (160°F) for 25 minutes, but overall the same A_0 requirements would apply to textiles as described earlier. Temperature distribution is an important consideration and should be confirmed for a specific weight or load of textiles; remember, under- or overloading the washer may lead to negative effects (e.g. inadequate disinfection or drying). Following moist heat disinfection, hot air drying and ironing are also considered effective to reduce microbial loads in textiles. Lower temperatures can be used in combination with chemical biocides. Chlorine (specifically the addition of bleach/sodium hypochlorite at ~50–150 ppm) and the use of alkaline detergents (at high pH, >10) at temperatures ranging from 20 to 50°C are traditional examples. It is important to note that high-alkaline applications need to be adequately neutralized (to a neutral pH) if used for cleaning (prior to disinfection with another biocide) or on completion of the cleaning–disinfection cycle during rinsing. Other types of chemical disinfectants that have become popular in recent years, due to their cleaning/disinfection effects or reducing the consumption of water/energy, including direct application of PAA or ozone. PAA is added in as a liquid or solid-generation type of disinfectant and then rinsed to remove any residuals (and odors, as PAA has a strong associated vinegar smell). Ozone (O_3) is a popular alternative, being produced in a generator (e.g. based on passing dried air or an oxygen source through a corona discharge or UV light) and directly injected into the washer water (e.g. by bubbling/diffusion) for the desired concentration/contact time (Figure 9.21). In general, chemical applications are used at lower temperatures to reduce energy costs and for optimal antimicrobial activity.

Antiseptics

Antiseptics are disinfectants that are used on the skin and mucous membranes. They include hand washes, hand rubs, surgical scrubs, pre-operative preparations, and various other types of preventative and therapeutic products (e.g. mouth rinses, biocide-containing creams, etc.; Figure 9.22). They are generally low-level disinfectants, being specifically designed to remove and/or inactivate microorganisms (particularly bacteria) but also not to irritate the skin. The most widely used antimicrobials are alcohols, iodine, chlorhexidine, and certain types of phenolics like triclosan. The role of antiseptics in infection prevention and control is discussed in Chapter 5 and further consideration given to their use in Chapter 6, in the section on antiseptics.

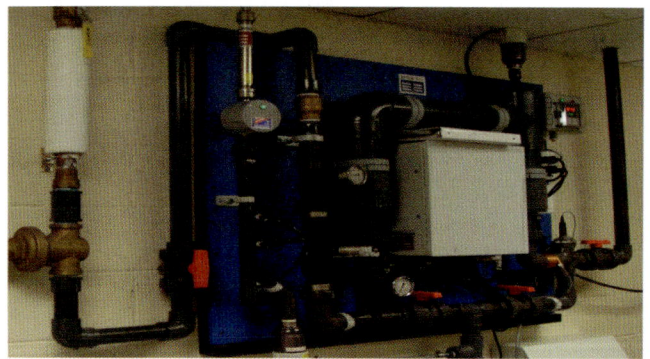
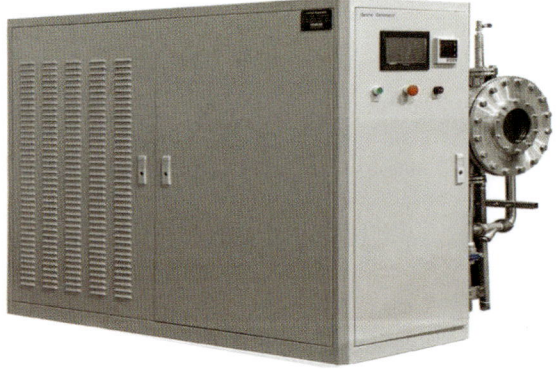

Figure 9.21 Examples of ozone generators used for laundry applications.

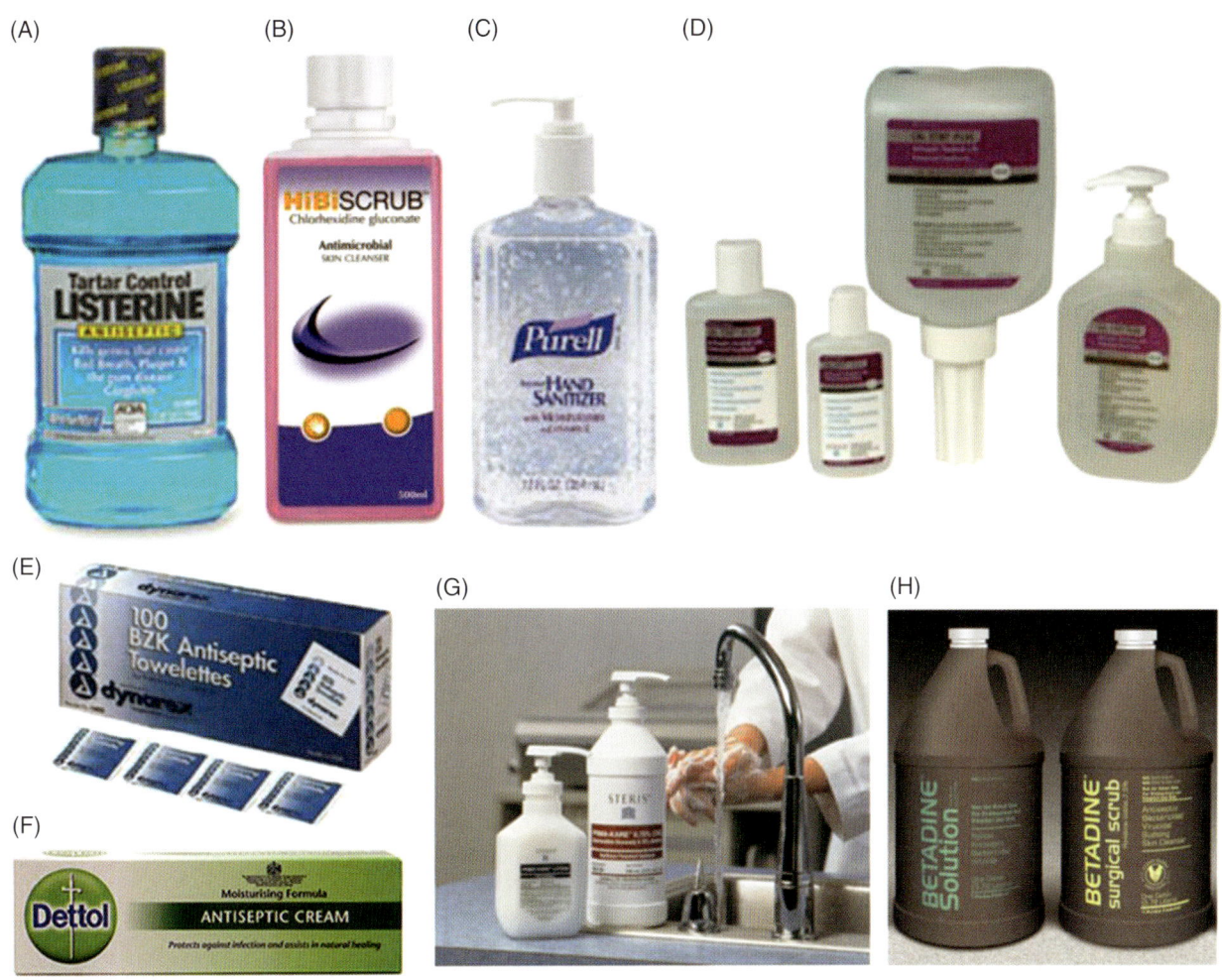

Figure 9.22 Examples of various types of antiseptics. (A) With permission of JNTL Consumer Health Middle East FZ-LLC. (B) With permission of Lagaay Medical. (C) With permission of GOJO Industries, Inc. (D) With permission of Thermo Fisher Scientific Inc. (E) With permission of Dynarex Corporation. (F) With permission of Reckitt Benckiser. (H) With permission of Emerson Betadine Solutions.

Environmental disinfection

Environmental disinfectants are specifically used for the disinfection of a variety of hard surfaces such counter-tops, beds and bedrails, wheelchairs, floors, toilets, phones, computer keyboards, and other types of non-critical devices such as non-invasive monitors and other general medical equipment. These surfaces can be a source of unseen contamination, particularly within a healthcare facility, for the transfer of microorganisms to patients (see Chapter 5, in the section on infection control and prevention strategies). This can be expected to occur directly by patients themselves (by touching a contaminated surface and cross-contaminating themselves, such as by eating, accidentally contaminating a wound, etc.) or by contact with medical/surgical staff and visitors (contaminating their hands/gloves and transferring the microorganisms to a patient).

Some equipment can be removed from its normal location for clinical use and routinely cleaned/disinfected in washer-disinfectors that use thermal or chemical disinfectants (as discussed earlier in this chapter). But in some cases it is subjected to manual cleaning–disinfection using chemical disinfectants at the point of use or at a centralized location, which can also include repair or calibration of such equipment. Examples of commonly used chemical surface disinfectants are formulations that include phenolics, QACs, alcohols, chlorine-based solutions (such as "bleach," being preparations of sodium hypochlorite that release chlorine), iodophors (which release iodine), hydrogen peroxide, chlorine dioxide, and PAA. They can also be provided in a variety of forms such as in concentrates (requiring dilution in water for use), ready-to-use preparations, two-component chemistries requiring mixing (activation) prior to use, disinfectant-impregnated wipes, and even fumigation systems (where gas- or liquid-based disinfectants are automatically distributed around an area/room).

Overall, environmental disinfectants will be similarly labeled for use to device disinfectants, but with specific consideration to their recommended environmental use. It is important to note that it is extremely rare for a disinfectant to be labeled for use as both a device and an environmental disinfectant. In fact they are most often considered different products and, as a rule, should only be used according to their specified label claims. Environmental disinfectants are often also classified as low-, medium-, or high-level disinfectants, but more often will have specific antimicrobial claims provided with their recommended conditions of use. These include claims such as bactericidal, viricidal, germicidal, and sporicidal. Care should be taken to closely inspect any such label claims and how they have been verified (as highlighted previously). For example, in the United States the term "germicidal" only refers to antimicrobial activity against certain types of bacteria, specifically *Staphylococcus aureus*, *Salmonella enterica*, and *Pseudomonas aeruginosa*, in a standardized test (noting that this excludes other bacteria with known higher resistance to inactivation such as *Mycobacterium tuberculosis*). Label claims (regulated and unregulated) can vary significantly from country to country, based on various test methods and exposure conditions (such as exposure time, presence/absence of interfering soils, etc.).

Environmental disinfectants are often not used correctly to ensure that they are safe and effective. A typical use pattern will be applying the disinfectant to a surface and wiping it off immediately. The disinfectant may not have even contacted all required surfaces or had any time to be effective against the target microorganisms. The presence of soil will also significantly affect the ability of the disinfectant to provide the desired antimicrobial activity. As highlighted for other disinfectants, the disinfection efficacy will only be as good as how it is used (see the first two sections of this chapter). Most importantly, the disinfectant needs to be prepared (if applicable) and used in accordance with the manufacturer's instructions. An important consideration is the contact time for disinfection. Typical test conditions can range from five minutes to three hours for certain types of standardized test methods and associated disinfection claims. Overall, disinfectant label claims should be closely inspected, and manufacturer's instructions for use should be followed to ensure the optimal use of environmental disinfectants.

It is not necessary that all surfaces in a healthcare environment are regularly disinfected. In many cases (such as floors and ceilings) cleaning (or the physical removal of microorganisms and visual soiling) is considered sufficient and will itself adequately reduce patient safety risks. But care should be taken to ensure that many high-touch or high-risk surfaces are routinely and adequately disinfected. This includes high-risk surfaces around the patient such as bedrails, emergency call buttons, and potential food-contact surfaces, as well as surfaces that are routinely used by healthcare workers such as computer keyboards, touch surfaces on patient monitoring equipment, and even door handles. In certain microbial outbreak situations, where there is a sudden increase in the number of cases of an infection putting other patients/staff in the vicinity at risk, more detailed consideration of environmental disinfection is often considered necessary (see Chapter 5, in the section on the role of infection control and prevention). Within a device-processing area, routine environmental surface disinfection should be particularly considered in any manual cleaning or soiled device handling areas (e.g. as described in Chapters 7 and 8), where the risks of microbial contamination and accidental transmission to staff can be a concern.

Prion disinfection

Prion disinfection has been the subject of investigation since prions' description as transmissible agents. Traditionally prion disinfection (and/or sterilization) methods have included the use of harsh, oxidative chemicals. Examples of these, as recommended by the WHO in 1999, include:

- Immersion in 1–2M NaOH (sodium hydroxide, a strong alkali; see Chapters 6 and 15) for one hour at 20°C. Equally effective was immersion of the device in 1M NaOH and subjecting this to an extended steam sterilization cycle (e.g. a gravity displacement cycle at 121°C for one hour) or disinfection temperatures (e.g. boiling for 10 minutes). "Steam sterilization" in this case refers to a mechanism of heating only, as these experiments consisted of prion material immersed in NaOH solutions and did not consider what exact temperature was achieved, air removal, etc. that are required for a typical steam sterilization process (see Chapter 11). It is noted that recent experiments have shown that lower concentrations of NaOH, other alkalis, and some alkaline cleaning formulations may be effective at higher temperatures.
- Immersion in ≥20,000 ppm (~2%) NaOCl (sodium hypochlorite, the major component of household "bleach") for one hour at room temperature (~20°C).

Some of these methods are not only considered to be effective against prions but will also have significant activity against bacteria, fungi, and viruses; however, in both cases significant damage may occur on device surfaces with the use of such chemical procedures, and they are generally not recommended by device manufacturers. These aspects are considered in further detail in Chapter 15 in the section on devices known or suspected to be contaminated with prion material. More recently, alkaline cleaning and disinfection processes have been shown to be effective (depending on their formulation and process conditions, such as concentration, exposure time, and temperature). Similarly, some other chemical formulations and process conditions have been described as effective against prions, including gaseous hydrogen peroxide, some phenolic disinfectant formulations, and other formulation mixtures. Any claims associated with such products should be carefully inspected and understood.

To date the typical conditions of thermal disinfection have been shown to have little effect on prion decontamination. In general, much higher temperatures are considered to be required and longer exposure times than those typically used for sterilization (e.g. 121°C for 1 hour or 134°C for 18 minutes; see Chapter 15). Chemical disinfectants or disinfection processes may or may not have some effect. Some types of biocides are not recommended due to their known mechanisms of action. Examples include aldehydes and alcohols, in that they may even increase the risks of transmission due to their cross-linking or protein-fixation effects. Others such as the oxidizing agents, including chlorine, PAA, and hydrogen peroxide (particularly in gas form), may have some benefit, but this will depend on the product formulation or process conditions. It is incorrect to conclude that oxidizing agents can reduce the risk due to any potential claims of protein degradation or removal from a surface alone.

Overall, chemical disinfectants should not be considered to have any beneficial effect in reducing the risk of prion contamination unless specific testing is completed to demonstrate that the product is safe for such use (see Chapter 15, in the section on devices known or suspected to be contaminated with prion material). Unfortunately, this may or may not be predicted based on the type of chemical biocide.

Troubleshooting disinfection problems

Many of the considerations discussed in the section on troubleshooting problems with cleaning (Chapter 8) are also applicable to disinfection. Unlike cleaning, where a visual examination of the device may be acceptable to say whether the device has been cleaned or not, evaluation of the success/failure of disinfection is difficult. Microorganisms may be present but will not be seen. Therefore, the successful application of a disinfectant or disinfection process, along with any associated verification checks, is essential to ensure a safe process.

The greatest risk for device disinfection lies with manual disinfection (thermal and/or chemical), therefore it is recommended that any variables of the disinfection process are monitored and, if possible documented. These include exposure times, temperatures, preparation methods for the disinfectant, CIs for use with chemical disinfectants (to verify the MEC, as discussed earlier), and so on. Thermal disinfection will only be achieved if all parts of the device are contacted for the minimum specified temperature and contact time; equally, chemical disinfection requires the correct formulation/biocide concentration (including preparation when applicable), contact time, and exposure to all parts of the device, but may also depend on temperature, pH, and so on. The same concept applies to any risks of residual toxicity remaining on the device in the use of chemical disinfectants, for example number and times of rinses.

These risks can be reduced but not eliminated with automated washer-disinfector or disinfectors. These machines need to be correctly designed, used, and maintained to ensure a reproducible and adequate disinfection process. Modern washer-disinfectors, in particular those compliant with ISO 15883 (as discussed earlier), are provided with the means to verify that important variables of the process have been achieved. In such cases, known as independent monitoring, variables such as temperature, pressure, dosing volumes, and contact times are controlled by the machine but independently verified by a separate set of monitoring sensors. The data collected from these sensors may be checked directly by the machine and compared to the control sensors, providing an instantaneous alarm if the process is detected to be incorrect; in other systems the data may need to be downloaded from the washer-disinfector (e.g. onto a computer or printed out) and manually checked to ensure the process is correct. In addition to these sensors (known as parametric sensors), chemical indicators are also used in automated systems to ensure that the disinfectant has been present during the process (although it is important to note that these will not confirm that the disinfectant has actually contacted all surfaces of the device/load). Although these automated systems can reduce the risks of inadequate disinfection, they still need to be used (loaded) and maintained correctly, as highlighted in Chapter 8 in the section on troubleshooting problems with cleaning. Overall, in both manual and automated systems, human error can be an important variable; the best way to reduce this risk is by having written procedures, routine training of staff, and periodic assessment of staff competency and inspections.

Disinfection, both by heat and particularly with chemical disinfectants, can be compromised by the presence of patient soils (blood, lipids, fats, proteins, etc.) that have not been adequately cleaned from device surfaces. This is due to the protection of microorganisms within these soils from the effect of the disinfectant and the reaction of the biocide with the soil preventing contact with the microorganisms. Aldehydes, for example, can potentially fix soils onto device surfaces, thereby protecting any internal microorganisms from disinfection, and oxidizing agents can be rapidly inactivated (depending on their concentration) by the presence of organic soils. Further negative effects can be due to the presence of cleaning chemistry residuals (e.g. enzymes used in cleaning formulations are proteins and can remain on inadequately rinsed devices following cleaning) and poor water quality (e.g. where the presence of water hardness or chemicals such as heavy metals can compromise the activity of the disinfectant formulation). In conclusion, if the device is not cleaned it cannot be assumed to be disinfected (or even sterilized; see Chapter 11).

A limited but increasing number of devices cannot withstand the typical thermal disinfection conditions, such as flexible endoscopes (see the earlier section on flexible endoscopes). It is obvious that these devices should not be heated to over 60°C to prevent damage. Heat tolerances are usually described by the device manufacturer in its instructions for use or processing guidelines. Device compatibility is often an important consideration in the use of chemical disinfectants. As highlighted in the section on flexible endoscopes, aldehydes often provide better device compatibility with such devices/materials but are difficult to rinse away, while oxidizing agents can range considerably based on their use and formulation. Therefore, when considering chemical disinfectants, it is optimal for the device manufacturer to provide a statement of compatibility with a given product (not a type of biocide); but as this is not always practical a written assurance of compatibility should at least be provided by the disinfectant/washer-disinfector manufacturer.

Water quality can also play a role with both thermal and chemical disinfection techniques (as previously highlighted in Chapter 8 in the section on troubleshooting problems with cleaning). This includes:
- Interference with the activity of chemical disinfectants (e.g. high levels of water hardness and "heavy" metals such as copper, chromium, and lead).
- Filter damage, leading to breakthrough of bacteria and other microorganisms over time (e.g. with high levels of chlorine).
- Device damage and rusting (due to chlorine and other chemicals, particularly when heated).
- Build-up of various deposits and color changes on device and equipment surfaces (these were highlighted in Chapter 8). Examples include water hardness (white, grainy deposits), phosphates (orange-brown staining), and acids (black staining).

The importance of water quality and troubleshooting problems associated with it are discussed in further detail in Chapter 15.

10 Inspection, assembly, and packaging

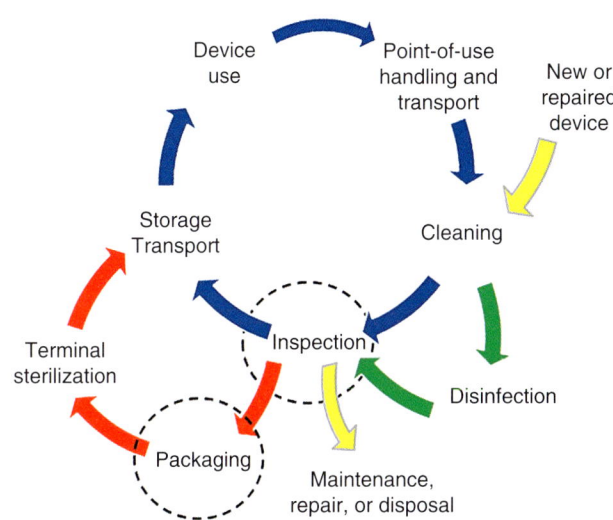

Reusable devices can be subjected to cleaning and disinfection and/or sterilization (see Chapter 1 on the decontamination process). Inspection (and when appropriate the disposal or repair of devices) may be conducted as a single or in many step(s) during the processing cycle. As an example, non-critical devices can be inspected immediately following cleaning/disinfection and may also be inspected immediately prior to patient use. Most critical (and many semi-critical) devices are also packaged in a way that prepares them for sterilization and sterile storage prior to a patient procedure. In some unique cases, critical devices may not be packaged but must be used immediately following sterilization (no sterile storage). This chapter considers the inspection of devices prior to patient use, and packaging when this is applicable prior to sterilization.

As discussed in Chapter 1 (in the section on the design of a decontamination area), processing facilities should be designed to prevent the inadvertent mixing of contaminated/soiled devices with decontaminated/clean devices. Following cleaning and disinfection (if applicable), devices should be held in a designated "clean" area where decontaminated devices are checked for cleanliness and functionality. Following this the device(s) can be correctly assembled (if required), safely transferred (to prevent recontamination) to a patient area for use in a procedure, or prepared for further sterilization. In a busy processing department, thousands of devices may pass through these areas daily, and each device has the potential to significantly influence the patient's outcome. Devices that are not correctly cleaned can pose a serious risk of infection or other patient adverse effects (e.g. toxicity; see Chapter 8). Likewise, if devices are not disinfected correctly, microorganisms or other contaminants may be transferred to a patient with significant health consequences (see Chapter 9).

Area design

The design of "clean" areas can range from a designated part of a single room or, preferably, to a physically separated room of a facility design that includes a dedicated air-handling system.

Devices that only need to be cleaned (e.g. non-critical devices) and/or disinfected (non-critical or semi-critical devices) should be handled in a designated "clean way," ensuring a flow from dirty to clean to prevent mix-ups, but this does not generally need to be conducted in a specifically designated room; however, it is best practice to have a dedicated room or at least an area for equipment or device processing. With increasing concerns regarding the use of certain semi-critical devices (such as flexible endoscopes that may often be used for semi-critical or critical procedures), such dedicated facilities are often considered necessary. For critical devices, which need to be prepared for subsequent sterilization, a dedicated inspection, assembly, and packing room should be considered. Such rooms are designated "controlled environments." A controlled environment is defined as a zone in which sources of contamination are controlled by specified means. It is distinct from a "cleanroom," which may require a higher level of environmental control that may not always be necessary for a sterile processing area, but is certainly best practice. Such rooms are controlled to prevent contamination with air contaminants that may come from "dirty" areas (e.g. cleaning areas), other hospital or external areas, and even from staff and materials that are present. Cleaning "dirty" areas is designed to keep contamination within a given risk area, while clean areas or rooms should be designed to keep contamination out. Ideally these dedicated rooms are maintained at a differential, positive pressure (e.g. at a 10 Pa pressure difference to the cleaning or external areas) and are physically separated from the cleaning area, with restricted access.

Specific air-handling systems can be employed to maintain these conditions and to circulate the air in such a way as to maintain a low particle count in the area. In such designs, the circulation of air can be controlled, but also the quality of the air can be maintained by passing the air continually through designated filter (high-efficiency particulate air or HEPA filter) systems that will remove contaminants above a certain size. Examples of air contaminants that may cause concern include bacteria, fungi, hair, skin cells, dust particles, lint, and other materials. Regular air particle counts can be determined in this area (to ensure the air-handling system is working effectively) and staff should wear low-linting clothing to ensure that specifications are met. In addition to controlling the presence of contaminants, area designs should also consider temperature and humidity controls for the comfort of those working in the area and to ensure that conditions are not excessive in respect to the various different label claims of the equipment or materials used in the area (e.g. packaging materials).

In summary, design criteria for designated "cleanroom" areas should include:
- Separation of "clean and dirty" (preferably physical or a separate room).
- Controlled, limited access.
- The clean area must meet specific temperature, humidity, and air-exchange controls.
- Controlled, monitored air quality and environment, such as 10 air exchanges per hour.
- Positive pressure to reduce the presence of airborne microorganisms (e.g. 10 Pa with respect to external areas).
- Comfortable working environmental temperature (18–23°C or 66–73°F).
- Comfortable and compliant air humidity levels (e.g. 40–60%).
- Adequate space for inspection, handling, maintenance (if applicable), and packaging of devices.
- Adequate availability of materials for packaging, sterilization, and process monitoring.

Despite the design of clean areas, the effective management of microbial and particulate quality levels in these areas is dependent on the people who work there following facility guidelines. Guidelines should be in place to protect both workers and patients and to maintain a clean environment. Entry and exit procedures should be defined, including attire and best practices while working in the area. Routine cleaning/disinfection of all work area surfaces and equipment will assist in controlling the spread of microorganisms. A maintenance schedule must be in place to ensure that the temperature, humidity, and air control is kept constant, as well as routine maintenance of the air-handling system (e.g. periodic changes in HEPA filters). On installation and periodically, the air-handling system may be checked for the adequate flow of air through the system/room (e.g. using air-flow visualization tests such as smoke tests) and air microbiological or particle counts should be conducted (e.g. using air particle sampling systems) to ensure they are correctly maintained.

Personal attire and other material considerations

As discussed in Chapter 8 on cleaning, personal attire (including personal protective equipment, PPE) is designed to protect staff from various microbiological and chemical risks encountered during the receiving, sorting, and cleaning of devices/materials. In the clean area, personal attire and materials should be suitable to prevent any microbiological or chemical risks from being transferred from the technician to the patient. The following should be considered:

- Wear and use only low-linting materials; linting materials, such as cotton, can lead to complications if introduced into a patient during a surgical procedure.
- Defined clothing only to be worn within the clean area (e.g. surgical scrubs). Staff and visitors should wear these on entering the room and remove them on leaving, usually in a designated anteroom.
- Hair (including beard) covering should be worn when applicable.
- Closed shoes should be worn and shoe covers may be considered (to reduce transfer of floor contamination from outside into the area).
- Gloves may or may not be worn; if they are used, it is recommended that they are powder-free and non-latex. Latex gloves can lead to severe allergic reactions in some people and powder is an unnecessary source of contamination (particularly on cleaned devices). Although the use of gloves can be debated, it should be remembered that the skin is a source of microorganisms and protein contamination (see Chapter 2 on the integumentary system). If gloves are not used, frequent washing of hands is recommended to reduce cross-contamination risks.

Guidance

It is important to understand and employ best practices when inspecting, assembling, and packaging devices to ensure that the devices are maintained safely for patient use. Inspection, assembly, packaging, and labeling policies and procedures should be established within the facility. These procedures should define the facility practices regarding the handling of devices within these areas and the monitoring of the care and use of devices and equipment. Guidelines and standards regarding facility design can vary from region to region. Examples of such guidelines include:

- The ISO 14644 series of standards define cleanroom and associated environment requirements, including classifications based on air particulate levels. ISO 14698 is a series of standards on recommended controls, including decontamination, in clean rooms and associated controlled environments. These and similar standards/guidelines are published by ISO and local organizations such as the Association for the Advancement of Medical Instrumentation (AAMI) in the United States.
- Health Building Notice (HBN) 13 on Sterile services departments, Department of Health and Social Care, United Kingdom.
- ANSI/AAMI ST79, a guide to steam sterilization and sterility assurance in healthcare facilities, including inspection and packaging area requirements.
- Australasian Health Facility Guidelines Health Planning Unit B.190 Sterilizing Services and Endoscope Reprocessing Unit.

Inspection

Each device should be individually examined and inspected for cleanliness, functioning, and signs of damage. Other criteria may apply, depending on the devices, associated instructions for use (IFU), and stage of processing. For example, following a washer-disinfector drying process (Chapter 9), critical devices should be inspected for dryness, and if moisture is detected this should be addressed at the inspection phase (e.g. manual or automated drying processes). Where possible the inspection and functional testing should be carried out independently at the workstation. All non-conforming products should be removed from service; for example, devices that are dirty or stained should be rejected and returned to the wash area for recleaning or for specific remediation (e.g. for stain removal). If any device is found to be defective or malfunctioning, it must be replaced with a functioning one. Defective devices must not be returned to the set and should be identified for replacement or repair.

Only trained personnel familiar with the manufacturer's instructions and/or local policy should carry out inspections. Inspection criteria should be defined in standard procedures to ensure quality. For staff safety, it is recommended that devices are only tested for function once cleaned and preferably disinfected.

Manufacturer's instructions should be followed at all times when handling and inspecting devices. Disregarding the manufacturer's recommendations may damage or shorten a device's life, as well as impacting patient safety. Device manufacturers should supply guidelines on the use, safety considerations, care, and maintenance of their products (see Chapter 1 on where to start). Such written instructions and any other technical documentation should be provided by the manufacturer on delivery, to ensure that the device will be used in a safe and effective manner, and to minimize the risk of harm to either the user or the patient. Legally, this document absolves the manufacturer of liability in the event that the guidelines are not followed. The liability for the functioning of the device then transfers to those who process it, which is why it is important that all processing staff are aware of the instructions and trained in the appropriate use and care of each device. If these guidelines are not adhered to then the manufacturer's warranty will generally become null and void. The appropriate manufacturer's guidelines should be directly accessible to all staff working in the processing area at any time. If these documents are lost or unavailable, a new set needs to be obtained from the manufacturer. Most IFU are now available online, but care should be taken to ensure that the correct current version of instructions specific to the devices being used is being referenced.

The manufacturer's guidelines or IFU should include the following important information on the proper use and care of the device:

- Definition of the intended use of the device.
- Provision and explanation of safety-related information regarding proper handling, use, and operation of the device.
- What may constitute misuse, including any particular warnings.
- Limitations and restrictions on processing.
- Functional and safety tests.
- Cleaning, disinfection, and/or sterilization instructions (where applicable). It is recommended that at least one method of manual or automated processing has been validated by the device manufacturer. Preference is clearly given to providing automated methods.
- Types of physical or chemical processes/products that may or may not be used during device processing or maintenance.
- Lists of accessories and consumables that may be used with the device.
- Requirements for safety inspection of the device/equipment.
- Requirements for planned maintenance (e.g. lubrication, repair, etc.).

Ignoring, not fully recognizing, or not understanding the manufacturer's instructions may result in decreased efficiency of the device, deterioration of the equipment, or harm to the user or patient. It is essential that appropriate staff training is given and that the training program is documented and regularly reviewed for new equipment and/or new employees.

In many cases, as with complex devices, training should preferably be given by the manufacturer with regular refresher courses.

Cleanliness

The objective of cleaning is to remove or significantly reduce the presence of contaminants, including microorganisms (bioburden), from an item to an acceptable level so that it can be safely used or safely disinfected/sterilized. Inadequate cleaning may result in damage to the device such as rusting, corrosion, and pitting, and the transfer of toxic residues to a patient. There are many different types of methods that can be used to determine that a device has been adequately cleaned. Ensuring a consistent cleaning process overall provides a further level of security that sufficient cleaning has been performed. Visual cleanliness is a minimum requirement following cleaning. Other endpoints of cleaning (for semicritical and critical devices) are also in use and include determination of the levels of bacteria/fungi (microbiological methods) and biochemical and chemical tests. The most common biochemical marker used is protein. Protein-detection methods can be very detailed, generally requiring a biochemical laboratory to evaluate; however, various types of readily available test kits have been developed for routine healthcare facility use. These are considered in this section and in more detail in Chapter 8 on cleaning guidelines, standards, and testing, as well as in Chapter 14 on management and quality.

Visual inspection

Visual inspection is the most common method used to provide evidence of cleaning and proper functioning of most devices. Inspection using the naked eye alone, however, may not always be effective as it relies on the individual's eyesight and ability to detect residual soil. Further, visual inspection is not practical with any device that has internal components, such as cannulated (lumened) devices, or where parts of the device cannot be seen. The original condition of the item before cleaning will have a significant effect on how adequately it can be cleaned. Devices that are subjected to prior rough handling (during either surgical/medical procedures, processing, or transport) will develop scratches and roughened surfaces that can harbor materials that are difficult to detect. Damaged surfaces will allow dirt and microorganisms to collect, and also be potentially dangerous for both staff and patients. Therefore, visual inspection is not limited to inspecting the device for cleanliness but also ensures that it is not damaged and is fit for use (see the later section on functionality testing).

The processing manager (or designee) is responsible for having a basic visual/enhanced visual inspection policy and determining the type of medical devices to be visually inspected using some type of enhanced magnification, like an inspection scope (borescope) or other means according to that specific medical device's IFU. In cases where the manufacturer's IFU state that inspection should be done under magnification, devices should be inspected in this manner every time they are processed. Inspection results should be recorded. This allows the processing staff the ability to monitor and improve their cleaning process based on the data from their inspection (this is problem analysis; see Chapter 13 on the importance of this to physical and emotional health).

Optical aids are available to assist with the inspection of devices: lighted magnifying glasses with interchangeable lenses and small magnifiers are ideal (Figure 10.1). Adequate

(A)

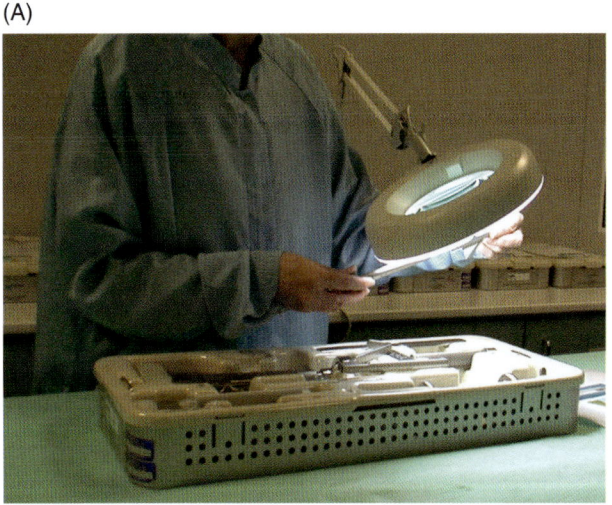

(B)

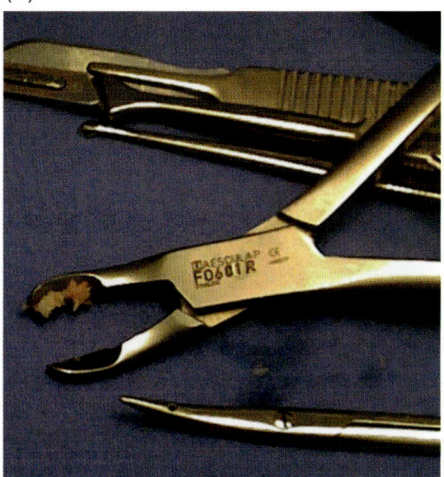

Figure 10.1 (A) Use of an optical aid (lighted magnifying glass) to inspect devices for cleanliness and damage. (B) An example of a soiled device (note the jaws on the bone nibbler).

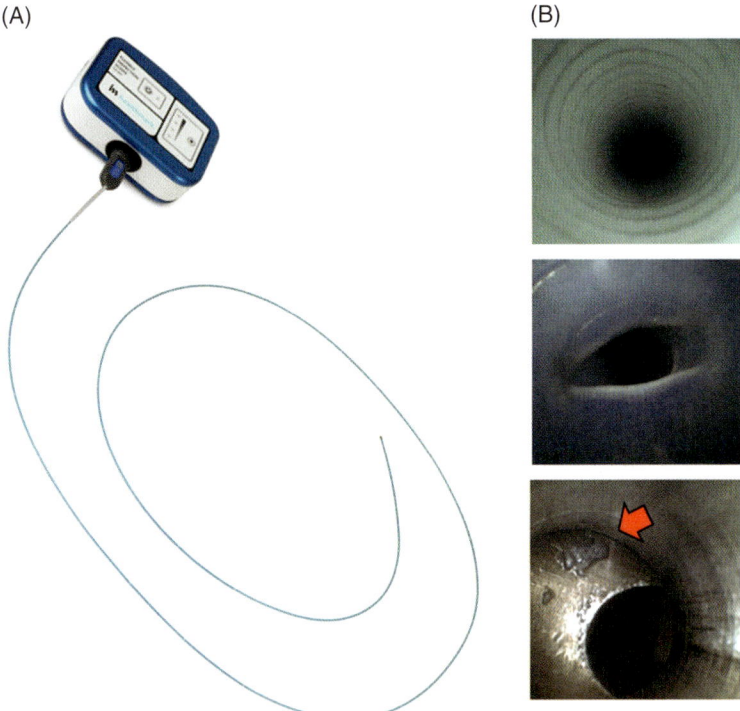

Figure 10.2 (A) Example of a borescope for inspection of lumens. (B) Examples of a new, clean lumen (top), a damaged (crushed) lumen (middle), and soil present in a lumen (arrow, bottom).

lighting is critical when staff are attempting to identify small details and should not be undervalued. Some bodily fluids that contain no obvious color are transparent (e.g. cerebrospinal fluid; see Chapter 2 on the nervous system) and create more of a challenge as they cannot be seen easily with the naked eye. The processing manager (or designee) is responsible for ensuring initiation, completion, documentation, and analysis of the enhanced visual inspection policy. When writing inspection procedures, use the manufacture's IFU, standards, and guidelines as well as peer-reviewed article(s) to support the practice. Implementation will only be successful if the staff are properly trained not only on the equipment being used but on what is acceptable or non-acceptable concerning visual cleanliness for each medical device being inspected. Visual inspection alone might not be sufficient for assessing the efficacy of cleaning processes; the use of methods that are able to measure or detect organic residues that are not detectable using visual inspection should be considered in facility cleaning policies and procedures.

Other technologies, such as microscopes and borescopes, will increase quality in any department's inspection practices. Borescopes in particular may be used to inspect channels such as in endoscopes and other difficult-to-see areas and their findings may highlight defects that require repair, additional cleaning, or other action. The value of such inspections is dependent on image quality, but is also impacted by the skill and technique used by the operator of the inspecting device, hence training is critical. An example of a borescope and various images are shown in Figure 10.2.

Biochemical tests

Biochemical or chemical tests are used as they are more sensitive and less subjective than visual inspection (see Chapter 8 on cleaning guidelines, standards, and testing and Chapter 14 on quality management and monitoring cleaning). But this may not always be the case. Consider, for example, how the device is tested: Is the whole surface sampled or is only part of the device tested? Is the method of testing effective to remove what may or may not be present on the device? What is the detection method specifically detecting? These aspects should be considered and be defined by the manufacturer of the method or kit being used to detect soil. It is also important to highlight that as for any indicator, it may be useful to verify that a cleaning processes has been conducted but this may not ensure that the device(s) has been cleaned. Overall, while biochemical tests are not a replacement for visual inspection, they may provide a more sensitive method for the detection of soil and of whether a device is clean. At the time of writing, as discussed in the introduction to Chapter 8, visual cleanliness is considered adequate to indicate that cleaning has been effective, but in some parts of the world more sensitive methods are recommended for use with semi-critical and critical devices. The most common biochemical markers used are test methods for protein (see Chapter 8, Table 8.4). Proteins are one of the four major types of molecules that make up cellular structure and function (including human and microbial cells) and are therefore a key component of soils found on devices. Laboratory studies that have investigated the different soil components found on devices after patient use have highlighted the presence of protein; it is not only a major component of soiling on a device but is also considered a sensitive marker as to whether a device has been cleaned or not. Protein-detection methods can be very detailed, generally requiring a biochemical laboratory to evaluate them; however, various types of test kits have been developed for routine healthcare facility use. These are generally swab-based tests, where the swab is used to wipe the surface (note: without touching the hands or other surfaces that can themselves contain high levels of protein) and is then exposed to a chemical that detects the presence/absence of protein at a certain level. These may range from simple color-change reactions to more sophisticated light-emitting types of assays (where the level of light equates to the level of protein). Examples of various types of protein test kits are shown in Figure 14.10 and are further discussed in Chapter 14 in respect to quality management and monitoring cleaning. These kits can vary in the methods they use for protein recovery and detection, guidelines on how they should be used/controlled, and protein-detection levels. Some of these systems use different types of chemicals to aid in the detection of protein on devices, and the removal of such chemical residuals should be considered in order to reduce any patient safety risks. As a general guide, the level of protein that may be considered "clean" has been suggested to be about $\leq 6.4\,\mu g/cm^2$ protein on a device surface (see Table 8.4 and the associated discussion in Chapter 8).

Other types of biochemical tests are used to aid in soil detection. These relate to the following types of soil:
- Adenosine triphosphate (ATP) is a molecule that is present in most living cells, including human and bacterial cells. Therefore, the detection of ATP can be an indirect indicator of the presence of contamination (including bacteria/fungi and patient soil) on a surface. ATP test kits are available based on surface swabbing and detection of ATP within a monitoring device or simple color-change types of indicators.
- Blood/hemoglobin detection can be achieved using hydrogen peroxide; various different types of enzymes that are found in blood cells break down the peroxide to release oxygen, shown as bubbling. Kits are available for the sensitive detection of blood contamination, such as swab-based tests that give a color change in the presence of low levels of blood.

Functionality tests

As well as checking that devices have been properly cleaned, all items should be subject to functionality testing to ensure that they will perform the tasks for which they are designed. It is the duty of the processing area also to manage the inventory of devices, which involves knowing how to care for devices, which individual parts must be tested, and when devices should be repaired, refurbished, or even replaced. Devices that are not cared for and handled correctly can have a shorter life span, which leads to an increased requirement for repair or replacement, and higher costs. It is the responsibility of processing staff to ensure that devices are functional, available, and assembled in the right sets to meet the demands of surgery and the wards. For patient safety it is crucial that all devices are maintained in optimal working condition. Damaged devices can cause clinical delays or cancelations and, if the damage is undetected, can even cause patient injury.

Only trained staff familiar with the manufacturer's instructions and/or local policy should carry out inspections, which include checking for damage and ensuring that the medical device is functioning. To ensure staff safety and reliable functioning, it is recommended that instruments are only tested for function once they have been cleaned and preferably disinfected. If any problems are noted during the inspection process, the item may need to be sent for repair or disposal, depending on the problem observed.

Each instrument should be individually examined and inspected for cleanliness, proper functioning, and damage to surfaces. The following general guidelines are given for the inspection of devices (for reference on instrument/device types, see Chapter 4):
- Ensure that devices with serrations or inserts on the jaws are free from any visible materials and are not damaged (e.g. chipped or missing parts).
- Check devices for corrosion (rusting, surface damage) that may lead to further damage or device breakage. While visible stains and rust can be removed using commercial stain removers (acid cleaner; see Chapters 6 and 8), the underlying device damage is already present and will likely continue to be further damaged at this site, leading to permanent damage.
- Open and close ratchets using one hand and feel whether they move easily. Stiffness in the joint is an indication of debris in the joint; if it is not cleaned, over time the joint will fail.
- Check that the tension is being maintained on instruments with box locks or ratchets.
- Check hinged devices such as clamps and forceps for stiffness.
- Test devices that grip or clamp for their holding strength.
- Check devices with cutting edges such as scissors, rongeurs, or curettes for sharpness. There should be no dull spots, chips,

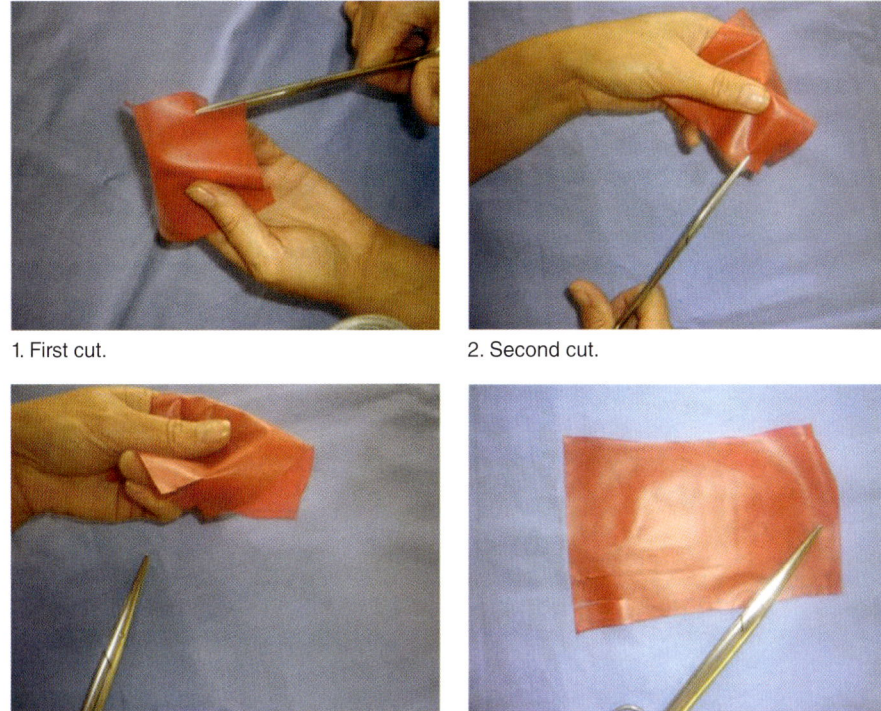

Figure 10.3 Sharpness testing with red THERABAND.

or dents. THERABAND test material can be used for checking the sharpness of scissors and rongeurs (Figure 10.3).
• Check that moving parts (such as hinges and box locks) move smoothly throughout the intended range of motion. Lubricate hinges, threads, and other moving parts with a commercial, water-based, surgical-grade device lubricant ("instrument milk") to reduce friction and wear. Follow any specific manufacturer's guidelines regarding lubrication.
• Check that tips are properly aligned, jaws meet perfectly, and joints move easily.
• Run your fingers down device shafts to feel for dents. Check for bends and dents in devices with lumens, including trocars.
• Check that where individual parts form part of a larger device assembly, all parts are present, matching, and can be assembled.
• Check the presence and condition of device identification/marking systems, for example devices with marking tape or those that have coating rings. These easily become brittle after multiple processing cycles and particles fall off. This is very likely to occur during surgery, resulting in adverse patient issues. Generally, both of these device identification methods are discouraged in most countries, as they may not have been considered during the design and processing validation of the device. If they are used, then they must be routinely replaced when they are chipped, torn, and rough, or if the edges of the tape start to curl or come off, or if there is an excess of glue residue at the edge of the tape. It is recommended to consult the manufacturer's technical data regarding such marking methods to verify that sterilization testing was performed.
• Check insulated devices carefully, ensuring that there is no breach in the insulation.

Examples of specific device inspections
Scissors

Scissors are designed to cut tissue and suture materials and should not be tested on any paper, types of tubing, or similar. All scissors are designed to be resharpened, with the exception of those with serrated edges, which are replaced when found to be blunt. Scissors dull first at the distal tip, where most of the cutting occurs. Inspection covers the following steps:
• Check the scissors' cutting action by opening and closing them to ensure a smooth glide that is not too loose, too tight, grinding, or jumping. The cutting blades should glide smoothly past each other.

- When testing scissors for sharpness use a THERABAND test material. Depending on the scissors' manufacturer, red THERABAND can be used for scissors larger than 4.5 inches and yellow THERABAND for scissors smaller than 4.5 inches (Figure 10.3). Make at least two cuts in the test material. The scissors should cut all the way through to the top of the blade. Check for catching or snagging and ensure that the scissors cut all the way through to the tip.
- Check that both tips are present and not damaged. Device tips are rounded and should not have burrs, which could cause puncturing and tearing.
- Check the distal ends (surgeon handling end) for bent blades or damage.
- Inspect for chips or burrs on cutting surfaces.
- Inspect tungsten carbide inserts for cracks, and check for pitting where the tungsten carbide meets the stainless steel. Tungsten carbide blades cannot be repaired and should be discarded if damaged.
- Do not over-sharpen scissors; if the carbide coating is ground off then the scissors will no longer be useful.
- Inspect both sides of the hinge for cracking, staining, or bioburden trapped inside the screw or screw head.
- Inspect the finger rings for cracks, which could cause the handles to break.
- Inspect the jaws for blood or bioburden.
- Check that the jaws are in alignment and fit together, not overlapping.
- If box joints are present, check for soil and cracks on both sides of the hinged area (in particular the closed sides).

Tissue and dressing forceps

Forceps inspection covers the following steps:
- Check the tips (jaws) to see that they are even and undamaged.
- Check that there is no overlap and that tips meet evenly.
- Check that teeth are not broken and inter-fit smoothly.
- Check distal serrations for blood or baked-on debris.
- Check proximal ends (handle, spring, and forceps link) for cracks.

Hemostatic forceps

These are used primarily to occlude vessels and control blood flow. Hemostats are designed to clamp blood vessels and should not be tested on any type of tubing. A typical inspection covers the following steps:
- Check that tips are rounded and do not have burrs, which could cause puncturing and tearing.
- Check that both tips are present.
- Check distal ends for bending or damage.
- Check that the forceps do not stick abnormally.
- Inspect for chips or burrs on tissue-holding surfaces.
- Check tips of serrated hemostat forceps – Crile, Kelly, etc. – for alignment; they should meet equally, with no overlap.
- Check that the teeth of hemostat tissue forceps – Allis, Kocher, etc. – are intact, straight, and that jaws inter-fit. Check the space between the teeth for tissue.
- Inspect teeth and any serrations for soil.
- If box joints are present, check for soil and cracks on both sides of the hinged area.
- Test the ratchets by opening and closing. The action should be smooth and the ratchet should hold on each engagement (click). The tips should meet just before the ratchets engage and as the ratchets engage the entire jaw should mesh, clamping closed.
- To test the spring, set the clamp on the first ratchet and gently tap the device on a flat surface. If the instrument is "sprung" the ratchet will pop open.
- Check the spring area for cracks and soil.

Needle holders

These are used for holding suture needles and should not be tested on any type of tubing. Inspection covers the following steps:
- Check that tips are rounded and do not have burrs, which could cause puncturing and tearing.
- Check that both tips are present.
- Inspect for worn or chipped edges.
- Check the tread for wear on the tips.
- Check that cardiovascular needle holders are demagnetized by holding a needle against the tips; if the needle is drawn to the tip the holder must be demagnetized.
- Check smooth jaws for wear and tear by holding them up to the light. If light is seen the needle holder is worn and will not hold a needle.
- Check that shanks are not bent or misshaped.
- Check for cracked/missing inserts.
- Inspect the neck for cracks – the larger the crack, the longer it has been there.
- Inspect tungsten carbide inserts for cracks, and check for pitting where the tungsten carbide meets the stainless steel; tungsten carbide blades cannot be repaired.
- Inspect both sides of the hinge for cracking, staining, or soil trapped inside the screw or screw head.
- Inspect the finger rings for cracks, which could cause the handles to break.
- Inspect the jaws for blood or other soils.
- Jaws of needle holders must be able to hold a suture needle. Check that the jaws are in alignment and fit together, not overlapping.
- If box joints are present, check for soil and cracks on both sides of the hinged area.
- Test the ratchets by opening and closing. The action should be smooth and the ratchet should hold on each engagement

(click). The tips should meet just before the ratchets engage and as the ratchets engage the entire jaw should mesh, clamping closed.
- Check the spring area for cracks and soil.
- To test the spring, set the clamp on the first ratchet and gently tap the device on a flat surface. If the instrument is "sprung" the ratchet will pop open.

Suction nozzles

These are used to extract fluids from a surgical site or area of the body. Inspection covers the following steps:
- Inspect for sharp or abraded edges and for dents.
- Inspect the holes/cannula for blockages and trapped debris.
- Inspect the shaft for bending or dents, visually and by running your finger down the shaft to feel for dents.
- Check the suction control is unblocked, clear of debris, and working. Check any soldered areas of the device for cracks and soil.
- Check that the stylet can be inserted at the proximal end of the device.

Hooks and spatulas

These are used for retracting skin in various procedures. Inspection covers the following steps:
- Inspect the entire area, in particular the edges, for cracks and chips.
- Check for any buckling or bending on the device.

Self-retaining retractors

These retractors are used to open up the working space and improve visualization of the operative site for the surgeon. Tissue damage may result from mismatched retractor blades or points, causing tissue healing problems. Inspection covers the following steps:
- Check that flexible retractors are in their original shape and flat.
- Check that any small accessories with the device (e.g. washers, screws) are present – these systems cannot be used if such parts are missing.
- Inspect all parts to ensure that they are completely clean.
- Check that all parts are in proper working order.
- Particularly inspect any screws and springs for cracks/soiling.
- Check that all parts are moving freely – lubricate according to manufacturer's guidelines using an approved lubricant that is compatible with the device and any subsequent processing stages (e.g. sterilization).
- Inspect distal ends for bent blades and prongs.
- Check the release lever – when the release lever is "flicked" it should spring back into place.
- Retractors should open and close smoothly.
- Check that the ratchets hold in the open position by opening the retractor and simultaneously applying pressure to both shanks. The ratchet should unlock with minimal pressure.

Microsurgical instrumentation

Various types of microsurgical devices were considered in Chapter 4. They are used for particularly delicate surgical/medical procedures. Because of the high risk of damage, such devices should be handled with extra care. The tips of delicate and sharp medical devices should be protected to avoid unnecessary damage. These devices can be extremely fragile and must be inspected before and after every endoscopic procedure. Some eye micro-instruments can be unhinged to ensure proper cleaning (confirm with the manufacturer). Ensure that all devices are reassembled correctly after cleaning. Very delicate or sharp devices may have their tips covered with device caps (Figure 10.4).

Rigid endoscopes and accessories (such as trocars)

It is recommended that after cleaning, endoscopes are visually inspected for defects such as rough surfaces, sharp edges, or prominent parts, as these defects could harm the end user or patient. Endoscopes should also be inspected for any soil residues, but this is not easy, depending on the design of the endoscope (e.g. for endoscopes that are black in color, visually inspecting internal lumens is virtually impossible), unless using a borescope (Figure 10.2). Inspection covers the following steps:
- Inspect the telescopes for scratches, dents, protrusions, distal tip burrs, or other surface irregularities by running your fingers down the length of the endoscope.
- Pay attention to dents or defects due to high-frequency or laser surgery devices as well as cracks at the ocular (patient) end of the endoscope.
- Check that the surfaces of the light inlets and outlets are smooth and clean. If the surfaces show deposit layers, or rough fibers can be felt, this could lead to decreased illumination. If the endoscope is used or prepared in this condition, it may be continuously damaged over time.
- Test any moving components to ensure they are functional.
- If present, check the eyepiece and its seal on the device for visible signs of damage. Inspect and detach the eyepiece of the lens if it is detachable.
- Do not touch the telescope's ocular lens or the objective lenses to avoid fingerprints and debris that will impair the view and possibly cause scratches.
- Endoscopes with damaged glass surfaces (e.g. cracks), impaired image quality, or noticeable surface damage or distortions should not be used. In some cases they may be checked by directly viewing through the endoscope (with or without a light source).
- Check any proximal or distal glass surfaces, which must be clean and free from deposit layers.
- Check the image through the endoscope, which should be sharp and clear. This can be done by looking at a piece of

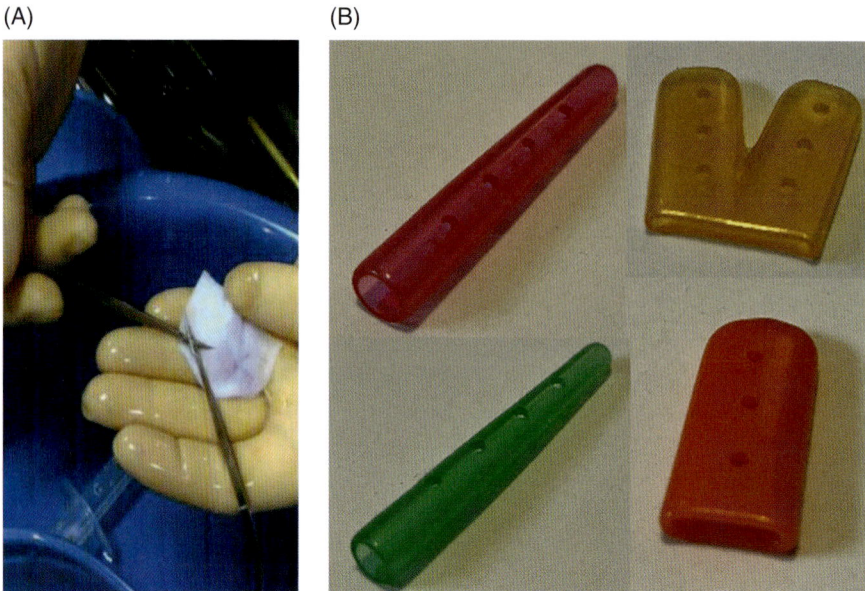

Figure 10.4 (A) An example of a delicate microsurgical device; note that this device should be closely inspected, e.g. tip inspection. (B) Various device caps, flat round and twin, that encapsulate and protect delicate tips.

non-glare white paper with printing. Start with the endoscope's distal tip about 3 inches from the paper and move the tip until it is about a ¼ inch from the paper. The printing should appear crisp and clear, with minimal distortion. Discolored or unclear print could be due to improper cleaning, disinfectant residue, a cracked or broken lens, moisture within the shaft, or external shaft damage that has broken some fibers.

• Check the light transmission through the fibers by holding the light guide connector against a light (not a cold light source). If numerous black spots appear on the distal end, the light output is insufficient. The black spots are broken fibers and the scope should be sent for repair (Figure 10.5). There are specialized test systems that can detect the percentage of broken light fibers in a device.

• On inspection of the proximal and distal lenses, they may be further cleaned with a lint-free cloth/swab saturated with 70% alcohol; repeat the inspection process. Some manufacturers may recommend the use of specific cleaning wipes. If the view through either lens remains cloudy or distorted after cleaning, the endoscope is damaged and should be sent for repair.

• Before reassembling, any stopcocks provided with the device may need to be treated (on their sliding surfaces) with a small amount of lubricant according to the manufacturer's instructions.

• Reassemble the endoscope according to instructions.

• Check and disconnect any associated light cables. These may be reprocessed separately from the other parts of the device.

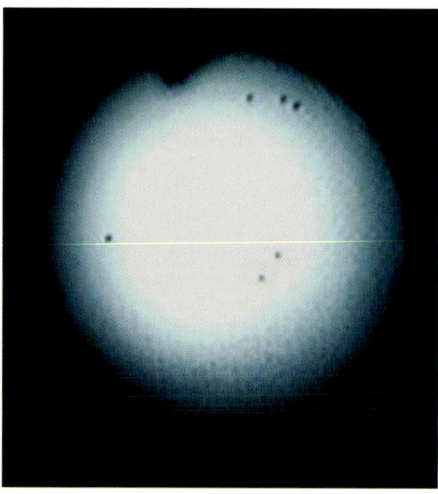

Figure 10.5 Checking endoscope light transmission. Broken light fibers are shown by black spots within the field of view.

Flexible endoscopes

Flexible endoscopes are very delicate devices with unique complexity. Close attention should be paid to the inspection of such devices prior to patient use or further processing. Inspection covers the following steps:

• Inspect for any extraneous materials or cracks at the working end of the endoscope (tip), including any moving mechanisms. A particular example is with the distal tip of a duodenoscope

(see Chapter 4, Figure 4.56) that contains an elevator mechanism; this area of the endoscope is particularly difficult to clean and soil can get trapped within the moving mechanism.
- Check the seals around the various parts of the distal tip lenses and other components. These are generally held in place by adhesives and may become loose or detached over time.
- Visually inspect the entire shaft of the device for nicks and cuts, as well as kinks or other irregularities along the length of the device.
- Physically check the device for any obvious damage and functionality. Ensure that all moving parts are moving freely.
- Ensure that all detachable buttons, valves, or caps are free of soiling and move freely. These parts will need to be reassembled with the device for patient use.
- Inspect any electrodes and light cables for damage.
- Inspect the connection post for the light source.
- Lightly pull back on the insulation; if you can slide it (or it becomes detached), the insulation needs to be replaced.
- Inspect that all channels are clear. Passing sterile or medical-grade air down each lumen is a widespread practice in many parts of the world. The introduction of borescope examination, which is now recommended in many endoscope processing guidelines, further enables visualization of structural damage, foreign material, and moisture within endoscopes. Such inspections are normally conducted during cleaning/disinfection and are also checked on setting the device up for a patient procedure (see Chapter 15 on endoscopy).

Electrical equipment

Electrical equipment should be handled with care and tested according to manufacturer guidelines. Failure to adequately inspect these devices can be dangerous for both patients and staff. Inspection covers the following steps:
- Reusable appliances should be disconnected from any mains current before cleaning and inspecting.
- Check for corrosion – electrical equipment (and indeed any device/equipment) should never be cleaned with saline as this causes corrosion.
- Move any control switches and check that they are operating.
- All insulated devices should be visually inspected for breaks in the integrity of the insulation each time the devices are processed to avoid possible injury to the patient and/or surgical/medical team. Devices that have an outer insulation coating, for example diathermy forceps, require close inspection to ensure that the insulation remains intact. Check that the insulating material and electrical cables are not damaged in any way and look for cracks and splits due to damage or wear. There are specialized test systems that can be used to verify that the device and cables are free from defects that allow leakage of electrical current.
- Check the battery pack if the equipment is battery driven.

- Lubricate all powered equipment and attachments according to the manufacturer's written instructions.
- Check that attachments fit firmly – improperly fitting attachments can be thrown from powered equipment, resulting in injury to patients and personnel.
- Check that any trigger handles are in the safety position to prevent accidental activation of powered equipment, causing injury to patients or personnel.

Maintenance, repairs, and replacements

All devices should be accompanied by instructions on routine and periodic maintenance and repair in order to maintain their safe and effective use. These instructions should give information on the type and frequency of maintenance, safety, and calibration check requirements, and should be directly accessible to the processing staff as well as those in charge of maintenance. It is recommended that a maintenance plan is put in place and that all maintenance or repairs performed are recorded; these may be performed by in-house staff (e.g. by trained biomedical engineers), an external third-party group, and/or the device manufacturer.

Devices are often damaged during their intended use or suffer from general wear and tear for a number of reasons, but are more often damaged due to inappropriate use, poor handling, or contact with corrosive chemicals/processes. Devices may be physically damaged due to being dropped on the floor or rough handling, or as a result of contact with agents during surgical/medical use, for example iodine or saline solutions. Damage typically seen with the naked eye can include rusting, pitting, or general surface corrosion (Figure 10.6).

If during inspection and function testing items are found to be faulty or damaged, or if a fault is identified by surgical/medical staff, the items should be taken out of use and either repaired or replaced. A written procedure should be in place describing which procedure to follow when a device is found to be damaged. The procedure should be agreed by both the processing staff and the users. It should include details about who should be notified, how the damage will be recorded, how replacements can be obtained, who should be notified if a replacement is not immediately available, whether the set can be packaged and sterilized without the missing item, and, finally, if an incomplete set is approved for sterilization, how it will be labeled so that the user is made aware of the missing device before the surgical procedure begins.

Devices identified as needing repair should be placed in a dedicated tray in the preparation room following the wash/decontamination procedure and recorded in a "damages" or "repairs" file. A decision must be taken on whether it is viable to repair the device or whether it needs to be disposed of and replaced. Devices for repair must be clearly marked, then

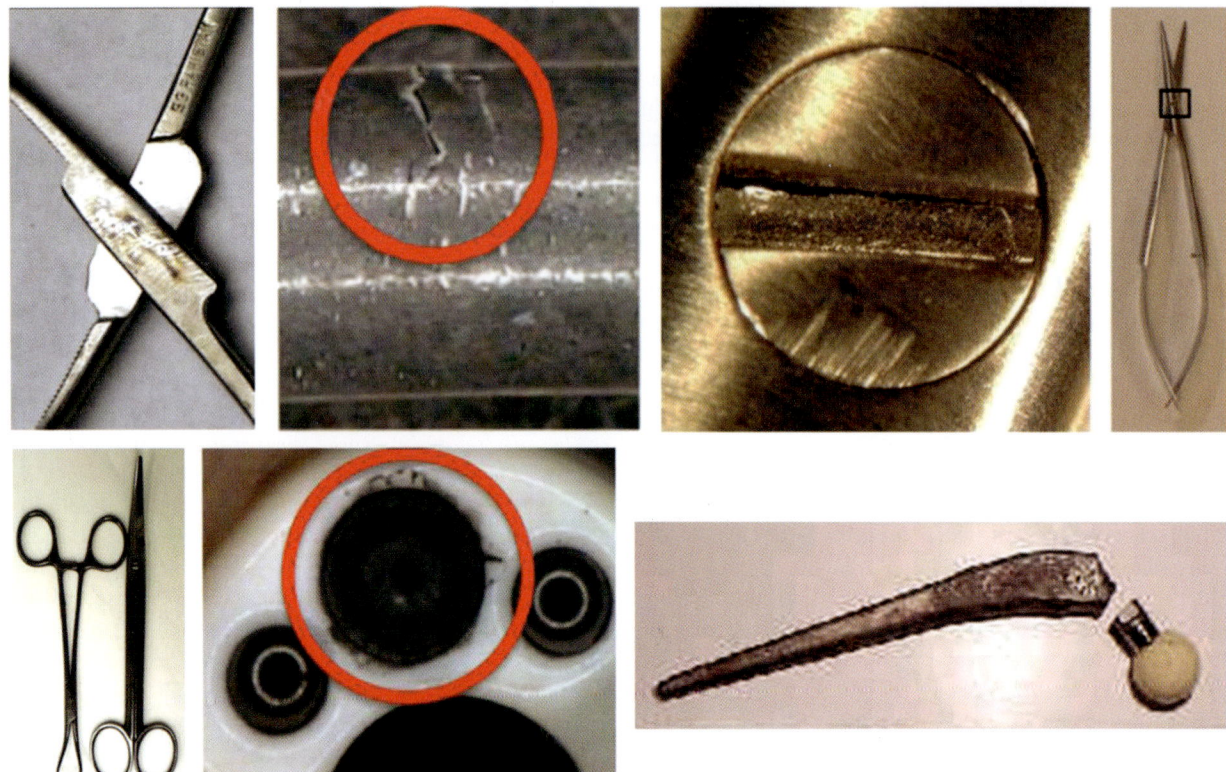

Figure 10.6 Examples of device damage. Rusting (top left) and staining (bottom left), cracking (top middle) and erosion of adhesives on flexible endoscopes, and stress cracking on devices (right). Some of these effects may be very obvious while others are not.

cleaned and disinfected or sterilized before being sent for repair, in order to protect the engineers. Devices for repair should be returned to a trained biomedical engineer/maintenance department, the manufacturer, or a reputable repair company.

Items sent for repair should be identified on the checklist (see the next section) and on the set to which they belong or, in the case of individual devices (for example endoscopes), that particular device noted on the list. If only parts of an instrument are sent for repair, the device should be held in a quarantine area until the repair has been completed and then reassembled/prepared for reuse.

Devices that cannot be repaired should be removed from use and if a replacement is not available, a note should be made on the device checklist to alert users. When devices that are part of device sets are taken out of use, the whole set should ideally be removed from use until the device has been repaired/replaced and returned to the set. This should be agreed with the surgical/medical personnel concerned.

After a device has been returned from repair, it is essential that it is exposed to all necessary processing procedures before being used for patient care.

If the manufacturer has limited the number of times that a reusable medical device can be processed, then accurate records must be retained in order to achieve compliance. The device must be discarded once that usage limit has been reached and the item replaced (see Chapter 4 on single-use, limited use, and reusable medical devices).

Device and tray assembly

Medical and surgical devices are used for a variety of procedures in healthcare facilities (see Chapter 3). These procedures can range from the use of a single device to a whole complicated set of devices used with many types of equipment (as is the case with most surgical procedures). In all cases, ensuring that the proper types of devices (and any accessories) for a given procedure are ready and available is important, particularly in endoscopic, surgical, and robotic procedures. It is therefore an important role of the processing staff to ensure that devices/sets are correctly prepared for patient use. For non-critical and semi-critical devices this is most often a direct or combined role of staff available within designated departments/facilities; but with critical (and sometimes semi-critical) devices that are processed by centralized departments, the devices are organized into sets for particular procedures according to the surgical/medical needs, packaged, and sterilized prior to distribution/use within the facility.

General considerations

Surgical devices are organized into trays, and then into sets, if applicable, to meet specific requirements for specific procedures. Each set will contain those devices that are required to perform a specific procedure. Sets may also contain basins, bowls, receivers, drills, implants, and other items that may be needed for that particular procedure. Therefore, trays/sets can range in complexity and in the number of devices that are needed for different procedures. This section provides guidance on how these trays/sets are assembled for sterilization and then subsequent patient use.

Given the range of devices that can be used for a given surgical procedure, the weight of device trays should be controlled. Consider, for example, an orthopedic set that may contain particularly heavy devices such as mallets. By limiting the weight of devices in a tray, this can reduce the risk of damage to the devices and also reduce any staff injury risks (as an ergonomic precaution). Note: ergonomics is the design of procedures, work areas, and equipment to reduce operator fatigue, discomfort, and injury, and is covered further in Chapter 13 in the section on physical and emotional health). Heavy trays can lead to back or arm strains and even more serious injury. The guideline weight for an object being carried using extended arms is 7 kg for a female and 10 kg for a male. Overall, it is best practice that instrument sets and trays prepared for sterilization should not exceed 11.5 kg (or 25 lb). As part of best practice and for the safety of staff, these weights should form the basis for how heavy the trays should be in assembly.

When assembling device trays/sets it is critical that staff understand what the devices are used for, that they are functioning correctly, and that each set is assembled in the proper manner for any given procedure. Training of staff is therefore important and can be assisted by the use of assembly aids, such as a "pick list" or "tray checklist" or a similar computerized system (Figure 10.7). Tray or set checklists provide a list

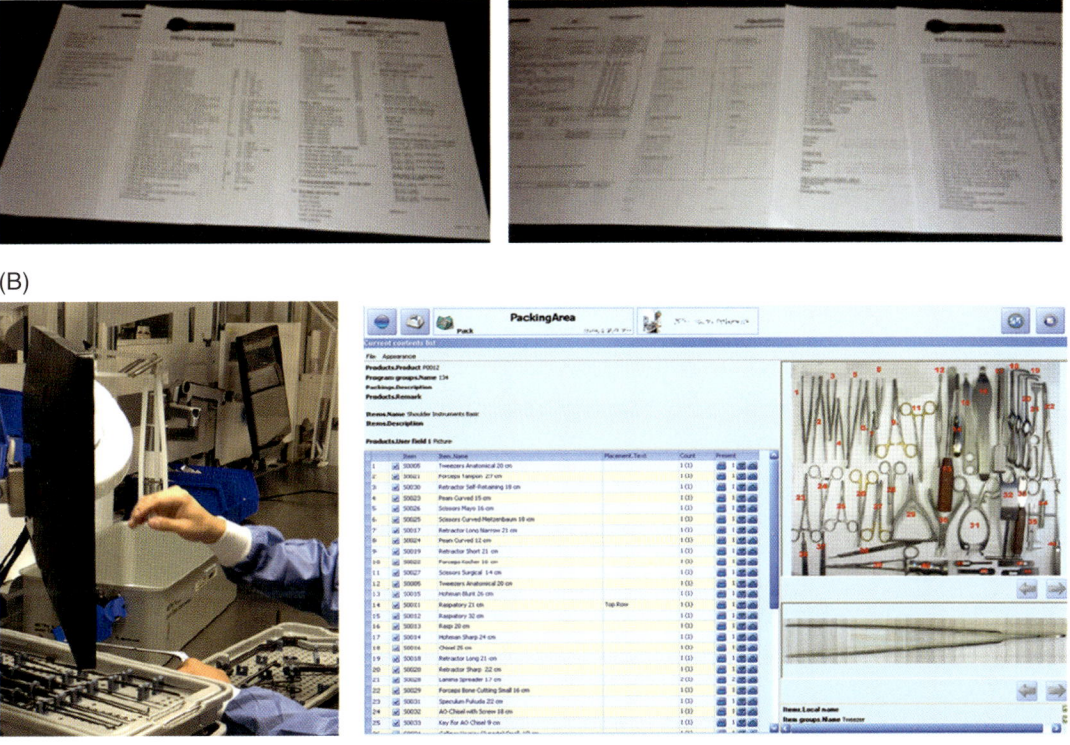

Figure 10.7 Examples of device tray and set checklists. A variety of different formats may be used. (A) Traditional paper-based checklists; the lists are completed by the member of staff assembling the tray/set and are usually signed on completion. (B) Examples of modern computerized systems for assembling device sets for surgery.

of devices that should be in the tray/set and can include pictures, device identification codes/numbers, item descriptions, quantity of devices, and so on. These may be paper or computer-based systems that assist staff in assembling the tray/sets correctly and in a standard manner. In computer-based systems the device may be scanned (to read a unique identification code) and confirmed as being in the applicable set (including, for example, particular checks, assembly, or maintenance that need to be conducted on the device at that stage).

These checklists can form the basis of a tracking and traceability system for devices within a facility. After verification in a central processing/assembly area, the set will be signed off by staff responsible for checking/packing, the checklists kept with the set/tray during sterilization and transport/storage, and then further verified by staff receiving, opening, and preparing the devices for surgical/medical use. Further, the same tray/set checklist should be used to verify that all devices are accounted for following a procedure and on transfer to a processing area. It is recommended in these cases that each responsible person in this cycle should indicate and sign that the quantities are correct and that nothing is missing. This allows sets or devices to be traced back to a specific person and located if applicable. It is not uncommon for devices and accessories to go missing, which includes removal of devices from one set to replace those in another set (instead of introducing an entirely new device to the incomplete set), accidental loss by mixing with linens or waste following a procedure in an operating room, or, in extreme though unfortunate cases, where a device is accidentally left within a patient following a procedure. Ultimately, the checklists can be archived, depending on whether they are used as a patient safety document or for inventory control; this may include them staying with the device set throughout (from processing to procedure and back to processing) or being filed with the patient's records post procedure.

Operating rooms use the greatest number and variety of devices and are by far the largest users of processed and particularly sterile items in a healthcare facility. Accuracy is thus vital when assembling devices in sets. The contents of device sets are usually decided by the surgical team. The assembly of a tray should be agreed by both the processing area and operating suite managers, as best fits the clinical need. However, it should be remembered that how a tray is assembled may have some safety (e.g. weight) restrictions and may also be crucial for effective sterilization. For example, overloading or inappropriate placement of certain items in trays can affect the outcome of the sterilization process. Overloaded and heavy trays/sets may not be adequately conditioned/sterilized by pre-programmed steam sterilization cycles (see Chapter 11) and may in some cases remain wet; this can lead to residual moisture (water) remaining in or on the pack ("wet-pack"; see Chapter 11 on troubleshooting steam sterilization problems), which can lead to them being subsequently rejected when presented in an operating room for use. Distributing devices evenly within a tray will enhance the drying process.

Trays are usually packed in the order in which the devices will be used. When the scrub person sets up for a case in the operating room (see Chapter 3 on the operating room set-up), the following may be typically prepared:

- The sterile trolley/surfaces to work from. Drapes and trolley covers will be needed to cover these surfaces.
- The devices that will be required laid out on the surface in the order of use. Depending on the type of surgery the following are most commonly used first: BP handle and scalpel blade (for cutting), diathermy (bleeding control), scissors (cutting/dissecting), retractor/dilators, and forceps.
- A skin antiseptic solution bowl and often a device to aid in cleaning the patient's skin (e.g. a swab holder), if applicable.
- Towel clips and drapes that are needed for prepping and draping the patient, unless self-adhesive disposable drapes are used.
- The sterile core is established by all staff assembling on and around the operating table. Sterile light handles will be applied, and suction, diathermy, drills/camera light sources, and so on will be attached by operating room staff.

These steps should be considered in the preparation of sets/trays with the operating room staff to aid in an efficient process.

Overall, it is important that the following points are taken into consideration when choosing a tray/set and packaging method:

- The type of pack.
- The size and weight of items to be packed.
- The number of times the pack will be handled before use.
- The number and training of personnel who may handle the pack.
- The distances over which packs will be transported.
- Whether the storage system is open or closed.
- The condition of the storage area (cleanliness, temperature, humidity).
- Whether secondary packaging (e.g. dust covers) will be used.
- The method of sealing packs.

Once the tray and/or packaging system has been chosen, the following factors need to be taken into consideration when assembling the device trays (examples are given in the later section on assembling a tray):

- The correct type of carrier tray must be used (see the section on device trays and pouches). When choosing trays, allowances should be made for extra length or devices with an ungainly, heavy, or delicate design, all of which are more susceptible to damage than "regular"-shaped devices.
- Trays should be perforated to allow penetration of the sterilizing agent and efficient drying.

- The assembly should allow a subsequent user (e.g. an operating room scrub nurse) to remove the items aseptically without causing contamination.
- The weight of packs must be taken into consideration when assembling trays. As stated earlier, the guideline weight for an object being carried using extended arms is 7 kg (~15.5 lb) for a female and 10 kg (~22 lb) for a male. Some standards and guidelines may also provide recommendations, such as ANSI/AAMI ST77 (*Containment devices for re-usable medical device sterilization*) and ANSI/AAMI ST79 (*Comprehensive guide to steam sterilization and sterility assurance in healthcare facilities*), which recommend a maximum weight limit of 11.5 kg (25 lb) for device trays, which includes the packaging system.
- Device trays must be assembled to maximize device exposure to the sterilant as well as sterilant (e.g. water) removal.
- In order to allow the sterilant to touch all surfaces of the device, devices with ratchets or hinges should be held in an open/unlocked position, and sliding/extended/complex multiple-part devices should be disassembled or sufficiently loosened to permit the sterilizing agent to come into contact with all parts of the device (check the manufacturer's instructions for guidance).
- Devices should be in the open position to allow for sterilant penetration (unless otherwise recommended by the device manufacturer). Instruments locked or in the closed position during steam sterilization, as an example, can experience cracked hinges or other problems because of heat expansion. Accessories such as stringers (also used during cleaning processes) can be used for both organization and keeping the instruments open during sterilization (Figure 10.8).
- Unusually dense devices/trays or design characteristics that may create moisture problems (i.e. wet packs) should have appropriate tray liners. Items that could hold water during steam sterilization must be placed in a way that allows easy drainage.

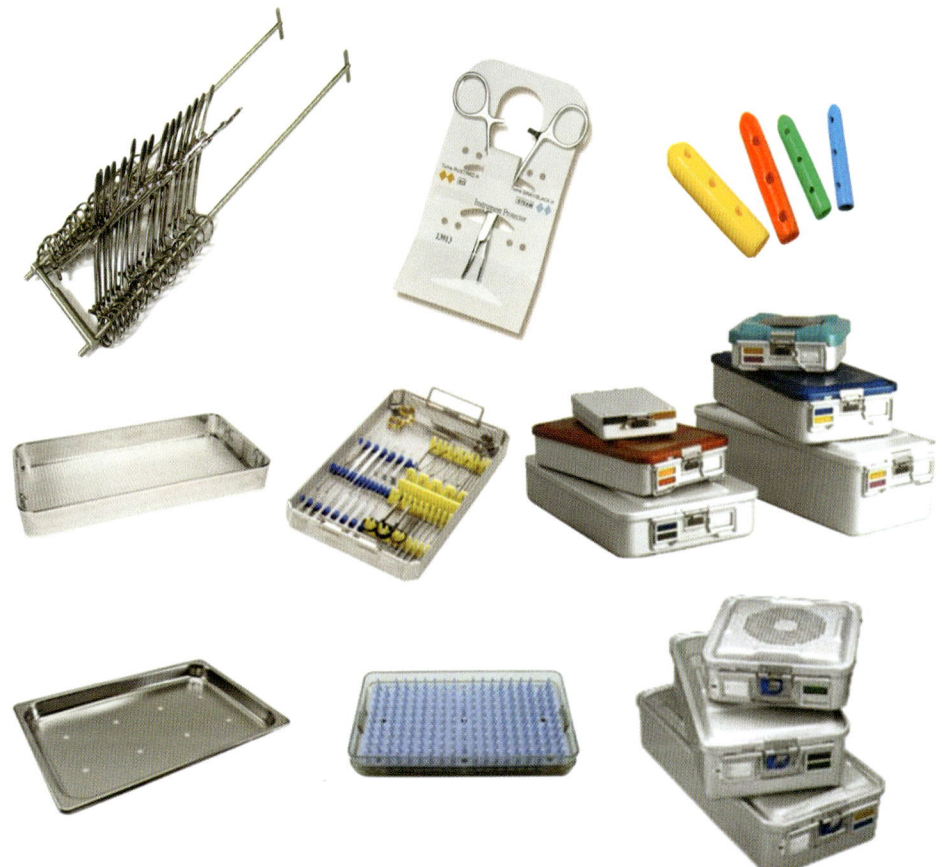

Figure 10.8 Various types of device accessories, trays, and containers. At the top are examples of accessories (e.g. stringers, device protectors, and tip protectors used during sterilization). On the middle left are a wire-mesh tray (upper) and a semi-solid (perforated; upper) tray, in the middle are example of specific types of set trays for holding delicate devices; and on the right are a variety of rigid containers.

- Heavy devices should be placed at the bottom of the tray, as the weight of heavy devices or retractors lying on top of or over other devices can cause the devices at the bottom to bend and become misaligned.
- The variety of angles and curvatures poses a challenge when assembling trays. It is difficult to organize unusually shaped devices, which can become damaged when they are "forced" to fit into trays. If trays are over-packed and devices do not lie flat, the tips of the devices can become entangled and easily damaged.
- Placing the devices in a single layer will provide more protection to them.
- Taller, rigid containers will permit segregation of delicate devices.
- The relative size of different devices must be the same, for example when using a 17.5 cm (7 in.) pair of scissors, a 17.5 cm (7 in.) needle holder and 17.5 cm (7 in.) forceps will also be used.
- The tips of devices should all be facing the same direction.
- Due to the fragile nature of distal tips, the use of tip protectors is often advised by the manufacturer. These should be intended for single use and should have been tested to ensure they are compatible with and safe to use for the designated sterilization process.
- Always make sure that all parts of the devices are present and trays are not overloaded. The inclusion of a tray checklist/device set count sheet is part of quality management and/or inventory control and is an essential communication strategy between processing staff and end users.
- In-pack chemical indicators should be placed in the most challenging part of the tray (see Chapter 14 on quality control). It is recommended that the indicator is placed in the densest part of the tray and it should be checked for the correct indicator change (e.g. change in color) by the operating room staff when opening the pack immediately prior to use.

Device trays and pouches (supplementary devices)

Choose a tray to suit the dimensions of the devices and the type of sterilization technique to be used. The various types of trays available should be specifically developed and tested to be compatible with the specified sterilization process (e.g. Figure 10.8). These trays may be provided by the device/device set manufacturer, the sterilization process manufacturer, or a third-party supplier. They may be open in design (therefore loaded with devices and wrapped with packaging materials for sterilization) in a mesh style rather than solid pans, or provided with rigid containers with lids that are locked/sealed in preparation for sterilization. They can be constructed from a variety of materials, such as stainless steel, anodized aluminum, or plastic.

When using trays that will be wrapped for sterilization, too much metal or plastic from solid or semi-solid trays may result in negative effects (e.g. in steam sterilization, leading to wet packs due to increased condensation). Edges should be smooth to prevent damage to packaging materials due to sharp edges that could cut or puncture the package. Some facilities may specifically use additional tray corner protectors that are designed for use on the bottom and/or top of the tray to create a barrier between the tray and the protector against rips, holes, and tears.

In addition to trays and containers, individual devices may also be prepared with medical-grade packaging pouches (Figure 10.9), which are designed for particular types of sterilization processes. These may be made of a variety of materials

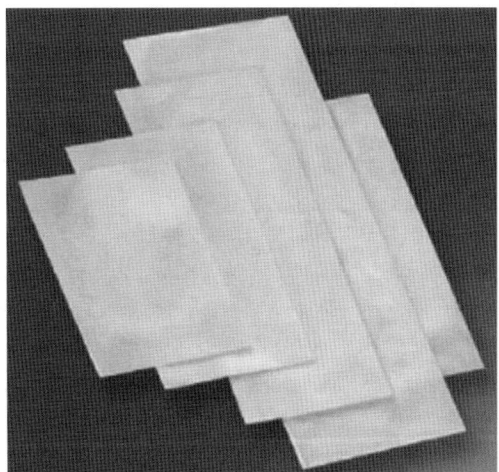
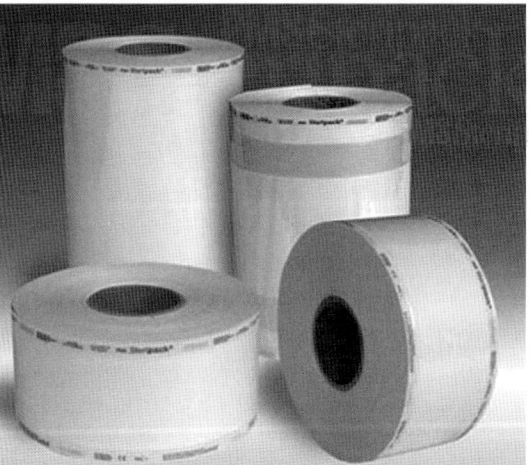

Figure 10.9 Various types of pouches and reels used as sterilization barrier systems.

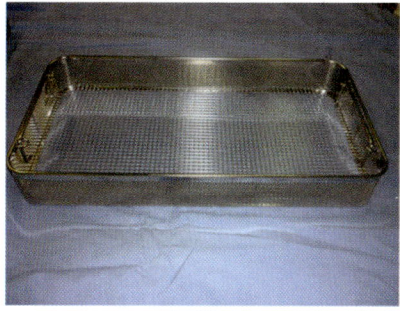
1. Select the appropriate tray

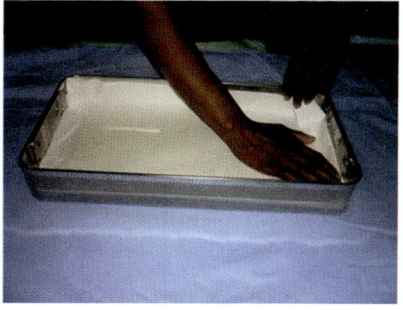
2. Place tray liner in the bottom of the tray

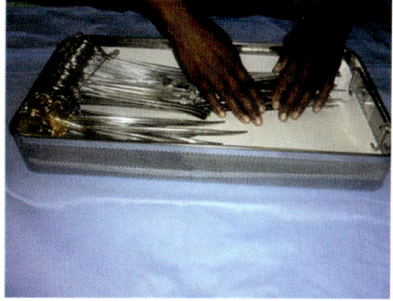
3. Inspect and pack instruments according to tray layout

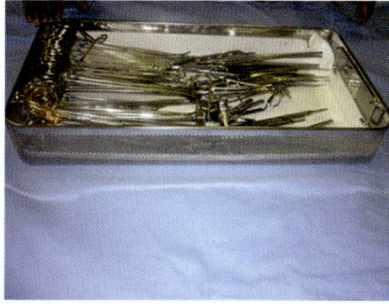
4. Complete packing instrument set

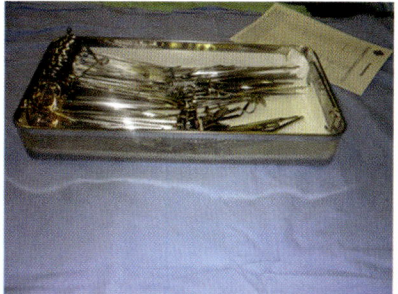
5. Check the type and quantity of instruments against a check list

Figure 10.10 A general guide in assembling a tray. Note: not all steps are required, depending on the tray load and sterilization process in use (e.g. it may not be necessary or advisable to use a tray liner).

such as paper and various types of plastics (a common material used for packaging for low-temperature sterilization is Tyvek®, a trade name for a strong type of material made of polyethylene fibers). Further consideration is given to the various types of packaging materials in the section on medical-grade packaging systems.

Assembling a tray

To assemble devices for surgical trays, the following steps should be performed:
- Make sure that all devices are clean, dry, and in the open position or disassembled to allow sterilant penetration.
- Place all hollow items face down.
- Place a tray liner in the bottom of the tray to assist with absorption of moisture (if applicable).
- Count the devices and place them into the tray according to the tray checklist.
- Place large devices such as retractors at the bottom and more delicate devices on top to prevent damaging the devices.
- Do not substitute devices.
- Place ring-handled devices on pins or stringers according to type to facilitate counting.
- Do not band flat devices together with rubber bands or in pouches.
- Use tip protectors for sharp or delicate tips.
- When packing single devices in pouches or bags, make sure that the handles are at the end that is open.
- Separate different metals, for example stainless steel and brass BP handles, as they may become discolored due to oxidation.
- Place cannulated devices such as suction nozzles at a slight angle (to allow for drainage of moisture during a steam sterilization process).
- Arrange the devices according to the checklist, usually in a pattern that will evenly distribute the weight, protect sharp edges, and facilitate their removal in the operating room.

The various steps in assembling a typical tray are summarized in Figure 10.10.

It is important to remember not to overload the tray (Figure 10.11). If too many devices are required for a particular procedure, they should be redistributed into a number of trays that are then provided as a set for surgical/medical use. Figure 10.12 shows examples of different types of device sets and assembled trays.

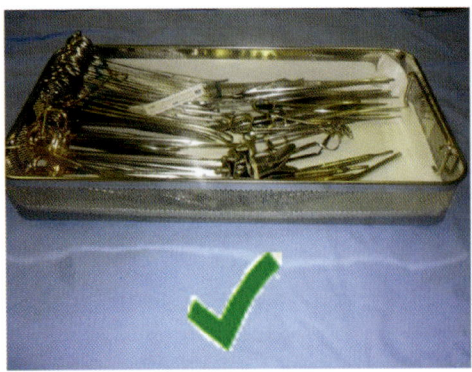 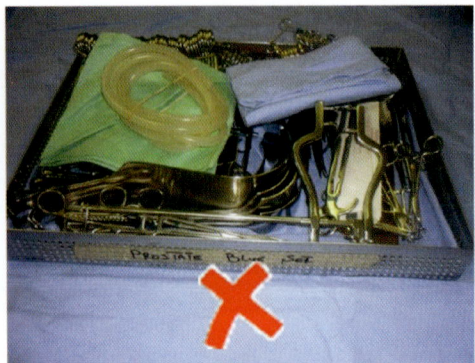

Figure 10.11 Do not overload device trays/sets.

Medical-grade packaging systems

Following the preparation and assembly of devices into trays/sets, the next step is to package the sets for sterilization and subsequent sterile storage. The term "sterility" implies that the devices have been subjected to a validated sterilization process *and* that the microbial barrier has not been compromised and the packaging is intact when being inspected for use. Therefore, sterilization packaging materials/containers have two main functions:
- To keep devices together in sets before, during and after sterilization.
- To maintain the sterility of the devices/sets during storage/transport until the time of use.

Creating ideal packaging conditions, where the sterility of the packaged and sterilized device/material is maintained until it is used is one of the day-to-day challenges that healthcare facilities need to consider. The purpose of a sterilization packaging system is to provide a safe and effective method of protecting sterile supplies and equipment while handling, transporting, and storing them, as well as allowing for aseptic presentation. The question of how many layers of wraps should be used, and whether this has been validated in the performance qualification of the sterilizers, should be asked when choosing a wrapping system. Most countries routinely use a minimum of two layers of wrap, the outer being the transport wrap and the inner the sterile field (allowing the tray to be opened and placed on a Mayo table/trolley; see Chapter 3).

Traditionally, sterile wrapping of individual items or trays consists of two separate layers of various different types of wrap materials, linens, see-through packaging, or a combination of different packaging materials. A variation on the same theme may be a container with or without an inner wrapping. In strict terms, a single barrier layer should be sufficient but is not ideal, since if the wrap is exposed to contaminants during its transport to the point of use, often through hospital corridors and operating rooms where the pack could be exposed to all sorts of bioburden, there is no additional layer protecting the tray/devices. The use of two layers of wraps reinforces the strength of the packaging, affording greater protection during handling, transport, and storage prior to its use in a surgical/medical situation. Folding the two wraps separately, one after the other, makes the pack more secure, as the greater the number of folds the more tortuous the path becomes for microorganisms to penetrate into the packaging. The double wrap with two sequential folds also affords a two-step unwrapping process, which assists in aseptic presentation and creation of a sterile field for users in the operating room; the outer wrap is removed before entering the operating room or by an assistant.

Inappropriate handling will cause contamination of the outer packaging. In the case of a single layer this means that the entire barrier has been contaminated; in the case of a double layer the inner pack remains sterile even on its outside until it is removed. In the case of a single layer there is also a risk that sterile goods can become contaminated, during opening, by microorganisms that cover the outside of the pack while the pack is opened. Therefore, whenever aseptic handling is necessary, especially in operating rooms, two layers are recommended in order to guarantee contamination-free removal, particularly after longer storage times.

In practice packaged materials will not become compromised due to the natural degradation of the packaging material but due to a specific event (e.g. damage to the packaging material such as ripping, wetting, etc.). It is therefore recommended (unless otherwise recommended by the packaging material manufacturer) that sterile packaged materials are not issued with a specific expiration time ("time-related shelf-life"), but that the shelf-life is based on any event that may recontaminate the device/set ("event-related shelf-life"). In this case, where no adverse event has occurred the device/set may be used at any time in the future. Storage times are limited because of any risk of recontamination, such as during handling, storage, transport, or opening the package. These concepts may often be challenged

Inspection, assembly, and packaging 275

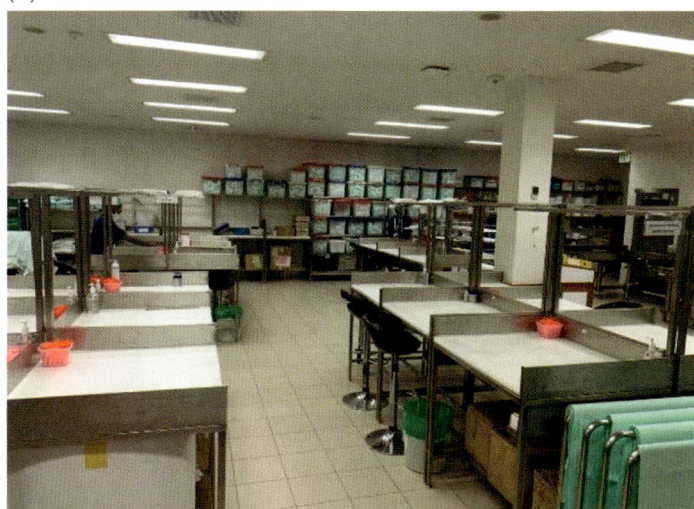
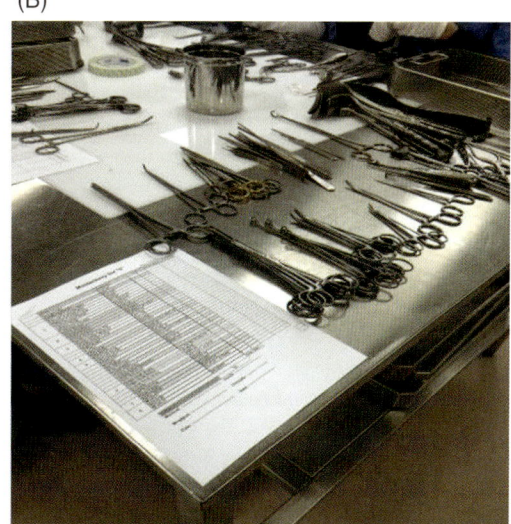
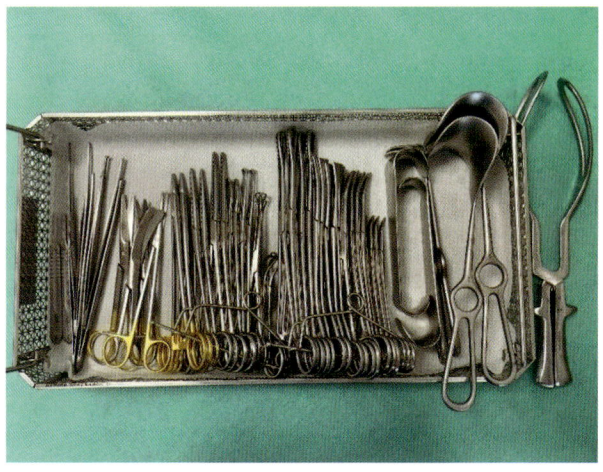
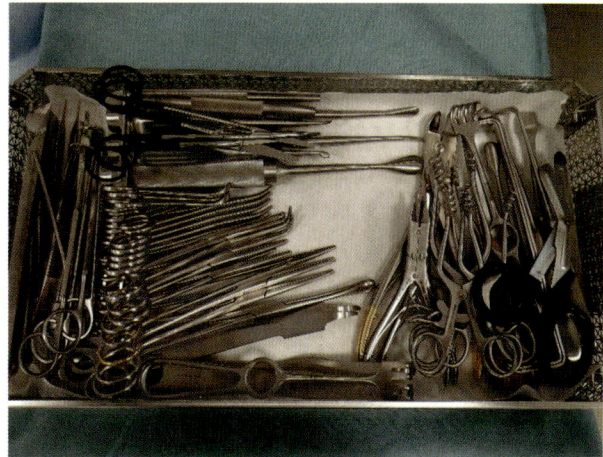
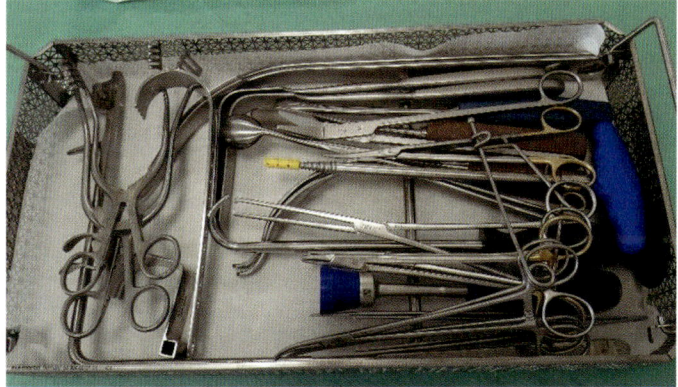
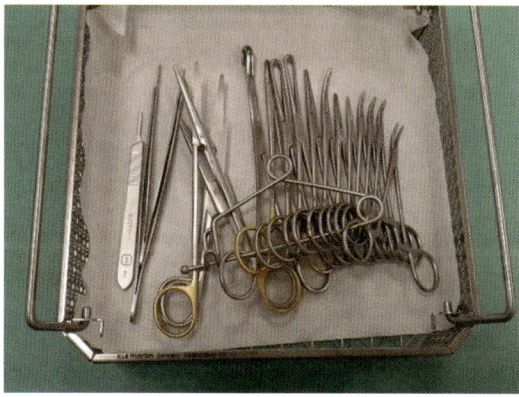

Figure 10.12 (A) Assembly and packaging workstations. (B) Devices inspected and counted for set assembly. (C) Examples of various device sets assembled in trays: C-section tray (middle left), orthopedic major set (middle right), hip instruments extra set (bottom left) and outpatient department minor procedure set (bottom right).

when new packaging materials or concepts are introduced; any such claims should be based on sound principles and scientific verification. The choice of packaging and how it is used within a facility should be based on that facility's own risk analysis. Healthcare facilities have traditionally used more than one packaging material/method, as all materials/methods have advantages and disadvantages. It is up to the facility to make an informed choice from the extensive range available, bearing in mind that the choice of packaging is extremely important, as it must meet the primary aim to guarantee the sterility and integrity of the contents until the time of use.

There are many different types of packaging materials and equipment available, with most healthcare facilities using a variety of these types. Items classified as critical devices should be packaged for sterilization (with the exception of immediate-use sterilization methods; see Chapter 11), transport, and storage. Developing a packaging and labeling system that meets patient safety and user requirements can be complicated, especially when issues such as cost, distribution, and storage facilities are taken into account. The packaging system chosen should be appropriate for the items being sterilized and compatible with the specific methods of sterilization being used. Packaging material used in steam sterilization, as an example, must be able to withstand high temperatures, allow for adequate air removal, be flexible in considering changes in pressure during the process, permit steam penetration to the pack's contents, and allow for adequate drying. Similarly, packaging materials used with low-temperature sterilization processes (e.g. ethylene oxide and vaporized hydrogen peroxide processes) must have similar properties, in particular being compatible with the sterilization chemicals, moisture, pressure changes, and temperature ranges. During and following such processes, whether heat or chemical based, the sterilization packaging systems should provide an effective barrier to microbes, particulates, and liquids, while maintaining the sterility of the contents until used. All these requirements should be supported by testing and validation by the packaging materials/container manufacturers, particularly to meet international and national standards and guidelines.

Choosing the correct packaging is therefore a critical component of sterility assurance and critical device processing, with each different type of packaging having advantages and limitations that must be understood by staff. High-quality sterilization packaging systems can optimize infection control and patient safety. Only validated products that protect the contents and provide a reliable barrier system against microbial penetration, during both handling and storage, should be considered for use.

Selection of packaging materials

When choosing a packaging system, turnover, ease of use, material compatibility, and storage space need to be balanced with patient and staff safety and device protection and cost.

The correct selection, care, use, and performance of sterile packaging systems is critical if sterilization of the contents is to be achieved and maintained until the package is opened for use.

When choosing a sterile packaging system, the following ideal properties may be taken into consideration. It should:
- Provide an adequate barrier to microorganisms, particulates, and fluids.
- Be compatible with the sterilization process.
- Be strong enough to withstand sterilization and subsequent handling.
- Be medical-grade packaging that will not cause any harm; that is, be non-reactive, stable, free of toxic ingredients and non-fast dyes, and non-odorous, ensuring product integrity and patient safety. An example of non-medical-grade packaging are cardboard boxes, which are not recommended.
- Permit adequate air removal.
- Allow the chosen sterilant (or sterilization process components) to penetrate and come into direct contact with all surfaces of the contents.
- Allow for removal of the sterilant, especially toxic biocides or their by-products.
- Securely and completely protect and enclose the contents.
- Provide adequate seal integrity and be tamper-proof.
- Be able to maintain sterility during handling, transport, and storage until use.
- Be easy to use.
- Be puncture and tearing resistant.
- Be easily disposed of and/or recyclable.
- Be available in various sizes.
- Have a low lint content.
- Allow for easy identification of contents.
- Be provided with manufacturer's instructions for use.
- Facilitate aseptic opening and allow for removal of the contents without contamination. When removing sterile items from the packaging, it should not be possible to accidentally touch the unsterile outer side of the packaging. Here, factors such as ease of peeling for opening such packaging materials without tearing are important.

Types of packaging

Traditionally, reusable packaging systems such as sterilizing drums and textiles were the only packaging choice available in most healthcare facilities. Due to a better understanding of packaging systems and advancements in technology this is no longer the case, and a wide range of packaging systems are now available, including disposable and reusable packaging materials (summarized in Table 10.1).

The choice of packaging will usually depend on the sterilization method being used. In general, packaging materials should only be used that have been tested to be compatible and safe for each sterilization purpose. This is true for both high- and low-temperature sterilization. It is important to note

Table 10.1 Summary of the various types of packaging materials/systems.

Type	Properties	Examples
Reusable woven textile	Textiles are supplied in sheets of woven materials and in a range of different fabrics	
Non-woven	Non-wovens consist of a bonded web made of textile and/or non-textile fibers They are usually supplied in sheets	
Paper	Paper wrapping materials come in several forms, including sheets of plain or crêpe paper and bags	
Paper–plastic	This combination is usually heat sealed together along the lengthwise edges to form peel-open packaging It is supplied as pouches or reels that can be cut to size	
Rigid containers	Rigid containers are usually made of aluminum or plastic and are often used for large or heavy items that require a robust form of packaging	

that packaging materials are only tested to be effective under claimed conditions and using them outside these claims may compromise the sterilization efficacy of the load, cause damage to the materials used (compromising storage), and pose other disadvantages.

Reusable woven textile wraps

Woven textiles were used almost exclusively for sterile packaging until the 1980s, when non-wovens that provided a more effective barrier against microbial contamination were introduced. Traditional woven textiles had a thread count of 140, which provided an ineffective microbial barrier, potentially allowing most microorganisms to pass through. Such woven textiles are still used to form sterile barrier systems in some countries, but they are generally not optimal for this purpose and should be actively discouraged. More modern woven textiles have now been developed and as long as they comply with international or national sterilization packaging standards (see the section on standards and guidelines for sterilization packaging systems), they are suitable to be used as wrappers for this purpose.

The advantages of woven textiles are that they are soft, reusable, inexpensive, and drapable (they have little or no "memory" and fall flat when opened). Reusable woven textile fabrics may be woven from cotton, linen, or blends of cotton and synthetic materials, such as polyester. Due to the nature of woven threads the textiles will degenerate over time the more often they are processed. The manufacturer should provide information about the number of laundering and sterilization cycles that the material can withstand.

Before use, such textiles should be laundered, delinted, and inspected, preferably over light boxes, for holes, worn spots, tears, and stains (for guidance on general laundering, see Chapter 15 on surgical and medical laundering and Chapter 8 on textiles and laundry). Any tears should be repaired on both sides with a vulcanized patch applied using heat. It is important to launder any previously sterilized textiles, as prior to processing woven textile will need to be rehydrated. Textiles should be thoroughly rinsed to ensure that they are free of detergents, bleaches, or other chemicals that may react with the sterilant and cause discoloration and/or adversely affect the contents of the pack. A laundry mark-off system should be used to monitor the number of times the wrap has been used.

Single-use, non-woven wraps

Various non-woven, single-use disposable products are available, for example spun-bonded olefin, fiber-reinforced tissue, spun-bonded polyethylene, and spun-laced, wood, and pulp-polyester materials. Non-woven fabrics are designed as single-use disposable products and *should not* be reused. Non-woven fabrics are not woven, they are made of fibers that have been pressure bonded together to form sheets of fabric. Special non-wovens have been developed for sterilization, to meet the requirements for primary packaging of sterile goods specified in standards. Non-wovens are suitable for steam, steam-formaldehyde, and low-temperature sterilization processes, such as ethylene oxide and vaporized hydrogen peroxide; they are considered to provide excellent bacterial barrier properties. However, not all non-wovens may be compatible with all types of sterilization methods as they contain varying amounts of synthetic material. For example, packaging that contains cellulose cannot be used in hydrogen peroxide or ozone sterilization.

Non-wovens are virtually lint free and due to the very small spaces between the fibers are generally resistant to dust penetration. Plastic polymers, such as polyolefins, provide excellent water vapor (steam) transmission, but some may resist liquid penetration altogether. Non-wovens generally repel liquids; they are hydrophobic ("water-hating"). Although these fabrics have the flexibility and handling qualities of woven materials, when used as wrapping they can be torn or punctured by the sharp edges of devices and/or device trays.

Non-wovens are available in a range of weights and a wide variety of sizes.

Paper

Paper is essentially a non-woven material intended for single use. Special papers have been developed to meet the requirements for primary packaging of sterile goods specified in various standards (see the section on standards and guidelines for sterilization packaging systems). There are many types and grades of paper, including:
- "Kraft"-type papers, which are generally smooth surfaced and are used in the manufacture of bags and peel-open pouches.
- Crêpe-type paper wrap, which has been specially treated to allow it to stretch and adapt to the types and sizes of items that it is used to wrap. It also makes the paper softer and easier to handle. This type of paper has "memory," which means that it tends to revert to the way it was folded and not lie flat when opened to form an adequate sterile field.

Prior to use, paper must be inspected for pin holes, tears, creases, or other flaws that would compromise the integrity of packaged items. Crêpe-type papers are easily penetrated by steam, ethylene oxide, and low-temperature steam/formaldehyde, and are suitable for these sterilization processes. They are not suitable for hydrogen peroxide gas or ozone processes, because of their cellulose content.

Disposable peel-open pouches and reels

Disposable peel-open pouches and reels are composed of paper or Tyvek/plastic combinations. They are designed to contain lightweight or small items and are available in various sizes, for single use only. Peel-open packaging should not be used for heavy or bulky items because the seals can become stressed and rupture. Pouches may be self-sealing or sealed by heat-sealing the open end (see the section on sealing pouches and reels). The open end of the pouch is closed with a sealing device, the heat sealer. It is essential that the heat sealer is functioning effectively in order to get an adequate seal. Both ready-made pouches and reels are available flat or with side gussets for packing bulkier objects. The user can cut reels to any size needed, in which case both sides of the pack will need to be sealed by the user.

Peel-open packaging is useful when visibility of the contents is important. When packaging items, care must be taken to leave a minimum of 2.5 cm (1 in.) of space around each side of the device and at the end of the item in order to facilitate sterilization and aseptic opening. To label, use a felt-tip, indelible, non-toxic ink marker on the clear plastic side of the pouch, outside the sterile window area. Peel-open pouches should be placed upright or tilted on edge in a grid basket or container during sterilization. Also they should not be tightly packed together, as this may prevent expansion of the package during the air-removal stages and inhibit this process.

Double peel-open packaging is not routinely required, but if items are double pouched they must be packaged paper against paper, plastic against plastic, in order to enable sterilant penetration. The inner pouch should be at least one size smaller than the outer pouch to prevent folding, which may entrap air and inhibit the sterilization process.

Paper/plastic peel-open packaging materials are suitable for steam, steam formaldehyde, and low-temperature sterilization processes such as ethylene oxide. They are not suitable for use in vaporized hydrogen peroxide and ozone sterilizers, again due to the paper (cellulose) content. The plastic front cannot be penetrated by steam or air, so removal of air and penetration of steam or gas are through the paper backing only.

Pouches made with non-cellulosic materials can be used for vaporized hydrogen peroxide and ozone methods of sterilization.

Reusable rigid container systems

Sterilization containers are a durable sterilization packaging system constructed of a rigid material such as metal or plastic. They are reusable, easy to use, cost-effective, and versatile. They provide excellent protection as they are rigid and cannot be easily crushed. A variety of sizes can accommodate a wide range of device sets. A container is a box-like structure composed of a lid and a base, carrying handles, and a latch or locking mechanism that secures the lid to the base (Figure 10.13). A gasket is used to seal the lid to the base. Inner baskets, trays, and various inserts organize and protect the devices within the container. Nameplates or tags identify the sets and disposable items such as filters, tamper-evident seals/locks, and load cards/external chemical indicators complete the system.

As such containers are manufactured from non-porous rigid materials they create a barrier to the sterilization process as well as microorganisms; therefore they need to have a means by which the sterilant can enter the container. This is achieved by either a filter or through a valve in the lid, which opens and closes with the varying pressure in a sterilizer (e.g. in a steam sterilization process). Filters can be single use or reusable.

Containers need to be disassembled and cleaned after each use, following the processing instructions supplied by the container manufacturer. Remember: such containers are classified as devices themselves and as such should be processed after each use in the same way as any other reusable device, not just wiped down. Following processing they should be checked to include:

• Checks of gaskets for fraying, cuts, missing pieces, bubbling, or compression.
• Cleaning reusable filters and inspecting them for cracks or chips.
• The number of uses also needs to be logged and the manufacturer's recommendations not exceeded.

Wrapping and sealing methods

Training should be provided on the correct methods of using the different types of sterile packaging systems. In all cases, attention should be given to any instructions provided by the sterile barrier system manufacturer. Three issues are highlighted in this section: standardization of tray-wrapping methods, securing of packs, and sealing of pouches/reels.

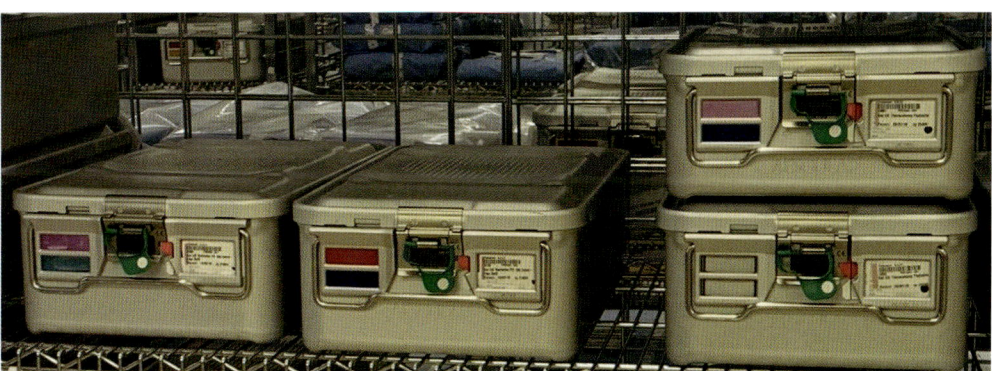

Figure 10.13 Examples of reusable, rigid containers with tamper-proof locks stored ready to use.

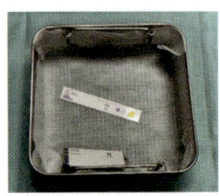
1. Select the correct size wrap for the tray to be wrapped. Lay two layers of wrap lengthways on a flat surface. Place the tray in the center of the wrap.

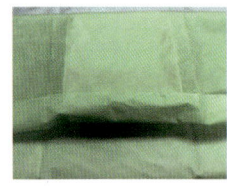
2. Fold the first side to cover the entire tray

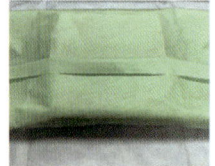
3. Fold back the first wrap to create a cuff ensuring the tray is still covered.

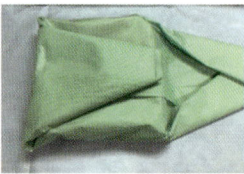
4. Fold both ends of the wrap to create a V shape.

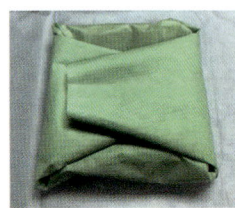
5. Fold the opposite side over the set, create the cuff to end in the centre

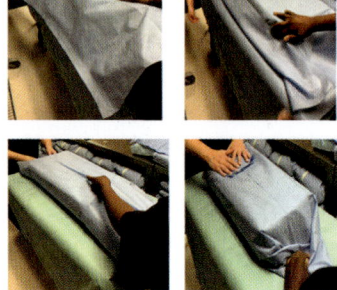
6. Repeat for the second layer of wrap. Wrap the set firmly but no too tight.

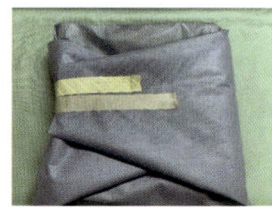
7. Secure the wrap with an adequate length of masking tape. Apply chemical indicator tape. Do not write directly onto wrap. Label pack according to hospital policy.

Figure 10.14 An example of the sequential square/parallel wrapping process of an open tray set.

Wrapping trays for sterilization

The delivery of sterile products depends not only on the effectiveness of the sterilization process but also on effective packaging of the tray. The wrapping procedure should be precise and performed reproducibly. Wrapping the devices incorrectly or using the incorrect type of wrap can lead to device recontamination. There are a number of wrapping options, including the envelope and the parallel/square fold that are described in standard ISO 17665:2024, *Sterilization of health care products – Moist heat – Requirements for the development, validation, and routine control of a sterilization process for medical devices*. The facility should agree on using a method that is compliant with national and specific institutional guidelines. An example of the sequential square/parallel technique using individual sheets of sterile barrier material is shown in Figure 10.14. The wrapping sequence should be done in such a manner as to avoid "tenting" or "gapping," which will allow the ingress of dust and microorganisms. Double layers remain common practice due to the rigors of handling within the facility, even though the barrier efficacy of a single sheet of wrap has improved over the years. The choice of single or double wrapping will depend on the packaging material manufacturer's claims and instructions, as well as the consideration of using the minimum of packaging materials (from sustainability and cost perspectives).

A sequential wrapping process uses two sheets of sterilization wrap, one wrapped after the other, creating a package within a package, thereby decreasing the risk of contamination (Figure 10.14). The non-sequential process uses two sheets wrapped at the same time so that the wrapping needs to be performed only once, but the risk of contamination in this case may be higher. Once the tray is wrapped it must be effectively sealed to prevent contamination. Likewise, if the package is packed too tightly the seal may loosen during sterilization, transport, or storage, leading to potential recontamination. The final step in the wrapping process is to seal and label the package.

Securing packs

Various types of adhesive tapes can be used, including specifically designed process indicator tape designed to change color on exposure to the sterilization process. Packages should be secured with a medical-grade adhesive tape (also referred to as masking tape) and/or a chemical indicator tape (Figure 10.15).

Figure 10.15 Examples of chemical indicator tapes used for steam sterilization. They can come in a variety of colors, but a typical black color change is shown on the right (in this case on exposure to steam sterilization).

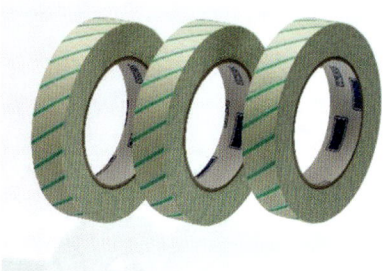
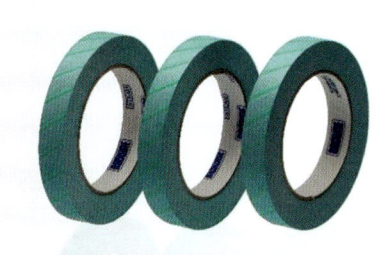
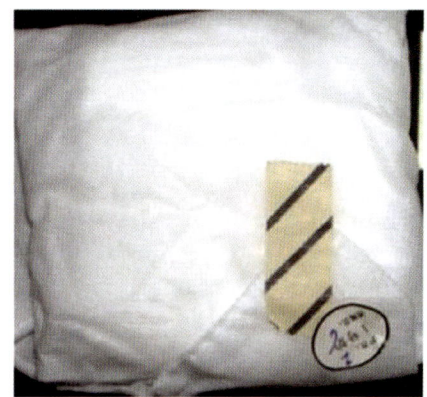

Chemical indicator tapes are useful to be able to verify whether a pack has been subjected to sterilization. Such process indicators are generally classified as being type 1 chemical indicators (see Chapter 14 on process indicators), in that they are simple indicators designed to demonstrate exposure to a process and/or to distinguish between processed/unprocessed devices. If the tape is designed as a chemical indicator, it should show a clear color change when exposed to a sterilization process.

The ideal tape should:
- Have good adhesive qualities.
- Be easy to remove.
- Not leave any glue or ink residues.

Sealing pouches/reels

Some pouches are provided with self-adhesive sealing tabs, where the devices are placed into the pouch and sealed for sterilization. Other pouches and reels are designed to be heat sealed as the final step before the packaged devices are loaded for sterilization. Examples of heat sealing machines are shown in Figure 10.16(A).

The heat sealer must be set to the packaging manufacturer's specifications, to include the correct:
- Pressure
- Temperature
- Sealing/hold time.

An example of a heat sealer and the sealing process are shown in Figure 10.16(B). The strength and integrity of the seal depend on the appropriate application methods, as well as the correct temperature and pressure being applied for the correct length of time. Device protector caps can be used to prevent sharp devices damaging the pack. These should not interfere with the sterilization process being applied. In some facilities, the contents of the package may be written on the external surface for identification purposes, specifically on the see-though side of the pack.

Devices in peel-open pouches should not be placed into wrapped sets or containers. This may create problems for sterilization outcomes (e.g. adequate air removal, sterilant contact, and drying, if applicable). Such devices should either be placed directly into the tray (unwrapped) or sterilized as a separate pack.

Standards and guidelines for sterilization packaging systems

Device packaging systems are regulated as an essential part of the process of maintaining the sterility of devices/materials through storage, distribution, and to the final site of use. The harmonized international standard for packaging is ISO 11607 *Packaging for terminally sterilized medical devices* – Parts 1 and 2, including the requirements for materials, sterile barrier systems, and packaging, as well as associated validation requirements. These standards have been adopted by many countries throughout the world and in this case the country adopting the standard will rename it to reflect this as follows:
- BS EN ISO 11607-1 (United Kingdom).
- ANSI/AAMI/ISO 11607-1 (United States).
- SANS ISO 11607-1 (South Africa).

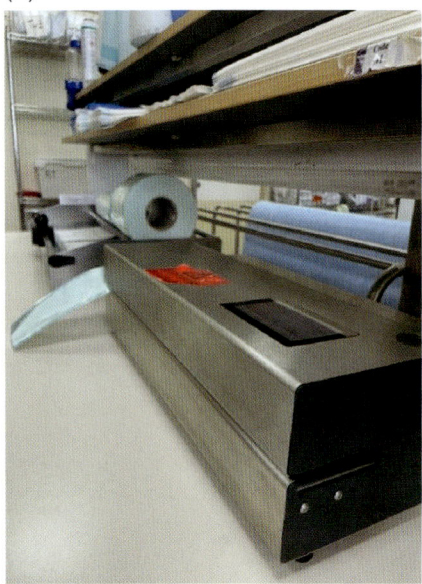
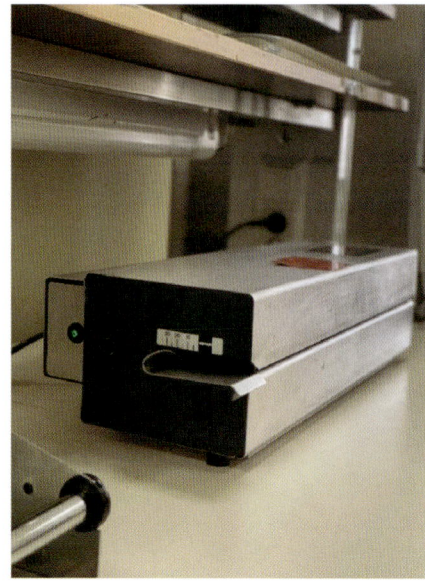
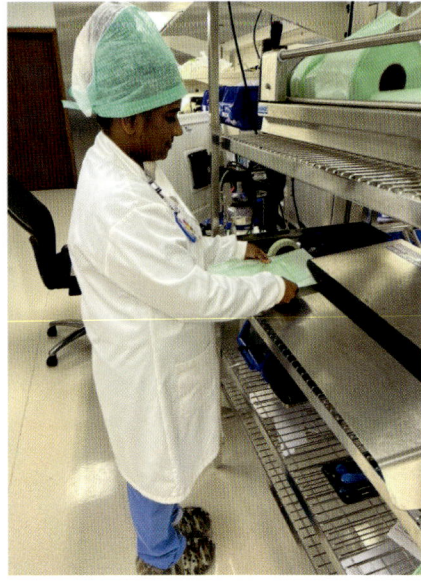
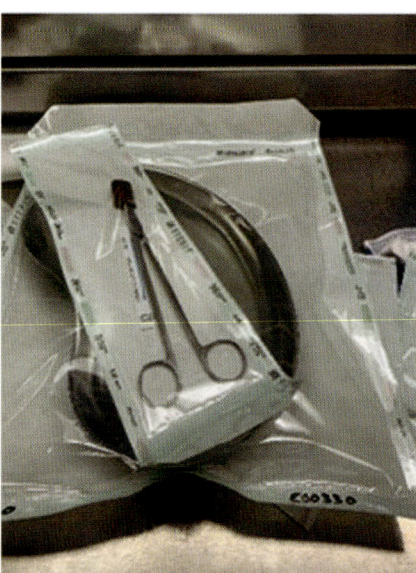

Figure 10.16 Examples of (A) heat-sealing apparatuses, benchtop design; and (B) the process of sealing a pouch and the final outcome of single devices sealed.

ISO 11607 has two parts: Part 1 focuses on materials and packaging structures and Part 2 covers validation requirements and provides detailed guidance to healthcare facilities on the requirements for material qualification, package system design and testing, and packaging process validation. Guidance on the use of these standards is defined in ISO/TS 16775 *Packaging for terminally sterilized medical devices – guidance on the application of ISO 11607-1 and ISO 11607-2*. Further regional standards and guidelines may also have been used in the past, such as the EN 868 series of standards that specify particular requirements for a range of commonly used packaging materials. This standard series was withdrawn in 2009 and harmonized to the equivalent ISO standards. A summary of packaging standards and guidance documents is given in Table 10.2.

Table 10.2 Examples of packaging standards and guidance documents.

Organization	Title	Description
International Organization for Standardization (ISO)	ISO 11607-1: *Packaging for terminally sterilized medical devices – Part 1*	Requirements and test methods for materials, sterile barrier systems, and packaging systems
ISO	ISO 11607-2: *Packaging for terminally sterilized medical devices – Part 2*	Requirements for development and validation of processes for packaging medical devices that are terminally sterilized
World Health Organization (WHO)	*Decontamination and reprocessing of medical devices for health-care facilities*	Guidance of preparation and packaging during processing
Association for the Advancement of Medical Instrumentation (AAMI)	TIR 22, *Guidance for ANSI/AAMI/ISO 11607, packaging for terminally sterilized medical devices – Part 1 and Part 2*	Guidance for the applications of ISO 11607-1 for materials, sterile barrier systems, and packaging
Association of periOperative Registered Nurses (AORN)	*Guideline for selection and use of packaging systems for sterilization*	Guidance for evaluating and selecting packaging systems, preparing items for sterilization, and verifying achievement of sterilization parameters
ASTM	ASTM F2096-11	Standard test method for detecting gross leaks in packaging by internal pressurization (bubble test)
ASTM	ASTM F1929-15	Standard test method for detecting seal leaks in porous medical packaging by dye penetration
Standards Australia/Standards New Zealand (AS/NZS)	AS/NZS 4187 *Reprocessing of reusable medical devices in health care service organizations*	Requirements and practices for reusable medical devices processing, including packaging and storage Note: replaced by AS 5369 in 2023 (*Reprocessing of reusable medical devices and other devices in health and non-health related facilities*)
Department of Health and Social Care, England	Health Technical Memorandum 01-01: *Management and decontamination of surgical instruments (medical devices) used in acute care. Part C: Steam sterilization*	General guidance on packaging in preparation for and following steam sterilization

Label identification of packaged devices

It is good practice for processing facilities to implement appropriate systems to allow for the tracking of reusable devices throughout the decontamination process and from patient to patient (see Chapter 14 on materials managemen*t*). Examples of manual methods include the use of checklists (see Figure 10.7) and appropriate labeling of packaged devices/device sets. Labels can be applied to the external packaging prior to sterilization to allow ease of identification. This is not only important in the loading and unloading of the sterilizer, but also in subsequent transport and storage, and also to correctly identify the contents of the package before it is opened for medical/surgical use. Proper labeling is important too for quality assurance, inventory control, and stock-rotation purposes.

In processing areas packaging should be labeled prior to sterilization in a way that does not compromise the integrity of the pack. Writing directly on the pack is not recommended as it may damage the sterile barrier material or cause leaking of ink through the barrier and onto the device. Instead, information may be captured on an adhesive label that is attached on the pack. In the case of a peel pack, attention should be paid that the label is attached on the see-through side and not on the paper/Tyvek side, which would interfere with sterilant penetration. Writing on the indicator tape should also be avoided. Never use a ballpoint pen on any packaging material as it can create holes in the material. Recommended labeling methods include:

- Soft-tipped, alcohol-based, felt marking pens.
- Pre-printed tapes.
- Pre-printed bags.
- Stamping systems.
- Pre-printed labels.
- Dedicated or automated labeling systems.

If using a manual system (Figure 10.17), the required labeling information must be written down on a sheet identifying the operator, the cycle printout, and any other monitoring devices linked to the particular load. An electronic system

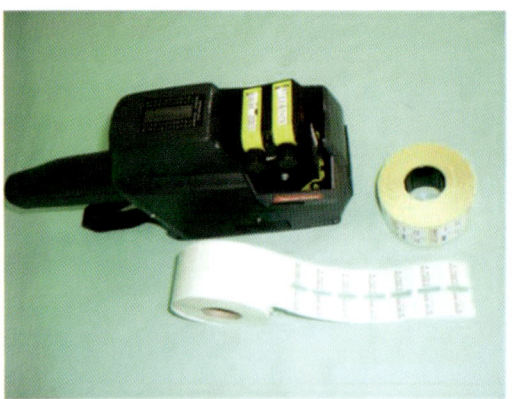 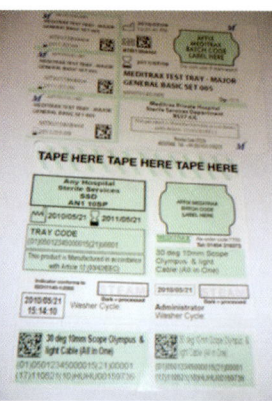

Figure 10.17 Examples of manual labeling systems.

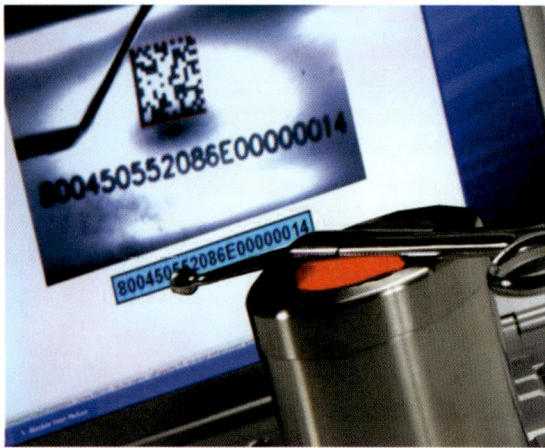 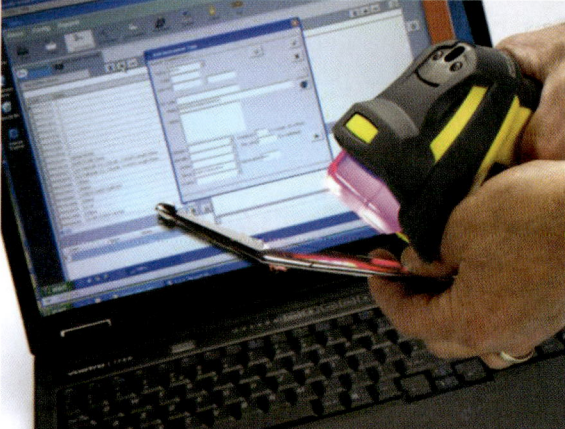

Figure 10.18 Examples of automated labeling systems.

allows the items to be scanned by a handheld scanner with the information downloaded to produce a batch report. Labels may be pre-printed directly onto packaging materials or packaging materials can be printed in-line. Often a combination is used, with generic information pre-printed and lot and date-specific information printed at the time of packaging. Alternatively, labels can be directly written and affixed to the packaging system. Automated systems can also be used (Figure 10.18). A common method involves the use of bar codes to identify packs (these are further considered in Chapter 14 on materials management) and device locations by a scanning process. More sophisticated systems scan digital photos into the system to provide visual assistance in tracking and identification.

It is recommended that packaging systems are labeled with a description of the package contents, the identification (e.g. initials) of the person assembling the package, and a lot control number. Further, the label may include other information such as:
- Date of sterilization.
- Sterilizer and cycle number.
- Any expiration date/shelf-life statement applicable to the facility policy (see Chapter 12 on storage and distribution).
- The procedure and department where the package is to be sent after sterilization.

Labels must be able to withstand exposure to the sterilization process, storage, and transport. Labeling must not:
- Affect the sterility or integrity of the pack.
- Become illegible.
- Transfer to pack contents.
- React with packaging.
- Interfere with the decontamination process.
- Become detached in sterilization or subsequent storage.

Loading and unloading sterilizers

An important part of processing that it is often underestimated is the correct loading and unloading of sterilizers. It is important to understand when loading a sterilizer that, in order to achieve sterility, all surfaces of the item must have direct contact with the sterilizing

agent for the prescribed amount of time. In order to achieve this, all items should be placed correctly in the sterilizer to allow contact of the sterilant with all surfaces. Specific guidelines and recommendations may be provided by the sterilizer manufacturer that should be understood and applied. Only trained and competent processing personnel should be responsible for the loading/unloading and operation of sterilizers. Sterilization itself is dependent on many parts of the decontamination process and associated procedures being undertaken correctly (considered in earlier chapters). These include:
- Adequate cleaning, inspection, packaging, and handling of items.
- Use of a defined, validated, and correctly installed sterilizer.
- Correct loading and operating of the sterilizer.
- Correct unloading of the sterilizer.
- Routine maintenance of the sterilizer and revalidation with any associated accessories.

Loading the sterilizer

Recommended PPE must be used when loading the sterilizer. An important example is with steam sterilizers, where the internal walls can be very hot to touch; therefore, special heat-protecting gloves or gauntlets may be needed in loading (and unloading) such sterilizers (Figure 10.19). In addition, safety glasses are important if there are risks of steam or chemical exposure in the area. Advances in the automation of loading and unloading technology will help in reducing these risks, including improving ergonomics (see Chapter 14 on physical and emotional health).

Whatever method of sterilization is being used, low or high temperature, the basic rule to consider in loading the sterilizer chamber is that all items need to be properly prepared and arranged in a way that will allow the process to be effective (e.g. present the least possible resistance to the extraction of air and the passage of the sterilant throughout the load). Always

(A)

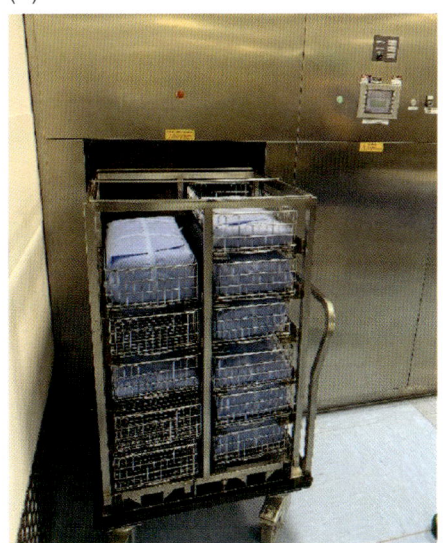
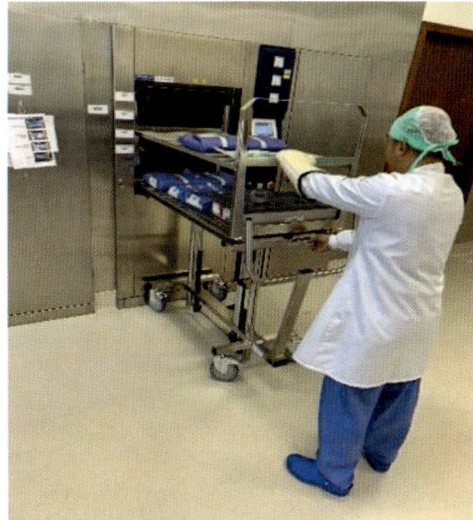

(B)

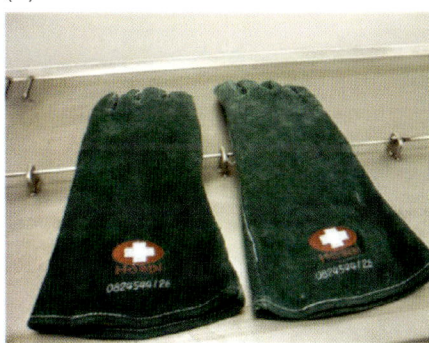

Figure 10.19 (A) Loading a steam sterilizer using (B) heatproof gauntlets/gloves.

follow the manufacturer's recommendations when loading the sterilizer. For example, most sterilization processes (such as steam, ethylene oxide, and vaporized hydrogen peroxide systems) recommend that devices are dry prior to sterilization, as they are not generally designed to remove excess moisture. Sterilizers should never be overloaded; there should be sufficient space between items to allow for the sterilant to permeate around each package and packages must not touch the top, bottom, or sides of the sterilizer. Overloading in both high-temperature and low-temperature sterilization processes can compromise the effectiveness of the process as it was designed for use. The correct load for a sterilizer is determined by the size of the sterilizer chamber and the number of items to be sterilized, their characteristics, and how they are prepared and positioned within the sterilizer. These requirements should be specified by the sterilizer manufacturer and may include material/device, positioning, and weight restrictions. A single large item, for example, may be the maximum load for the type of sterilizer being used. Large and small items can be included in the same load, but only if applicable. The sterilization process will be effective if items are properly prepared and positioned so that they get adequate contact with the sterilization process for the correct amount of time.

There are a number of general considerations when loading a sterilizer (see Figure 10.20):
- Verify the integrity of packaging before loading (e.g. seals, no tears, packaging correctly, etc.).
- Load according to manufacturer's recommendations or local operating procedures that have considered this and other best practices. Do not overload.
- Place peel pouches on their edge so they can expand and contract during the cycle. These can expand considerably

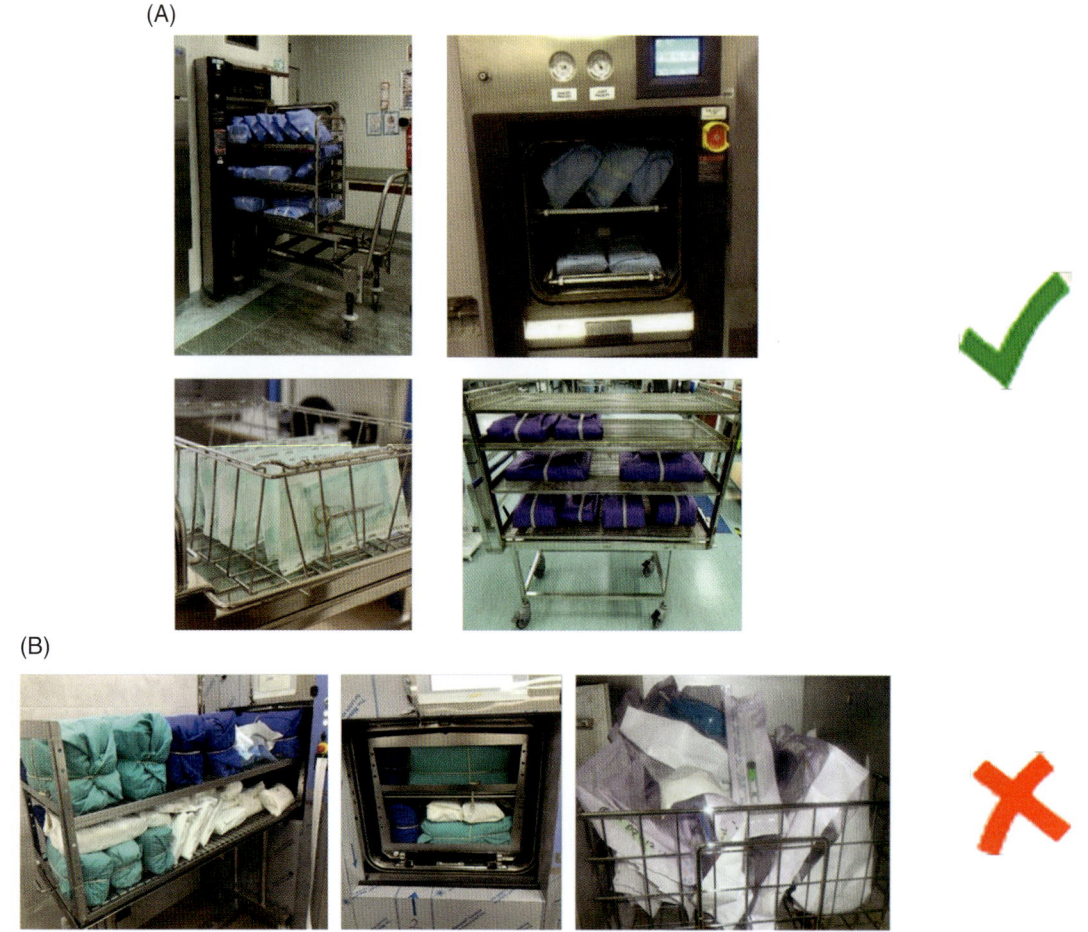

Figure 10.20 Examples of (A) good and (B) poor loading of a sterilizer. The basic principles apply irrespective of the type of sterilizer. Items should be loaded loosely. Leave space between packs. Do not layer packs, or touch the walls or base of the sterilizer. Place small packs in holders. Do not overload.

during a steam/gas-based process. Arrange so that the plastic of one pouch touches the paper side of the next for penetration and aeration.
- Use only perforated or wire-mesh bottom trays, wire baskets, or specially designed pouch baskets. Do not use plastic-coated baskets unless designed and validated for sterilization and aeration.
- Load items in a loose fashion to facilitate air removal, humidification (if applicable), circulation and penetration of all surfaces, and removal during aeration.
- Load baskets and carts so that hands will not touch packs if you need to transfer them to an aeration cabinet.
- If using approved rigid containers, follow the manufacturer's validated loading instructions.
- Packages should not touch the walls, floor, or ceiling of the chamber, otherwise package damage from heat, moisture, or other effects may occur.
- Never place items directly on the floor of the sterilizer chamber as this could block the discharge of air from the sterilizer, or allow air and sterilants to be trapped in pockets, resulting in sterilization failure and "wet packs" in the case of steam sterilization. Packs touching the chamber walls can be scorched or contents damaged due to excessive heat of the metal walls, or become wet due to excessive moisture on the walls in the case of steam sterilization. Always allow 7–8 cm (3 in.) of space between the top-most package and the top of chamber. This allows displacement of air and free flow of the sterilant.
- Loading racks or holding trays will help establish package separation. In combination loads of soft packs and device trays, place soft packs on top shelves and trays on lower shelves. In the case of steam sterilization this prevents condensation forming when the steam initially comes into contact with the cool metals and dripping onto soft packs below.
- Soft packs, for example linen bundles, should be placed on their sides/edges with folds perpendicular to the shelf. This makes it easier for the sterilant to penetrate by flowing down through the folds than through flat, compressed surfaces.
- Never place packages directly on top of each other; this will compress the packages, limiting air removal and sterilant penetration.
- Place solid utensils (basins/bowls) on their sides in a draining position. Nested packs of hollow-ware should be positioned facing the same direction to help prevent air pockets, so that condensation can drain and steam can circulate freely. Slatted trays, mesh baskets, or a loading cart must be used to ensure proper loading.
- Device trays should be placed flat on the shelves.
- Liquids (for steam sterilization) must be sterilized by themselves in a separate dedicated cycle according to manufacturer's instructions. The length of the sterilization cycle will be determined by the amount of liquid in the bottle. Use only heat-resistant glass (Pyrex®) and automatic self-sealing caps for closure, as there is always a possibility that solutions will explode.
- Liquids should not be sterilized in gas-based sterilization processes.
- Place all empty bottles and empty rigid containers on their sides with lids held loosely in place. This will allow air to drain out and sterilant to take its place.
- Rigid containers should be spaced about 2.5 cm (1 in.) apart from each other. Stacking should not be performed unless the container manufacturer gives specific information on this process.
- Peel packs should be placed on their edge in a basket.
- Always place the heaviest trays on the lowest shelf of the carriage.
- Special requirements are often provided for the use of gas sterilization processes, including limits in the number and types of devices that can be sterilized in different cycles, limits of weight, excluding certain types of materials (e.g. paper or other cellulosic materials in hydrogen peroxide-based sterilizer), that devices must be dry, inspection of devices/packaging following sterilization to ensure they are dry and no residual moisture is present (which can contain chemicals), and additional (extended) aeration times following ethylene oxide sterilization.

Unloading the sterilizer

Recommended PPE must be worn when unloading the sterilizer. For chemical-based sterilization processes, protective gloves should be worn as required to minimize the risks of chemical exposure that may occur due to errors in loading or equipment malfunction. As already mentioned, additional drying or aeration may be necessary depending on inspection or manufacturer's requirements (e.g. following ethylene oxide sterilization).

For heat-based processes, the processed load and inner sterilizer/rack surfaces may be hot at the completion of the cycle and this could result in serious burns. In the case of high-temperature sterilizers, the load cart should be removed from the sterilizer and transferred to the cooling zone at the completion of the process cycle. All sterilizers should be unloaded in such a manner as to maintain the sterility of the items that have been processed. The cooling zone should have no open windows/fans/air-conditioning vents in close proximity as there may be residual humidity in the packages, and dust and dirt could be forced through the wrappers, contaminating the contents. Hot packs should not be placed on cold metal surfaces as condensation will occur, resulting in an unsterile or rejected pack. The actual time for cooling should be based on professional judgment, experience, and the environmental conditions of the area. Only handle packs once they have reached room temperature or can be handled safely. The most important rule to follow is to allow the packs to cool and dry completely before handling.

Sterilized packs should be handled gently and as little as possible to avoid contamination. If a pack is dropped, tears, or comes into contact with moisture, it must be considered contaminated and subjected to repeated processing. If there are water droplets or visible moisture on the inside or outside of the package, extended drying and investigation of the cause will be necessary and in some cases the pack may be considered unsterile. When unloading, packs should be checked to verify that they are not incorrectly wrapped, that seals are intact, that the process indicator on the outside of the pack has changed, that a tracking date/label is present, and that the package is in a good condition. The use of carrying trays or baskets when loading the sterilizer will reduce the amount of handling when unloading.

11 Sterilization

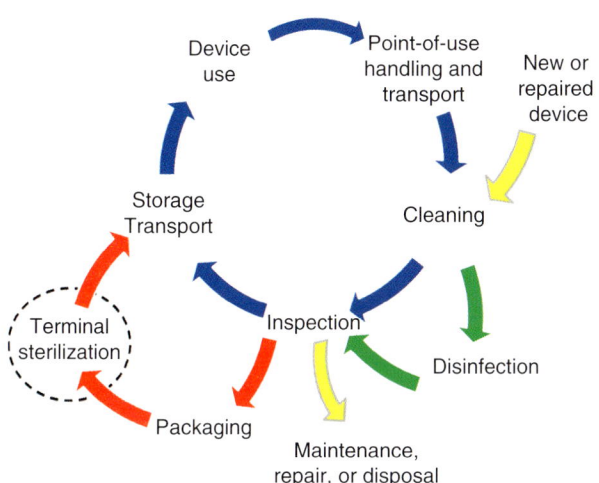

Sterilization is defined as a validated process used to render an item free from viable microorganisms (including dormant forms such as bacterial spores). Disinfection and sterilization products/processes are both antimicrobial, but while disinfection may only provide a reduction in microorganisms (see Chapter 9), sterilization processes are designed to completely destroy all viable microbial life that may be present (i.e. to render a product "sterile" or having been "sterilized"). As previously defined in Chapter 1, reusable devices can provide different levels of risks to a patient and therefore various levels of disinfection or sterilization are recommended to reduce these risks. In the Spaulding classification, disinfection (ranging from low to intermediate and high levels) is widely used for the safe processing of non-critical and some semi-critical devices (see Chapter 9; Figure 11.1); however, critical and many semi-critical devices that may penetrate skin or mucous membranes or enter a sterile body cavity, including blood contact, pose the highest risk to patient safety and should be sterilized.

How can sterilization assurance be provided and confirmed? Although the term "sterilization" may be commonly used, it is a condition that can be difficult to achieve and hard to guarantee. In fact, sterilization is only the result of a well-defined, repeatable, and measurable process in a well-organized and well-operated processing department. This process must at a minimum be shown to be effective against all types of microorganisms, including bacterial spores that are considered highly resistant to inactivation (Figure 11.1). The only current exception to this requirement is for efficacy against prions, which is considered separately and may or may not be shown for individual sterilization processes (see Chapter 15). But the demonstration of antimicrobial effects against all representative types of microorganisms is not sufficient. Consider, for example, that many of the disinfection products/processes described in Chapter 9 may also be effective against the same range of microorganisms (certain types of high-level disinfectants) but they are not used for sterilization. It is important to remember that "sporicidal" or even "sterilant" refers to a biocidal product/process that is effective against spores, but this is not in practice the same as sterilization. Further, it cannot be assumed that a product is sterile merely because it has passed through a sterilization technique; the process may only be effective if designed for that application, and if the sterilizer is installed/maintained according to instructions, correctly used by staff, and the process verified to have taken place correctly. These aspects will be further considered in this chapter.

Given the wide range of antimicrobial chemicals/processes available (see Chapter 6), only a limited number of technologies have been widely used in sterilization processes. Like the discussion of disinfection, these may also be classified as being physical or chemical in their main mechanisms of antimicrobial activity. The most widely used physical method is based on moist heat (steam sterilization), which is also the most used method of sterilization worldwide for processing of reusable devices. Other physical methods such as dry heat, radiation, and filtration have limited applications in healthcare facilities today and are only discussed briefly in this chapter. Chemical sterilization methods have traditionally only been used as low-temperature alternatives to steam for the processing of devices that are temperature sensitive or otherwise not compatible or

---

Decontamination and Device Processing in Healthcare, Second Edition. Gerald McDonnell and Georgia Alevizopoulou.
© 2025 John Wiley & Sons Ltd. Published 2025 by John Wiley & Sons Ltd.

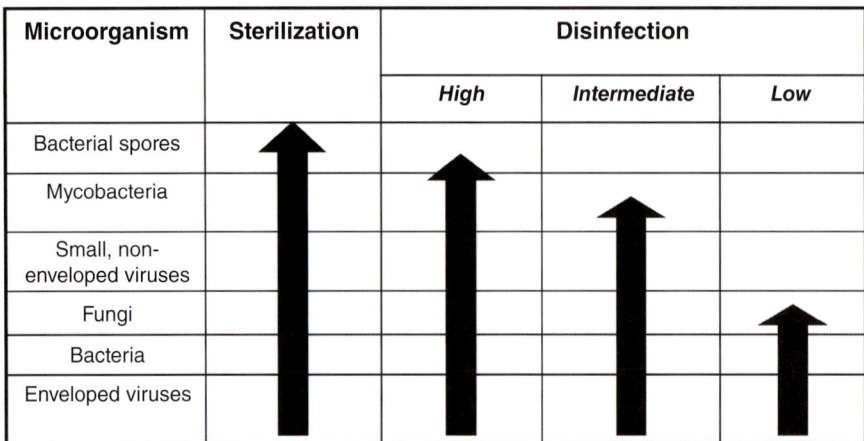

Figure 11.1 A commonly used classification system for disinfection and sterilization, based on the antimicrobial activity of the product/process. The different types of microorganisms are shown on the left (from those that are considered the least resistant to inactivation at the bottom and most resistant at the top), with the expected levels of activity shown for each product/process on the right. In the case of sterilization processes, the minimum criteria is that they are effective against bacterial spores, but the ability to be effective against all microorganisms (including bacterial spores) is only the beginning of defining a sterilization process.

practical to be used with steam processes. These technologies are based on chemicals such as ethylene oxide (EO) gas, formaldehyde gas, hydrogen peroxide gas (which may or may not employ plasma generation as part of the overall process), liquid or gaseous peracetic acid (PAA), and ozone gas. These are all based on effective, broad-spectrum antimicrobials, but are used in well-defined processes to ensure their safe and effective use for sterilization. Most large healthcare facilities will employ at least two or more types of sterilization systems to allow for the processing of different types of devices. Staff training is always important to ensure that such processes are used correctly, according to the manufacturer's instructions, and in compliance with any written facility policies (concerning loading, unloading, process monitoring, safety, maintenance, etc.). The choice of an unsuitable process for a device could cause damage to the item and possibly even compromise the achievement of sterility, with increased risks of patient complications and increased costs.

As discussed for disinfection (Chapter 9), assurance of sterilization occurs even before the sterilization process itself. Any effective decontamination process is dependent on effective cleaning, as the higher the level of soil and microbial load that may be present on a device or load, the lower the probability of achieving sterility can be. The effective cleaning of a reusable item that is to be sterilized is important, with failure to clean potentially resulting in failed sterilization (the survival of microorganisms) and other significant patient risks (see Chapter 8). Remember, if you cannot clean a device you are unlikely to be able to sterilize it. Cleaning and disinfection can both play a role in reducing the numbers and types of microorganisms present; this may be important even though the sterilization process is actually designed to provide a significant "overkill" of microorganisms (see the following section on the basic principles of sterilization). Further, sterilization may be achieved but the item may not be maintained sterile by the time it is used on a patient (e.g. the packaging may be compromised or the device accidentally recontaminated). Therefore, sterilization and the provision of a sterile device for a patient procedure are dependent on the whole cycle of processing, including cleaning, packaging, sterilization, storage/transport, even to the point of preparing and using the device on a patient.

Basic principles of sterilization

As for disinfection (Chapter 9), any sterilization process needs to be effective against microorganisms and be safely applied to devices. Efficacy and safety are the minimum requirements, but to these other considerations may be added such as practical issues (installation and maintenance, ease of use, sterilization time, etc.), regulatory approvals, water quality/purity (water is an important part of many of these processes, particularly steam sterilization), staff training, and even environmental concerns (such as energy costs, water consumption, chemical safety, etc.). The choice of a sterilization process for a particular application will depend on the needs (today and in the future) of any facility. An ideal sterilization process will include:
- Demonstrated broad-spectrum antimicrobial efficacy.
- Demonstration as being a reliable sterilization process within controlled process conditions (e.g. sterility assurance

level or alternative in compliance with international/national standards or guidelines).
- Compatibility with a range of devices and materials (i.e. not damaging).
- Being capable of penetrating a range of loads, packaging materials, and complex devices.
- Being safe for staff to use with minimal risks.
- No toxic residues that could present a risk to staff or patients.
- Rapid cycle time (and not requiring additional holding times before or after use).
- Allowing for sterile storage, if required, following sterilization.
- Good environmental profile.
- Sterilizer equipment available in a range of sizes to accommodate various types of loads.
- Being economic to acquire, use, and maintain.
- Being easy to install.
- Methods available to monitor and confirm that the sterilization process has been adequately applied to a load.
- Compliance with international and any national standards or requirements (including local registrations or clearance from regulatory agencies).

This is not an exhaustive list, but no ideal process exists for all situations. This list highlights that there are strengths and weaknesses to all true sterilization processes, which is why it is important to understand the needs of the facility when defining sterilization needs, but also to understand any limitations of the various types of sterilization processes that may be available for use.

Further consideration should be given to defining the minimal criteria for any sterilization process, in particular efficacy. It is important to note that the first requisite when designing a sterilization process is that the process can demonstrate effectiveness against all types of microorganisms (see the introduction to Chapter 9 and Figure 11.1). This will include at least a representative number of bacteria (Gram-negative and Gram-positive bacteria), viruses (enveloped and non-enveloped forms), fungi (molds and yeasts, vegetative forms), protozoa, mycobacteria, and bacterial spores (see Chapter 5). A variety of test methods, including those used to establish and register disinfection claims (see Chapter 9 on disinfection guidelines and standards), are often used to verify the effectiveness of such processes. Bacterial spores are particularly highlighted as they generally represent those microorganisms with the greatest resistance to inactivation due to their structure (see Chapter 5 on bacteria). But the specific strain (or type) of bacteria from which the spores are made, which is considered the "most-resistant organism," can be different depending on the sterilization process (Table 11.1). For example, *Geobacillus stearothermophilus* spores are considered the most resistant to steam and hydrogen peroxide gas (including gas plasma) processes, while *Bacillus atrophaeus* is considered the most resistant to EO sterilization methods.

Table 11.1 A list of different sterilization methods and their most resistant organisms. Note: other microorganisms may show unusually high-level resistance to the sterilization method, but this may be due to other factors such as presence of soils rather than true resistance to the sterilizing agent. These microorganisms are widely accepted and used for the testing of their respective sterilization methods.

Sterilization method	Most resistant organism
Steam under pressure	*Geobacillus stearothermophilus* spores
Humidified ethylene oxide	*Bacillus atrophaeus*[1] spores
Hydrogen peroxide gas (with or without plasma)	*Geobacillus stearothermophilus* spores
Humidified formaldehyde	*Geobacillus stearothermophilus* spores
Liquid peracetic acid	*Geobacillus stearothermophilus* spores
Dry heat	*Bacillus atrophaeus*[1] spores

[1] Previously known as *Bacillus subtilis*.

On successful completion of these tests, the proposed sterilization process meets the first requirement in demonstrating broad-spectrum antimicrobial activity. The next step is to ensure that the process can provide a defined level of assurance of sterility. International standards, such as ISO 14937 *Sterilization of health care products – General requirements for characterization of a sterilizing agent and the development, validation, and routine control of a sterilization process for medical devices*, provide guidance on how this can be achieved. One approach, primarily used industrially, is based on knowing the types and numbers of microorganisms that are present on the device or load to be sterilized; given the range of surgical and medical procedures, this is not currently considered a practical method for defining a sterilization process for reusable devices. A more common method, which is typically used for defining sterilization processes for reusable devices, is studying the inactivation of the most resistant organism to the sterilizing agent (steam, chemical, etc.) and developing a process that provides an "overkill" of this organism. When this is studied by microbiological methods and analyzed by mathematical techniques, the survival of a microorganism can be expressed in terms of the probability of a single viable microorganism surviving after sterilization, or the "sterility assurance level" (SAL). The most widely used SAL in healthcare applications is an SAL of 10^{-6}, defined as the probability of survival following a sterilization process of 1 in a million. Any SAL can theoretically be used (e.g. 10^{-1}, 10^{-3}, or 10^{-6}), as they can all give a minimal assurance of sterility when the relationship between the exposure to a sterilization process and how it kills the most resistant organism to that process is understood. Note that a

10^{-6} SAL is considered a *higher* level of SAL than 10^{-3}: where 10^{-3} is a 1 in 1000 probability of survival, 10^{-6} is a 1 in 1,000,000 probability of survival. Why is 10^{-6} so often used? It is traditional and has been widespread since the concept was first proposed. The use of such SALs provides a level of overkill to ensure that following the sterilization process the items can be considered "sterile."

The correct definition of an SAL is "the probability of a single viable microorganism occurring on an item after sterilization." We will investigate a typical method used to demonstrate an SAL of 10^{-6} in order to understand the level of safety that is associated with these processes. Consider a surface with a known population of bacterial spores at 10^6 or 1 million (1,000,000) spores. This can be exposed to a sterilizing agent (under the conditions proposed as the minimum for its use in a sterilization process) over time and the level of microorganisms remaining at different times shown by microbiological techniques. An example of this data is given in Table 11.2.

These results can also be shown in graph form (Figure 11.2). It can be seen that the sterilization process provides a rapid reduction in the number of spores, but it is the structure of the graph showing the results in log form that we are particularly interested in, as it shows a "straight-line" or, to the mathematician, a "linear" response. The graph shows a 6-$\log_{10}$ reduction of the test spores in about 40 minutes, but because the rate of kill is linear (shows a straight-line response over time), this allows us to predict the time for an additional theoretical 6-$\log_{10}$ reduction (Figure 11.3).

Therefore, in this example, when starting with a population of the most resistant organism of 1 million (10^6, 6 $\log_{10}$) and testing under the minimum process conditions for the sterilizing agent, a 6 $\log_{10}$ reduction is shown in about 40 minutes and a 12 $\log_{10}$ reduction is predicted mathematically to occur within 80 minutes. Therefore, for a SAL of 10^{-6} the process time would be at least 80 minutes; equally, an SAL or 10^{-3} would take about 60 minutes. Remember that in most cases with critical devices following use on a patient the device is cleaned (see Chapter 9) and usually disinfected (see Chapter 10) prior to sterilization. These processes can remove and inactivate most of the microorganisms that may or may not be present; therefore the level of microorganisms on a device is generally considered to be very low when it is placed into a sterilizer (but note that this is not always the case depending on how the device was used). With these initial processing steps, the level of overkill and therefore the safety level to ensure that the device is sterile following a sterilization process are considered exceptionally high with most critical devices.

Further analysis of the data, as presented in Figure 11.3, is often done when defining a sterilization process. An example is determining the D-value, which may be defined as the average time (in seconds, minutes, etc.) to give a 1 $\log_{10}$ reduction of a test organism. In the example shown in Figure 11.3, the D-value for the test organism in the sterilization process would be approximately 6.7 minutes (total time for a 12 $\log_{10}$ reduction was 80 minutes, and therefore the time for a 1 $\log_{10}$ reduction would be ~6.7 minutes). Further experiments can look at other relationships, such as the effect of the D-value on the temperature or the concentration of a chemical sterilizing agent. The temperature relationship is particularly well described for steam sterilization; for example, a Z-value (defined as the average temperature change required for a 1-$\log_{10}$ change in the D-value) is often used to describe the relationship between the temperature and the average D-value. A typical Z-value for steam is 10°C/50°F. A further term used in steam sterilization is the D-reference at 121°C/~250°F ($D_{121°C}$), being the D-value of a population of spores when exposed to steam under pressure at 121°C/~250°F. When the $D_{121°C}$ and the Z-value are known for a population of spores, the D-value at any temperature of steam under pressure can be estimated and therefore the minimum time for sterilization under those conditions (i.e. for a SAL of 10^{-6}, this is the D-value at the sterilization temperature × 12). For example, at 131°C/~268°F a typical D-value would be 6 seconds, therefore a minimum sterilization time would be 72 seconds (just over 1 minute). In general, most sterilization times are well overstated to give an even greater overkill (e.g. 134°C/~273°F for 3 or 4 minutes is typical). In such a way, the minimum process

Table 11.2 An example of results from studying the antimicrobial activity of a sterilizing agent/process over time. The number of microorganisms (usually bacterial spores) remaining on a test surface is determined over exposure time to the sterilizing agent. The number of spores remaining can be given as the actual number counted or, for the purpose of mathematical analysis, converted into a "$\log_{10}$" scale. This mathematical scale expresses the actual number in a scale of 10; as an example, 10 spores would be a $\log_{10}$ of 1 (or 1×10^1), 100 is $\log_{10}$ 2 (or 1×10^2), 1000 is $\log_{10}$ 3, etc. Therefore 300 is 3×10^2 or about $\log_{10}$ 2.5.

Exposure time (min)	Number of microorganisms remaining	
	Number of spores	$\log_{10}$ number of spores
0	1,000,000	6
5	500,000	5.7
10	100,000	5
15	10,000	4
20	1,000	3
25	200	2.3
30	30	1.5
35	5	0.7
40	0	0

Figure 11.2 The spore reduction results in Table 11.2 shown in graph form, with the number of spores surviving (Y or vertical axis) at various exposure times (X or horizontal axis). At the top is a graph showing the actual number of spores surviving and at the bottom $\log_{10}$ (the number of spores surviving).

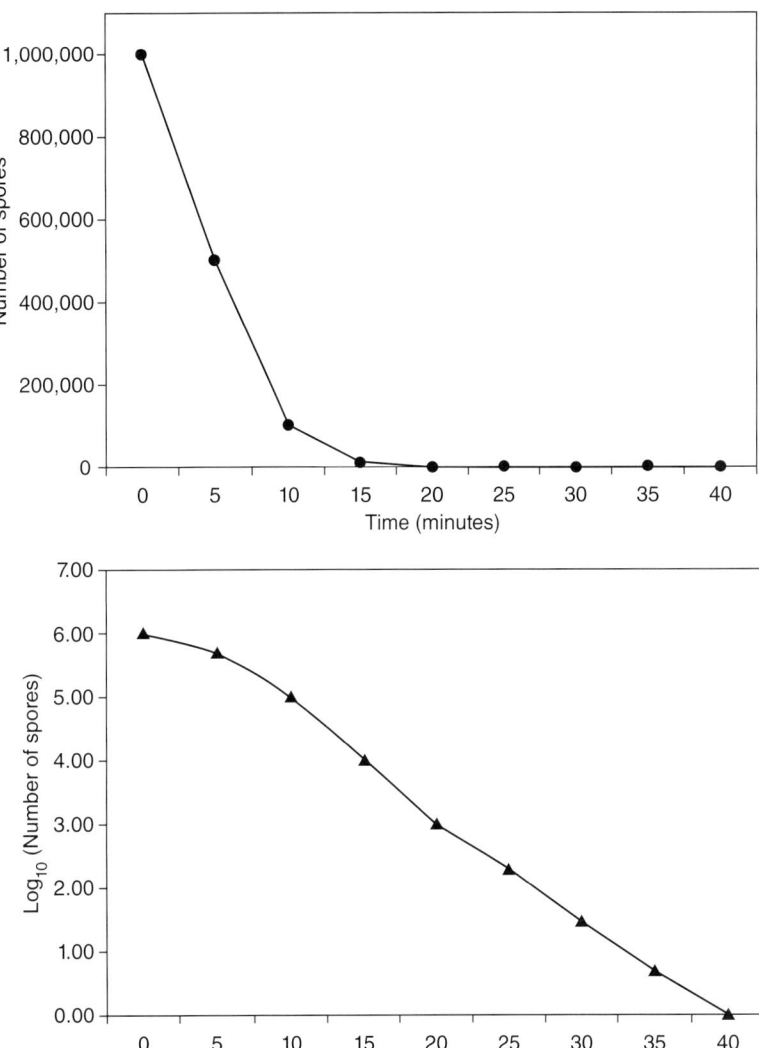

conditions (e.g. temperature, time, concentration of chemical, humidity, etc.) are defined to provide a minimum SAL of 10^{-6}. During this analysis, these process variables and their effects may also be studied and further understood.

When this is complete, the sterilization process itself needs to be developed that allows these minimum process conditions for sterilization to be achieved in the various types of loads ("product") that the process will be used to sterilize. This will define the type of equipment necessary to be able to apply and control the sterilization process. The number, type, design, and packaging of different types of devices can provide different challenges to any process. An example is with air removal from the load, as air can prevent the penetration of the sterilizing agent(s) to all areas of the load. Devices that have internal lumens ("cannulas" or cannulated devices) are examples of instruments that are considered difficult to remove air from and/or to allow a sterilizing agent to fully penetrate. Other variables, depending on the sterilizing agent, may include temperature as well as the antimicrobial chemical and humidity distribution within the load. It is therefore important that examples of such loads are tested and confirmed to be sterilized by the chosen process.

In addition to the antimicrobial efficacy, the process is also tested for any material effects on the devices to be sterilized ("compatibility"), including the different types of materials used to make the devices as well as the devices themselves, and for safety aspects. The process should not damage the devices or may be restricted from being used on certain types of materials or device types. Safety aspects will include staff safety when using or working in the same area as the sterilizer,

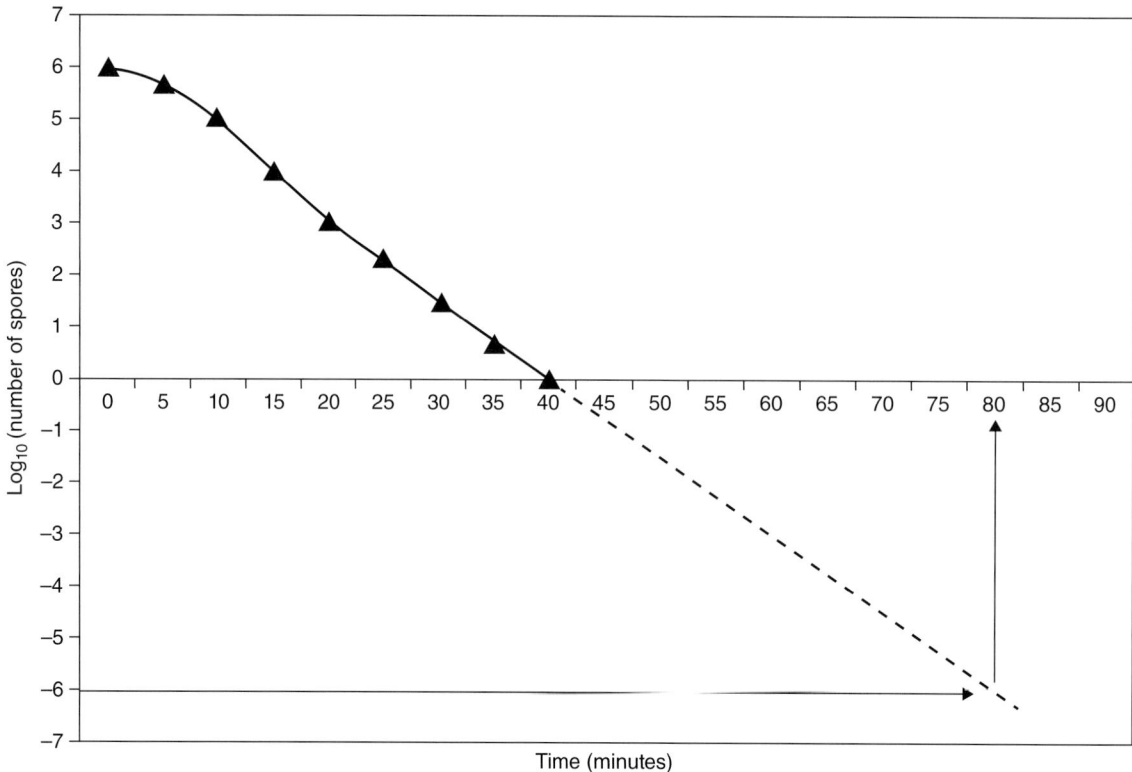

Figure 11.3 Demonstration of a sterility assurance level (SAL) of 10^{-6}. In this case, an SAL of 10^{-6} (or a predicted 12 $\log_{10}$ reduction from a starting population of 6 $\log_{10}$) would be defined for this sterilizing agent, under the process conditions tested, at about 80 minutes. Equally, an SAL of 10^{-1} would be about 47 minutes and 10^{-3} about 60 minutes.

patient safety to ensure that there are no toxic residues present after the process from the sterilizing agent and any associated by-products, as well as safety of the environment. All of these aspects should be considered and verified through testing in the design of the final sterilization process and associated equipment.

A typical sterilization process will typically include three stages:
- Conditioning, ensuring that the load is correctly prepared to be sterilized under defined conditions. This can include air removal, adequate temperature distribution, drying, and chemical agent distribution (under the conditions required for it to be effective as a sterilizing agent). The specific requirements that need to be verified during conditioning will depend on the sterilization process.
- Sterilization, where the minimal SAL of 10^{-6} is ensured.
- Safe release of the load. This can include removal of toxic chemicals (aeration or ventilation), which is typical of chemical sterilization processes, and drying/cooling (as required following steam sterilization). In some cases, such as certain designs of EO and formaldehyde gas sterilizers, additional and often extended aeration may be required in a separate equipment design to ensure that the load does not contain high levels of these antimicrobials or their by-products.

Monitoring

It is important to remember that the proper instructions and tests need to be provided to ensure that the equipment is installed, operated, and performing correctly at the healthcare facility, including requirements for routine monitoring of the process and maintenance of any associated equipment. There are many standards and guidelines that may need to be considered during the design, testing, and routine monitoring of sterilization processes. These may be specific to the mechanism of sterilization (e.g. steam under pressure or humidified EO) or general in considering any newer sterilization method. The specific methods used to routinely monitor sterilization processes can vary depending on the sterilization process, country-specific requirements (or traditions), and the individual preferences/needs of the healthcare facility. Each facility should have a written policy regarding how and when these various methods and indicators are used, as well as describing the action steps to be taken in the event of a fail result being detected.

There are three main methods used to routinely monitor sterilization processes: parametric release, biological indicators, and chemical indicators.

Parametric release (or control)

Parametric release refers to the monitoring of the important conditions (parameters or controls) during the sterilization process and verification that they have been achieved during that process cycle. The official definition is the declaration that the product has reached a desired microbiological quality state based on records demonstrating that the process variables were delivered within specified tolerances. Steam is a useful example, as its successful application for sterilization is dependent on reaching the correct temperature (which can only be achieved by steam under pressure; see the section on steam (moist heat) sterilization). Therefore, the physical monitoring of the temperature and time of the process is a good indicator that the process has been correctly applied. Others monitors may include various types of air detector systems, as effective air removal is an important consideration for steam sterilization. Steam is, however, somewhat more complicated than this (as discussed later in this chapter). For a chemical sterilization process, this may include the concentration (directly or indirectly) of the sterilizing agent, humidity levels, temperature, pressure, and other process variables, depending on the sterilization process. Overall, these various types of sensors can be used for monitoring the effectiveness of the process and can provide this information immediately for inspection/control. There are limitations, though, and the sensors are often complemented by chemical indicators (CIs) and/or biological indicators (Bis).

Biological indicators

BIs are defined as test systems containing viable microorganisms providing a defined resistance to a specified sterilization or disinfection process. Various examples are shown in Figure 11.4. For sterilization processes, BIs usually contain a known population of bacterial spores (e.g. 10^5 or 10^6) placed onto a carrier material (e.g. paper or a stainless steel disc). The bacterial spore type is usually the defined most resistant organism for the process, such as *Geobacillus stearothermophilus* spores for steam sterilization and *Bacillus atrophaeus* spores for EO (Table 11.1). A BI is designed to be able to show

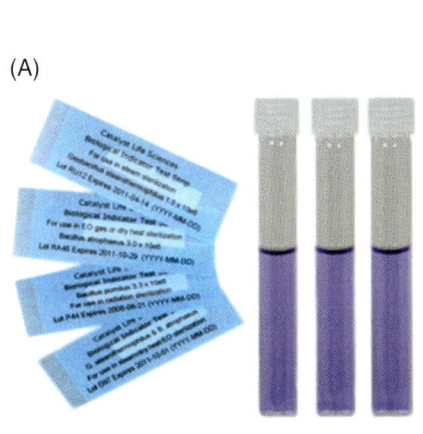
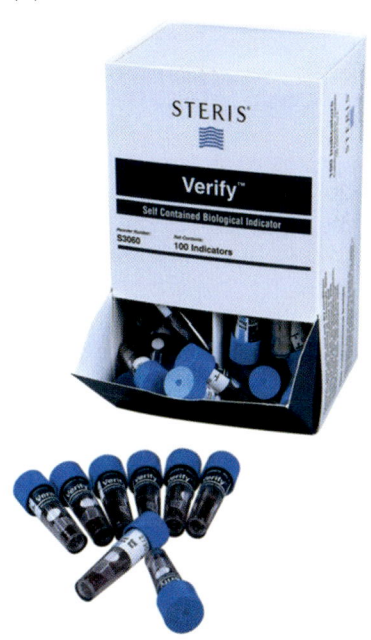

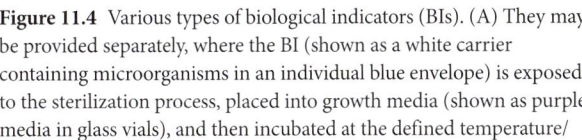

Figure 11.4 Various types of biological indicators (BIs). (A) They may be provided separately, where the BI (shown as a white carrier containing microorganisms in an individual blue envelope) is exposed to the sterilization process, placed into growth media (shown as purple media in glass vials), and then incubated at the defined temperature/ time to show growth or no growth. (B) In other more commonly used examples, known as self-contained BIs (SCBIs) the indicator is contained in an all-in-one pack that is exposed to the sterilization process and mixed directly afterward with little handling by the operator. Courtesy STERIS Corporation 2024. All rights reserved.

growth or no growth following its incubation on exposure to a sterilization process. Growth would be a failed result and no growth a pass result. This can take time, with the incubation time ranging from 1 day (24 hours) to 7 days before the result is known.

Some BI designs (known as "rapid-read") can include various technologies that allow for the detection of growth or no growth much quicker than traditional methods. One example is the use of an indirect CI of this result such as a color change (based on a change in pH in the growth media). Others are more specialized, depending on the presence of enzyme activity (indicated by the production of light) suggesting that spore growth is occurring. In both cases, these early indications are considered preliminary and require verification of growth/no growth for the final result, and must be verified at a later stage according to the manufacturer's instructions. But these technologies have become widely used and accepted in comparison to traditional BIs. Examples of widely used rapid-read BIs are shown in Figure 11.5.

BIs may also be included in specially designed challenge packs (known as process challenge devices or PCDs, see later) to further challenge a sterilization process. BIs are discussed in further detail in Chapter 14 on monitoring sterilization.

Chemical indicators

CIs were briefly introduced in Chapter 9, in the section on disinfection guidelines and standards, and will be discussed in more detail in Chapter 14. They are defined as test systems (usually in the form of test strips) that reveal a change in one or more pre-defined process variables based on a chemical and/or physical change resulting from exposure to the process. They are generally provided as color-change indicators and are widely used in monitoring sterilization processes (Figure 11.6). They are classified and defined by ISO 11140 *Sterilization of health care products –Chemical indicators. Part 1: General Requirements* into six types, previously referred to as "classes" (Table 11.3).

For sterilization monitoring, type 1 indicators are widely used to indicate on the outside of a pack that it has been exposed to a sterilization process; they are usually applied during packaging (see Chapter 10) and provide a visual color change to differentiate sterilized from non-sterilized packs. An example of a type 2 indicator is a Bowie–Dick (B–D) test,

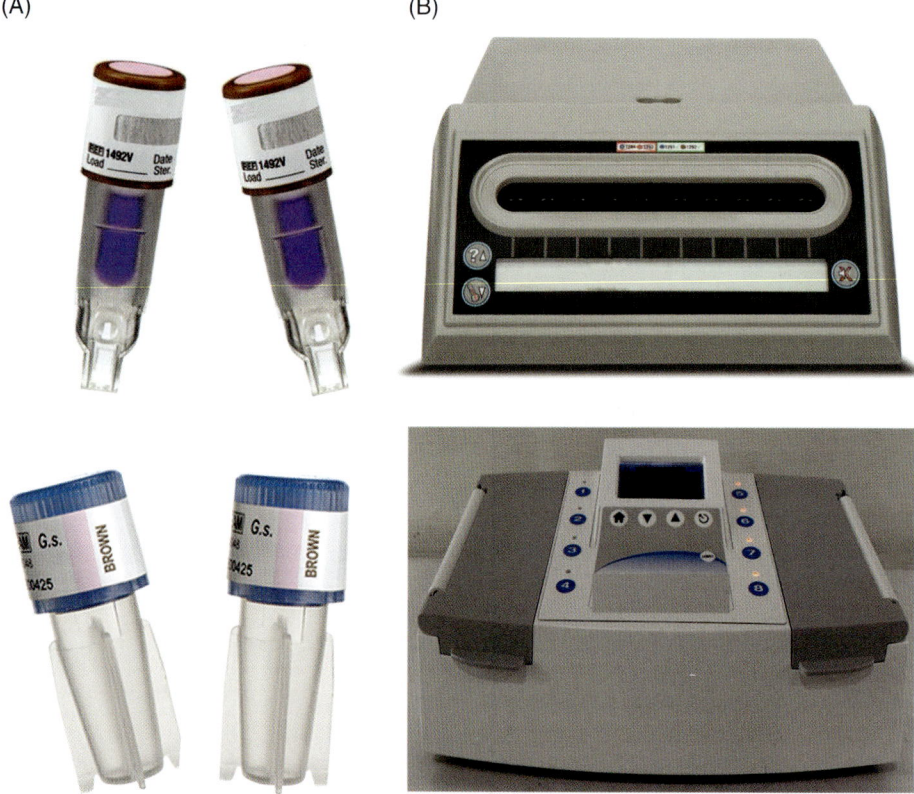

Figure 11.5 Example of widely used, self-contained, and rapid-readout biological indicators used to monitor steam sterilization. (A) Self-contained indicators and (B) indicator incubators.

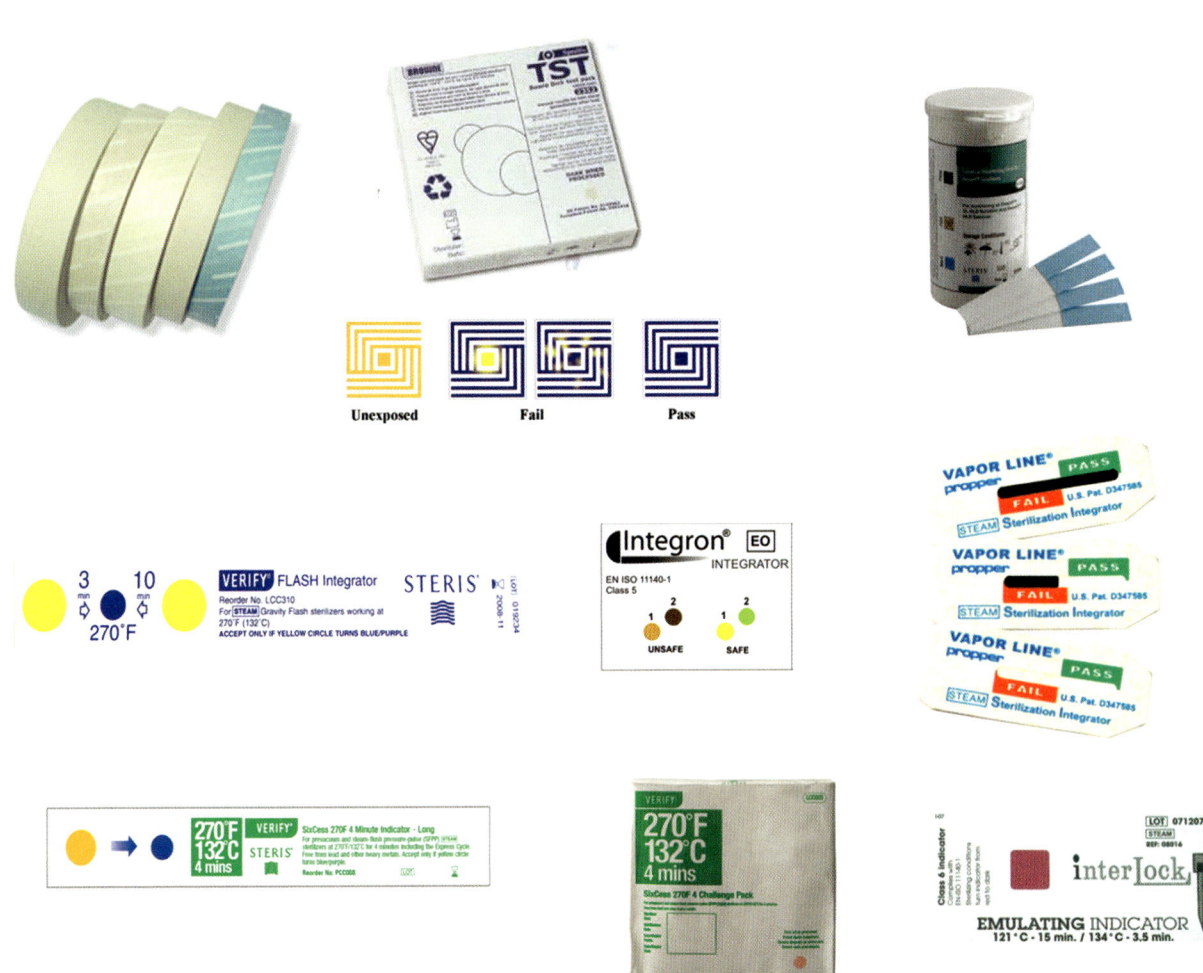

Figure 11.6 Various types of chemical indicators used for monitoring sterilization processes.

Table 11.3 The classification of chemical indicators. Defined based on ISO 11140 *Sterilization of health care products – Chemical indicators. Part 1: General Requirements.*

Type	Indicator type	Description
Type 1	Process indicator	Simple indicators to demonstrate exposure to a process and to distinguish between processed/unprocessed units A pass result may not mean that the process has been achieved
Type 2	Indicators for use in specific tests	Used to indicate a specific type of test, generally established in another standard An example is a Bowie–Dick test to test for steam penetration/air removal in a steam sterilization process
Type 3	Single-variable indicators	Designed to respond to only one critical process variable (e.g. concentration of a biocide or temperature)
Type 4	Multi-variable indicators	Designed to respond to two or more of the critical variables (e.g. temperature, time, and concentration of a biocide)
Type 5	Integrating indicators	Designed to respond to all critical variables of the process, to be equivalent to a biological indicator (e.g. indicators containing bacterial spores used to test sterilization processes)
Type 6	Emulating (or cycle verification) indicators	Designed to react to all critical variables for a full specified cycle (which may be over and above that matching a biological indicator)

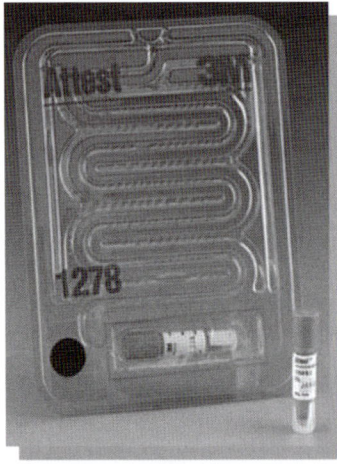 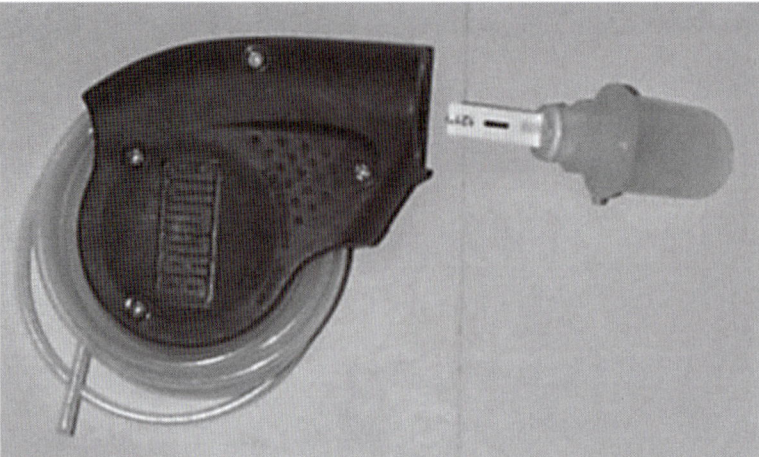
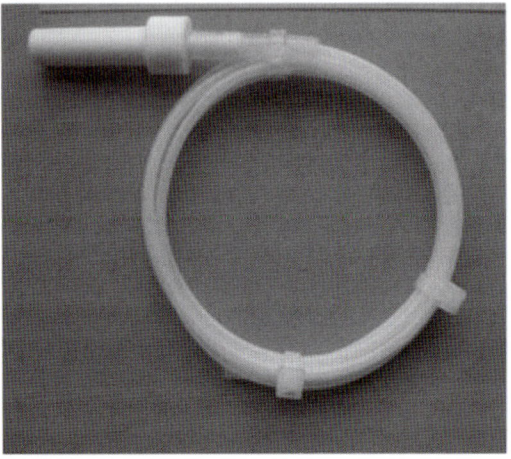 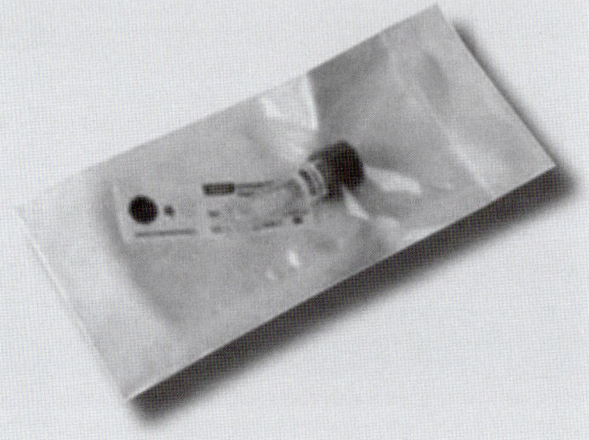

Figure 11.7 Various types of process challenge devices.

which is specifically used to monitor air removal from and steam penetration into a "porous load" in a vacuum-assisted steam sterilizer (see the section on steam (moist heat) sterilization); the test simulates a towel pack that can be difficult to remove air from with a chemical indicator in the center of the pack to detect that air removal/steam penetration has been effective. Types 3, 4, 5, and 6 indicators may also be used. They are usually placed inside packs to be sterilized and can be checked on opening just prior to use in a surgical/medical procedure. The most widely used internationally (in particular for steam sterilization) are type 5 and 6 indicators. Type 5 indicators simulate the response to a BI (but without the need for incubation) and type 6 are designed to indicate that all critical parameters of the sterilization process have been met, including the full exposure time for the process. CIs have the advantage over BIs that they give an immediate result and are sometimes used in combination with BIs as dual indicators.

Process challenge devices

A PCD is designed to be able to provide a specific challenge (e.g. penetration challenge) for a sterilization process, and is used as a more robust method to monitor the performance of that process. Examples are shown in Figure 11.7. They are usually combined with a CI, BI, or even both as the indication system(s), but provide a defined additional challenge unique to a sterilization process.

Physical sterilization

The most widely used method of sterilization in healthcare facilities today is based on steam (or specifically steam under pressure). Other physical methods are less commonly used and are briefly considered in this section, including dry heat, radiation, and filtration.

Steam (moist heat) sterilization
Principles of steam sterilization

High-temperature steam (steam under pressure, commonly known as moist heat) is the most widely used and well-studied method of sterilization. As introduced in Chapter 6, water can be present as a solid (ice), liquid (water), or gas (steam) depending on the energy (e.g. temperature) provided to it. Under atmospheric pressure conditions, at sea level, water forms steam at ~100°C/212°F. We can see this by boiling water to produce steam. As a gas, steam follows the gas laws, therefore if you have a fixed amount of steam in a fixed volume (such as a sealed sterilization chamber), there is a direct relationship between the temperature and the pressure. As the pressure increases the temperature of the steam increases (Figure 11.8).

Therefore, higher temperatures of steam can be achieved by increasing the pressure of the steam in a dedicated chamber (steam sterilizer). This is achieved during the steam sterilization process by the introduction of steam into the chamber, controlling the amount of steam that is released to cause an increase in pressure and continuing to provide heat to a defined point. The point at which steam forms under controlled conditions of pressure and temperature is considered the most efficient for sterilization (referred to as being "saturated"). Typical sterilization times, pressures, and temperatures are summarized in Table 11.4.

When steam at these high temperatures comes into contact with cooler surfaces (such as a load of devices to be sterilized) it immediately condenses (goes from being a gas to a liquid) as water on the surface. Condensation has two powerful effects:

- It releases the thermal energy of the steam with a tremendous antimicrobial activity on any microorganisms present as well as heating the surface.

- It causes an huge reduction in the volume of steam present as it changes into water, causing further steam to be drawn toward the items being sterilized.

Under such conditions, saturated steam is extremely efficient, with an enormous heating and penetrating capacity. This direct application of energy/heat destroys microorganisms, but this destruction is made even more effective by the addition of moisture, as steam is a much more efficient carrier of thermal energy or heat than air (or dry heat). Steam can have many direct effects on the structure and function of microorganisms that culminate in their death or loss of viability. One of the major mechanisms of action is the destruction of proteins, which are essential to the structure and function of microorganisms; heat causes proteins to denature ("unfold") and coagulate. Steam will also have negative effects on all the other molecules that make up these structures, such as lipids and nucleic acids.

If the steam contains too much water it is considered too "wet," and if it contains less water it is considered too "dry," also known as "superheated." Wet steam already has a lot of condensed water present, so will be less efficient at transferring its antimicrobial effect to a surface. Superheated steam may be formed by temperatures higher than those required to generate steam at a specified pressure, therefore it has less water available to condense and essentially acts like dry heat (which is known to be a much less efficient sterilization method). Therefore, although the concept of steam sterilization at defined temperatures and pressures is straightforward, the control of such processes is important to ensure that they are optimal for sterilization. In fact, the essential process conditions for adequate steam sterilization are:

- The absence of air (or specifically non-condensable gases (NCGs) that can interfere with the process). Note that air may be present in the sterilization chamber, in the load to be

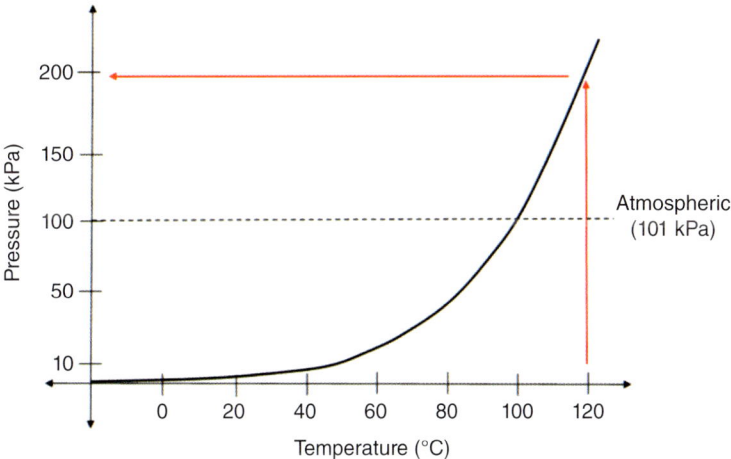

Figure 11.8 The relationship between temperature and pressure of water according to the gas laws. The line in the graph represents the point at which steam is formed from water at a given temperature and pressure. Atmospheric pressure (101 kPa) is shown by a dashed line. As the pressure is increased the temperature at which steam is formed also increases, giving it more energy. Therefore, as an example, steam at 120°C can be made at a pressure of 200 kPa.

Table 11.4 Typical steam sterilization conditions. The related temperatures and pressures are shown, with the estimated minimum time for sterilization (providing a sterility assurance level (SAL) of 10^{-6} with a population of bacterial spores at a $D_{121°C}$ of 1 and a Z-value of 10°C) and typical examples of exposure times used.

Temperature[1]		Pressure[2]			Minimum exposure time (minutes)[3]	Actual exposure times used (minutes)[4]
°C	°F	kPa	Bar	psi		
121	249.8	205	2.05	29.7	12	15–30
125	257	232	2.32	33.7	6	10–15
132	269.6	287	2.87	41.6	1	3–5
134	273.2	304	3.04	44.1	0.6	3–5
138	280.4	341	3.41	49.5	0.2	1–18[5]

[1] To convert from °C to °F, use the following formula:

$$°F = (1.8 \times °C) + 32$$

$$°C = (°F - 32) \times 0.5555$$

[2] 1 kPa is equivalent to 0.01 bar (or 10 millibar), 7.5 mmHg, 7.5 Torr, 0.145 psi.
[3] Estimated to provide an SAL of 10^{-6} with a population of bacterial spores at a $D_{121°C}$ of 1 and a Z-value of 10°C.
[4] Note that these exposure times generally provide a significant overkill, in excess of the minimal requirement of an SAL of 10^{-6}; they are given only as traditional times used.
[5] 134°C for 18 minutes conditions are often used as specific steam sterilization cycles to reduce the risk of prion contamination.

sterilized, and even in the water used to make the steam. As introduced in Chapter 6 (in the section on mixtures, formulations, and solutions), air is a mixture of gases, consisting of about 78% nitrogen, 21% oxygen, and a range of other gases at much lower amounts (e.g. carbon dioxide, CO_2, and water vapor). Water also can contain an amount of air and therefore types of gases, particularly carbon dioxide and oxygen, but also others such as nitrogen, hydrogen, helium, chlorine, and sulfur oxide. Water likes to be a liquid at room temperature and atmospheric pressure, and when in gas (steam) form it is known as a "condensable" gas, being defined as condensing to its liquid form (water) under the typical conditions of pressure/temperature used during steam sterilization. The gases present in steam (and in the air) have different requirements and are therefore known as "non-condensable" gases under these steam sterilization conditions. They can remain in gas form and can impede the penetration of steam to or within the load. Therefore, it is important not only to remove air from the chamber/load but also to reduce to a minimum any NCGs gases present in the water used to make steam for the process.
• The presence of saturated steam, at the defined temperature and pressure. Remember, saturated steam is at the midpoint between condensation and evaporation of water (see Chapter 6, in the section on solids, liquids, and gases).
• The attainment of the minimum specified temperature in the load for the specified sterilization time.

Steam sterilization processes are designed to ensure that these conditions are met for specific types of loads. A typical steam sterilization cycle will therefore include several stages:
• Conditioning: air removal and pre-heating to the desired sterilization temperature. There are many different ways to remove air from the load, most often assisted by the use of steam (known as "displacement") that is used to heat the load to the desired sterilization temperature under pressure.
• Steam sterilization: the steam temperature and pressure are maintained at a "constant" level for the desired sterilization time ("holding time").
• Cooling and drying (often optional in the sterilizer depending on the load and sterilizer design). Cooling is essential to ensure that the materials can be safely unloaded and transported for storage/use. Drying is also important, as if water remains in the pack it may be suspected as being compromised when opened for a patient procedure (referred to as a "wet-pack"). Excessive water present within a pack can be due to excessive wetness in the steam and the product may not have been sterilized correctly (see the section on troubleshooting steam sterilization problems).

Steam sterilization processes are developed and tested by the manufacturer for a variety of different applications, including:
• Wrapped devices/instruments (often referred to as non-porous loads or cycles).

- Textile packs (sometimes referred to as "porous" loads or cycles). Porous refers to the ability to trap air/liquid within the structure of such materials due to their structure. Examples of porous materials are textiles, woven and non-woven fabrics, paper, and even some types of plastics. These are often some of the more difficult materials/loads to sterilize with steam.
- Lumened or hollow devices (e.g. rigid endoscopes and dental handpieces, which sometimes require special cycle conditions).
- Utensils and glassware.
- Mixtures of all different types of wrapped devices and instruments, including lumened or hollow devices, utensils, glassware, and textile packs.
- Liquids and solutions. These items have become infrequently sterilized in healthcare facilities, being supplied pre-sterilized by manufacturers (e.g. sterile water or saline). Note: specific cycle conditions are required to ensure the correct sterilization of such materials.
- Immediate-use (known as "flash" historically) sterilization, which refers to the sterilization of devices/items for immediate use on a patient (not being stored sterile). Specific immediate-use steam sterilization cycles may be designed for certain types of items (e.g. porous or non-porous materials) and are usually for quick sterilization (e.g. in the case of a dropped instrument during a surgical procedure that is required and there is no replacement available). Items are usually unwrapped, as most immediate-use cycles have no or an abbreviated drying cycle. In some cases a specifically designed and labeled-for-use rigid container can be used for the purpose of exposure during sterilization and maintaining sterility during temporary transport to the sterile field. Such sterilization processes are designed for immediate use of the device and items should not be stored prior to use but aseptically transferred to the patient for use. Immediate-use sterilization is further discussed as a special consideration later in this chapter.

Overall, specific cycles will be defined and tested by the sterilizer manufacturer, not only to include the types of materials but also the recommended loads and loading practices. Care should be taken to ensure that the right cycles are available/selected for the various types of loads to be sterilized, as well as confirming that the sterilizer chamber is correctly loaded to ensure that the defined process is effective (see Chapter 10, in the section on loading and unloading sterilizers).

Steam sterilization processes are performed in specific sterilizers capable of handling the pressures and temperatures required during the steam process. These are referred to as steam sterilizers, "autoclaves," or pressure vessels (Figure 11.9–11.11). They are designed in a variety of ways to provide the required steam sterilization process, including ensuring that the air can be efficiently removed from the load being sterilized. Steam sterilizers can be classified based on the methods used for air removal such as upward displacement, downward displacement, pressure pulsing, and vacuum assisted. These are discussed in further detail in the next section. In many cases, in particular large steam sterilizers, multiple steam processing cycles including different methods of air removal (e.g. pre-vacuum and gravity displacement cycles) are provided in the same sterilizer design to accommodate the variety of different types of materials to be sterilized.

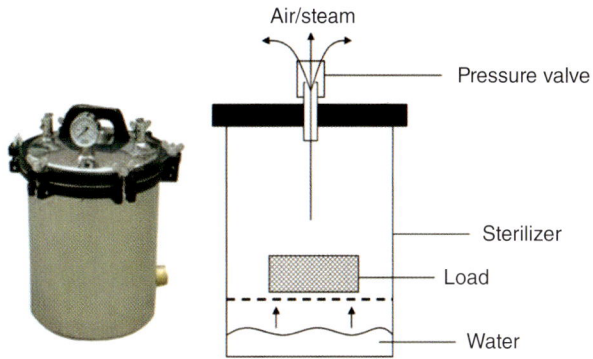

Figure 11.9 An example and the basic design of an upward displacement steam sterilizer. Water is placed at the bottom and heated, to produce steam that rises to push the air out from the top of the vessel.

Overall, steam sterilization has many advantages, being a simple process (with three key variables: time, temperature, and moisture), well described, easy to monitor, rapidly effective against all types of microorganisms (including prions, but generally recommended at longer contact times), and with a variety of sterilizers (sizes, types, etc.) available. Once installed, these sterilizers are economical, providing a low cost per cycle and relatively short sterilization times (with the longest times of a typical process taken up by conditioning and cooling/drying). Despite these advantages, steam sterilization is not appropriate for temperature- or moisture-sensitive materials/devices and may not be applicable to certain types of pressure-sensitive items. Successful steam sterilization is dependent on an adequate supply of water, with water quality and purity being important considerations to reduce any negative effects (see the section on water purity and steam quality).

Types of steam sterilization processes, based on air removal

The removal of air is important to ensure an efficient steam sterilization process. Air can prevent the penetration of steam into a load and contact with all surfaces. While hot air can have some antimicrobial effects, it is a much more inefficient sterilizing agent than saturated steam. Due to the physics and thermodynamics of steam, air, and water mixtures, each air removal method can be

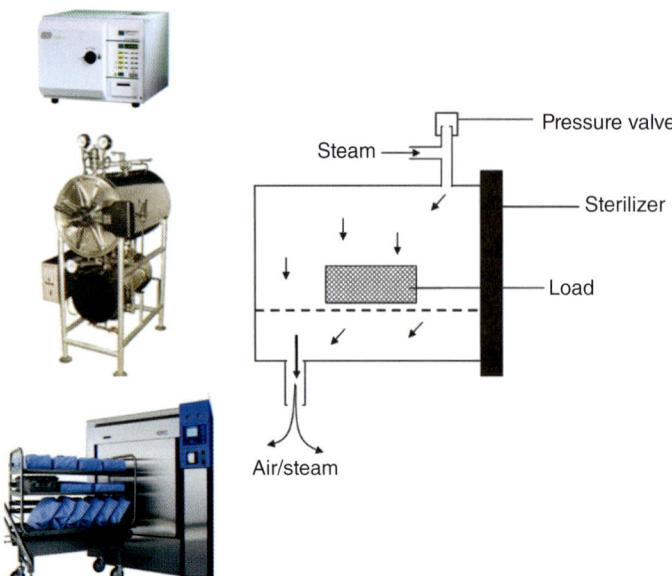

Figure 11.10 Examples and the basic design of a downward displacement steam sterilizer. The lower steam sterilizer offers downward displacement and vacuum-assisted steam sterilization cycle options. Steam enters at the top of the vessel that falls by gravity ("gravity displacement") to force the air out from the bottom of the vessel.

non-porous loads. In these designs (shown in Figure 11.9), water is placed at the bottom of the sterilizer and heated. As steam is generated it rises to push the air/steam out of the top of the chamber (therefore the air is displaced by upward displacement). Once air has been removed for the desired length of time, a pressure valve can be manually placed at the point of steam/air exit (or controlled automatically); this will allow the steam pressure to build up to the desired pressure/temperature for sterilization. Such designs are often used for simple devices, in particular for immediate-use sterilization, but overall have poor air removal capabilities. They are not widely used by healthcare facilities.

Downward displacement

Downward (or gravity, non-vacuum) displacement sterilizer designs and steam sterilization cycles work on the opposite principle to upward displacement but have the benefit that steam is lighter than air (Figure 11.10). During a typical cycle, the steam is introduced slowly into the top of the sterilizer and as more steam enters the chamber it will begin to push the air down (due to the weight or mass of steam present). As more steam is introduced the air is continually displaced downward and out through the bottom of the vessel. When the air removal phase is complete and the correct steam/pressure is achieved, the load is held for the desired sterilization time. Downward displacement sterilizers, when designed and operated correctly, are more efficient at air removal than upward displacement designs, but are generally less efficient at air removal from porous loads and lumened devices. Note that steam sterilization processes based on gravity displacement air removal cycles can be designed for non-porous, lumened

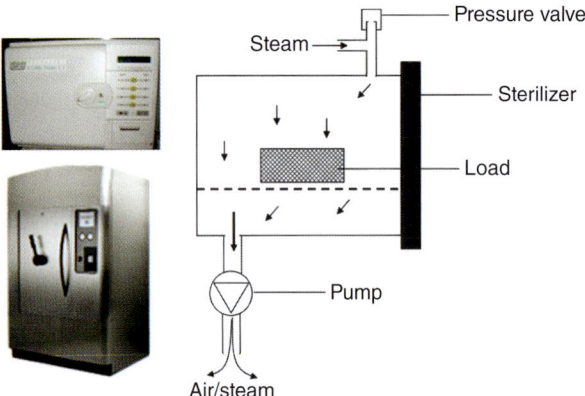

Figure 11.11 Examples and the basic design of vacuum-assisted steam sterilizers. The lower steam sterilizer offers downward displacement and vacuum-assisted steam sterilization cycle options. Air is removed by pulling a vacuum (low pressure) within the chamber. Steam then enters at the top of the vessel and increases to the desired pressure for sterilization.

used in certain circumstances but has its own deficiencies. Further, while the general types of air removal cycles are discussed here, the specific cycle conditions can vary in air removal/steam penetration efficiency and care should be taken to review all the manufacturer's instructions regarding their use.

Upward displacement

These are simple yet older designs of steam sterilizers based on the concepts used in pressure cooking. They are usually smaller-type sterilizers and are recommended for smaller, devices and porous loads, depending on the manufacturer's cycle and testing conditions.

Vacuum assisted

Vacuum-assisted air removal cycles and sterilizer designs are examples of dynamic air removal processes, using a vacuum pump to extract the air prior to the introduction of steam (Figure 11.11). In the simplest form, the air is forcibly removed by pulling a vacuum (a low pressure) within the vessel and then steam is introduced to replace the air. When the correct temperature and pressure conditions are met, the steam sterilization process proceeds. Such cycles are particularly effective at removing air from porous loads (such as fabrics and towels) and lumened devices. Some types of loads/devices may be restricted from such cycles due to being pressure (vacuum) restricted by the manufacturer. Note that many sterilizer designs will be programmed with both downward displacement and vacuum-assisted types of conditioning cycles to meet the needs of the variety of load/device types that may need to be sterilized. The vacuum levels, number of vacuum pulses, and so on can vary from manufacturer to manufacturer and design to design (as shown in Figure 11.12), therefore care should be taken to closely inspect the instructions regarding the load configuration/restrictions for each type of defined cycle. In general, the lower the pressure/vacuum, the more air is removed from the load, but this may also be compensated by various vacuum/steam-pulsing cycles. Vacuum-assisted cycles are the basis for many other types of dynamic air removal cycles (see the next section on variations). In addition to conditioning advantages, vacuum conditions may be useful in assisting with drying and cooling following the steam sterilization cycle.

Variations of pressure and/or vacuum pulsing

The role of steam sterilization conditioning cycles is to remove air and pre-heat the load to the desired temperature for sterilization. Many different types of efficient conditioning cycles have been described and used for these purposes, in order to minimize the overall sterilization process time, optimize air removal for various types of loads, and reduce sterilizer costs. Examples of such steam sterilization processes are shown in Figure 11.12. They can include pulsing conditions of high pressure and low pressure (vacuum) to various extents to optimize air removal. As in the other cases, care should be taken to understand any instructions, restrictions, or limitations of such defined cycles to ensure that they are used correctly. Even efficient conditioning cycles may be compromised if not used according to the manufacturer's instructions.

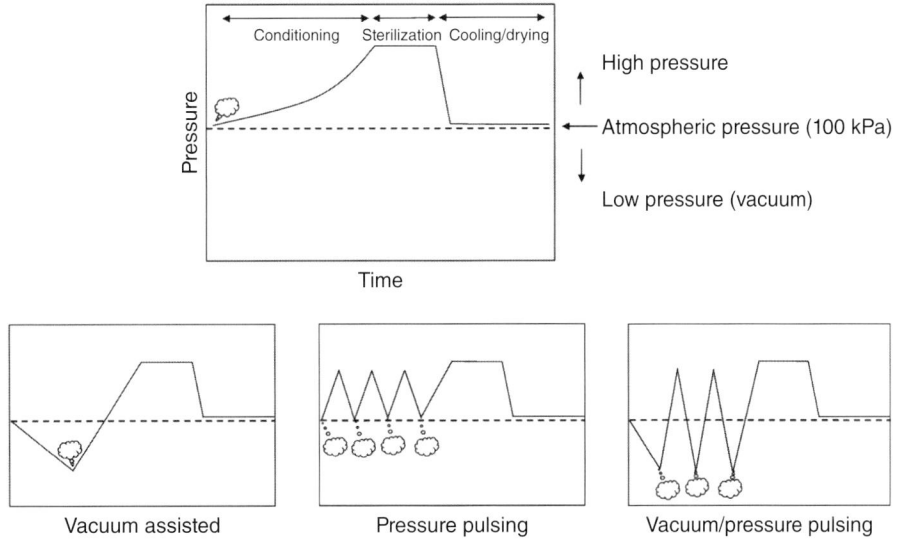

Figure 11.12 Simplified examples of different types of steam conditioning cycles, as part of the overall sterilization process. A typical steam sterilization process will include conditioning, sterilization, and cooling/drying phases. The upper cycle shows these phases in a typical gravity displacement cycle (with steam introduced at the start of the cycle); the dashed line indicates atmospheric pressure. Examples of vacuum-assisted, pressure-pulsing, and vacuum-pressure pulsing cycles are shown below, with steam introduction times shown during the cycle. Note that the cycle times are not drawn to scale, but in general gravity displacement cycles are the longest, followed by vacuum-assisted cycles, and then the various types of pressure/vacuum dynamic cycles. Such cycles and their efficiencies will vary from manufacturer to manufacturer.

304 Decontamination and Device Processing in Healthcare

Steam sterilizer design

Although steam sterilizers can vary in size, shape, and complexity, they can all be described as having the same essential design features (Figure 11.13). This section should not be considered as an exhaustive introduction to the various design criteria and sterilizer types that are available, but it does provide an understanding of some of the basic components of a steam sterilizer.

The major components include:

- The sterilization chamber, also known as the pressure vessel. The chamber is commonly constructed of a high grade of

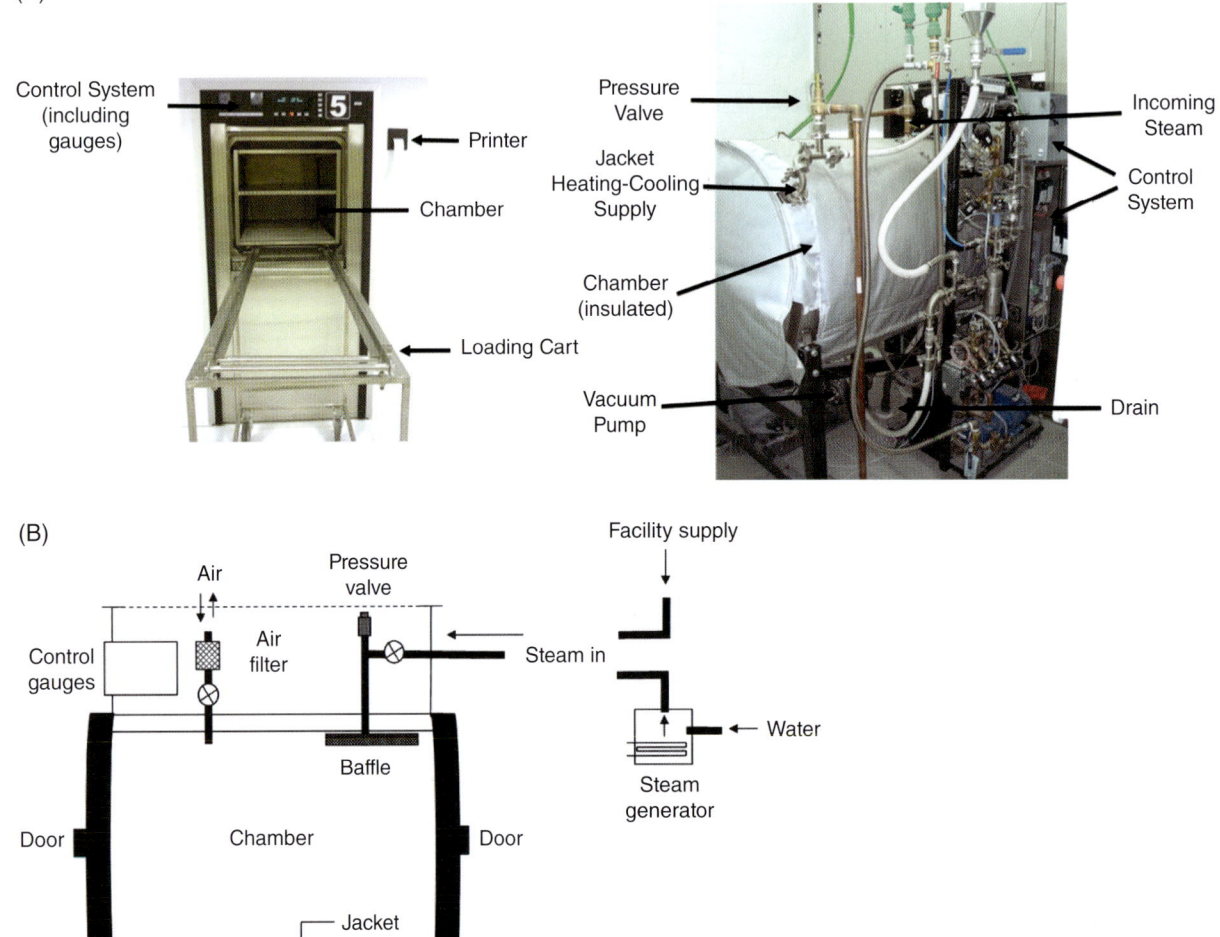

Figure 11.13 (A) Typical design of a medium-sized steam sterilizer, showing the user interface (on the upper left; entrance to the chamber/door, loading mechanism, control system, and, optionally, a printer) and the working mechanisms shown from the side (on the upper right). Smaller or larger sizes will have many of the same features. (B) The major components of a typical, larger steam sterilizer are shown (showing a double-door, jacketed sterilizer with a vacuum pump and optional steam generator).

stainless steel and needs to be designed (and verified) to meet various safety codes as a pressure vessel (a chamber designed to withstand high pressures). There may be one or two entry doors into the chamber in single- or double-door designs, respectively. In single-door designs the load is placed into and removed from the chamber through the same door, while in double-door designs the load is placed into the chamber on one side and removed following sterilization from the other (allowing for physical separation of unsterilized and sterilized packs). In addition, the chamber may be designed with an external "jacket" that allows the walls of the sterilizer to be heated (e.g. with steam) during the process. Jacketed sterilizer designs have advantages over non-jacketed such as improved cycle time (as the heat-up time for the load and even the drying time may be quicker) and preventing excessive condensation during the cycle (which can lead to "wet-packs" or loads that require extended drying in order to ensure there is no residual moisture remaining during storage/transport).

- A steam supply. Steam can be injected into the chamber via an internal steam source within or close to the sterilizer (such as an integral steam generator) and/or it can be supplied separately, usually from a main facility supply. In both cases, the volume of water provided is controlled within a steam generator or boiler. With main hospital steam supplies, the steam is produced in large boilers and piped to the sterilizer "plant room." Pressures in these systems can be very high (e.g. 1000 kPa), much higher than the actual pressure required by the sterilizer (e.g. ~260 Kpa), and are therefore reduced using a pressure-reducing valve. An isolating steam valve is used to shut off the steam to the sterilizers for maintenance. In other designs, or as a back-up to the facility supply, a steam generator may be built into the design of the sterilizer or closely associated with it. In further designs, water is introduced directly into the base of the sterilizer chamber and heaters are provided that heat the water until it boils and produces steam directly within the chamber. Most steam sterilizers are designed with a system that will decrease the amount of condensed water present in the steam and direct only saturated steam into the chamber. An example is a baffle plate located at the entrance of steam into the chamber. Another example is the use of a "steam separator" or "steam trap" to remove condensate from the steam pipework. Remember, increased water content in the steam means that the transfer of thermal energy to the load can be compromised, resulting in ineffective sterilization and possibly result in wet loads (or packs). Wet-packs are a sign of an inefficient or ineffective sterilization process for the type of load being sterilized, which increases the risk of packs being contaminated during storage/transport (see the section on process failures).
- Piping systems to aid in conditioning, sterilization, and drying/cooling, which may be made from high-grade stainless steel (preferred) or other metals. These pipes transfer steam/air in and out of the chamber by a system of control (including pressure) valves, generally under an automated control system. In vacuum-assisted sterilizers this may also include a vacuum pump that assists during the conditioning and drying phases of the cycle, as well as various temperature or other monitoring systems. Sterilizers are often designed to conserve the use of water and energy, e.g. by reusing water and using heat-recovery systems.
- An air venting system. This allows air to be vented into the chamber at various times during the cycle, where the air is passed through a microbial (bacteria/fungi) retentive filter to prevent microbial cross-contamination.
- Control system and gauges. The control system automatically controls the pre-programmed cycle when selected by the user and may be associated with various sensors and gauges (for variables such as temperature and pressure) that aid in controlling and/or monitoring the process. In addition to controlling temperature/pressure, safety limits are also set to avoid over-temperature or over-pressurization. An example is a "jacket over pressure switch" that is used to shut off the steam supply to the jacket should the temperature probe fail and the pressure go too high in the jacket; if such a switch fails there is often a further safety valve that will release if the maximum safe working pressure is exceeded. In such extreme cases, where a sterilizer safety valve blows, the machine must be turned off and the steam supply isolating valve shut off immediately.
- A printer/recorder, to provide a simple or detailed description of the cycle and sterilization parameters. This may be part of the sterilizer design or connected separately to a computer/recording system. In some designs an independent monitoring system may be provided, which independently monitors the different cycle parameters (e.g. temperature, time, pressure) in parallel with the control system to ensure that the process is performing within specified limits.

Maintenance and quality control

Regular maintenance, quality control, and performance testing are essential to ensure that the sterilizer is functioning correctly. This can include daily, weekly, monthly, quarterly, and annual tests, and should be carried out according to department policy, local regulatory requirements, and manufacturer's guidelines.

Maintenance refers to the routine care of equipment to reduce the malfunction of critical components that could cause sterilization failure and downtime. Manufacturers should provide clear written care and maintenance schedules and instructions that must be adhered to by the user, as only a properly maintained sterilizer will consistently provide sterile packs. Maintenance may be routine or preventative, performed by in-house or outsourced staff. Maintenance instructions are usually recommended by the manufacturer

in its instruction manual, but as examples they should include:
- Wiping and checking the door sealing gasket (seal).
- Removing debris or foreign bodies from the chamber, trays/rack, and drains, as these may block filters or damage sterilizer parts (e.g. vacuum pump and door gasket).
- Regularly inspecting, cleaning, and/or replacing filters such as water, air, and drain filters.
- Regularly confirming the calibration of the sterilizer sensors (e.g. temperature and pressure sensors).
- Checking and, if applicable, replacing pressure relief valves.
- Performing vacuum leak tests and steam penetration tests (such as B–D or Helix tests).

Regularly scheduled preventative maintenance is required for safe and reliable operation of steam sterilizers. When undertaking maintenance, appropriate safety procedures must be always followed. Before commencing maintenance work always follow lockout/tagout and electrical safe work practice standards by disconnecting all utilities to the sterilizer. Any recommended, routine cleaning should only be performed by trained staff and maintenance, repairs, and adjustments should only be performed by fully qualified service personnel. It is important that the sterilizer chamber and accessories are allowed to cool to room temperature before any cleaning or maintenance procedures are performed. Maintenance and cleaning by inexperienced or unqualified staff could result in personal injury or costly equipment damage.

A standard cleaning procedure for the steam sterilizer chamber should be in place in the decontamination facility. Remember to make sure that the chamber is not hot before cleaning. Not only is it easier to remove stains when the machine is cold, it also ensures that accidental burns do not occur. The manufacturer's recommendations should be followed when choosing any types of cleaning detergents, brushes, and equipment. The frequency of cleaning can vary depending on the extent of use and water purity used in the sterilizer. This can range from daily to weekly, monthly, and even yearly. The inside of the chamber should be cleaned with a mild detergent-containing cleaning solution, using equipment (e.g. a mop or brush) that is kept especially for the purpose. Strong abrasives or steel wool should not be used on the chamber walls as they may scratch the surface and allow corrosion (rusting) to develop. It is recommended to wipe the door gasket clean daily with a lint-free cloth. While doing so, it is important to check for any defects or signs of wear and tear, especially if the sterilizer utilizes vacuum as part of its sterilization cycles. Any associated carts and loading baskets should also be frequently washed with a mild detergent and any castors and rollers cleaned, checked, and lubricated when necessary. The drain strainer at the bottom of the chamber (check the manufacturer's design/instructions) should be removed daily and cleaned thoroughly; this may be done by cleaning under running water using a brush and mild detergent. If debris has been allowed to build up, it may be necessary to soak the strainer (e.g. in an acid cleaner) before further cleaning.

The sterilizer should also undergo periodic maintenance inspections, as recommended by the manufacturer, where the correct functioning of all valves is checked, filters are replaced, and the temperature/pressure sensors are calibrated. This should be conducted by trained service engineers (from the healthcare facility, the manufacturer, or an applicable third party). It is also recommended that to trace any vacuum leaks, the sterilizer has a maintenance plan and is checked to make sure that it is leak proof. This is typically done using a pre-programmed sterilizer vacuum leak test. These can often indicate potential failure over time if closely inspected.

Whereas maintenance deals with routine cleaning and care to reduce malfunction of critical equipment, routine quality control deals with individual load or process monitoring (see Chapter 14 on monitoring sterilization, and the section on the basic principles of sterilization at the beginning of this chapter). The sterilization process is typically monitored through a combination of parametric, chemical, and biological indication methods that are intended to evaluate the sterilizing conditions and process effectiveness. These include:
- Parametric monitoring of the cycle time (including the sterilization exposure phase), temperature, and pressure during the process. These conditions must be monitored as part of the process and independently monitored by a parallel set of sensors/gauges, if included. In some cases of independent monitoring the sterilizer control system will compare these sensor readings to ensure an effective process (e.g. if two temperature sensors give significantly different results, one or both sensors will require recalibration); in other cases the data is collected but needs to be manually inspected for accuracy. Other parametric monitors may also be included in the steam sterilizer design, such as a mechanical air detector.
- BIs, using the most resistant microorganism for steam (i.e. a known population of bacterial spores of *Geobacillus stearothermophilus*), are often used for individual load monitoring as well as for routine (e.g. weekly) monitoring. Recommendations for process monitoring can vary depending on the location/region. They can include traditional growth–no growth indicators or, more often, rapid read-out indicators (discussed earlier in this chapter). BIs are more widely used in some geographic locations than others depending on local or regional guidelines.
- CIs are also widely used for monitoring steam sterilization processes, both internal and external to individual packs. These can range in classification from type 1 (e.g. steam sterilizer tape) to type 5 or 6 (see earlier in this chapter and

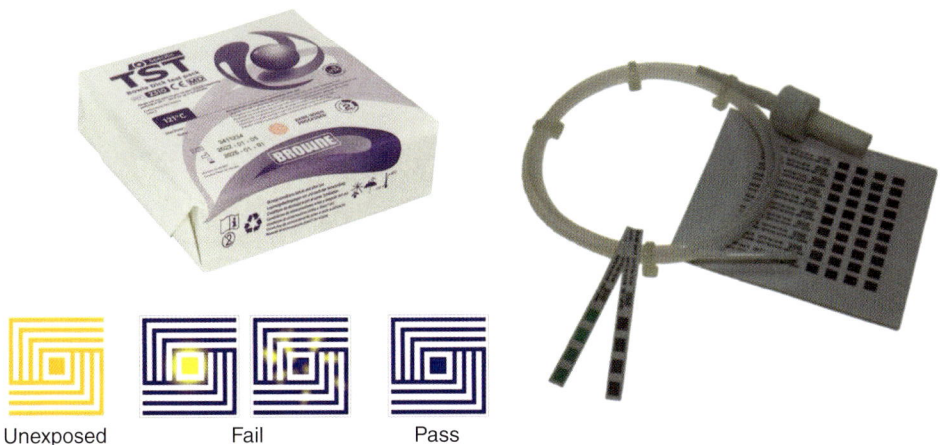

Figure 11.14 Examples of air removal tests for dynamic (including vacuum-assisted) air removal steam sterilizers, including a Bowie–Dick-type test (left) and a hollow load (lumen penetration) test (right) with their associated chemical indicators. The Bowie–Dick test example shows examples of various fail and pass results following exposure to a steam sterilization test cycle.

Table 11.3). In some cases, type 5 or particularly type 6 indicators are used as replacements for BIs.

- PCDs are used in steam sterilization to test for steam penetration and air removal capability. Air removal and steam penetration tests are recommended to be conducted daily within the steam sterilizer. CI test systems are available for this purpose. The most common example is the B–D test, which is classified as a type 2 CI (Figure 11.14). This test simulates a load containing porous materials, consisting of a pile of cotton towels in the middle of which is a CI. It is designed to meet rigorous test conditions (based on ISO 11140-3 *Sterilization of healthcare products – Chemical indicators – Part 3: Type 2 indicator systems for use in the Bowie and Dick-type steam penetration test* and ISO 11140-5 *Sterilization of health care products – Chemical indicators – Part 5: Type 2 indicators for Bowie and Dick type air removal tests*). A specific cycle is programmed into the steam sterilizer to be able to conduct such a test under defined process conditions. A positive (pass) result of a B–D test will indicate that air has been removed and steam penetration has taken place in the test package. Failure of the test will result in the presence of air in the test package, which can be caused by poor air removal, a leakage of air during a vacuum phase, or the presence of excessive air in the steam. Another example is the hollow load ("Helix") test, which is used to check the air removal/steam penetration of a lumened device.

Special considerations in steam sterilization
Immediate-use (flash) sterilization

Immediate-use (previously known as "flash") sterilization may be defined as a process designed for the sterilization of patient care items for immediate use. It should ensure the shortest time between a sterilized item's removal from the sterilizer and its aseptic transfer to the sterile field. A typical example of the traditional use of flash sterilization was when an essential instrument has been dropped onto the floor during a surgical procedure, and following cleaning a rapid sterilization process is used to resterilize the device quickly before its continued use on the patient. It is common for the device to be unwrapped, but this will depend on the sterilizer manufacturer's instructions (which may include the use of sterilization wraps or specific types of rigid containers). Immediate-use sterilization should not be used for convenience or in cases of poor planning prior to surgery.

Like any sterilization process, safe and effective immediate-use sterilization requires that all processing steps have been correctly adhered to before each cycle and during sterilization, and maintained up until the point of use. Shortcuts should not be taken as improper sterilization (i.e. contaminated instruments) can result in serious consequences such as surgical site infections (SSIs). Each immediate-use sterilization cycle should be routinely monitored according to a written facility policy; physical monitors, as well as CIs and BIs, should be considered to verify that the required parameters for effective sterilization have been met. Immediate-use sterilization of certain devices (such as implantable devices) is generally not recommended.

Good practice when using immediate-use sterilization should include an effective cleaning and inspection process before sterilization. Inadequate cleaning and lack of correct documentation regarding the process can result in increased risks of human error and to patient safety. The sterilizer must be maintained as per the manufacturer's instructions and hospital policy, and all routine sterilizer monitoring must be documented. Typical steam sterilization times range from 3 to

10 minutes, depending on the type of device being sterilized and the type of immediate-use sterilizer (i.e. pre-vacuum or gravity displacement). The manufacturer's instructions for use (IFU) should be reviewed and always followed. It is important that staff using immediate-use sterilization are trained how to operate the equipment, to decrease the possibility of operator error during the process. Following immediate-use sterilization items should be transported to the point of use in a manner that minimizes the potential for contamination; ideally the sterilizers to be used for immediate-use sterilization should be located in close proximity to the surgical suite or treatment site. Staff must wear PPE such as heat-protective gloves when handling items, as the tray and the items within it will be hot. Immediate-use sterilized items cannot be stored; they must be used immediately. If the immediate-use sterilizer allows the item to be wrapped with a single wrapper or other packaging, these packs must be clearly marked as being immediate-use sterilized in order to differentiate between them and conventionally processed trays and sealed devices. As most immediate-use sterilization cycles will only have a very brief drying time, the device and/or any associated packaging material should be considered as being wet.

Staff should be trained on facility policies and procedures for immediate-use sterilization based on relevant regulations, standards, and recommended practices. In these situations, it is recommended that sterilization is only performed once all of the following conditions have been met:
• Work practices ensure proper cleaning, inspection, and arrangement of instruments before sterilization.
• The physical layout of the department or work area ensures direct delivery of sterilized items to the point of use (e.g. the sterilizer opens into an area either within or directly adjacent to the procedure room).
• Procedures developed, followed, and audited to ensure aseptic handling and personnel safety during transfer of the sterilized items from the sterilizer to the point of use.
• Items always used immediately following immediate-use sterilization.

In most sterilizers the immediate-use cycle is preprogrammed to a specific time and temperature setting established by the sterilizer manufacturer. It is critical that staff check the device manufacturer's guidelines to make sure that the device is compatible with the cycle, as the specific cycle will vary depending on the type, age, and model of the sterilizer (including the method of air removal). Selecting the correct cycle parameters for the devices to be sterilized is critical if sterility is to be achieved and to prevent damage to the device. It is also important to follow the manufacturer's instructions regarding the types of devices that are suitable for a particular sterilizer cycle, as in some cases instruments with lumens, power equipment, and porous items may not be processed by this method (due to potential difficulties with air removal and steam penetration). In some cases manufacturers explicitly recommend that immediate-use sterilization is not used.

Extended steam sterilization cycles

An "extended" sterilization cycle is a cycle that is longer than would typically be expected from the sterilizer manufacturer's standard cycle time. Steam sterilization cycles with exposure times greater than 4 minutes in a 134°C/274°F dynamic air removal sterilization cycle (or indeed any typical steam sterilization cycle described earlier in this chapter) are commonly referred to as extended cycles. Extended steam sterilization cycles have been recommended in two traditional cases:
• As defined by the device manufacturer to sterilize complex devices and their containers. Most device manufacturers recommend standard sterilization cycle times, such as 4 minutes at 132–135°C/270–275°F in a dynamic air removal sterilizer. Extended exposure times were often recommended in the past for larger orthopedic and neurological instrument sets that are considered a more significant challenge to air removal and steam penetration. Such loads are often heavier or denser and may incorporate a complex and/or difficult-to-sterilize design, such as lumened devices. Longer cycle times were often recommended to compensate for these types of loads, but overall indicated inefficient steam sterilization cycle design, testing, or product limitations. It should be noted that heavier sets are typically more difficult to dry during routine steam sterilization cycles, therefore manufacturers may recommend longer or additional drying cycles to ensure drying (also see the section on troubleshooting steam sterilization problems and Table 11.5).
• For the inactivation of prions, when reusable devices are known to be used in high-risk surgical procedures on patients with known or suspected prion diseases (such as Creutzfeldt-Jakob disease, see Chapter 15). As an example, neurological devices are often considered to present a high risk of contamination when used on patients with known or suspected prion diseases. Typical recommended prion sterilization cycles include a pre-vacuum cycle at 134°C/274°F for 18 minutes and a gravity displacement cycle at 121°C/250°F for 1 hour. Prion sterilization with steam is considered in more detail later in this chapter.

The extension of sterilization times should be followed if recommended by the device manufacturer but can create some concerns within a facility. Specific extended cycles will need to be programmed into the sterilizer and staff trained on when they are to be used. It is critical to check with the device, packaging, and sterilizer manufacturers before using an extended cycle, to ensure it is safe and will not have a negative effect on the product. Most stainless steel instruments may routinely undergo extended steam sterilization times without affecting their functionality, but this may not be the case for all devices.

Table 11.5 Common steam sterilization problems, causes, and potential solutions.

Problem	Cause	Solution
Failed chemical or biological indicators	Inadequate sterilization The fault may be with the sterilizer (mechanical or electrical), steam supply (superheat or wet), and/or the load being sterilized Always confirm that the correct indicator has been used for monitoring the steam sterilization cycle in use	Confirm that the sterilizer is operating correctly A common cause is the way the sterilizer chamber has been loaded It is essential that packs are not too dense and are loosely loaded into the sterilizer to ensure that air is not trapped and can easily circulate
Failed Bowie–Dick-type test	Incomplete air removal Trapped air may be due to human error, mechanical failure, and/or water quality Typical causes include: • Faulty door seals/gaskets • Problems with the vacuum pump • Clogged drain • Low steam pressure or high water pressure • High levels of dissolved gases (non-condensed) in the feedwater/steam	A routine maintenance schedule should be followed to ensure the sterilizer is operating correctly, to include daily inspections by staff (e.g. ensuring the sterilizer chamber drain is not blocked) and maintenance of the sterilizer/utilities (such as routine maintenance of the vacuum pump and any steam/water pre-treatment)
Wet-packs, where a pack/load contains an appreciable amount of moisture after a sterilization cycle	Intermittent operation (chamber cold) or jacket heating not working (e.g. steam supply line malfunctioning) Steam supply is wet Sterilizer installation, including improper insulation of steam pipes or excess water in steam (wet steam) Insufficient drying time Improper loading or cycle for the load Large overweight packs/sets (in particular metals) Overloading may not only cause improper sterilization (insufficient air removal/steam contact) but may promote excessive condensation Clogged or malfunctioning drain or steam supply systems	Pre-warm the sterilizer before using and check steam supply valves/traps (chamber and jacket) Confirm steam supply; test steam quality (see the section on water purity and quality) Check that steam pipes are insulated Review manufacturer's instructions or consider additional drying methods (e.g. adding drying time to the cycle or the use of a drying cabinet) Review procedures and train staff on how to pack, load correctly, pack size, pack weight or pack density, and proper packaging (wrapping) technique Review sterilizer manufacturer's recommendations on proper loading Inspect and, if applicable, clean debris from the chamber drain daily Ensure any associated valves/traps controlling incoming or draining steam are functioning A preventative maintenance schedule should be established to ensure these are functional
Material damage (e.g. rubber deterioration or textile/paper/packaging material scorching) or steam pressure too low for the desired steam temperature	Superheated (unsaturated or super-dry) steam This is steam at a very high temperature for its saturation pressure (see the section on water purity and team quality) Superheated steam can act as hot air, which is less efficient as a sterilization medium	Test for superheated steam (see the section on water purity and steam quality) Confirm that the steam supply is correct (e.g. steam pressure, not only to the chamber but also to the jacket) and associated supply/drain valves are functioning correctly Check calibration of pressure/temperature sensors

(*continued*)

Table 11.5 (cont'd).

Problem	Cause	Solution
Variations in pressure	Persistent or dangerously high pressure is rare and is controlled by safety valves High pressure usually indicates a blockage (e.g. in the drain line) or a malfunctioning valves (in the steam supply or drain valves) Low pressure can be attributed to many causes such as inadequate steam supply (e.g. boiler heater is broken or there is a clogged water/steam line/filters), leaks (chamber or associated pipework), out-of-calibration pressure/temperature gauges, broken/malfunctioning valves, and the presence of non-condensable gases	Safety valve – sterilizers have a safety valve to prevent over-pressurization; this valve can get stuck open and leak Other supply and drain valves should be checked to ensure they are functioning correctly By observing the sterilizer as it pressurizes, steam may be detected as escaping from a particular location (e.g. around the door gasket) Particularly check the door gasket for signs of wear, cracks, chips, etc. Ensure that the sterilizer is correctly maintained/serviced according to manufacturer's guidelines Check steam quality
Instrument staining	Improper instrument cleaning procedures including incomplete removal of soil, inadequate rinsing, or rinsing with water of high mineral content Inadequate cleaning/rinsing can be detected prior to sterilization but not always (e.g. change of color observed after steam treatment or when surfaces are dry) Poor steam purity, where any chemicals present in the steam will react with or precipitate out on surfaces Sometimes the color or types of instrument staining may help in understanding the cause (Table 11.7)	Standardized cleaning procedures and post-cleaning inspections should be established (Chapter 8) Check for any deviations Check the water quality used in the generation of steam (including the dosing of any chemicals used in the boiler) Remember the water purity can vary seasonally and often from day to day
Excessive rusting of stainless steel devices	Damage of stainless steel surfaces that allows for the development of Fe_2O_3 (ferric oxide or "rust") as a reddish-brown material on the surfaces of instruments (particularly on any moving parts) This will also be observed as "pitting" or the development of small pin holes on the surface of the device	The main causes of rust are wear and tear on the device and the presence of high levels of chlorine/silica-based chemicals in the water used to generate steam (but also from other sources) Check for the levels of chlorine/chlorides and/or silicates in the feedwater to the steam generator Note: chlorine is widely used for the disinfection of water It is also considered good practice not to sterilize stainless steel instruments together in the same pack with aluminum, brass, copper, or chrome-plated instruments because of the risk of "galvanic" corrosion that may result The visual signs of rust can be removed by immersing the device in an acid-based cleaner (Table 11.7), but it should be noted that this only removes the visual signs of rust (by dissolving the ferric oxide) and does not resolve the existing damage; further, overuse of acids can unfortunately enhance the damage to the device surface
Packaging materials show signs of staining but not the instruments	The wrap may act as a "filter" to keep various chemicals (as specified above or in Table 11.7) away from the instruments If the wrap shows signs of staining but the instruments are clean, or if unwrapped instruments are consistently dirtier than wrapped ones, steam purity/quality is the major cause of the problem	It is likely that the sterilizer in question has a deficiency in steam purity/quality Review Table 11.7 for typical causes of various stains Wet steam can particularly show these problems (as an early warning sign)

For example, textile products, devices containing lenses, and delicate instrumentation can become damaged (warped or brittle) during such cycles. The extended conditions of pressure and temperature can also lead to premature aging of the device. Extended pressure/temperature conditions may even compromise packaging materials (if not tested for such purposes). For example, it is possible that extended exposure of packaging materials (peel pouches, wrap, etc.) to steam may break down the barrier properties of these materials, therefore their compatibility should be confirmed (in writing) with the supplier/manufacturer.

Various types of CIs and BIs used to monitor defined steam sterilization processes may not be validated to be used in extended cycles. It is important to note that indicators should only be used under their label claims, to include their use and validation in specific steam sterilization cycles. This should be confirmed with the CI/BI suppliers. Historically existing CI and BI challenge packs and indicators have been designed for and labeled for use in shorter steam cycles (e.g. 3- or 4-minute pre-vacuum cycles at 132°C–135°C/~270°F–275°F) and may not be reliable to be used to monitor cycles that are longer. As examples:

- CIs designed to indicate shorter steam sterilization cycle times will give no assurance that longer cycle times have been achieved.
- The growth media or growth indication methods used in BIs are also designed for shorter exposure times, and may become damaged on extended exposure conditions that would fail to allow the test spores (if they survived) to grow or to identify growth.

As a final consideration, extending the steam exposure time for sterilization is more than often indicative of the need to optimize the conditioning phase of the steam sterilization cycle. Conditioning should be designed to ensure that air removal and steam penetration are adequate prior to the sterilization holding phase (at the sterilization temperature and pressure). Therefore, modification of the steam sterilization cycle (conditioning phase) or the device set (into sub-sets) may be necessary to ensure adequate conditioning and sterilization in typical steam cycles.

Prion sterilization

Prions are unusual infectious agents and are reported to be highly resistant to many sterilization methods, including steam. A more detailed discussion of prion decontamination of devices (including the use of sterilization techniques) is given in Chapter 15 on special interest topics. Initial laboratory investigations to study the inactivation of prions, under worst-case and grossly soiled conditions, showed that longer steam sterilization cycles should be considered, to include:

- A pre-vacuum cycle at 134°C/274°F for 18 minutes.
- A gravity displacement cycle at 121°C/250°F for 1 hour.

Such extended cycles were recommended by the World Health Organization (WHO) in 1999 due to the high level of resistance of prions to physical and chemical inactivation. These steam cycles (in particular 134°C/274°F for 18 minutes) have become widely recommended and used in healthcare facilities as a precaution against prion contamination. They are considered also as extended steam sterilization cycles. As discussed earlier, extended pressure/temperature conditions may not be recommended by the device manufacturer (due to the risks of damage) and any packaging materials may become compromised (unless specifically labeled for such use). Further, CIs and BIs should only be used to monitor such processes if they have been validated and are labeled for those uses. These points are important to confirm prior to considering the use of any, including prion-specific, extended steam sterilization conditions.

Other recommendations (including the WHO 1999 guidelines) have included the immersion of suspected or known prion-contaminated devices into strong chemical solutions (such as 1 N NaOH, a strong alkaline chemical) and then exposing them (in the chemical) to a steam sterilization process. Although this may be considered an effective process, this treatment is not recommended by device or steam sterilizer manufacturers due to the risks of damage and may void any manufacturer's warranty.

The initial laboratory experiments conducted to study the resistance of prions to steam sterilization did not consider the cycle of device processing used in healthcare facilities, such as cleaning followed by sterilization. For example, many of the experiments did not test surfaces contaminated with prions or the effects of cleaning prior to steam sterilization. In recent years these aspects have been considered in more detail, with the following conclusions to date:

- Steam sterilization is an effective process to reduce the risks of prion contamination. Even in the absence of cleaning, standard steam sterilization cycles (such as 134°C/~273°F for 4 minutes) can significantly reduce this risk and efficacy is further improved by extending the exposure conditions (such as 134°C/~273°F for 18 minutes).
- If contaminated devices are required to be pre-treated by a steam sterilization process prior to routine cleaning, disinfection, and sterilization, this should be performed under conditions where the devices are placed into water and then exposed to steam sterilization. Note that this is not a sterilization method, as it may not have been validated as such for that purpose by the manufacturer. But maintaining "wet" conditions when there is gross contamination has been shown to be more effective than direct exposure to a normal steam sterilization process.
- Cleaning of contaminated surfaces can also reduce the risk (see Chapter 15) when followed by steam sterilization. A note of caution: the choice of cleaning chemistry and the cleaning

process used are important. Specific types of cleaning chemistries and their effects on prion inactivation/surface removal are considered in Chapter 15. In some cases, normal cleaning processes with some cleaning chemistry formulations followed by standard steam sterilization cycles (134°C/~273°F for 4 minutes) were effective, but with other cleaning formulations this was not the case. There is also evidence that some cleaning chemistries can have a negative effect, reducing the ability of steam sterilization to be effective. Therefore, the cleaning chemistry used should be considered in addition to the steam sterilization process. It is recommended that such decontamination processes are tested and supported in writing by the manufacturer before being made part of any facility policy for reducing the risks associated with prion contamination.

Local guidelines and standards for the handling of prion-contaminated (or suspected) situations can vary significantly from country to country, and can periodically change. It is also true that local prion decontamination recommendations may not be recommended by the device or steam sterilizer manufacturer for various safety reasons. Therefore, a facility policy (to include requirements for steam sterilization) should be developed and maintained based on local guidance to ensure the correct handling of any known or considered high-risk prion-contaminated devices (see Chapter 15).

Water purity and steam quality

Water is the basis for the generation of steam and any steam sterilization process. Chemically it is a simple molecule (H_2O), but the chemistry of water (liquid H_2O and, when heated, its gas form, steam or gas H_2O) can be complicated (see Chapter 6). Water is rarely pure but is found to have a range of different chemical, microbial, and other contaminants. These include various types of dissolved materials (such as calcium, chlorine, iron, etc.) and gases (e.g. oxygen and carbon dioxide), as well as suspended materials (such as microorganisms and larger particles; see Chapter 6, Table 6.3). In considering steam sterilization, two terms are frequently used in relation to water/steam:
- Water/steam purity. "Purity" refers to the levels of chemical (and microbiological) contaminants that may (or may not) be present in water or steam. It is important to note that any chemical contaminants present in the water can carry over into the steam produced from that water. Depending on the chemical, this can lead to device damage as well as potential toxic effects in patients (following condensation onto a device during the steam sterilization cycle). Further, although most microorganisms in a water source will be inactivated when converted into steam (depending on the temperature and time), parts of the microorganism can remain intact and biologically active (such as endotoxins; see Chapter 5, Table 5.4). Such toxins can also be carried over in the steam and can cause adverse patient reactions if they are deposited onto a device (during condensation).

- Steam quality. In this case, "quality" refers to the physical properties of steam such as its saturation, presence of NCGs, and dryness (these are defined in further detail later). These properties are indicative of the ability of steam to perform optimally in a steam sterilization process (i.e. when provided as saturated steam and to ensure that air/NCGs do not impede the penetration of steam to all surfaces of the device/load).

Water and steam purity is an important variable to understand and control (for more detailed discussion of water purity, see Chapter 15). For steam sterilization, good-quality potable (drinking) water may be used to generate steam, but it is highly recommended to confirm the following purity guidelines:
- "Hardness" levels of <20 mg/L (the official term is mg $CaCO_3$/L), which is typical of softened water. Water hardness is defined as the concentration of calcium and magnesium in water. It is typically given as milligrams per liter (mg/L) or parts per million (ppm) of calcium carbonate ($CaCO_3$) in the water. "Hard" typically refers to water containing high levels of hardness, in excess of 120 ppm, and "soft" water is considered less than 60 ppm $CaCO_3$. Therefore, softened water (<20 mg/L) should be considered for steam generation. Softened water can be generated by passing the water through a water softener (see Chapter 15). The levels of hardness can range considerably depending on where you live and even the time of the year. Hardness cannot be seen by the eye as the chemicals are dissolved in the water, but when the water is heated it causes the deposition of often visible water-insoluble precipitates (known as limescale, a white grainy substance consisting of chemicals such as calcium carbonate). Water hardness can cause problems by precipitating on device surfaces (known as spotting or as a fine white or otherwise colored precipitate) or building up as scale within boilers, steam generators, and pipework (Figure 11.15). Over time it can cause steam generation and handling systems to fail.
- Conductivity <10 μS/cm. Conductivity is an overall measurement of chemicals (particularly those that are dissolved) in the water and is a simple method of determining the purity of the water. In this case, high levels of chemicals such as chlorides or silicates in the water can lead to device damage (e.g. rusting, seen as a brown deposit; Figure 11.16). For example, when chlorine is present in water and is heated it can form chlorine gas, which can be damaging to stainless steel surfaces (in the steam sterilizer and on many reusable devices). As an estimate, a conductivity level of below 10 μS/cm is equivalent to a chloride level of below 5 mg/l. If it is suspected that specific chemicals may contaminate the water source, other tests for individual compounds may be carried out (e.g. silicates, iron, copper, phosphates, etc.) using other chemical analysis methods (such as inductively coupled plasma–optical emission spectroscopy or ICP-OES analysis).
- pH in the range of 5.0–9.2 (measured from steam condensate). If the water is too acidic (<pH 5) or too alkaline (>pH 9) it can lead to damage to devices/materials but is also not considered potable (see Chapter 6). A further test for total

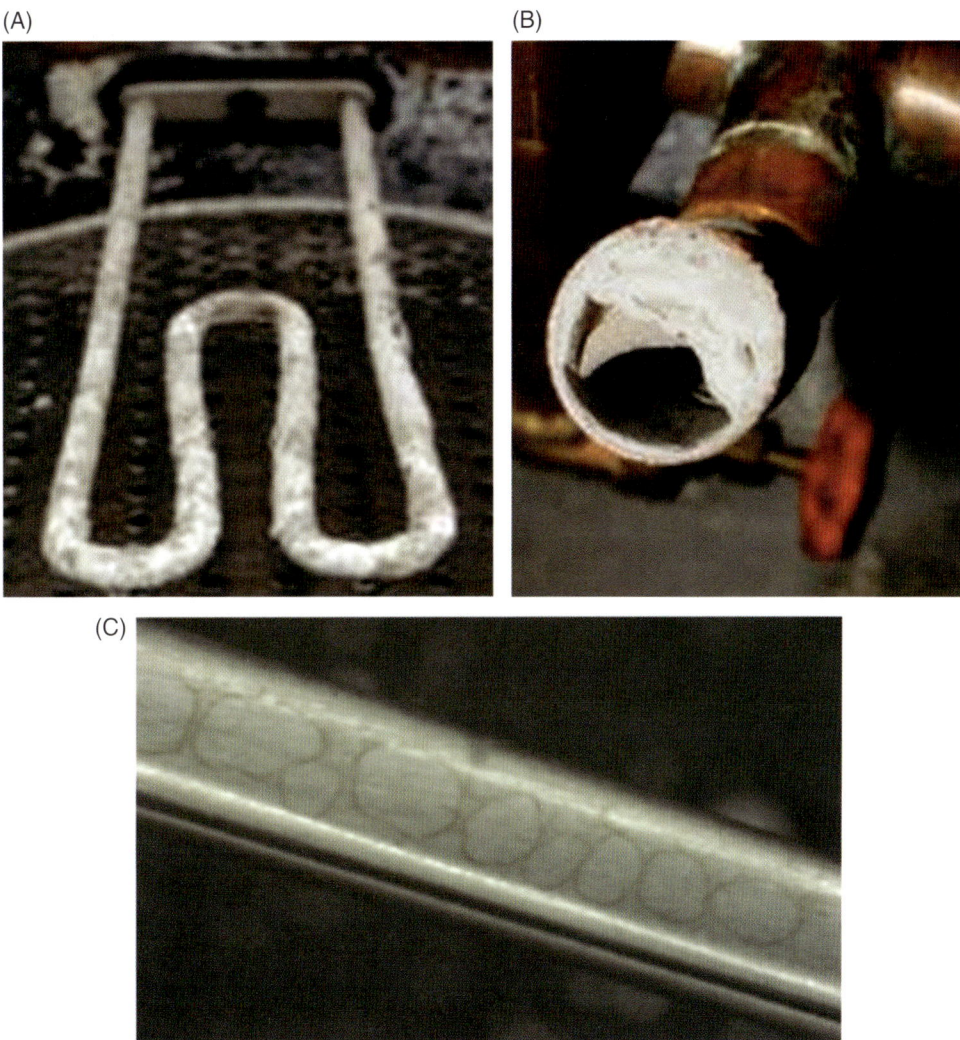

Figure 11.15 Examples of water hardness deposits associated with steam. (A) White scaling seen on a heating element and (B) in a supply pipe. (C) Water hardness-associated "spotting" observed on a device surface.

alkalinity, at <8 mg $CaCO_3$/L, is also recommended. Total alkalinity is a measure of certain types of dissolved solids that are alkaline in nature (e.g. bicarbonates, carbonates, and hydroxides). These are important as they increase the ability of hard water salts present in the water to form scale (see the earlier discussion of hardness).

- Total organic carbon (TOC) <1 mg/L. TOC is a measure of any organic (carbon-containing) materials in the water, including microorganisms. It is an overall indicator of water quality. An example of an organic concern with steam is endotoxin, a particular type of toxin found associated with Gram-negative bacteria (see Chapter 5). Endotoxins may be carried over in steam and if deposited at high concentrations onto a device may lead to a toxic reaction when used on a patient. Endotoxin levels are generally recommended to be <10 EU (endotoxin units)/mL and may be separately tested for.

If the water purity levels are higher, this may affect the safety of steam sterilization and particularly lead to device damage or build-up of residues. In many cases the water quality may need to be improved, either by using specific methods to remove specific contaminants (e.g. carbon filtration for chlorine and water softener for hardness) or by providing pure water quality, by reverse osmosis (RO), deionization, or distillation (see Chapter 15). RO is generally the most practical method but

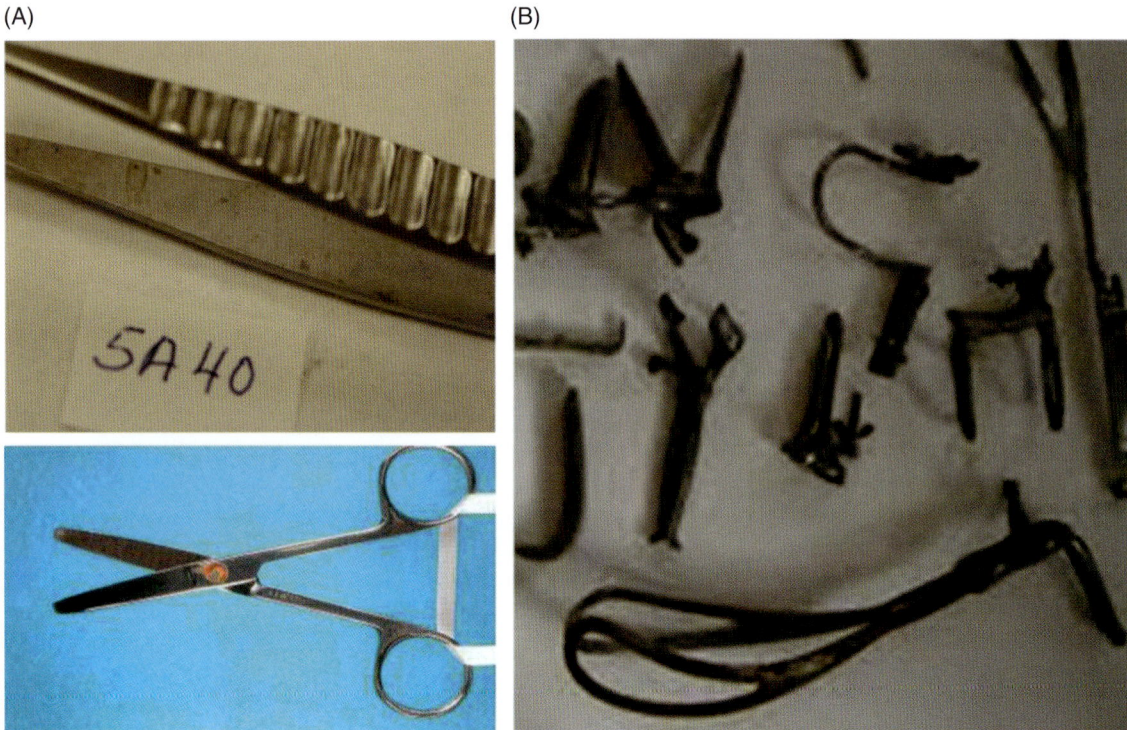

Figure 11.16 Examples of (A) minor and (B) excessive rusting observed due to high levels of chlorine in steam.

requires close inspection/controls to ensure that the process is operating correctly. If the method for pure water production is correctly operating and maintained, the typical levels of acceptable contaminants in steam should be:
- pH 5.0–9.2 in steam concentrate or 5.0–7.5 in water used for steam generation.
- Conductivity $\leq 10\,\mu S/cm$.
- Hardness $\leq 1\,mg/L$.
- TOC $\leq 1\,mg/L$.
- Total alkalinity $\leq 0.5\,mg/L$.
- Chloride $\leq 8\,mg/L$.
- Silicates $\leq 1\,mg/L$.
- Phosphates $\leq 0.5\,mg/L$.
- Endotoxins $\leq 10\,EU/mL$.

Note that the specific requirement can vary between different guidelines and standards.

Testing of water purity can be conducted directly from the water used to produce the steam (e.g. within or being fed to a facility or plant room boiler or integral steam generator) or more specifically by the collection of water from the steam being provided to the steam sterilizer (e.g. using a condenser system that rapidly cools the steam by passing it along a cold water–treated surface, causing the steam to condense into water and then collected for analysis). The second method reflects the final steam being provided for sterilization (including any potential boiler/generator feedwater, boiler treatment, and supply pipework contaminants/chemicals that may be present). This may be a more suitable method for testing the complete steam generation and handling system. But different guidance and standards may only focus on testing the feed water and may be acceptable.

A separate issue is steam quality, referring to the physical properties of the steam. These are important to ensure that saturated steam is provided and that air/NCGs are sufficiently removed so that they do not impede the penetration of steam to all surfaces of the device/load. The typical measurements of steam quality are:
- Non-condensable gases. High levels of NCGs can prevent the penetration of steam to all areas of the load, like the presence of air. These gases can be present in the water and therefore their main source is the water being used to generate the steam, but they may also be present due to the design of the steam generation/supply system. NCGs are removed by degassing the water (preheating the water to temperatures at or above 80°C/~176°F, such as by boiling, which drives off the gases). A typical recommendation for the level of NCGs is $\leq 3.5\%$ in water. This is determined using a NCG test, which determines the volume (in mL) of gas collected from a volume of water/condensed steam (expressed as a %, where

3.5% refers to 3.5 mL of NCGs in 100 mL of condensed water). Examples of test methods for non-condensable gases are specified in EN285 – *Large sterilizers* and EN13060 – *Small sterilizers*.

- Saturated steam. This is the point at which steam forms or condenses under controlled conditions of pressure and temperature, and is considered the most efficient for sterilization (see earlier discussion). At a given pressure/temperature, if too little moisture is present the steam is "superheated" and is less efficient for steam sterilization (acting more like a dry heat process). Equally, when excessive moisture is present the steam is considered "wet" (or oversaturated) and can also lead to problems such as wet loads (requiring extended drying post sterilization). The two tests that can be used to check that saturated steam is present are:
  - Dryness test: tests for the amount of moisture present in steam and is typically expressed as a dryness value or fraction. Typical recommended dryness factors range from 0.90 to 0.99 (therefore 90–99% steam and 10–1% water); a dryness factor for healthcare (including metal) loads is often given as ≥ 0.95.
  - Superheat test: a temperature-based test. When steam is taken from its supply line at a certain pressure and suddenly is exposed to atmospheric pressure, the observed temperature should not exceed 25 K when measured with a specific superheat test apparatus (Figure 11.17).

Examples of test methods for dryness and superheat are specified in EN285 – *Large sterilizers*. Examples of apparatus used for the testing of steam quality are shown in Figure 11.17.

Further consideration is given to water used during the decontamination cycle, including for sterilization, in Chapter 15.

Steam sterilization process failures

There are many different causes of steam sterilization process failures, from procedural errors that are easily remedied (like overloading) to mechanical problems that can take a sterilizer out of service. A sterilization process failure may be detected by any of the process monitoring tools used in or with the sterilizer as part of any quality control program, including physical, mechanical, chemical, and biological indicators. These can range from an event within a single pack (in-pack CI) or load (PCD) or a complete sterilizer (B–D test, BI test, or any of the types of parametric monitoring mechanisms within the sterilizer). Many of these are first-line (often immediate) monitoring tools that assist in detecting that the sterilization process may not have occurred correctly. Steam sterilization failures are most commonly due to human error, such as incorrect packaging material or techniques being used, improper loading, and incorrect cycle selection for the load contents resulting in an inadequate cycle temperature, inadequate time at that temperature, and incomplete air removal. But sterilizer

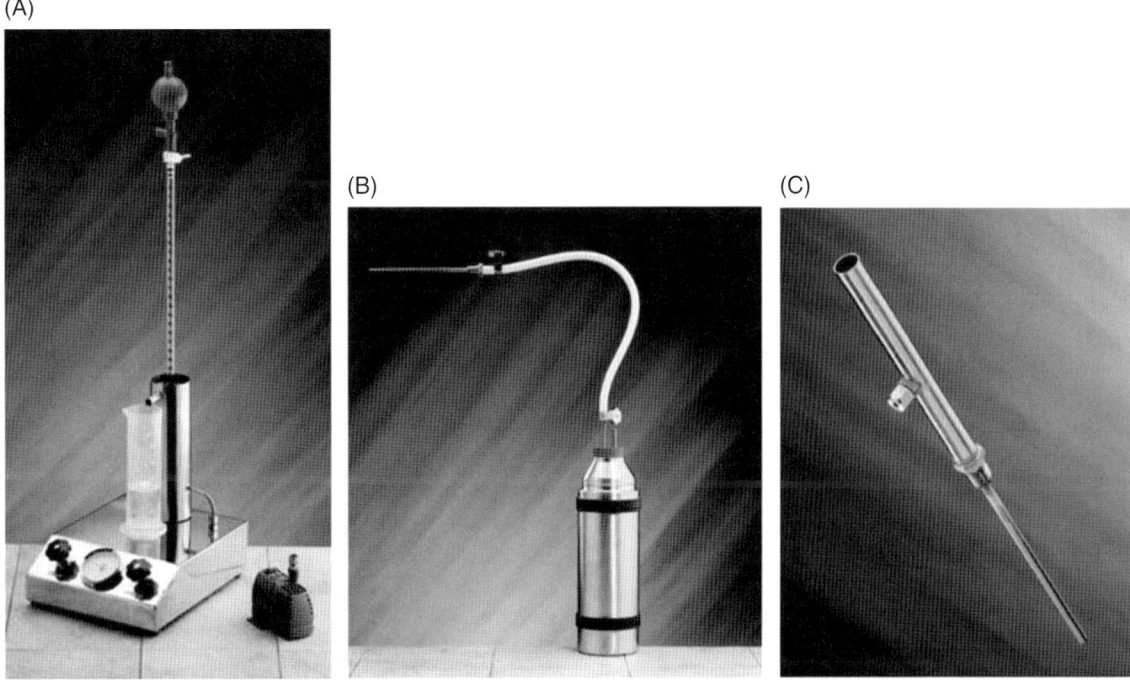

Figure 11.17 Examples of test apparatus used for testing (A) non-condensable gases, (B) dryness value/fraction, (C) and superheat.

equipment, including the steam generation and supply systems, is often to blame (e.g. due to being out of calibration, lack of maintenance, air leaks, inadequate steam supply, etc.).

In the event of a failed process indicator(s) the first step should be to quarantine the load (avoiding its accidental use in a patient procedure) and prevent the sterilizer from being used until the extent of the failure is known. It is important that a suspected faulty sterilizer should not be made operational without identifying and correcting any underlying problem. A well-planned, systematic, and written procedure should be in place at the facility to address any of these potential situations, since they can occur at any time. An investigation will need to take place to identify the failure and the sterilizer needs to be taken out of service while the investigation is taking place. This investigation is critical in assisting the supervisor to decide whether to recall just the one load or potentially an entire day's work. The decision will be based on all the available evidence used for monitoring the effectiveness of the sterilization cycle (i.e. physical monitors, CIs, and BIs). All process monitors used in parametric and routine monitoring of the sterilizer should be reviewed to aid in solving the problem.

A logical first step is to ensure that the pack/load actually passed through a sterilization cycle and that the cycle was initiated by the operator by comparing the cycle sequence from the printout tape or graph recorder against the number of loads documented in the sterilization load log. Inspect what packaging material/wrap and indicator(s) were used to ensure that the correct steam sterilization materials/indicators were employed. It is also possible that there may have been an operator error in loading or packaging that may have resulted in sterilization failures in only one or some of the items in the load. Always follow the manufacturer's recommendations when loading the sterilizer. The basic rule to consider when loading the sterilizer chamber is that all items need to be properly prepared and arranged in a way that will present the least possible resistance to the extraction of air and the passage of the steam throughout the load (see Chapter 10 on loading and unloading sterilizers). Steam sterilizers should never be overloaded (Figure 11.18). Packages should not touch the top, bottom, or sides of the sterilizer, as this may result in sterilization failure and "wet-packs" in the case of steam sterilization (see the later discussion and Table 11.5).

A single non-responsive or inconclusive CI should not be considered definitive proof that the entire load is non-sterile. If, however, the sterilization failure is due to a procedural/human error, all affected devices will need to be packaged and resterilized. A large percentage of sterilization failures are due to human error. Although there are many ways in which human error can play a part, the most common errors are incorrect cycle selection, overloading or improperly loading the sterilizer, failing to initiate the cycle once the sterilizer has been loaded, and change in procedure or personnel. Procedural errors occur when improper sterilization procedures are being used, for example processing a device in the wrong cycle or even according to a departmental procedure that does not comply with the device manufacturer's or equipment manufacturer's instructions. The facility's written operating procedures should be reviewed and compared with the sterilizer and device manufacturers' instructions to ensure that they are consistent. Make sure that all staff are trained on how to operate and interpret monitoring equipment, selecting the correct cycle for load contents (devices and device sets, including weight), choosing the correct packaging materials/techniques, operating the equipment, and following the medical device manufacturer's instructions. If the failure is due to human error and no equipment repairs are necessary, the sterilizer can be immediately returned to service. If there is no obvious cause identified from this review, the investigation will need to be expanded and it may be necessary to seek outside assistance.

Once procedural errors have been ruled out, the investigation continues by reviewing all sterilizer monitoring (parametric and other indicators) that has been collected in at least the last 24 hours. Review any sterilizer printout tapes or records, such as computerized data collected from the sterilizer control systems(s), to determine whether the appropriate sterilization parameters have been met (in this case, temperature/time/pressure). Sterilizers that have independent monitoring systems have two sets of data that can be compared: from the control system and from the independent monitoring system. In some cases the results from such systems need to be visually inspected for differences, while in others this is performed by the sterilizer. Overall, independent monitoring systems are useful to ensure that various sensors used for controlling the process are adequately calibrated and functioning. If the physical monitoring results have changed or differ from what is expected, the sterilization process should be considered incomplete, and the load(s) not released for patient use. Physical monitors provide a real-time assessment of each individual sterilization cycle and assist in the early detection of sterilizer malfunction.

A next step is to review the results of any air removal tests, the most common of which is the recommended daily B–D test. The B–D test is designed to ensure that air removal is sufficient within the steam process, which is noted to be affected not only by the programmed conditioning phase of the test cycle but also the quality of steam (see the section on water quality/purity). Steam sterilization failures often result from incomplete air removal, including poor steam quality/quantity. Inadequate air removal, sterilization temperatures, and/or times can also be indicated by failed BIs or CIs used during routine testing of the sterilizer. Note that there are different classifications of chemical indicators, with different stringencies in their capabilities to detect a passed/failed cycle (Table 11.3). In the case of a failed B–D or BI test, it is

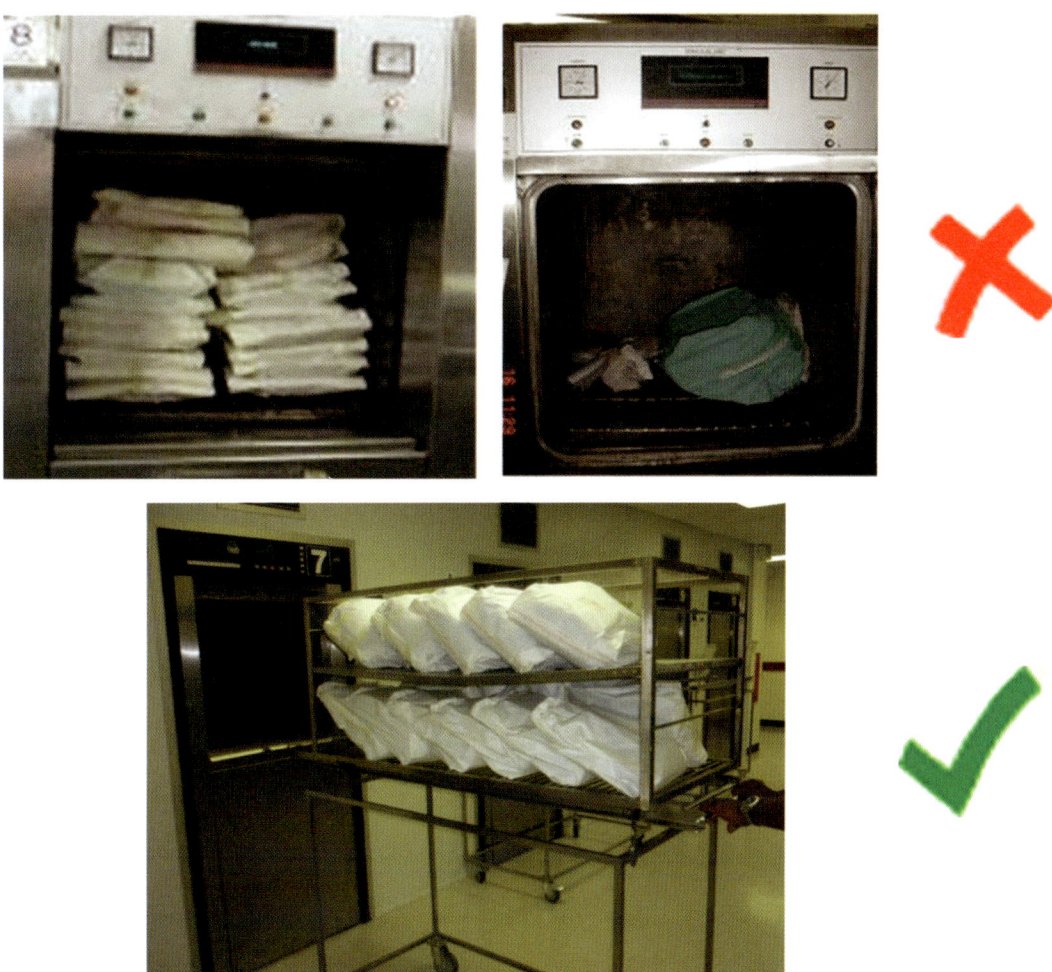

Figure 11.18 Examples of incorrect and correct loading of steam sterilizers.

recommended to repeat the test (if possible using a different product batch) to confirm the result. The indicator manufacturer's instructions should be consulted, and it may also be necessary to confirm that these are performing as intended, for example by confirming that the indicators have been used according to their instructions and are within any stated shelf-life. If the repeated tests indicate a "pass" result suggesting that the sterilizer is operating effectively, facility procedures will need to be reassessed to identify what went wrong (e.g. training on correct use). In the case of a "fail" result, the sterilizer and/or the utilities that supply the equipment will require further investigation.

Factors that can often affect the efficiency of a steam sterilizer include the air seal of the door, the quality of the steam, and the characteristics of the load. It is the responsibility of the processing area manager to establish a periodic maintenance procedure to ensure correct operation of the sterilizer and its utilities. Many common problems associated with steam sterilizers are due to lack of maintenance. Such malfunctions will require further investigation from a trained engineer, manufacturer, or other process/equipment expert. When a mechanical failure is identified, this may immediately cause an investigation and potential recall procedure. It may be necessary to recall affected loads (prior to patient use) identified during the investigation. All such packs should be retrieved, quarantined, repackaged, and resterilized (if necessary) under the standard facility quality procedures (see Chapter 14).

In the case of any inconclusive results from the inspection of internal pack CIs, other packs associated with the same sterilizer load should be identified and inspected if possible. If an individual CI has failed, there is a possibility that the entire batch/load is also compromised. These are often identified at the site of surgical/medical use; therefore, staff handling devices in these areas should be trained on the correct inspection procedures prior to patient use (see Chapter 12). First verify that the correct internal CI was selected for the items that were sterilized. All other packages should be opened to check their internal indicators and then reprocessed. If no other packs have been affected, this is probably a procedural failure. If all the other packs in that load are affected, it could be a mechanical or process monitoring product failure, and further investigation will need to be carried out. Verify that all monitoring products are within their manufactured expiration date and have been stored properly.

If BIs are used as the only load control monitoring test, then items from all loads since the last passed biological test may need to be recalled. Similarly, if type 5 or 6 indicators or PCDs are used, then all items from all loads since the last passed result may also need to be recalled.

After any major repair has been performed, the sterilizer should not be used until the necessary quality monitoring tests have been completed in accordance with facility policy. For steam sterilizers, this will typically include a vacuum or leak-rate test, B–D type tests, and CI/BI tests (sometimes in multiple test cycles). If all the test results are satisfactory and the mechanical monitoring results are acceptable, the sterilizer should be considered in good working order and can be put back into service.

There are many potential hidden process failures that can occur. These are difficult to detect and are dependent on having proper controls in place for the whole processing cycle. They are often the case when procedures that should take place prior to sterilization are not properly followed. Examples include incorrect cleaning methods (soil remaining on a device), detergents or other chemicals that are not dosed or correctly rinsed from devices or during laundering, damaged or malfunctioning valves associated with devices, damaged filters used with rigid sterilization containers, or incorrect loading and wrapping techniques, all of which may compromise sterilization. Such failures can lead to adverse patient reactions and can only be minimized as part of a quality assurance system within a facility, such as by ensuring that staff are correctly trained and that devices undergo inspection. Further failures can occur when environmental conditions cause a sterilized device to become recontaminated, such as during storage, transport, or preparation for a surgical/medical procedure (see Chapter 12).

Troubleshooting common steam sterilization problems

Troubleshooting can be defined as the identification of problems and their cause(s) in order to prevent or minimize any negative effects. Troubleshooting requires patience and often in-depth investigation. A variety of problems can be observed following steam sterilization, most often related to the quality/ purity of water used during processing (see earlier in this chapter). A summary of the most common problems, causes, and recommended solutions is given in Table 11.5.

A common complaint with steam sterilization processes is the gradual or sudden onset of changes in color on or the appearance of devices. These problems are most often associated with inadequate cleaning/rinsing of devices or water purity. Sudden changes in observed device coloration and/or damage (such as rusting) often indicate varying purity of water over time. It should be noted that these effects may only visually be observed after a while. The problem may be due to water used in washer-disinfector and/or steam generation systems. As a note, if the problem is not observed following cleaning/ disinfection but is observed following sterilization (usually on opening and inspection of the pack prior to patient use; see Chapter 12), this usually indicates a problem with inadequate rinsing of cleaning agents from the devices prior to sterilization. These effects may be seen not only on the devices but also on the steam sterilizer chamber walls if the source of the problem is the sterilizer. Common examples are given in Table 11.6.

Steam sterilization guidelines and standards

Steam is the most widely used method of sterilization and there are many guidelines and standards associated with steam sterilization processes and equipment. The specific recommendations can vary from country to country and although there may be many similarities, there are also many specific requirements that need to be considered locally. Table 11.7 lists some examples of the guidelines and standards related to steam sterilization and monitoring used worldwide, but this list should not be considered exhaustive.

Dry heat sterilization
Principles of dry heat sterilization

Dry heat methods are used for sterilization applications. These are based on the principles of directly applying heat or heated air for sterilization. Heat is transferred to the devices through conduction, convection, and radiant heat. Typical applications include the use of incinerators and dry heat ovens.

Incineration refers to "burning to ashes," where contaminated materials and devices are directly burned in specifically designed furnaces (known as incinerators) at excessive temperatures (such as >800°C/~1472°F). Burning (also known as combustion) is one of the oldest described methods of sterilization, but is essentially destructive. This is a commonly used method for the destruction of clinical waste materials that are no longer required (including many single-use or discarded devices). Waste can include infectious and non-infectious waste, and the management of this waste is an important consideration in healthcare. In addition to being an effective sterilization method, incineration is useful to reduce the volume of waste for disposal, up to a 95% reduction.

Table 11.6 Examples of problems frequently associated with color changes on devices and their causes. This list is given only as a guide and the specific cause of such problems may be due to more complicated reasons than those specified. Many of the examples given may be identified following sterilization but are caused by other effects earlier in the processing cycle.

Observed color	Typical cause	Solution
Brown/red residues	Incomplete removal of soil (in particular blood) Development of rust, in particular due to the presence of chlorine in the water used to make steam This may come directly from the feedwater (where it is used for the control of microorganisms in water-distribution systems) A further common sources of chlorine in water is due to the incorrect installation/maintenance of a water softener system (used to reduce water hardness); these systems exchange (swap) hardness in the water (e.g. calcium carbonate) with sodium chloride (NaCl) and can therefore be a source of chlorides if not balanced correctly A build-up of iron deposits from water and/or supply lines (e.g. from old iron-containing pipes in water-delivery/circulation systems)	Soil (material from a previous patient procedure) can be generally removed using an alkaline cleaning Inorganic deposits (such as rusting or iron deposits) generally require treatment with an acid-based cleaner to dissolve/remove Check the purity of the water/steam, in particular for high levels of chlorine/chlorites and chlorides High levels of chlorine can be removed by installing/maintaining an activated carbon filter Ensure that any water softener systems are correctly installed and maintained Check the purity of the water/steam and inspect the associated water/steam lines with the facility engineering or maintenance team
Brown residues	Excessive heat (e.g. superheat) due to the development of chromium oxide on stainless steel surfaces	Check the steam quality, in particular for superheat
Fading of colored device surfaces over time (in particular on aluminum-based devices)	Chlorine (and other oxidizing agents) in the steam supply or highly alkaline (pH > 8) products in the cleaning chemistry These will cause a reaction with colored surfaces, causing fading over time	Check the purity of the water/steam, in particular for pH and presence of chlorine This is sometimes observed with the use of reverse osmosis water, which naturally happens over time and may indicate a limited number of processing cycles with such devices (note these effects are typically cosmetic only)
Orange/brown staining	Presence of phosphates (from water/steam or as a residual from the cleaning chemistry on reaction with heat) Note: an orange-brown color may also come from the use of iodine/iodophor-based antiseptics on the device, which should be discussed with the operating room and such practices discontinued	Check the purity of the water/steam, in particular for phosphates Water treatment systems should reduce these levels if present
Black staining	Overuse of acid-based cleaner or inadequate neutralization of such cleaners during a cleaning process May also occur due to the use of bleaching agents on devices (e.g. bleach solutions for cleaning), which should be identified and discontinued	Ensure that acid-cleaning solutions are either correctly neutralized (as required by the manufacturer) or correctly rinsed from device surfaces Discontinue the use of bleaching agents during device decontamination
Multi-colored, "rainbow" effect	Excessive (in particular) dry heat, often associated with superheat (see above) or excessive drying phases	Check the steam quality, in particular for superheat Discuss with the sterilizer manufacturer or steam sterilization cycle development expert

(continued)

Table 11.6 (cont'd).

Observed color	Typical cause	Solution
White or otherwise colored grainy precipitate	Often seen first as a build-up over time on the chamber walls (particularly close to steam entry ports into a chamber), but also in excessive cases on devices/container surfaces Will eventually cause the failure of valves and steam-generation systems, and even pipework clogging in excessive cases Is due to the presence of water hardness in the water/steam Other causes may include high levels of silica- or sulfur-containing water contaminants Also observed as spotting on device surfaces (Figure 11.38)	Check the purity of the water/steam, in particular for hardness (but also other minerals such as copper, iron, and chromium that may also be present) Consider installing and maintaining water softeners for pre-treating feedwater for steam generation Further pre-treatment may be required to reduce levels of silica- and sulfur-water contaminants if present
Gold tinting	High chlorine levels	Check the purity of the water/steam, in particular for pH and presence of chlorine Chlorine levels may be reduced by installing carbon filters in the incoming water lines prior to steam generation
Purple/blue colors	Over-dosing of amines, commonly used to reduce the risks of corrosion within water/steam boilers/lines	Review for amine or other dosing systems associated with boilers/steam generators

Table 11.7 Examples of steam sterilization guidelines and standards.

Guidelines/standards	Title	Description
ISO 17665-1: 2006[1]	Sterilization of health care products – Moist heat. Part 1: Requirements for the development, validation, and routine control of a sterilization process for medical devices	Specifies requirements for the development, validation, and routine control of moist heat (steam) sterilization processes for devices
ISO/TS 17665-2: 2009[1]	Sterilization of health care products – Moist heat. Part 2: Guidance on the application of ISO 17665 Part 1: 2006	Provides general guidance on the understanding and implementation of ISO 17665-1
ISO/TS 17665-3: 2013[1]	Sterilization of health care products – Moist heat. Part 3: Guidance on the designation of a medical device to a product family and processing category for steam sterilization	Provides guidance about defining product families for the purpose of validation of a sterilization process under ISO 17665-1 A product family is a group or subgroup of devices characterized by similar attributes determined to be same (or "equivalent") for evaluation and processing of steam sterilization loads
EN 285: 2015 + A1: 2021	Sterilization – Steam sterilizers – Large sterilizers	This European standard specifies requirements and the relevant tests for large steam sterilizers primarily used in healthcare for the sterilization of devices and accessories
EN 13060: 2014 + A1: 2018	Small steam sterilizers	This European standard specifies requirements and the relevant tests for small steam sterilizers primarily used in healthcare for the sterilization of devices and accessories
ISO 11138-3: 2017	Sterilization of health care products – Biological indicators. Part 3: Biological indicators for moist heat sterilization processes	Provides specific requirements for test organisms, suspensions, inoculated carriers, biological indicators, and test methods intended for use in assessing the performance of steam sterilization processes

Table 11.7 (cont'd).

Guidelines/standards	Title	Description
ISO 11140-3: 2007	Sterilization of health care products – Chemical indicators. Part 3: Type 2 indicator systems for use in the Bowie and Dick-type steam penetration test	Specifies the requirements for chemical indicators to be used in the steam penetration test for steam sterilizers for wrapped goods, e.g. instruments and porous materials (an example of a type 2 indicator as described in ISO 11140-1)
ISO 11140-4: 2007	Sterilization of health care products – Chemical indicators. Part 4: Type 2 indicators as an alternative to the Bowie and Dick-type test for detection of steam penetration	Specifies the performance for a type 2 indicator to be used as an alternative to the Bowie–Dick-type test This type of indicator is intended to identify poor steam penetration but does not necessarily indicate the cause
ISO 11140-5: 2007	Sterilization of health care products – Chemical indicators. Part 5: Type 2 indicators for Bowie and Dick-type air removal tests	Specifies the requirements for type 2 indicators for Bowie–Dick-type air removal tests used to evaluate the effectiveness of air removal
ISO 11140-6: 2022	Sterilization of health care products – Chemical indicators. Part 6: Type 2 indicators and process challenge devices for use in performance testing of small steam sterilizers	Specifies the performance requirements and test methods for both hollow and porous devices and the chemical and/or biological indicators used in these devices for the purpose of establishing effective steam penetration in small steam sterilizers
WHO: 2016	Decontamination and reprocessing of medical devices for health-care facilities	Guidance on processing, to include steam sterilization
AS 5369: 2023	Reprocessing of reusable medical devices in health and non-health related facilities	Guidance on processing of medical devices, including requirements for steam sterilization in Australia
ANSI/AAMI ST79: 2017 (amendments A1: 2020, A2: 2020, A3: 2020, A4: 2020)	Comprehensive guide to steam sterilization and sterility assurance in health care facilities	Provides recommended practice on steam sterilization in healthcare facilities in the United States ANSI/AAMI ST 79 is a consolidation of a previous series of guidelines
CDC/HICPAC: 2008	Guideline for disinfection and sterilization in healthcare facilities	General recommendations on methods for cleaning, disinfection, and sterilization of patient-care medical devices in the United States
HTM 01-01, Part C	Management and decontamination of surgical instruments (medical devices) used in acute care Part C: Steam sterilization	The UK HTMs are published in five parts, with Part C dedicated to steam sterilization, including the design, testing, and use of steam sterilizers Was previously known as HTM 2010
CSA Z314: 23	Canadian medical device reprocessing in all health care settings	Canadian standard of device processing including requirements for steam sterilization
WS 310.1: 2016	Central sterile supply department (CSSD)	Industrial standard of the People's Republic of China on device processing, including steam sterilization Published in three parts, for management, operating procedures, and surveillance requirements

[1] At the time of writing, the three parts of this standard series are in the process of being combined into a single standard (ISO 17665).

Incinerators can range in design and capacity, from simple burners to high-capacity furnaces and batch to continuous systems (Figure 11.19). High-capacity incinerators usually consist of a feed system, a primary chamber (in which the waste is incinerated), a secondary chamber/furnace (particularly for burning off waste gases that may be toxic), and a cooling/feed-out system. Typical temperatures for primary incineration are in the 400–980°C/750–1800°F range and for the secondary furnace 870–1100°C/1600–2000°F. They may also include heat-recovery systems that can be used to heat a water supply. Exposure times will vary on the volume of the load but can be up to several hours.

A concern with incineration is the release of highly toxic (even carcinogenic) and particularly persistent chemicals released on burning of plastic and other materials. These include dioxins, a series of fluorine-containing chemicals, and various gases such as carbon monoxide and carbon dioxide. For this reason, alternative systems such as hot-alkaline digestion and other heating/chemical treatment/shredding systems have been adopted. As an example, electro-thermal

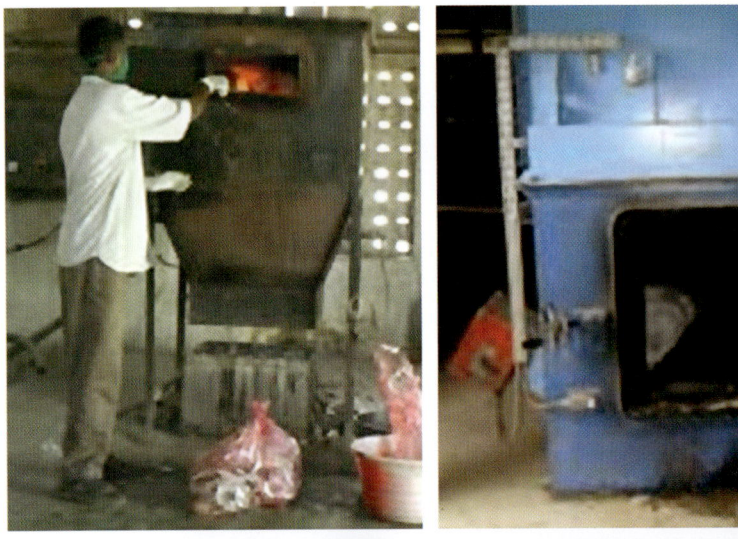
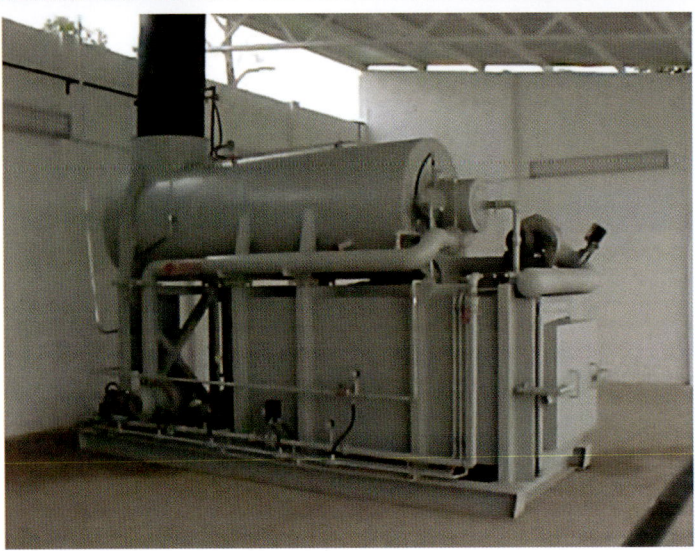

Figure 11.19 Examples of incinerators, ranging from simple burning furnaces to more complicated two-stage incinerator designs.

deactivation (ETD) employs an electrically heated oven in combination with low-frequency radio waves as a rapid dry heating method, but without melting of plastics; in such systems the waste is treated and shredded to reduce volume up to 80%. Incineration and similar systems are destructive and are only used for waste-disposal methods; these are not considered in further detail.

Dry heat sterilizers (also known as hot air or oven sterilizers) are rarely used clinically for sterilization and are often restricted to certain types of materials such as glassware, oils, powders, and instruments that for various reasons cannot be routinely sterilized by steam (e.g. moisture-sensitive materials/devices). Many of these items are provided as single-use (often sterile) materials/devices and are not subjected to processing. Therefore it is rare to see the use of dry heat sterilizers in clinical practice today. Dry heat sterilizers should not be confused with drying cabinets that are only designed to remove water (i.e. for drying) using dry, heated air (although sometimes at disinfection temperatures (>70°C/158°F; see Chapter 9). Although drying cabinets may provide some antimicrobial effects, including restricting the ability of certain types of microorganisms to grow such as bacteria, fungi, and protozoa, they are not designed (or validated) and should not be considered for use as sterilizers.

Dry heat sterilization applications use air heated to a high temperature, generally in excess of 150°C/~302°F, for its antimicrobial effects and therefore uses much higher temperatures than those used for steam sterilization. The presence of some moisture (e.g. as humidity) may assist in the efficacy of the process, but this will be inconsistent. There may or may not be various levels of water (humidity) present during such processes (e.g. within the load or air), but this is not specifically controlled as part of the process. It is of interest to note that the less humidity that is present, the longer the time required for dry heat sterilization. Therefore, the conditions for effective dry heat sterilization can depend on the amount of water present in the materials to be sterilized and in the environment/air of the sterilizer. To compensate for this variability, dry heat sterilization cycle times can be overall quite long.

As for other disinfection and sterilization methods, all items to be sterilized must be cleaned, dried, and prepared for dry heat sterilization. Items may be wrapped with foil, packed into a closed metal container, or placed unwrapped onto a tray or sterilizer shelf. They should remain in the sterilizer at the correct temperature for the required time, including cooldown, as a safety precaution.

The mechanisms of action of dry heat are predominantly due to direct heating and oxidation effects on various molecules present and essential for life in microorganisms; the overall mechanisms are similar but considered distinct to those observed with steam (as discussed earlier in this chapter). The only parameters that need to be controlled during a typical dry heat sterilization process are the air temperature and exposure time, therefore they are relatively simple processes in design. A typical sterilization process will include pre-heating of the air and load to the desired sterilization temperature (pre-conditioning), holding it at a set temperature for sterilization, and then allowing the load to cool prior to handling/patient use (typically to <80°C/~176°F). There are variations in times and temperatures in dry heat sterilization cycles based on the sterilizer design itself and the volume, density, and packaging recommendations for the load. The heating process is generally slow, and traditionally long sterilizing times are required. Sterilization times at specified temperatures are not described in ISO 20857, but specifications for temperature and exposure times may be described in various national standards. They can range from a 30-minute exposure at 180°C/~356°F to a 6-hour exposure at 121°C/~250°F or higher temperatures, not including times for conditioning (pre-heating) and cooling the load. Traditionally used sterilization phase temperatures and exposure times are:

- 180°C/~356°F 30 minutes
- 170°C/~338°F 1 hour
- 160°C/~320°F 2 hours
- 142°C/~288°F 2.5 hours

There are no standard cycle times, as this will depend on the sterilizer design and indications for use. At such high temperatures (>150°C/302°F) and contact times, dry heat is considered effective against microorganisms, with the most resistant organism to such processes widely accepted to be *Bacillus atrophaeus* spores. These spores are therefore used in the design, validation, and routine testing of dry heat sterilization processes (in compliance with standards such as ISO 20857; see Table 11.8). Following such long sterilization times, cooling of the load can take some time before the devices can be

Table 11.8 Examples of guidelines and standards considering dry heat sterilization.

Guidelines/standards	Title	Description
ISO 20857: 2010	Sterilization of health care products – Dry heat –Requirements for the development, validation, and routine control of a sterilization process for medical devices	Specifies requirements for the development, validation, and routine control of a dry heat sterilization process for devices (including for depyrogenation)
ISO 11138-4: 2017	Sterilization of health care products – Biological indicators Part 4: Biological indicators for dry heat sterilization processes	Provides specific requirements for test organisms, suspensions, inoculated carriers, biological indicators, and test methods intended for use in dry heat sterilizers
ANSI/AAMI ST40: 2004 (R2018)	Table-top dry heat (heated air) sterilization and sterility assurance in health care facilities	Provides guidelines for dry heat sterilization in US healthcare facilities
ANSI/AAMI ST50: 2004 (R2018)	Dry heat (heated air) sterilizers	Labeling and performance requirements for dry heat sterilizers used in US healthcare facilities
AS5369: 2023	Reprocessing of reusable medical devices in health and non-health related facilities	General guidance on processing, and includes reference to dry heat sterilization in Australia
WHO: 2016	Decontamination and reprocessing of medical devices for health-care facilities	Guidance on processing, to include dry heat sterilization

safely handled/used, sometimes up to eight hours depending on the load and sterilizer design.

In some older designs, the control of the sterilization process is conducted manually. Care should be taken to ensure that these processes are effective for their defined use. Under such conditions, defined load configurations should be specified in a written procedure (in collaboration with the sterilizer manufacturer), timing for sterilization should not begin until the oven/load reaches the desired temperature, and care should be taken to allow the load to cool prior to handling/use.

Dry heat sterilization is not recommended for items that could melt or burn at higher temperatures. These can include rubber, many plastics, elastomers, devices containing certain types of adhesives, and even some devices that may be considered heat resistant (such as stainless steel devices that can be damaged by stress cracking). In all cases, devices or material (including packaging) manufacturer's instructions should be reviewed to ensure they are compatible and can be safely used in dry heat sterilization processes. Given such high temperatures (and times used) and lack of consideration in most IFU, the clinical applications for dry heat sterilizers are limited at this time.

Dry heat sterilization methods are effective by penetrating the load over time, due to the convection transfer of heat. Convection, in this case, is defined as transfer of heat by the movement or circulation of air. In comparison to steam sterilization dry heat is also considered to have a low corrosive profile and not to be associated with many of the common water quality/purity problems reported with steam sterilization (as discussed under steam sterilization). It is often the only option for the sterilization of moisture-sensitive materials such as powders and oils. Dry heat sterilizers are typically available at low cost and are not associated with the complexity of installation/utility requirements of steam sterilizers. Dry heat is an effective method to neutralize endotoxins (see Chapter 5), but is more widely used industrially for such applications. The term "depyrogenation" refers to the specific inactivation of the toxic effects of toxins such as endotoxins, but dry heat is rarely used clinically for such purposes. Dry heat sterilizers do, however, have many disadvantages, such as the length of time required for sterilization and the restrictions on the types of materials/devices that can tolerate dry heat sterilization processes.

Design

There are two essential designs of dry heat sterilization systems: dry heat ovens and incinerators. Incinerator designs were briefly introduced earlier in this section. Dry heat ovens consist of a chamber (generally made of stainless steel) within which the air is electrically heated (not unlike a kitchen oven). More efficient designs will typically include fans to allow for the circulation of air during the process, to optimize even heat distribution. The process is often conducted under slight pressure and the ovens are vented through high-efficiency particulate air (HEPA) filters to prevent the ingress of contaminants during the sterilization process. HEPA-filtered air can be used to assist with cooling during the sterilization process.

Dry heat sterilizers can be designed for batch sterilization (like other sterilizers, where a load is placed into the sterilizer, sterilized, and then removed) or as a continuous design (a tunnel or conveyor system). Batch sterilizers are generally used for packaged materials, while continuous systems are for non-packaged items and depyrogenation. The sterilizer design should have calibrated thermometer(s) or temperature gauge(s) to make sure that the designated temperature is reached, distributed, and maintained for the desired time. Overall, the sterilizer may be automatically (microprocessor) controlled or operated manually. It is recommended that any sterilizer process records (manually or automatically produced by the sterilizer) should be maintained as verification that the process was correctly completed.

Standards and guidelines

Table 11.8 lists some examples of widely used guidelines and standards relating to dry heat sterilizers, sterilization processes, and monitoring.

Radiation

Radiation and various forms of light can have disinfection and sterilization properties (see Chapter 6, in the section on light, radiation, and the electromagnetic spectrum). Low-energy radiation methods, such as ultraviolet (UV) and infrared (IR) light, are used for various disinfection applications (see Chapter 9, on the section on radiation). High-energy radiation sources are widely used as industrial sterilization methods, but not for reusable device processing or for routine use in healthcare facilities. High-energy radiation sources and generators are more widely used for the sterilization of single-use materials within healthcare facilities, such as bandages and types of single-use devices.

Radiation sterilization is mostly used for contract sterilization of single-use devices and materials that are then supplied to a healthcare facility pre-sterilized and discarded following use. They all consist of exposing a load to a given dose of radiation (over time). Typical radiation technologies are:

- γ-radiation. This form of radiation is released from unstable forms of certain types of elements (see Chapter 6) known as "radioactive isotopes." Examples include ^{60}Cobalt and ^{137}Caesium. Being unstable, they break down (or "decay") over time to release energy (in the form of γ-radiation) that is a very powerful antimicrobial.
- X-ray radiation. Also a source of high-energy radiation (X-rays are less energized than γ-radiation, see Chapter 6), but in this case are generated from specific X-ray–producing tubes/systems.
- E-beam radiation. A different form of radiation (β-particles or "electrons") that is generated and focused in systems known as "accelerators," also producing a powerful antimicrobial effect.

Table 11.9 Examples of radiation sterilization standards used for industrial purposes.

Guidelines/standards	Title	Description
ISO 11137-1: 2006	Sterilization of health care products – Radiation Part 1: Requirements for development, validation, and routine control of a sterilization process for medical devices	Specifies requirements for the development, validation, and routine control of a radiation sterilization process for medical devices. Covers radiation processes employing irradiators using the radionuclide ^{60}Co or ^{137}Cs, a beam from an electron generator, or a beam from an X-ray generator
ISO 11137-2: 2013	Sterilization of health care products – Radiation Part 2: Establishing the sterilization dose	Specifies methods of determining the minimum dose needed to achieve a specified requirement for sterility

Specific facilities are designed to ensure the safe handling/production of radiation and its use for sterilization. For this reason, they are not covered in detail here. The various different forms of radiation were identified in Chapter 6.

At the time of writing, there are no specific guidelines or standards regarding the routine use of radiation for sterilization of reusable devices in healthcare facilities. There are, however, a number of industrial standards that may be referenced if applicable (Table 11.9).

Filtration

Filtration is commonly used as a physical removal mechanism in disinfection and sterilization, especially with gases (e.g. air) and liquids (such as water). For this reason, it is often used as a part of various device sterilization processes. Examples include:
- For the introduction of air during steam and low-temperature gas sterilization methods. The most commonly used filters are HEPA filters of various grades. Typically these filters have the capacity to retain particles down to a 0.5–1 µm range (thereby removing most bacteria), but this will depend on their specific design. They can also cause removal of smaller particles due to attachment to/interaction with the filter material.
- As part of the treatment of water used for rinsing of devices during disinfection or following liquid chemical disinfection/sterilization. Examples include sterile water filters (0.1–0.2 µm), RO systems, and sterile water filter/UV light combination treatment systems, depending on their design and integration as part of the sterilization process/sterilizer.

Filters are used to physically remove various microorganisms due to their size. This is discussed in further detail in Chapter 9, in the section on filtration. The use of filters as part of a sterilizer design needs to be controlled to ensure their safe and effective use. This will include the design of the filter(s) and how they are used/tested within the process, as well as maintenance/replacement recommendations. In such cases, care should be taken to follow the sterilizer manufacturer's instructions.

Chemical sterilization

Ethylene oxide gas

Ethylene oxide (C_2H_4O), or more commonly EO or ETO, is a colorless gas at 20°C (68°F) and atmospheric pressure. It is possible to smell EO at about 500 ppm of the gas in air, described as a sweet, almond-like odor, but at lower concentrations it is essentially odorless. EO is a hazardous substance, so exposure to levels of EO gas where the odor is detected should not routinely occur. Note that in gas 500 ppm is approximately (but not exactly) equal to 500 mg/L, therefore these levels are within the range used for sterilization.

EO dissolves easily in water, alcohol, and most organic solvents. It is one of the most widely used industrial chemicals in the manufacture of plastics, detergents, polyesters, and antifreeze (glycols). A minor fraction of the total amount of EO used is for antimicrobial processes and particularly for low-temperature sterilization. It is primarily used for industrial sterilization (e.g. for single-use devices provided sterile and even for certain types of foods) and, to a much lesser extent, in hospitals or contract sterilization facilities for the sterilization of reusable, heat-sensitive devices. As a biocide, it demonstrates broad-spectrum antimicrobial activity including against bacterial spores when controlled as part of a sterilization process (depending on the chemical concentration and presence of high humidity). Its main mechanism of action is by a process called alkylation, which attacks the various types of macromolecules (such as protein) leading to the loss of structure and function, resulting in microbial death.

EO is used to sterilize items that are heat or moisture sensitive. The ability to process plastics, electronics, and many complex products of diverse material composition accelerated the development and evolution of many of these types of devices, including flexible endoscopes. EO readily permeates commonly used packaging materials, porous materials, and various types of devices (including lumened devices) at low temperatures; it is also used to sterilize other materials such as paper and types of fabrics. Further, EO is generally considered non-corrosive and non-damaging to a variety of materials, including those used in devices and packaging systems. But on the negative side, it can be flammable and explosive in the presence of air (at or above 3% air), is irritating, and is carcinogenic (associated with causing cancer). Therefore, close control of the use of EO is important for staff and patient safety.

Principles of ethylene oxide gas sterilization

EO sterilization requires the chemical concentration, water (humidity) level, temperature, and contact time to be controlled during any such process (Table 11.10):

- EO concentration at ranges typically from 300 to 1200 mg/L. In general, the higher the concentration the more efficient the sterilization process, but it is also considered that concentrations >400 mg/L do not appear to provide any further significant increase in activity against bacterial spores.
- Temperatures can vary, but for most hospital applications will be between 30 and 65°C/86–149°F, with higher temperatures found to be more efficient than lower. The temperature range of such processes is generally limited to at or below 55°C/131°F, as higher temperatures are considered damaging to many types of materials/devices (for which a temperature of <60°C/140°F is recommended).
- Humidity (specifically the "relative humidity," which is the amount of water in air at a specific temperature) is recommended to be 40–80%. Lower and higher levels may be recommended depending on the sterilizer/process manufacturer. Note: 100% relative humidity is considered water "saturated" at a given temperature (see Chapter 6).
- Exposure times, which will depend on the EO concentration, temperature, and humidity, as defined by the manufacturer to meet an SAL of 10^{-6} or equivalent.

Overall, these are the minimum required variables for sterilization to be achieved. Individual sterilization processes are defined and verified to be effective within these ranges using bacterial spore preparations of *Bacillus atrophaeus* (previously known as *Bacillus subtilis* subspecies *niger*). *B. atrophaeus* spores are considered one of the more resistant organisms to EO sterilization processes, although certain types of fungal spore formations (e.g. of the type known as *Pyronema*) have been shown to have unique tolerance profiles to EO depending on the process conditions.

Similar to other sterilization processes, there are various different phases of the process to ensure that these conditions are achieved within the types of loads that are being sterilized, as well as to ensure that such loads are safe for use following sterilization. A typical EO sterilization process will therefore include (Figure 11.20):

- Conditioning, to ensure that the load is correctly humidified, heated, and mixed with EO gas to meet the defined conditions for sterilization. In some cases, although rare, preconditioning may be conducted in a separate chamber to preheat and humidify the load prior to placing it into the EO sterilizer. It is important during conditioning to ensure that air is adequately removed, for two reasons: air can inhibit the penetration of humidity/EO to all surfaces within the load;

Table 11.10 Examples of ethylene oxide (EO) gas sterilization processes, highlighting the gas concentration, relative humidity range, temperature, and typical exposure times for sterilization.

EO concentration (mg/L)	Temperature (°C)	Temperature (°F)	Relative humidity (%)	Exposure time (hours)
700–900	37–38	98–100	50–80	4–4.5
700–900	55	131	50–80	1
550–650	55	131	30–70	2
350–450	55	131	30–80	7.5

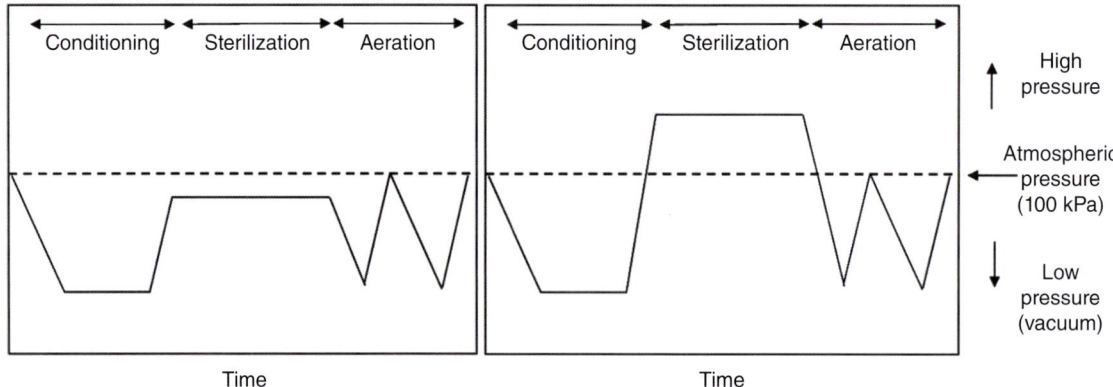

Figure 11.20 Examples of ethylene oxide sterilization processes. On the left is a sterilization cycle under vacuum (negative pressure), specifically the gas exposure phase of the cycle, and on the right a pressurized (positive pressure) cycle.

and EO is explosive in the presence of as little as 3% air. This is generally achieved by pulling the air out of the chamber/load using a vacuum pump ("drawing a vacuum" to a predetermined low pressure). Steam is also introduced (or generated directly within the chamber from water) under these conditions to act as both a heating and a humidification mechanism; remember from the discussion on steam (see principles of steam sterilization) that while steam can be generated at higher temperatures by increasing the pressure, it can also be made at lower temperatures under lower pressures. In this way, steam (under vacuum/low pressure) can be used to precondition the load at lower temperatures prior to sterilization. Steam introduction and air removal may be assisted by repeated pulses of pulling a vacuum and introducing steam to given controlled pressure set points. Generally, as a final part of the conditioning cycle, EO gas is then introduced into the chamber and allowed to diffuse within the load. As EO is a gas at temperatures above ~11°C/~52°F and at atmospheric pressure, in accordance with the gas laws it can be maintained as a liquid at lower temperatures or higher pressures. EO is therefore generally provided as a liquid in single- or multiple-use pressurized canisters (Figure 11.21). The canister is provided to a delivery system within or associated with the sterilizer (an example of a single-use canister loaded within the sterilizer chamber is shown in Figure 11.21); the gas is then generated during the process (under vacuum or negative pressure;

Figure 11.20) by heating (e.g. at 60–70°C/140–158°F). EO can be provided as a 100% preparation, typically in single-use canisters or vials containing low volumes of EO (e.g. 10–100 mL). Such canisters are designed for specific sterilization processes, as defined by the manufacturer. But because of the flammable nature of EO in the pure form, EO preparations are also provided mixed with an excess of inert gases such as carbon dioxide (CO_2) or, in the past, could be mixed with hydrochlorofluorocarbons (HCFC) as non-flammable blends. Traditional examples include 10% EO, 90% HCFC (commonly referred to as 10–90) or 8.5% EO, 91.5% CO_2. In general, these preparations are usually provided in larger canisters for use in multiple EO sterilization cycles. Conditioning is complete when the required conditions of temperature, humidity, and EO concentration are achieved.

- Sterilization, where the temperature, humidity, and EO gas concentration are maintained within the sterilizer for the defined time (e.g. to provide an SAL of 10^{-6} as defined by the manufacturer). It is typical for processes using 100% EO to be maintained under a vacuum (negative pressure) and the same when EO blends are used as the sterilant supply to which loads are exposed under pressure; however, the specific process variables will vary depending on the manufacturer and cycle definition. In both cases the processes are designed to ensure adequate distribution and penetration of the gas. Typical cycle conditions are summarized in Table 11.10.

(A)

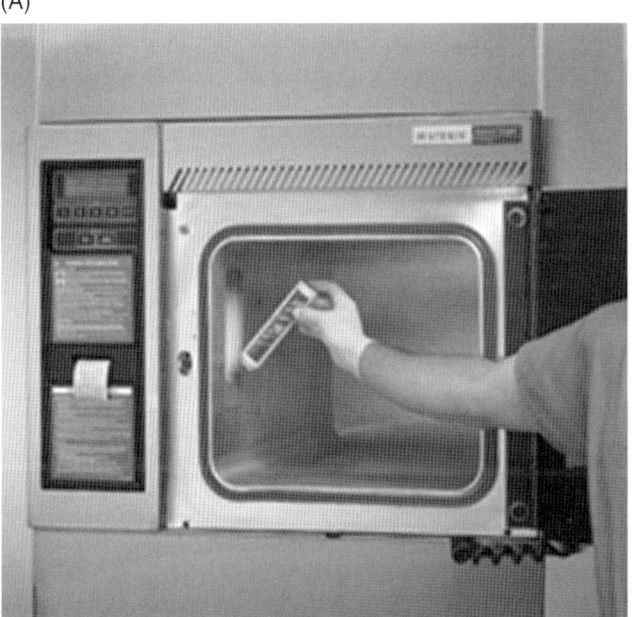

(B)

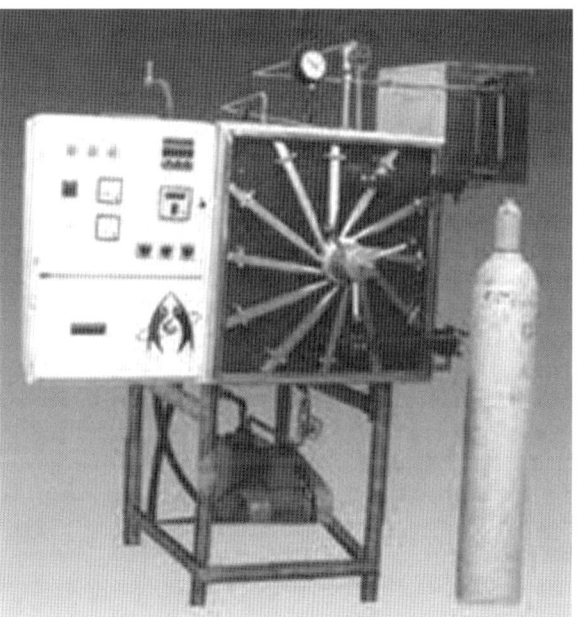

Figure 11.21 Examples of ethylene oxide (EO) sterilizers and supply canisters/tanks (providing liquid EO under pressure). (A) A canister (100% EO) being placed into a sterilizer chamber. (B) An older larger sterilizer provided with an EO blend canister.

- Aeration, in which EO is removed from the chamber and associated load by one or several vacuum pulses (sometimes including the aid of steam or heat to improve the aeration time). The gas is passed through a system (e.g. an abater or catalytic converter) to break down the gas safely into water and carbon dioxide. Safe aeration of the load is the longest part of a typical EO sterilization cycle; depending on the load materials and size, it can be typically 8–12 hours (depending on the aeration process, including the temperature) but may even be longer. An example of an aeration cycle would be 12 hours at 50°C/122°F, although device manufacturers should provide information supporting the safe aeration cycle conditions for their specific device types. Aeration can be achieved in the sterilizer itself (depending on the type of load and sterilization process defined by the manufacturer) and/or more commonly in a separate aeration chamber/cabinet that holds the load at a constant air flow and temperature (e.g. 35–60°C/95–140°F) to aid in the removal of EO toxic residues.

As discussed, there are essentially two main types of EO sterilization processes: those that use EO blends and those using 100% EO. They both have advantages and disadvantages:
- 100% EO: generally provided in single-use EO cartridges used directly within the sterilizer. These require no additional supply tanks, valves, or fittings that could leak on providing EO to the sterilizer. Such sterilizer designs ensure that the used cartridges are safely aerated with the load, rendering them non-hazardous and safe to discard (in a safe manner according to the gas manufacturer/supplier's instructions and healthcare facility's policy). One canister is typically used per sterilization cycle. Most sterilizer chambers are limited in size but do operate under negative pressure (vacuum); therefore, if a leak did accidentally occur the gas should remain in the chamber and not vent into the room.
- EO blends: typically provided as multiple-use gas tanks, which can offer greater flexibility in the number of types of cycles that can be programmed with the sterilizer. Such blends are safer in handling and storage due to their non-flammability; but it is important to ensure that they are connected correctly to the sterilizer and that the connection system does not leak during use or over time. Sterilizer designs can be smaller or larger, able to accommodate smaller or larger loads, respectively (as specified by the manufacturer). Sterilization cycles using blends are most often designed to operate under pressure, which may increase the risk of leaking from the sterilizer during processes; as with all sterilizer designs, routine maintenance and periodic servicing according to the manufacturer's instructions should minimize such risks.

EO sterilization processes are used as low-temperature alternatives to steam sterilization. EO, under the correct exposure conditions (particularly temperature and humidity), is a reliable and well-described sterilizing agent. As it is a very stable gas, it demonstrates good penetration capabilities into loads and specifically challenging devices (such as long-lumened or porous instruments); however, it is important to note that the antimicrobial effects are dependent on the presence of the gas and humidity (therefore also the consistent removal of air). EO demonstrates exceptional device and material compatibility. Overall, these benefits are due to the non-reactive nature of EO with various types of metals, plastics, electronics, and other materials (including various types of sterile packaging materials and containers); despite this, it is recommended to only use packaging materials that are labeled for use with EO sterilization processes. Typical loads can include temperature-sensitive materials and devices, including flexible endoscopes and plastic ware.

When handled properly, EO is a reliable and safe agent for sterilization, but the risks of gas emissions and residues of EO present hazards to personnel and patients. A safe work environment must be maintained for employees when working with EO. Many countries have strict regulations in place governing its safe use. Adequate ventilation, air exchanges, and environmental monitoring are required. EO is a toxic gas even at very low concentrations and is listed as a carcinogen (cancer associated). As an example, the typical recommended average exposure limit over an 8 hour day is 1 ppm (although 0.2 ppm has become widely used), but the short-term exposure limit is 5 ppm for 15 minutes; remember that under these conditions the gas cannot be readily detected by smell and these levels are under review at the time of writing. The first safety limit is often referred to as the time-weighted average (TWA), referring to the personnel exposure concentration measured over a specific period of time, usually eight hours. Personnel exposure is usually expressed as a TWA based on environmental exposure, measured by wearing a personal monitor (Figure 11.22). These recommended safety levels are periodically reviewed and may change depending on the individual country or region. Further terms that are used include:
- Permissible exposure limit (PEL), the maximum EO exposure allowed per worker. It is the employer's responsibility to ensure that employees are not exposed to airborne concentrations of EO in excess of this limit. The required maximum exposure level is usually set at 1 ppm over a typical eight-hour working day, but may be lower in some countries.
- Excursion limit (EL), workers' short-term exposure limit. No more than four exposure periods within this range are permitted within an eight-hour work day. This exposure is typically task related (transferring a load to the aerator, removing indicators from an unaerated load, changing cylinders, performing maintenance, etc.).

Low concentrations can lead to irritation of the eyes and mucous membranes, with higher concentrations being more damaging to health as well as posing a flammability risk. EO installation requirements can vary regionally, but generally require a dedicated exhaust, emission controls, enclosed

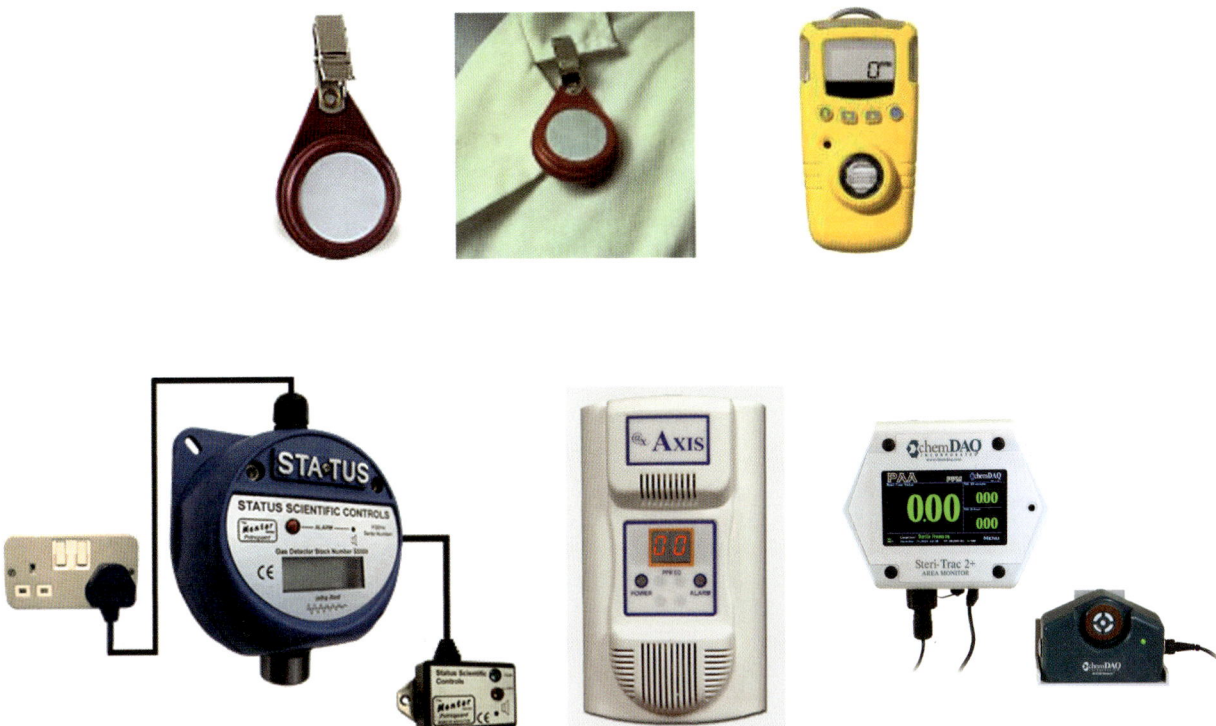

Figure 11.22 Ethylene oxide gas sensors and monitoring equipment. These include personal monitors (upper left), hand-held, and wall-mounted sensors (upper-right and lower sensor examples).

controlled EO sterilizer/aerator room, and monitoring systems. Gas manufacturer/suppliers' instructions (including safety sheets) should be consulted regarding EO storage conditions. These will include storage in a well-ventilated area under controlled conditions (including temperature, flammable gas safety cabinets, etc.; Figure 11.23).

The levels of EO present at any point in time and over time can be reliably monitored using a range of sensor systems (Figure 11.22). These include personal monitors that are recommended to be worn (as badges or pins) during a normal working day near to the "breathing zone" (on a lapel or upper pocket, as shown in Figure 11.22). The monitoring discs are collected and sent to an external laboratory for analysis, which provides a final result of the exposure to EO during the time worn (within a range). They have the advantage of providing information regarding the actual exposure to EO over a period of time within an area, but the results are not available until after the analysis (sometimes days or weeks after being worn). Therefore, as an additional safety precaution, real-time monitors or sensors are also recommended; these can range from simple hand-held monitors (providing a digital display of the EO concentration) to wall-mounted systems of various complexity. It is common for such systems to provide visual (flashing light) or audible (siren) alarms at various warning or danger levels. Procedures should be in place and staff trained on the emergency procedures (including evacuation and area re-entry) that need to take place in the event of an alarm. Correct installation and maintenance of such systems are therefore important. In some countries the results from personal monitoring and any excursions (including investigations and resolutions of any problems) are required to be maintained (archived) with personnel history files.

Policies must be in place to ensure that sterilization loads are adequately aerated prior to storage and/or direct patient use. Even low levels of EO remaining on devices or within packaging can lead to patient and staff toxicity risks. For example, EO can be released over time from exposed loads within a storage area and, without adequate ventilation, can cause toxicity problems to staff working in that area. In addition to EO gas residuals, the gas can react with other chemicals present in/on the load and can form other toxic chemicals. For example, in preparation for sterilization, it is recommended that residual soil or excess liquids (e.g. water) should not be present as they will not only hinder sterilization efficacy but

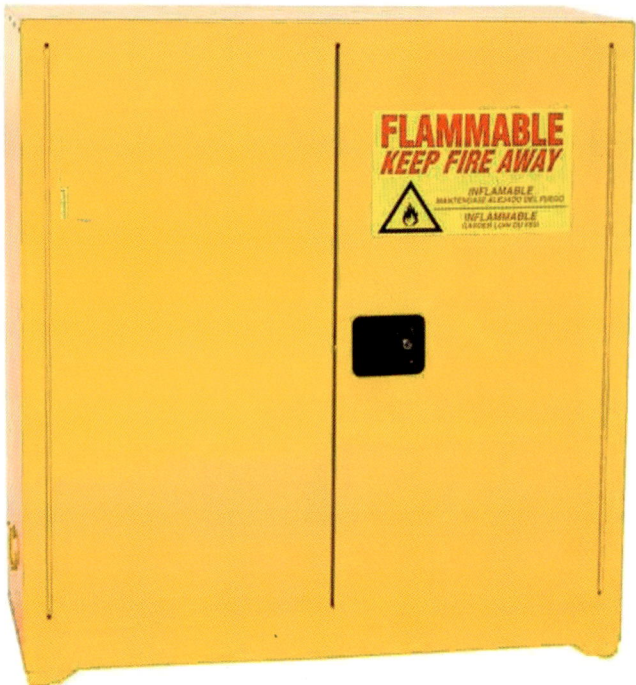
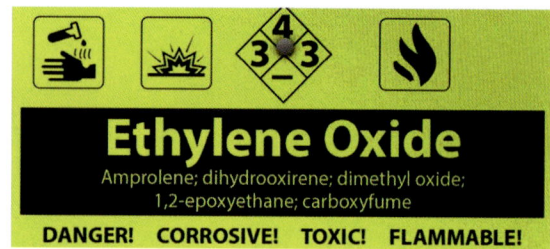
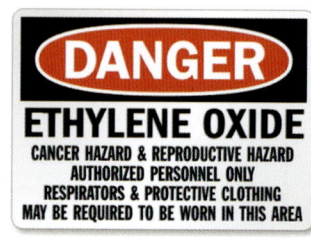

Figure 11.23 A gas safety cabinet and typical warning signs used for ethylene oxide gas storage.

may also result in further harmful residuals being formed. For instance:
- Water and EO can generate ethylene glycol residuals,
- Saline and EO can generate ethylene chlorohydrin, which is also a toxic chemical.

Therefore, efficient aeration is required to remove not only residuals of EO but also any other toxic by-products. This is initially conducted within the sterilizer (during the aeration phase of the cycle) and may be completed by further, extended aeration within the sterilizing chamber or in a specially designed aeration chamber. Aeration is achieved by holding the load at a given temperature and time under a controlled number of air exchanges per minute (e.g. 4–6 air volume changes/minute). Aeration may also be assisted by drawing a vacuum within the chamber and pulsing steam/air into the chamber during the aeration process. The aeration requirements (time, temperature, number of air pulses/changes, etc.) should be specified by the manufacturer and defined for different types of loads. Staff should consider the correct aeration conditions not only for the devices but also any other associated sterile packaging materials. If using a separate aeration chamber, the contents of the sterilizer need to be safely transferred to the aeration cabinet after completion of the sterilizer cycle (including initial aeration). Before transferring items, it is important to confirm that the aerator has sufficient room to handle the load and is turned on (and working) at the appropriate temperature. Typical aeration conditions (specified as a time–temperature relationship) are:
- 8 hours at 60°C/140°F
- 10 hours at 54°C/130°F
- 12 hours at 49°C/120°F
- 20 hours at 38°C/100°F

It is important to note that the overall aeration time/conditions will depend on the EO sterilization process and aeration system used (including the air exchanges provided), the thickness of the sterile barrier systems used, the design and weight of the load, the size and arrangement of packages in the sterilizer/aerator or aeration cabinet, and the number/types of EO-absorbent materials within the load or being aerated at any given time.

Due to the required balance of efficacy and safety requirements with EO sterilization processes, it is important to ensure that EO sterilizers and/or aerators are not overloaded or contain materials/load descriptions that have not been defined as suitable for this process by the manufacturer. With the long times associated with such sterilization processes, there is often a tendency to attempt to maximize load capacity, but this can lead to inefficient sterilization and safety (toxicity) risks.

Typical sterilizer design

Similar to steam sterilizers, there are a variety of sizes and designs of EO sterilizers (Figure 11.24), ranging from

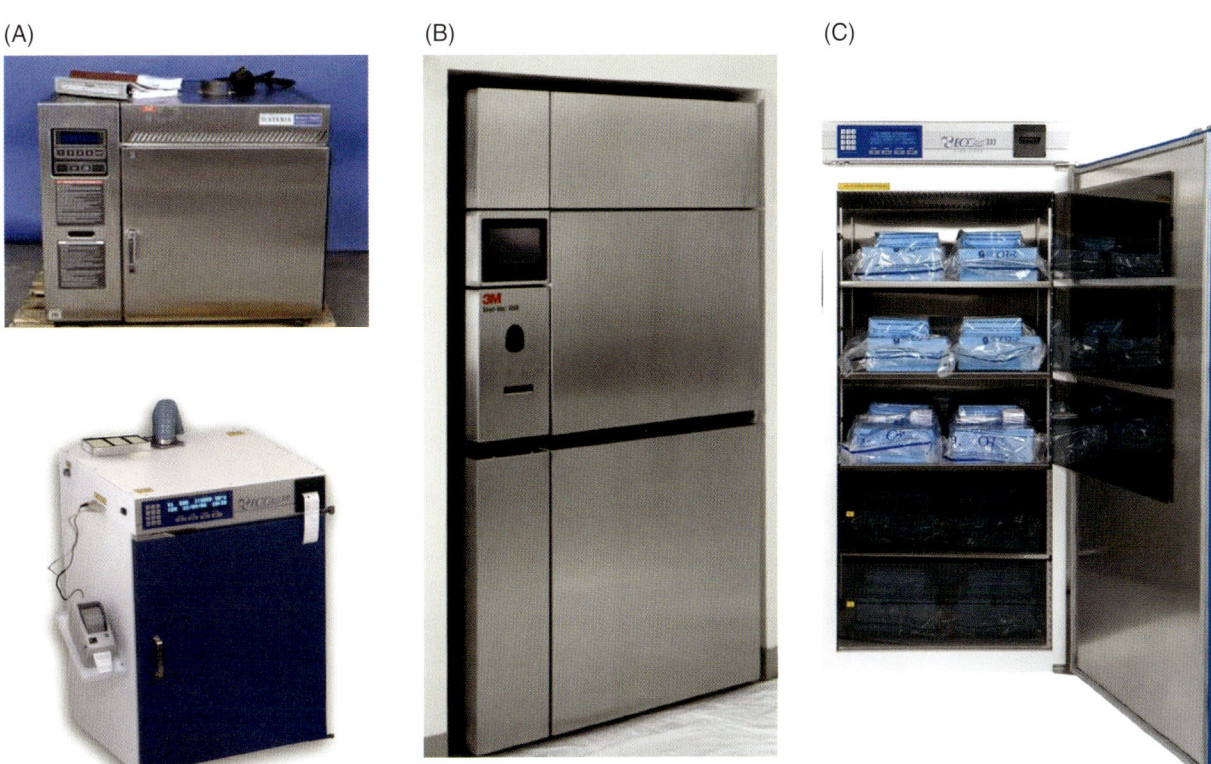

Figure 11.24 A variety of ethylene oxide (EO) sterilizer designs. They can come in a variety of sizes. (A, B) Traditional design sterilizers, where a load is placed into the chamber, exposed to the process, and then the full load removed. (C) A cabinet-based sterilizer, an example of a single-dose or sterilization in a bag–type application, where the devices and a supply of EO gas/humidity are placed into specially designed and sealed bags, and the sterilization process conducted within the bag but held within the exposure cabinet. The EO process is controlled in each individual bag within the exposure chamber. Both designs can range in size, shape, and sterilization cycle development.

bench-top to large-capacity sterilizers. Most systems widely used in hospitals are similar to small steam sterilizers, consisting of a sterilization chamber, associated piping system (including air venting and a vacuum pump), associated control system and gauges (where applicable), and a steam (or humidity) supply. In addition, the sterilizers will have an associated EO gas supply system, as well as a method of breaking down the residual EO as it is being removed from the chamber. Two essentially different types of systems are commonly used: traditional chamber-based systems (which may apply the EO sterilization under pressure or a vacuum; Figure 11.24) and sterilization in a bag–type systems.

The basic design of a traditional chamber-based EO sterilizer is shown in Figure 11.25. The chamber is designed to handle the required pressures associated with the process, including low pressures for vacuum-based stages of the process and high for pressurized EO processes. In some cases the chamber is also jacketed to allow for greater temperature control. EO sterilization chambers are more typically designed as single-door designs, although double-door designs are also available. In some designs fans may be present within the chamber to assist in the circulation of EO gas/humidity and air during the process. The chamber-associated pipework allows for the introduction of humidity (usually in the form of steam, which can both heat and humidify the load), EO gas, air, and their safe removal. EO gas is generated by passing the provided liquid EO over a heated surface and then introduced into the chamber. The chamber is usually associated with a vacuum pump that allows low pressures (e.g. during air removal) to be applied. As EO is a toxic chemical, the exhaust of the gas during the process is rendered safe by passing it through an abater/catalytic converter system, which degrades the gas into carbon dioxide and water (both naturally present in air). The whole process is controlled and monitored by a control system (which can be of various complexities), including a recording system that records the variables of the process conducted. In these designs the load is prepared, placed into the chamber, and sterilized in a batch-type process; the load is only released

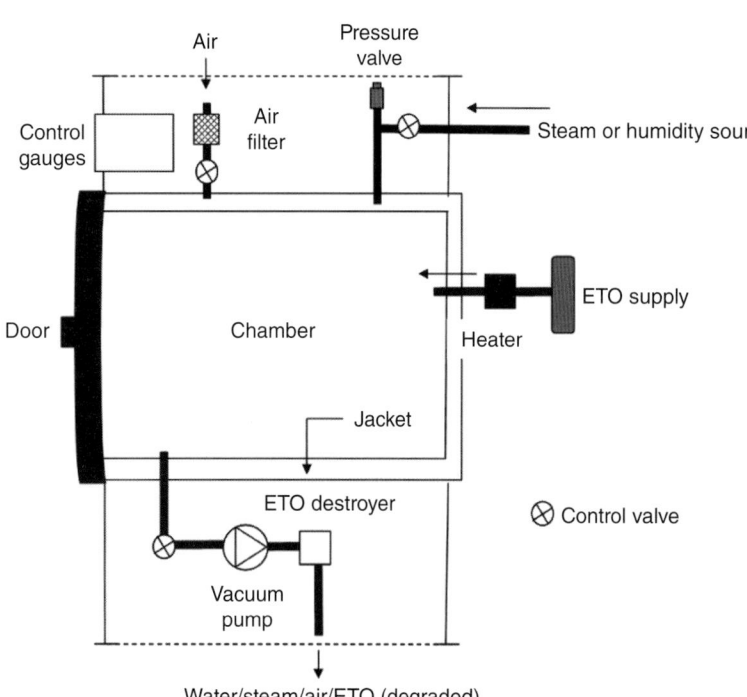

Figure 11.25 The basic design of a traditional, chamber-based or batch-type ethylene oxide (EO) sterilizer.

following the completed cycle and may or may not be subjected to extended aeration as part of a separate cycle within the same chamber or in a separate aeration system.

Alternative, cabinet-based sterilizer designs are also used that provide a chamber for the control of heat and provision of sterilization utilities (e.g. air, water supply, or exhaust system). In such designs the sterilization process is actually conducted within specifically designed plastic bags (generally made of heavy-duty plastics such as low-density polyethylene, LDPE; Figure 11.24). These are often referred to as single-dose or sterilization in a bag–type applications, where the devices to be sterilized and a supply of EO gas/humidity are placed into specially designed and sealed bags, and the sterilization process conducted within the bag but held within the exposure cabinet (for conditioning, including heating, and aeration control of the process). The cabinet is not sealed and allows the placement of a number of sterilization loads at different times into the chamber, depending on its capacity. The chambers can range from single (bench-top) to multiple (large, standing cabinet) load designs (Figure 11.24). They use 100% EO, provided in ampoules (e.g. containing 5 or 20 mL of liquid EO) specifically design for a given bag capacity (e.g. 7 or 35 L capacity, respectively) or similarly, for larger sizes, provided within EO-containing cartridges. The load is placed into the bag containing the EO source and, in some designs, a water supply (for humidification), heat sealed, and then placed into the holding chamber. Bag designs often allow for their connection to the utility supply/aeration system contained within the sterilizer cabinet design. Such sterilizer designs have the advantages of using less EO gas, often with minimal installation requirements, and are considered safer than the multiple-cycle gas tank systems described earlier. But they are also restrictive in load capacity (and load type), can require longer exposure times, and need the close attention of staff to ensure that the bags are correctly sealed during the process.

Standards and guidelines

Table 11.11 provides a list of guidelines and standards regarding sterilization with EO.

Formaldehyde gas

Formaldehyde (CH_2O), also chemically known as methanal, is a gas at room temperature and atmospheric pressure. It is generally provided as a white solid polymer (a molecule consisting of repeated single sub-units) known as paraformaldehyde (consisting of 8–100 repeated units of formaldehyde) or as a liquid (e.g. formalin solutions consisting of 34–40% of formaldehyde dissolved in water, often containing other chemicals such as methanol as chemical stabilizers). Formaldehyde is widely used in the chemical industry to make a variety of other chemicals such as resins (adhesives), plastics, and paints. It has been traditionally used as a disinfectant for a variety of applications, including as a gas for area/room fumigation and in liquids as a preservative (e.g. formaldehyde-releasing agents) and even as an antiseptic (e.g. for wart treatments). Formalin

Table 11.11 Ethylene oxide (EO) sterilization guidelines and standards.

Guidelines/standards	Title	Description
ISO 11135: 2014 (AMD 1: 2018)	Sterilization of health care products – Ethylene oxide Requirements for development, validation, and routine control of a sterilization process for medical devices	Specifies requirements for the development, validation, and routine control of an EO sterilization process for medical devices in both industrial and healthcare facility applications
ISO 11138-2: 2017	Sterilization of health care products – Biological indicators Part 2: Biological indicators for ethylene oxide sterilization processes	Provides specific requirements for test organisms, suspensions, inoculated carriers, biological indicators, and test methods intended for use in EO gas sterilization processes
ISO 10993-7: 2008 (AMD 1: 2019)	Biological evaluation of medical devices – Part 7: Ethylene oxide sterilization residuals	Specifies allowable limits for residual EO and ethylene chlorohydrin (ECH) on EO-sterilized devices Amendment 1 of this standard considered the applicability of allowable limits for neonates and infants
WHO: 2016	Decontamination and reprocessing of medical devices for health-care facilities	Guidance on processing, to include EO sterilization
ANSI/AAMI ST41: 2018	Ethylene oxide sterilization in health care facilities: Safety and effectiveness	Guidelines on the safe and effective use of EO for sterilization in the United States
CDC/HICPAC: 2008	Guideline for disinfection and sterilization in healthcare facilities	General recommendations on methods for cleaning, disinfection, and sterilization of patient-care medical devices in the United States
AS5369: 2023	Reprocessing of reusable medical devices in health and non-health facilities	General guidance on device processing, including EO sterilization in Australia
CSA Z314: 23	Canadian medical device reprocessing in all health care settings	Canadian standard of device processing including requirements for low-temperature sterilization

(a formaldehyde solution) is used in some hospital pathology departments for the treatment and mounting of tissue samples for microscopic investigations (in a discipline known as histology), but is rarely used as a solution or in formulation for disinfection or sterilization applications.

This section primarily considers the use of formaldehyde gas for the sterilization of reusable devices, particularly for hospital and dental use. Humidified formaldehyde gas is used on its own, or in combination with other biocides (such as alcohol), for low- (less than 60°C/140°F), intermediate- (60–80°C/140–176°F), and even high-temperature (e.g. at 134°C/273°F) application as an alternative to steam sterilization. It can therefore be used for temperature-sensitive devices/materials (which is its predominant use) or for temperature-resistant devices, depending on their design, process, and manufacturer's claims. Formaldehyde gas is recognized as a broad-spectrum antimicrobial, including activity against bacterial spores. The most-resistant microorganism to formaldehyde is recognized as *Geobacillus stearothermophilus* spores and these are therefore used in the development and routine testing of formaldehyde gas sterilization processes. Its mechanisms of action appear to be predominantly due to its toxicity to cells and viruses, by reacting with the various types of molecules that make up their essential structure and function such as proteins and nucleic acids. Formaldehyde reacts directly with these structures and can even cause them to cross-link to each other, leading to loss of the structures/function for viability. In this sense, formaldehyde is a considerably toxic chemical. Depending on the exact process used, formaldehyde-based processes can be considered very gentle on devices and materials due to the general lack of reactivity of the chemical with many of these surface materials; in particular, the humidified formaldehyde gas-only processes are considered non-damaging to materials, devices, and packaging. Despite this, some process conditions can be damaging to certain types of materials and devices; these should be specified by the process manufacturer.

Although formaldehyde sterilization has been described for many years, including the development of international standards for such sterilization processes (i.e. ISO 25424), it is not widely used internationally for device processing applications except in a limited number of countries. For this reason, it is rarely included as a potential method for reusable device sterilization in healthcare applications. The main disadvantages of formaldehyde sterilization processes can include longer cycle times, requirements for extended aeration, and particularly the associated toxicity of the chemical. Formaldehyde is toxic, an irritant, and is considered carcinogenic even at low exposure concentrations. Therefore, similar to the earlier discussion about EO, formaldehyde sterilization processes should be closely controlled, monitored, and maintained to ensure that they are safely used.

Principles of formaldehyde sterilization

Formaldehyde gas requires the correct gas concentration, water (humidity) level, temperature, and contact time for sterilization. Formaldehyde gas processes are optimized when condensation of formaldehyde in solution in water is formed on the surfaces to be sterilized; a similar condensation process is required for sterilization with high-temperature formaldehyde–alcohol-based processes. Formaldehyde gas–only processes are commonly referred to as low-temperature steam formaldehyde (LTSF). The variables of these processes include:

- Formaldehyde gas concentration: this can vary significantly from process to process, but is generally in the sporicidal range of 5–50 mg/L. The gas is commonly made by heating a liquid supply of formalin (ranging from 2% to 40% formaldehyde in solution). In some sterilizer designs other chemicals may also be used as part of the antimicrobial process, such as high concentrations of ethanol (70% ethanol with ~0.25% formaldehyde in water).
- Temperature of the process: this can also vary significantly between manufacturers and in specified sterilizer cycles. The typical range is between 50 and 80°C/122–176°F, depending on the specific process. Temperatures above 60°C/140°F, although considered "low temperature" in comparison to steam sterilization, may have limited application for certain types of devices (which have a limit of <60°C). The best way to attain and maintain such temperatures, in combination with the high humidity requirements for formaldehyde sterilization, is by using low-temperature steam (provided under vacuum, and as typically used for EO-based processes; see earlier in this chapter). There are limited types of sterilizers that use much higher temperatures (132°C/270°F) in combination with lower concentrations of formaldehyde, but note that these are high-temperature processes.
- High humidity levels: required for optimal formaldehyde sterilization. The required humidity levels are often cited at greater than 70% and up to 100%, but in most modern formaldehyde sterilizers 100% humidity at the required temperature is specified as the optimal for sterilization, in particular to allow liquid formaldehyde to condensate onto surfaces to ensure its antimicrobial effects.
- Contact time: specified by the manufacturer to meet at least the minimal requirements for sterilization, such as an SAL of 10^{-6}. Typical sterilization times depend on the process conditions, with shorter exposure times generally specified for higher-temperature cycles (such as 65°C/149°F for 30 minutes and 80°C/176°F for 10 minutes).

There are essentially two types of formaldehyde-based sterilization processes: those based on LTSF sterilization and alternative high-temperature formaldehyde/alcohol sterilization processes. LTSF processes have been well described but are not widely used, with the exception of certain countries in Europe, Asia, the Middle East, and South America. These are commonly larger types of sterilizers, often designed to provide low (formaldehyde gas) and high (steam) sterilization cycles within the same chamber design. LTSF sterilizers are used for lower-temperature sterilization of a variety of devices, including flexible/rigid endoscopes (and accessories), plastic materials (e.g. diathermy or other types of electrical cables), and other heat-sensitive materials/devices. High-temperature formaldehyde/alcohol chemical processes are even less used, perhaps in small table-top sterilizers for dental and medical clinics. A typical representation of such a process is shown in Figure 11.26.

A typical LTSF process will have three main stages:
- Conditioning: programmed to achieve air removal, heating, humidification, and formaldehyde gas distribution in the load as a requirement for sterilization. The load is first pre-treated by a series of low-pressure (vacuum) pulses, followed by the introduction of steam. This is to ensure air removal and steam penetration (for humidification and heating). Following these pre-treatment pulses, a similar series of vacuum pulses with the introduction of formaldehyde gas and steam is conducted to ensure that the formaldehyde gas/humidity requirements are obtained within the load. The gas is generally made from a liquid formaldehyde solution (e.g. ranging from 2% to 40% in water) that is heated and introduced into a chamber with steam to a pre-specified pressure setting. The number of formaldehyde pulse injections will depend on the specific cycle (e.g. up to 10 pulses).
- Sterilization: formaldehyde is a relatively stable molecule and is held as the pre-conditioned conditions for the length of the sterilization cycle (which can range from 10 to 60 minutes, or even longer). During this time the formaldehyde concentration, temperature, pressure, and humidity are considered to be constant, where the temperature can be maintained by a heating mechanism from the walls of the sterilizer chamber (as used with a jacketed chamber, similar to that described earlier for steam sterilization). Formaldehyde sterilization is generally conducted under low pressure, which will also prevent formaldehyde from leaking from the chamber.
- Aeration (also known as "desorption" or post-treatment conditioning): during this stage the load is treated to remove formaldehyde (or other associated) residues. This can be achieved by a series of vacuum pulses within the chamber

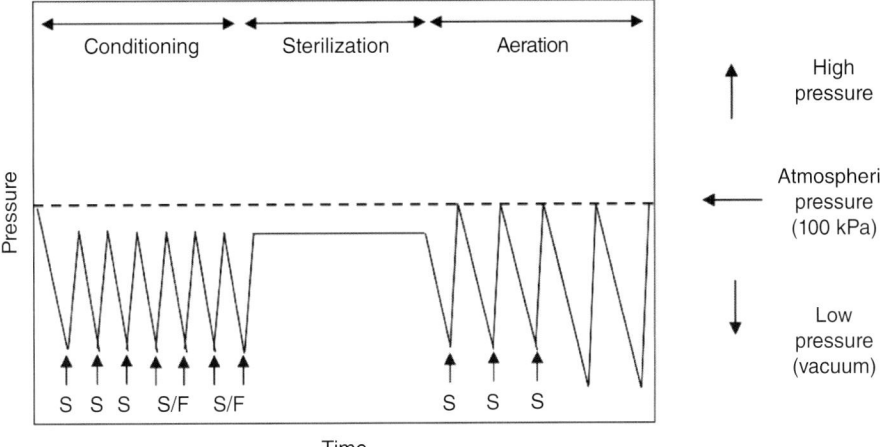

Figure 11.26 A typical low-temperature steam formaldehyde (LTSF) sterilization process. The cycle can be described under three phases: conditioning, sterilization, and aeration. The introduction of steam is indicated by S and steam/formaldehyde by S/F. Multiple steam, steam formaldehyde, and air introduction pulses can be specified by the manufacturer depending on the sterilization process.

followed by the introduction of steam as a flushing mechanism and/or by similarly pulling a vacuum and pulsing with air. The example in Figure 11.26 shows a series of vacuum/steam pulses followed by a series of lower (deeper) vacuum and air pulses. Such aeration cycles are developed to be efficient for the specified applications, although in the case of some types of materials/loads extended aeration of the load may be required prior to transport and direct patient use. The formaldehyde gas residues from the chamber are commonly removed from the air by condensation (cooling) and are diluted/flushed to the drain with water. Formaldehyde is considered biodegradable over a couple of hours in the environment. Following the process, the load may also need to be dried and may be assisted within the chamber by a series of vacuum pulses under controlled temperature or performed in a separate drying cabinet.

The other type of formaldehyde sterilizers described in certain countries are high-temperature chemical sterilizers combining heat (at 132°C/270°F), formaldehyde (at low concentrations, ~0.25%), and ethanol (72%). In these processes, the formaldehyde/ethanol liquid is heated to 132°C/270°F under pressure (138 kPa) to cause it to vaporize, be held in the presence of the load for the required exposure time, and then aerated to remove the chemical residues. In more modern and safer sterilizer designs, during aeration the air is passed through specific types of filter to remove any associated harmful chemicals/residuals.

Formaldehyde is known to be toxic, irritating, and an allergenic chemical; it is also referenced as a suspected carcinogen, but this is debated as it is also a naturally occurring molecule in the body. Like many chemicals, it may be naturally occurring from various sources at low concentrations but hazardous at higher or more persistent concentrations. Considering toxicity risks, tight controls are recommended regarding the safe use of formaldehyde. For example, the recommended full-day (eight-hour) working limit is 0.5 ppm (also known as the maximum allowable concentration, MAC), with a maximum limit of 1.1 ppm over 15 minutes (noting that 1 ppm is ~1.2 mg/cm^3 of formaldehyde in air). Formaldehyde has a pungent odor that can be detected by smell at ~0.05 ppm, with nose and eye irritation being sensed at 0.01–1.2 ppm (depending on the person). A variety of different types of sensors, hand held and wall mounted, can be used for the routine or contact monitoring of formaldehyde gas in a given area (Figure 11.27). These can be designed to be specific to formaldehyde or may be used to detect multiple types of gases.

Typical sterilizer design

Formaldehyde gas-based sterilizers can be provided in a variety of sizes, but in most cases bench-top sterilizers are used in limited applications for high-temperature formaldehyde/alcohol-based processes and larger-capacity sterilizers for LTSF systems (Figure 11.28).

The essential designs of formaldehyde sterilizers are similar to those described for EO-based processes (described earlier in this chapter) and are summarized in Figure 11.29. The chamber is usually constructed of stainless steel and, depending on the process, may be designed to withstand high pressure (i.e. a pressure vessel, like that described for steam sterilizers). Although this may not be required for low-temperature formaldehyde gas sterilization, many designs are provided as dual-process sterilizers being used for both high-temperature (steam) and low-temperature (formaldehyde gas) sterilizers. In such cases, a rapid cooling and/or heating

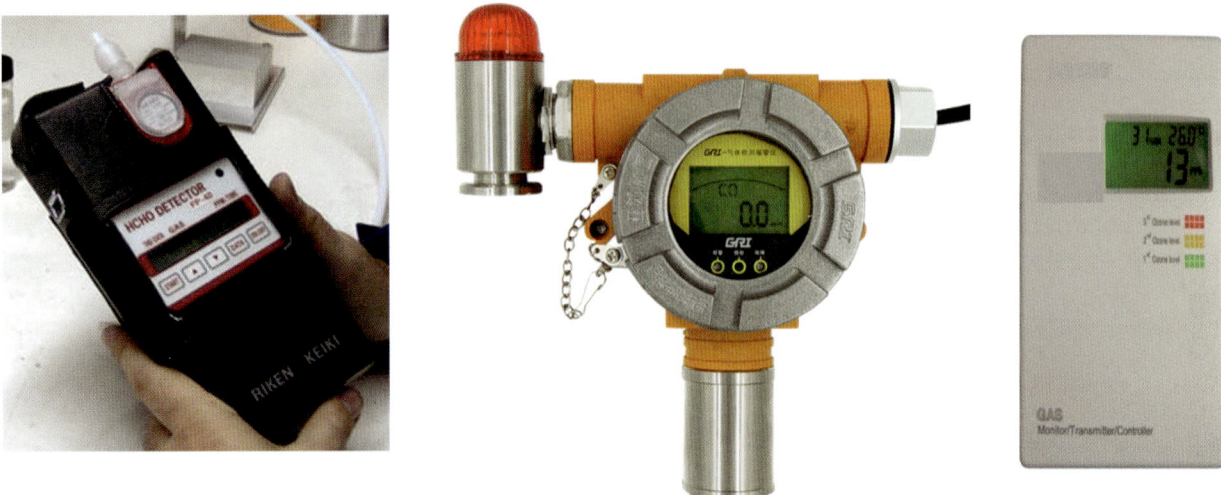

Figure 11.27 Various types of formaldehyde gas sensors.

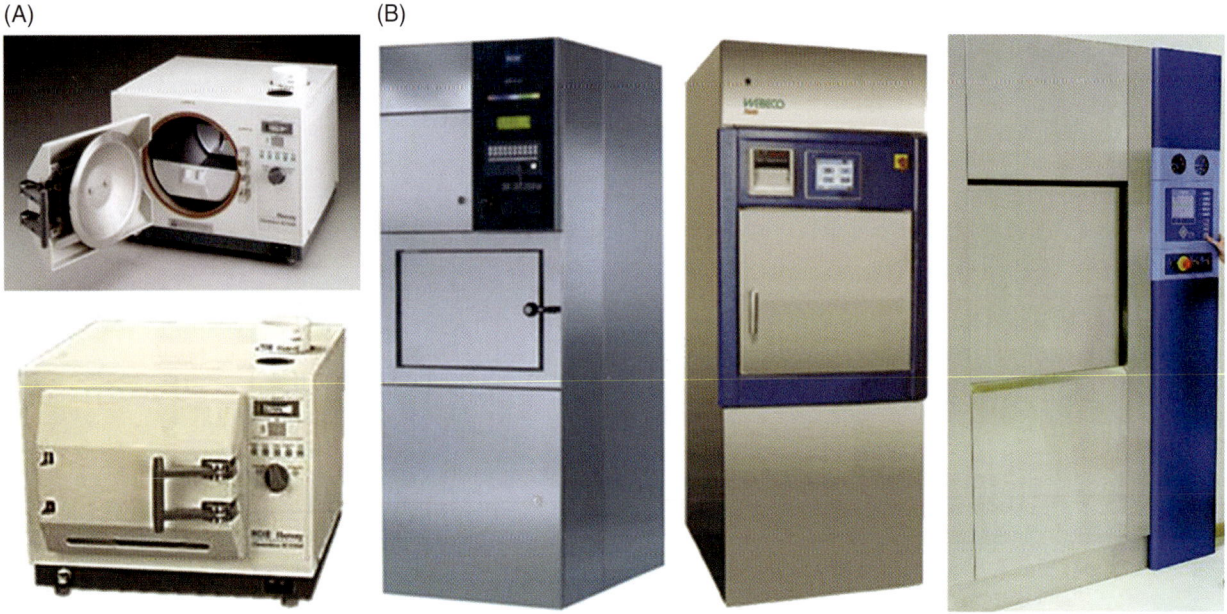

Figure 11.28 Examples of formaldehyde-based sterilization processes. (A) Bench-top sterilizers for high-temperature formaldehyde/alcohol processes; (B) larger LTSF sterilizers.

system may also be provided with or programmed into the sterilizer design to allow for alternate high- or low-temperature processes to be chosen without the need for extended pre-cooling or heating prior to placing a load into the sterilizer. Note: a cold chamber can cause excessive condensation to occur within a load during a high-temperature steam sterilization process and initial high temperatures within the chamber could cause some damage to certain types of loads designated for low-temperature sterilization. For high-temperature formaldehyde/alcohol sterilizers, these are required to be pressure vessels as the process is dependent on providing steam under pressure.

Steam, for humidification and load heating, is provided to the chamber either from an external source (house steam supply or separate local boiler) or through an integrated electrically heated steam generator within the design of the sterilizer

Figure 11.29 The basic design of a low-temperature steam formaldehyde (LTSF) sterilizer. A chamber jacket may or may not be present, the sterilizer chamber may be a single- or double-door design, and the formaldehyde supply may be mixed with other chemicals used as part of the process.

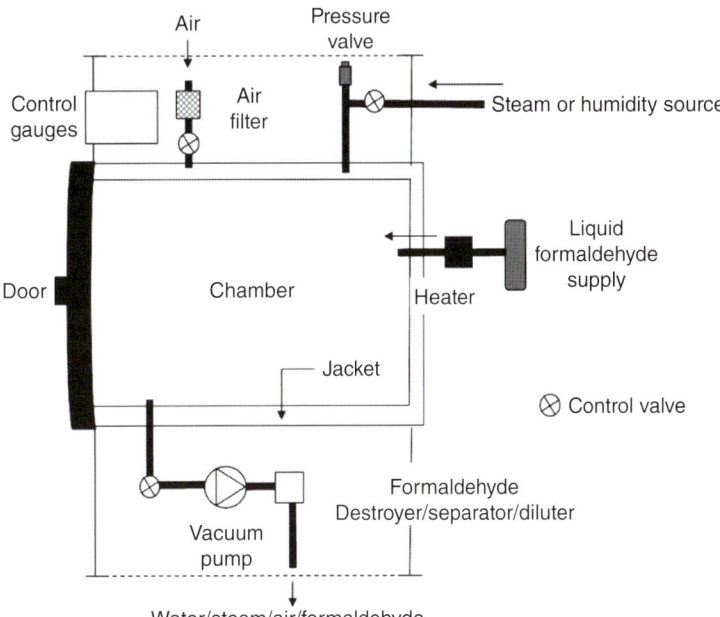

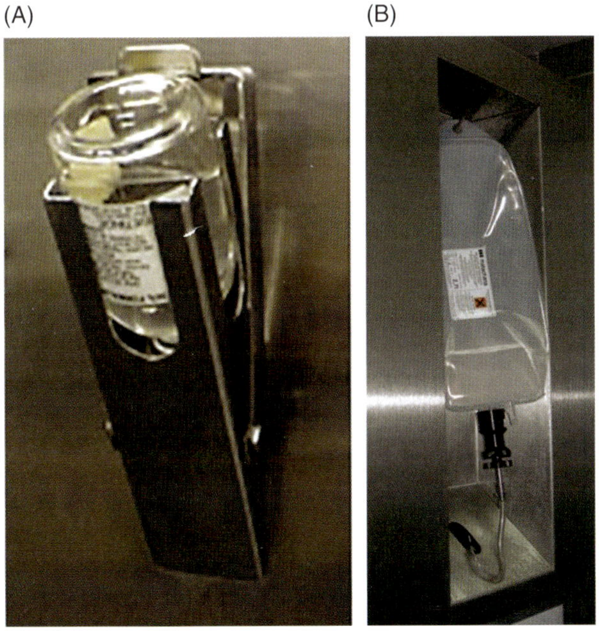

Figure 11.30 Examples of liquid formaldehyde solution delivery systems. (A) A formaldehyde solution containing a multiple-dose glass bottle and (B) a plastic bag.

itself. Formaldehyde-containing solutions are provided in single- or multiple-dose containers, being supplied to a heater to generate formaldehyde gas at the required stages of the programmed sterilization cycles (Figure 11.30).

Sterilizer designs will include an air vent, where air entering the chamber will pass through a HEPA filter to prevent the ingress of bacteria and other microorganisms during the process. The associated pipework will also include a vacuum pump, to be able to provide the necessary low-pressure requirement within the chamber for any applicable cycle stage (in both high- or low-temperature applications). Formaldehyde residues removed from the chamber are often simply diluted in water and flushed to drain; formaldehyde is generally considered unstable in the environment, being degraded over a number of hours into products such as water (H_2O) and carbon dioxide (CO_2). Alternative systems may include formaldehyde destroyers that degrade any formaldehyde residuals prior to release into the environment. The full sterilizer processes/cycles will be microprocessor controlled and may be associated with various process gauges, recorders, and/or cycle printers.

Standards and guidelines
Some examples of guidelines and standards regarding formaldehyde sterilization are given in Table 11.12.

Hydrogen peroxide gas (including plasma processes)
Hydrogen peroxide (H_2O_2) is a liquid at ambient temperature and atmospheric pressure. It is commonly used as a bleaching agent (e.g. for paper and hair), as a propellant, and industrially for the manufacturing of other chemicals. Its antimicrobial properties have been recognized for many years, and it was first used as an antiseptic and then as a disinfectant and sterilant. It is naturally produced in the body at low concentrations. For many

Table 11.12 Examples of guidelines and standards for formaldehyde sterilization processes.

Guidelines/standards	Title	Description
ISO 25424: 2018 (AMD 1: 2022)	Sterilization of medical devices – Low temperature steam and formaldehyde – Requirements for development, validation, and routine control of a sterilization process for medical devices	Specifies requirements for the development, validation, and routine control of a low-temperature steam and formaldehyde (LTSF) sterilization process for devices
ISO 11138-5: 2017	Sterilization of health care products – Biological indicators. Part 5: Biological indicators for low-temperature steam and formaldehyde sterilization processes	Specific requirements for test organisms, suspensions, inoculated carriers, biological indicators, and test methods intended for use in assessing the performance of sterilization processes employing LTSF as the sterilizing agent
EN 15424: 2007	Sterilization of medical devices – Low temperature steam and formaldehyde. Requirements for development, validation, and routine control of a sterilization process for medical devices	Requirements that will enable the demonstration that an LTSF sterilization process has appropriate microbicidal activity
EN14180: 2014	Sterilizers for medical purposes – Low temperature steam and formaldehyde sterilizers. Requirements and testing	Requirements for the design and performance of formaldehyde sterilizers
ISO 14937: 2009	Sterilization of health care products. General requirements for characterization of a sterilizing agent and the development, validation, and routine control of a sterilization process for medical devices	Specifies general requirements for the characterization of any sterilizing agent and for the development, validation, and routine monitoring and control of a sterilization process for devices
ANSI/AAMI ST58: 2013 (R2018)	Chemical sterilization and high-level disinfection in health care facilities	Guidelines for the selection and use of chemical sterilizing agents and high-level disinfectants that have been cleared for marketing by the US Food and Drug Administration for use in hospitals and other healthcare facilities, including some high-temperature formaldehyde chemical sterilization processes

applications (at lower concentrations) it is considered relatively safe for use, for example being used under certain conditions directly in the eye or on the skin (or in wounds), and is "generally regarded as safe" (GRAS) as an additive at certain concentrations for food applications in the United States. In contrast, at higher concentrations it can be dangerous.

As a disinfectant it is used in liquid (as direct solutions in water or as part of a formulated mixture with other chemicals) or in gas form (see Chapter 9, peroxygens) for device or general surface disinfection applications. For clinical sterilization applications it is predominantly used in gas form, referred to as vaporized (VH2O2), as the sterilizing agent. Hydrogen peroxide gas (or vapor) is generated by heating liquid peroxide; the temperature required will vary depending on the concentration of peroxide in the water, with examples being under atmospheric pressure at 108°C/226°F with 35% peroxide and 114°C/237°F with a 50% peroxide solution. In accordance with the gas laws (see Chapter 6), this can also be achieved at low temperatures under vacuum (low-pressure) conditions. In associated sterilization processes, the generation of the gas from a liquid source is typically achieved by flash heating (e.g. using a heated surface or other heating source) of a given volume of 35–60% liquid hydrogen peroxide. Pure samples of peroxide in water are very stable, but when generated into gas it can have a relatively short life and in particular in reaction on various surfaces, including devices, soils, and microorganisms. Note that a vapor and a gas are chemically similar, with the distinction being that a vapor is a gas that can readily revert to its liquid form (condense) under the right conditions (e.g. at a given temperature/pressure and depending on the concentration of the gas). In this sense, hydrogen peroxide and water gases are both considered vapors, while EO and formaldehyde in their own right may be considered "true" gases, as they have a preference to be in gas form under ambient temperature/atmospheric pressure. Hydrogen peroxide gas, depending on the process, may be used under condensed (over-saturated; gas and liquid present) or under-saturated (gas only) conditions for sterilization applications. The specific conditions within a given sterilization process may not always be known or described.

Hydrogen peroxide gas is a very powerful antimicrobial, being much more effective than liquid preparations at lower concentrations (e.g. 0.00001–0.001% in gas form are typically used in comparison to 2–6% or higher for liquid-based applications). This may be related to the increased reactivity of the gas form in comparison to a liquid solution in water. Depending on the concentration and contact time, peroxide gas is considered an effective antimicrobial, including demonstrating rapid bactericidal, fungicidal, cysticidal, virucidal, and sporicidal activity. In addition, the gas form (but notably not the liquid form, with the exception potentially of high-concentration >60% peroxide) has been shown to be effective under certain conditions against prions and toxins (including bacterial endotoxins; see Chapter 6 on bacteria) and to penetrate over time through organic soils (including blood). *Geobacillus stearothermophilus* spores are considered the most resistant organism to hydrogen peroxide gas and are therefore used for determining the minimal sterilization process conditions (e.g. in determining the conditions for a demonstrated minimal SAL of 10^{-6}) and for routine monitoring of the process (where BIs are used).

The mode of action of peroxide gas is due to its activity as an oxidizing agent, with effects on various molecules that make up microbial structure/function including proteins, nucleic acids, and lipids. These effects cause loss of function and structure, which culminates in death. It has been reported that the specific mechanism of action of liquid peroxide is distinct from gaseous peroxide, but the overall effects are antimicrobial.

In addition to being an effective antimicrobial, the gas can be safe for use on most device and material types, including electrical components and electronics, although this will vary depending on the process conditions (e.g. exposure time, concentration, temperature, etc.). Depending on the sterilization application/process, negative effects can include loss of color (bleaching) over time on certain types of materials (e.g. anodized aluminum), loss of antimicrobial activity on contacting certain types of materials (e.g. paper, wood, and brass/copper, by reacting with the surface to break down or neutralize the peroxide activity), and damage to some types of materials over time (particularly certain types of adhesives). Hydrogen peroxide gas has a good safety profile, but remember that exposure to peroxide under certain conditions can cause damage and is considered toxic even at concentrations as low as 1 ppm over time. Being unstable, it rapidly breaks down in the environment, which is often viewed as an environmental benefit.

Principles of hydrogen peroxide gas sterilization

Hydrogen peroxide gas sterilization is primarily dependent on the gas concentration and exposure time, but is also affected by the process temperature.

- Hydrogen peroxide has been shown to be sporicidal at as low as 0.1 mg/L gas concentrations, but typical concentrations used for sterilization processes are set at a higher range (e.g. 5–10 mg/L); however, the initial concentration of gas introduced into a chamber will degrade over time (particularly in the presence of a load for sterilization) and therefore the sterilization cycle should be developed at the lowest concentration found in the presence of a worst-case load for the manufacturer-defined process conditions. As the concentration increases, the sporicidal activity increases (the contact time for antimicrobial activity decreases), with a typical log reduction for bacterial spores (of *Geobacillus stearothermophilus*) being 10 minutes at 0.1 mg/L and 1 minute at 1 mg/L.
- Temperature can impact the activity of the gas in two ways. First, increased temperatures can improve the sporicidal activity of the gas, but can also accelerate the degradation of hydrogen peroxide over time (into water and oxygen, both ineffective as antimicrobials). Second, in accordance with the gas laws, maintaining peroxide in gas form is dependent on the temperature (therefore at lower temperatures peroxide gas will condense to revert to its preferred liquid state). In addition to temperature, condensation will be impacted by the pressure and the presence of humidity (water in gas form) in the load. But overall, hydrogen peroxide gas does not appear to have the same requirement as other antimicrobial gases, such as formaldehyde and EO, for high humidity levels to ensure sporicidal activity. Humidity is, however, always present as peroxide gas is generated from liquid peroxide solutions that contain water (e.g. at 50–60% peroxide in 50–40% water). Also, the level of water present will increase during the exposure process as peroxide degrades into water and oxygen, particularly on contact with target surfaces. It is therefore typical in sterilization processes with peroxide gas that pulses of gas are introduced and held in the sterilization chamber for a specific period of time, then removed and replaced with a fresh pulse of peroxide gas for the desired contact time and number of pulses to ensure sterilization. These variables are defined during equipment and process design, and associated validation by the manufacturer.
- The overall contact time for sterilization will depend on the conditions defined by the manufacturer in the design of the specific process. Typical exposure times for sterilization can range from 10 to 30 minutes, depending on the process with various levels of overkill (e.g. at or over an SAL of 10^{-6}). But remember that the peroxide exposure phase is only part of the overall sterilization process cycle.

Similar to other physical and chemical sterilization processes, a number of phases are defined during a hydrogen peroxide gas cycle in order to ensure that the load is prepared for sterilization, sterilized, and rendered safe for patient use (Figure 11.31). These include:

- Conditioning. This stage is designed primarily to remove air from the load, which may be simply facilitated by drawing a deep vacuum (low pressure, for example 0.053 kPa, equivalent

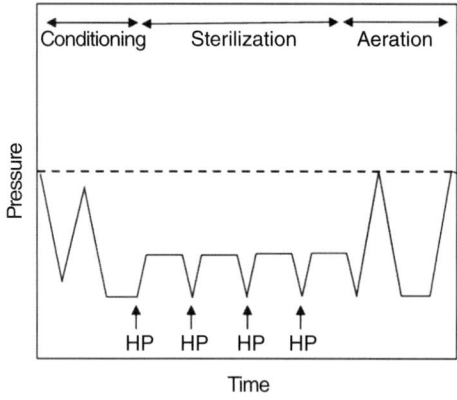
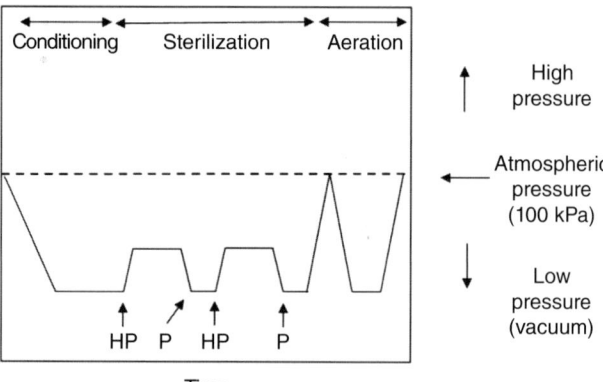

Figure 11.31 Examples of hydrogen peroxide gas (VH2O2) sterilization processes. Two examples are shown, with hydrogen peroxide gas alone (left) and peroxide gas utilizing plasma generation (right). On the left, a pulsing conditioning cycle is shown followed by a four-pulse sterilization phase with the introduction of peroxide gas, exposure, and then removal (by pulling a vacuum) in each pulse and aeration (by applying a vacuum to the load, assisted by heat). On the right is a similar cycle, with a simpler conditioning cycle, a two-pulse peroxide gas exposure (with exposure to peroxide gas, removal, and plasma generation in each pulse), followed by aeration.

to 0.0005 bar, 0.0077 psi, or 0.4 Torr). During this phase the load may also be further pre-conditioned by heating (within the chamber maintained at a given pressure) and/or drying. In general, drying at this stage should not be necessary as according to most manufacturers' instructions with these sterilization processes, loads should be pre-dried before placing them within the chamber, as excessive moisture can lead to cycle failure. Note that hydrogen peroxide gas, like other gaseous or low-temperature sterilization methods, is not used to sterilize liquids such as water. Conditioning, including air removal and drying, may be enhanced during this phase by pulsing the vacuum levels or by adding other heating methods (such as the generation of plasma during this phase, which is employed in some sterilizer designs).

- Sterilization. Hydrogen peroxide gas is generated from liquid hydrogen peroxide solutions (particularly in the 50–60%) range. Examples of different methods of liquid peroxide supply to sterilizer designs are shown in Figure 11.32. Gas is generated from liquid by vaporization, the rapid heating of liquid by applying it to a hot surface (a heating block, which can be of various designs) or a similar method, and then introduced into the chamber that is already under vacuum to allow rapid penetration of the gas. The introduction of the gas causes a rise in pressure within the chamber. The temperature at which hydrogen peroxide "boils" into a gas (boiling point) will depend on its concentration in water, e.g. 108°C/226°F with 35% peroxide and 114°C/237°F with 50% peroxide; as peroxide gas degrades at higher temperature, this can be minimized by vaporization at lower temperatures under lower pressures. Some systems will use alternative heating sources than heating blocks to generate the gas, such as the minimal use of plasma generation (see the next point) on the liquid as an energy source. In these designs to date, plasma generation is used as a heating source to generate peroxide gas rather than producing a true hydrogen peroxide gas plasma (for the difference between gases and plasmas, see Chapter 6 on solids, liquids, gases, and plasmas). As hydrogen peroxide gas degrades over time, including on contact with the load, it is generally held for a programmed exposure time, residual gas is removed by repulling a vacuum within the chamber, and then a further pulse of hydrogen peroxide gas is introduced. In some processes (known as gas plasma processes), a plasma is generated on any remaining liquid/gas within the chamber following the redrawing of a vacuum and prior to the introduction of fresh peroxide gas (Figure 11.31); the concept of plasma generation is discussed later, but it is used as a method to break down peroxide residuals. The number of pulses can typically range from two to four and exposure times can vary, but this will depend on the sterilization process and will be specified by the individual manufacturer (and for each cycle defined).

- Aeration. This phase is designed to remove any hydrogen peroxide (gas or liquid, if present as part of the process) residuals from the load. This is usually conducted in the heated chamber by pulling (and/or pulsing) a vacuum within the chamber/load; aeration may also be assisted by the generation of a plasma (which accelerates the breakdown of peroxide residuals into water and oxygen) during this phase.

Many types of hydrogen peroxide gas sterilizers are referred to as gas plasma sterilization systems. These describe the use or generation of a plasma at some stage (or stages) during the process of sterilization. As introduced in Chapter 6, there are essentially three states of matter: solids, liquids, and gases, depending on the energy provided to it. But plasmas are often considered as a separate state. In true chemical–physical

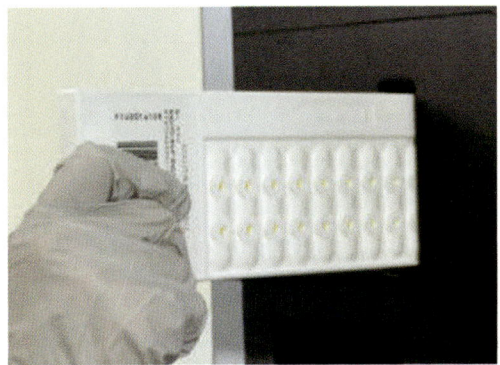
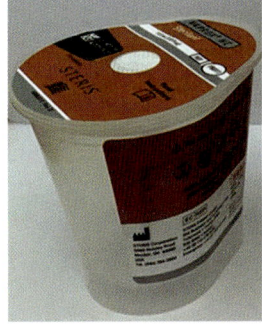
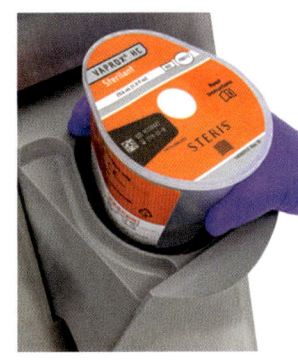
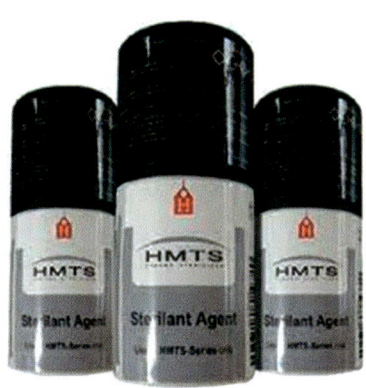

Figure 11.32 Examples of liquid hydrogen peroxide supply methods used in different types of peroxide gas sterilizers. All designs shown provide sufficient liquid hydrogen peroxide for multiple sterilization cycles in specific sterilizer designs. In the upper center is a supply cartridge system and in the lower center when it is placed into the sterilizer delivery system.

terms, a plasma is essentially a gas that has been further energized (or "ionized"). A plasma is therefore considered the fourth state of matter, being generated when sufficient energy is provided to a gas (e.g. hydrogen peroxide or indeed any gas) to break the gas molecules into its basic chemical parts. In the case of hydrogen peroxide (H_2O_2), this will essentially be hydrogen (H) and oxygen (O) in various reactive and unstable forms such as •OH (the "hydroxyl radical"; note the position of the •), OH^-, O_2^-, and H^+. This creates a very reactive mixture of chemicals/species, as well as releasing energy (in the form of light, such as UV light) that can all contribute to a potent antimicrobial effect. When the energy source is then turned off, the molecules will recombine to include various stable species, particularly water (H_2O) and oxygen (O_2). For these reasons, plasmas have been the focus of much research into their application as antimicrobial processes. Despite this, to date plasmas alone have not been used for their antimicrobial effects in standardized, routine sterilization processes. They are further discussed later in this chapter as new developments in low-temperature sterilization.

The use of plasmas in hydrogen peroxide gas sterilization processes is the subject of much debate. In these systems the primary antimicrobial effects appear to be due to hydrogen peroxide gas alone. Although the generation of plasma during the cycle may have a role as an antimicrobial, to date these effects have been shown to be minimal in the types of systems designed. Plasma generation does, however, play an important role as part of these processes. For example, the most widely used hydrogen peroxide gas plasma systems are the STERRAD® systems (Figure 11.33). Depending on the specific design and processes provided, plasma is used as a heating source (e.g. during conditioning) and primarily as a method of degrading residual peroxide (into water and oxygen) that remains following exposure to hydrogen peroxide gas. An example of such a process is shown in Figure 11.31, where following the introduction and exposure to hydrogen peroxide, the majority of the gas is removed by pulling a vacuum in the chamber and only then is the plasma generated; in such process conditions the plasma has been shown to have little antimicrobial effect as part of cycle but is an effective way of removing toxic residuals. Non-plasma systems use other methods for ensuring that such residuals are safely removed as part of the sterilization process.

Since the initial development of plasma systems, particularly in recent years, a range of alternative hydrogen peroxide gas plasma systems have been developed. These may use plasma in a similar manner to that discussed previously, but also as a method of generating peroxide gas from a liquid source (at lower energy levels), as a heating mechanism, as a

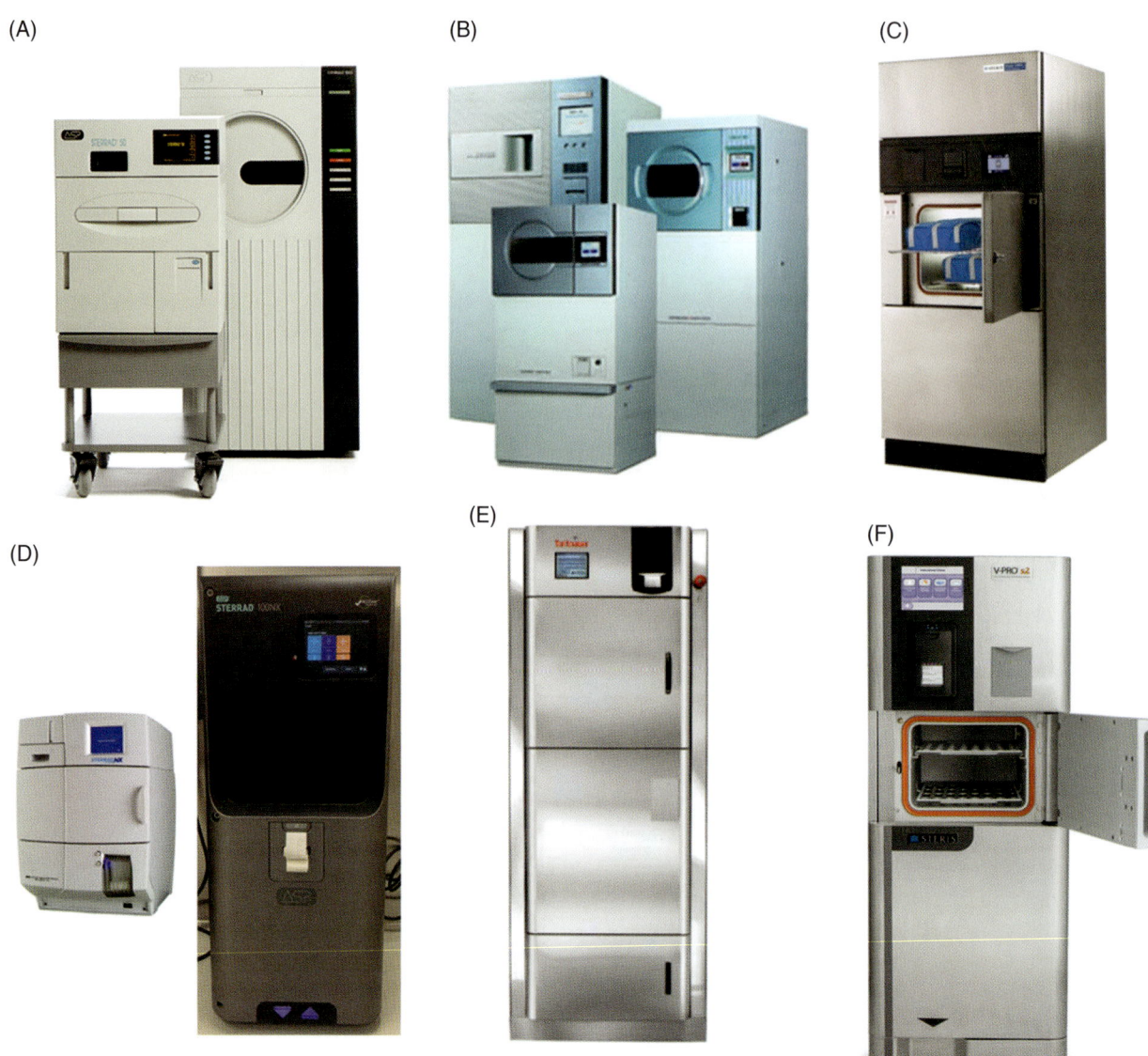

Figure 11.33 (A–F) Examples of hydrogen peroxide gas (VH2O2) sterilizers. They can be considered as using plasma or not as part of their sterilization processes. On the far left are examples of the STERRAD® series of plasma sterilizers (with older-type systems shown above and newer NX™-based processes below), various other designs of plasma sterilizers (center), and an example of a peroxide gas-only system (the V-PRO series that does not use plasma). Source: (A–C) with permission of ASP; (E) Courtesy STERIS Corporation 2024. All rights reserved.

drying method (to remove water from the load prior to exposure), and/or for enhancing aeration. In all cases, the sterilizer manufacturer should provide details regarding the specific sterilization cycle conditions/processes used.

An interesting topic regarding the development of hydrogen peroxide (or indeed other degrading biocide-based) gas processes is the ability to ensure that the gas can adequately penetrate the load and individual devices. As already described, the conditioning phase of such processes should be designed to ensure the adequate removal of air from the load/chamber prior to exposure. This can be a challenge in many situations, similar to the use of other gases for sterilization (including steam in some cases). For example, liquids such as water cannot be sterilized using hydrogen peroxide gas; this is particularly important when significant water residuals remain on a surface and can hinder the penetration of the gas into the surface. In many sterilizer designs the presence of water can be indirectly detected by the process conditions being controlled by the sterilizer (in particular the ability to draw low pressures/vacuum within the chamber); in such designs this can cause the cycle to abort or be extended to ensure that drying has occurred prior to sterilization. Another issue is to avoid the use of certain materials that could significantly absorb and/or break down the peroxide, with an example being paper or other cellulose-based materials. These can be used as packaging materials for steam sterilization, but when a significant amount of this material is present in a peroxide gas sterilizer it acts like a sponge to rapidly reduce the available gas concentration required for activity. Therefore, such materials should not be used, and alternative types of packaging material should be recommended by the sterilizer manufacturer. CIs specific to the sterilization process should be used to ensure that the correct concentration of peroxide is present in the load.

A final consideration is the penetration of gas through the lumen of a device such as rigid and flexible endoscopes (see Chapter 4). Lumened devices provide a challenge to all types of sterilization processes, due to the residual air that can remain within the lumen impeding the penetration of the gas. In all hydrogen peroxide sterilizer designs, the lumen penetration limitations are generally defined by the manufacturer based on their validation requirements. These are traditionally based on the diameter and length of the device lumen, but will also depend on the number of lumens and type of material the lumen is made from (e.g. plastic or stainless steel). Stainless steel lumens are a much greater challenge to sterilize in comparison to different types of plastics. Penetration claims should be inspected carefully and may be regularly updated or changed based on the manufacturer and/or local regulatory approval. Sterilizer, sterilization process, and accessory designs can be used to improve lumen penetration, such as pressure/vacuum pulsing mechanisms, number and process type of hydrogen peroxide exposure pulses, longer peroxide exposure conditions, and increased peroxide concentrations. As an example, the STERRAD NX process provides a different sterilization process to the older STERRAD series, in that the hydrogen peroxide gas concentrations are concentrated in the NX design and then exposed to the load. This is achieved by forming hydrogen peroxide gas from the liquid supply, removing the water (by a selective condensation process), and applying the concentrated gas to the load. Under these conditions it is shown that lumen penetration is improved, as defined by the manufacturer. Note that in many hydrogen peroxide sterilizer designs different sterilization processes are provided for various types of loads, including non-lumened devices, stainless steel–containing or rigid lumened devices, and flexible endoscopic devices, therefore care should be taken to ensure that staff are correctly trained on which cycle is correct for different types of loads. Overall, given the range of sterilizers and associated sterilization processes available, close attention should be paid to the manufacturer's instructions, particularly limitations on device/packaging materials and claims of sterilization with lumened and other devices.

Similar to all sterilant gases, hydrogen peroxide is considered to be toxic. It can be noxious at low concentrations (e.g. 5–10 ppm gas concentration) and a recommended safety level within an area is typically defined at 1 ppm over a typical eight-hour working day; a recommended short-term exposure limit is also defined at no more than 75 ppm for 15 minutes. Note: typical sporicidal concentrations of hydrogen peroxide gas are in excess of 75 ppm and for sterilization processes are generally greater than 1000 ppm. Hand-held and wall-mounted sensors are available for monitoring such low-level safety concentrations within a given area, and can include alarm systems that trigger a warning when excessive levels of peroxide gas are detected. Hydrogen peroxide gas is short-lived, rapidly degrading in the environment to water and oxygen; it is therefore considered safer for use as a sterilization agent than alternative EO or formaldehyde processes. Liquid hydrogen peroxide can also present a safety risk, particularly at the concentrations present in containers used in sterilization processes (Figure 11.32). Remember, at low liquid concentrations (e.g. 3%) peroxide can be safely used on the skin and hair, but at higher concentrations (such as in the 30–60% range) it can burn the skin, and at even higher concentration (e.g. >80%) is used as a rocket propellant! As with all chemicals, it should be handled with care. Liquid peroxide delivery systems can be designed to ensure that there is minimal risk of exposure, to include being tamper-proof and being empty following use in a sterilizer. Some sterilizer designs can also provide a mechanism for the safe disposal of expired peroxide containers/delivery systems prior to placing them in normal waste; others may require special handling and chemical disposal precautions. In addition, if any suspicious liquid is detected in the chamber or on a load following a sterilization cycle, it should always be suspected as being hydrogen peroxide and may be present at relatively high concentrations. In such cases the load should not be used, only handled with gloves and the sterilizer investigated to ensure that it is operating correctly.

Typical sterilizer design

Hydrogen peroxide gas-based sterilizers can be considered as two design types: those that use and those that do not use plasma as part of their design (Figure 11.33). Although these sterilizers can provide a variety of different and unique sterilization processes (Figure 11.31), their basic designs are very similar (Figure 11.34).

The chamber is typically made of aluminum, but other types of metals/materials can be used, and it is designed to be able to withstand and maintain vacuum conditions. Single- or double-door versions are available, which can be manual or automated for opening/closing. A chamber jacket may be

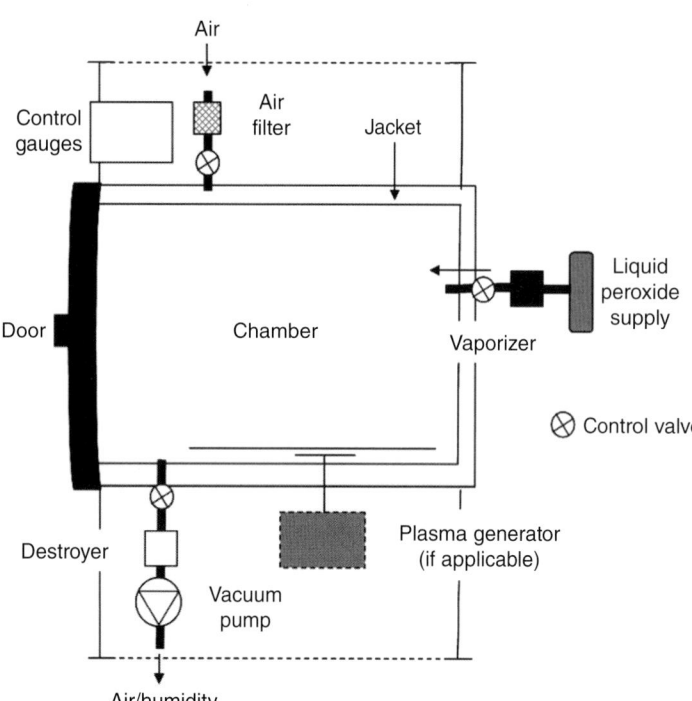

Figure 11.34 Typical basic design of a hydrogen peroxide gas sterilizer. A plasma source is only used in those designs that utilize plasma as part of the sterilization process and can include the generation of the plasma within and/or remote to the chamber. A vaporizer or other heating mechanism can be used to generate the gas at the appropriate stages of the programmed cycle.

present to optimize heating within the chamber. In gas plasma sterilizer designs, the plasma sources may be located within the chamber (along the walls), built into the chamber walls, and/or, depending on their use during a particular process, at a remote location from the chamber (e.g. as a method of vaporization or in destroyer designs). Depending on the specific design, when plasma is generated within the chamber it is recommended that the load (and particularly metal objects) is not allowed to touch the walls of the chamber/door due to the risks of arcing (sparking) during the cycle. A hydrogen peroxide gas generation system is included, providing the gas during the required stages of the cycle. This will include a system of peroxide liquid delivery, vaporization (at a specific temperature and pressure), and injection into the chamber. In addition, the chamber is connected to a vacuum pump for removal of air and/or peroxide gas; it is typical for the gas to be broken down (e.g. by passing through a catalytic converter) prior to being released into the immediate environment. Air can be introduced into the chamber, such as to relieve the vacuum stages of the process, passing through a HEPA filter to prevent contamination. The complete system is under microprocessor control, including different types of sensors for process control (such as temperature, pressure, and volume sensors).

Standards and guidelines

Table 11.13 provides a list of standards and guidelines associated with the use of hydrogen peroxide gas sterilizers.

Liquid peracetic acid

Peracetic acid (PAA, CH_3COOOH, also known as peroxyacetic acid) is a liquid at atmospheric pressure and ambient temperature. It is widely used industrially for the manufacturing of other chemicals/materials and is particularly used for disinfection and/or sterilization of surfaces in a liquid form. Gaseous peracetic acid–based sterilization has been developed (e.g. PAA plasma sterilization processes) and is used for industrial sterilization, but not currently for reusable device applications. PAA is supplied in liquid form (5–37% PAA in water) and is always found in the presence of its breakdown products (referred to chemically as being in equilibrium with) water, hydrogen peroxide, and acetic acid (Figure 11.35). For example, 35% PAA will contain 40% acetic acid, 18% water, and 7% hydrogen peroxide, with the concentrations of water and acetic acid increasing as the PAA degrades. The acetic acid component gives these preparations a strong "vinegar" odor (note: household vinegar contains 4–8% acetic acid), which can be quite noxious at high concentrations.

As an alternative to these commercial solutions, PAA can be generated by combining other chemicals in water such as sodium perborate or sodium percarbonate with acetylsalicylic acid, or tetraacetylethylenediamine (TAED) with hydrogen peroxide. When PAA is supplied on its own in solutions, they have a very low, acidic pH (e.g. pH 2.5), and under such conditions are considered very corrosive. For this reason, PAA is not used on its own but as part of a formulation (mixture of

Table 11.13 Standards and guidelines applicable to hydrogen peroxide gas sterilizers. Some standards remain under development at the time of writing.

Guidelines/standards	Title	Description
ISO 14937: 2009	Sterilization of health care products. General requirements for characterization of a sterilizing agent and the development, validation, and routine control of a sterilization process for medical devices	Specifies general requirements for the characterization of any sterilizing agent and for the development, validation, and routine monitoring and control of any sterilization process for devices
ISO 22441: 2022	Sterilization of health care products – Low temperature vaporized hydrogen peroxide. Requirements for the development, validation, and routine control of a sterilization process for medical devices	Provides requirements for the development, validation, and routine monitoring and control of low-temperature sterilization processes using vaporized hydrogen peroxide (VH2O2) as the sterilizing agent
ISO 11138-6 (in development)	Sterilization of health care products – Biological indicators. Part 6: Biological indicators for hydrogen peroxide vapour sterilization processes	Specific requirements for test organisms, suspensions, inoculated carriers, biological indicators, and test methods intended for use in assessing the performance of sterilizers and sterilization processes employing hydrogen peroxide vapor as the sterilizing agent
ISO 15882: 2009	Sterilization of health care products – Chemical indicators. Guidance for selection, use and interpretation of results	Provides guidance for the selection, use, and interpretation of results of chemical indicators used in process definition, validation, routine monitoring and overall control of sterilization processes
ANSI/AAMI ST58: 2013	Chemical sterilization and high-level disinfection in health care facilities	Guidelines for the selection and use of liquid chemical sterilants/high-level disinfectants and gaseous chemical sterilizers that have been cleared for marketing by the US Food and Drug Administration for use in hospitals and other healthcare facilities
AS5369: 2023	Reprocessing of reusable medical devices in health and non-health related facilities	Guidance on processing, including low-temperature sterilization in Australia
CSA Z314: 23	Canadian medical device reprocessing in all health care settings	Canadian standard of device processing including requirements for low-temperature sterilization
CDC/HICPAC: 2008	Guideline for disinfection and sterilization in healthcare facilities	General recommendations on methods for cleaning, disinfection, and sterilization of patient-care medical devices in the United States
GB YY/T 1266-2015	Evaluation of materials for medical devices suitable for hydrogen peroxide sterilization	Chinese national standard on the evaluation of device materials and their suitability for hydrogen peroxide sterilization
HTM 01-01, Part E	Management and decontamination of surgical instruments (medical devices) used in acute care: Part E: Alternatives to steam for the sterilization of reusable medical devices	The UK HTMs are published in five parts, with Part E dedicated to low-temperature (non-steam) sterilization processes, including the design, testing, and use of VH2O2 sterilizers
WHO: 2016	Decontamination and reprocessing of medical devices for health-care facilities	Guidance on processing, to include hydrogen peroxide gas (and gas plasma) sterilization

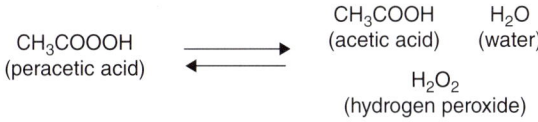

Figure 11.35 Typical components of a peracetic acid–based solution shown in equilibrium.

chemicals) for disinfection and sterilization applications (see Chapter 6 on mixtures, formulations, and solutions). The formulation effects can be designed to optimize the antimicrobial activity of PAA and minimize any negative effects, such as potential damage to surfaces; as an example, PAA-based disinfectants/sterilants generally have a pH within the 5–8 range. Therefore, these can range considerably in antimicrobial efficacy, safety, device compatibility, and practical application. They are widely used for high-level disinfection applications (as alternatives to traditional aldehyde-based disinfectants such as glutaraldehyde; see Chapter 9), but some PAA-based processes have been designed for liquid chemical sterilization applications. These are further considered in this section.

PAA is an oxidizing agent and has been shown to affect the structure/function of various molecules, including protein, lipids, and nucleic acids, which are essential to microbiological structure and function; these effects culminate to cause cellular death or loss of viral infectivity. PAA is considered an effective biocide with known broad-spectrum activity. PAA formulations are considered particularly effective, depending on the formulation and PAA concentration present, even in the presence of organic/inorganic soil that can interfere with the activity of other liquid/gas-based processes. But this does not mean that reliable antimicrobial activity can be achieved in the presence of soil.

PAA liquid sterilization processes can be very rapid (less than 30 minutes) and safe for use on water-immersible instrumentation, but do not allow for sterile storage of the devices following sterilization (as they use a liquid-based process). For this reason, they are often referred to as "just-in-time" processes, where the device is immediately used for the medical/surgical procedure following sterilization. In some system designs this can allow for immediate aseptic presentation but not storage of the device prior to use.

Principles of liquid peracetic acid sterilization

Although PAA is widely used as a disinfectant/sterilant, only a limited number of processes have been developed to date that provide sterilization claims (for example, in compliance with ISO 14937 and/or local regulatory approvals). Liquid chemical sterilization with PAA-containing formulations is dependent on the PAA concentration, formulation (including variables such as pH), temperature, and contact time.

- PAA concentration. Typical PAA concentrations range from 800 to 3000 mg/L. At such concentrations PAA can be shown to provide an SAL of 10^{-6}, depending on its formulation and exposure temperature. The most resistant organism to PAA has been shown to be *Geobacillus stearothermophilus* spores, which are therefore used to design and test such sterilization processes. Higher concentrations are known to be more effective than at lower concentrations, but lower concentrations can be enhanced by increasing the exposure temperature. PAA has the potential to degrade over time, with the rate of degradation depending on the water quality, presence of soil, temperature, and formulation. This should be considered in the development of any associated sterilization process, to ensure that the minimal SAL is achieved under worst-case test conditions (such as the lowest PAA concentration present during the exposure cycle).

- Formulation. This refers to the combination of ingredients, including active (antimicrobial) and inert ingredients, into a product for its intended use. PAA-based formulations will include ingredients such as buffers (for pH control), anti-corrosives (to reduce the potential of damage to surfaces), chelating agents (to aid in control chemical contaminants in water), and surfactants (e.g. to aid in penetration and even cleaning, depending on the formulation). In some formulations PAA can be used to enhance cleaning from a surface, but this may not always be the case and any claims should be supported with experimental evidence with that specific product.
- Temperature. This plays an important role in enhancing the activity of PAA. PAA-based processes can typically range from room temperature (20–25°C/68–77°F) to 50–60°C/122–140°F, where the higher the temperature the greater the antimicrobial activity. For example, at about 1000 mg/L PAA the typical time to kill one log of *G. stearothermophilus* spores (the D-value) at 30°C/86°F can be about 5 minutes (depending on the formulation), while at 50°C/122°F it is about 1 second. Therefore, at 50–55°C/122–131°F an SAL of 10^{-6} can be theoretically provided in less than 12 seconds.
- Exposure time for sterilization. This will depend on the SAL requirements, the PAA concentration, formulation, and temperature. It is typical for a significant level of overkill (greater exposure time under these defined conditions) to be provided in excess of the SAL (as seen in other sterilization processes). Typical sterilization processes will operate at ~2000 mg/L PAA, 50–56°C/122–133°F for 12 minutes, and ~2000 mg/L PAA, 46–55°C/115–131°F for 6 minutes.

A typical PAA sterilization process will consist of three phases: sterilant preparation, sterilization, and rinsing. In the sterilization processes designed to date, the PAA formulation is delivered in a single-dosed cup design (as shown in Figure 11.36). Each cup is designed with two compartments, an upper area containing liquid PAA (typically at 35%) and a lower dry solid–containing compartment with the other ingredients of the formulation. These cups are usually provided with a limited shelf life (e.g. six to nine months). The formulation cup is placed into the sterilizer and on initiation of the process the sterilant is prepared by mixing both compartments with water and heated to the desired sterilization temperature. The sterilant is then flowed through and over the load to be sterilized for the required sterilization time and within the defined temperature range. The external parts of the device(s) are sterilized by immersion in the sterilant, but special consideration is required for any lumened device. These are sterilized by flowing the sterilant solution through the respective lumens, for which purpose specific connectors are provided to allow the device lumens to be connected to the sterilant pumping systems within the process design (examples are shown in Figure 11.37). Such connectors are designed for use with defined individual and/or series of endoscopes; they should be

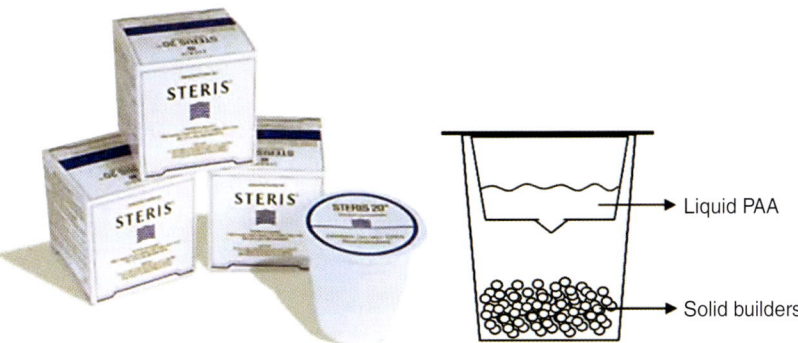

Figure 11.36 An example of a peracetic acid (PAA) sterilant formulation delivery system. The examples shown are known as STERIS 20™ and S40™. The single-use cup design (on the left) consists of two compartments (shown on the right, as a cup-within-a-cup design), consisting of an upper liquid PAA compartment and a lower area containing the dry components of the formulation. The cup components are mixed with water during the sterilization process to provide the final sterilant. Courtesy STERIS Corporation 2024. All rights reserved.

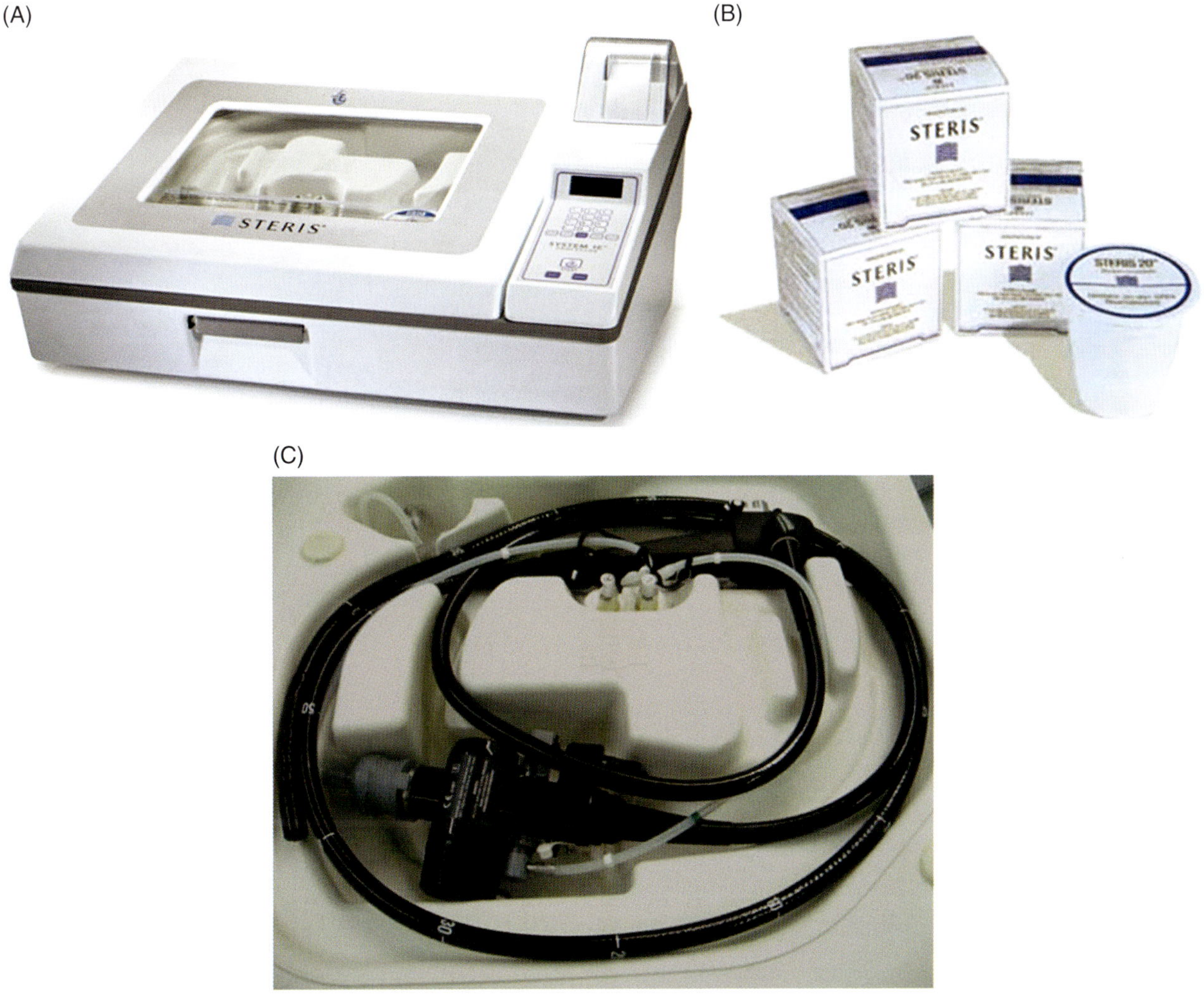

Figure 11.37 An example of a peracetic acid (PAA) sterilization process, including (A) the sterilizer, (B) PAA formulation source, and (C) other accessories. The accessories include support trays and device connectors that are required to allow the device internal lumens to be connected to the flow system in the sterilizer (an example of a connected device is shown). Source: (A, B) Courtesy STERIS Corporation 2024. All rights reserved.

designed to ensure that the correct flow is achieved through the lumen(s), as well as around the connection points to the endoscope to provide sterilization for the complete device.

Following the sterilant exposure, the devices are rinsed with the appropriate (sterile) quality of water (e.g. sterile filtered water and/or water that has been otherwise treated, such as with UV light) and for the process-defined number of rinse cycles (typically 2–4 rinses, depending on the process). To date, two such PAA sterilization processes have been developed, known as the STERIS SYSTEM 1® and SYSTEM 1 E™, which are similar in sterilizer/process design. It is important for the sterilization of lumened devices to ensure that the correct lumen connectors are used in accordance with the manufacturer's instructions, including confirming that connectors have remained attached during the process (Figure 11.37).

Peracetic acid can be a toxic, caustic, and irritating chemical, both on its own and in formulation. The greatest risk is with handling concentrations greater than 10% (such as in cup delivery systems that contain ~35% PAA), although such cup systems are designed to minimize any risks of direct exposure. The final formulation is only mixed with water when placed within the sealed sterilizer design (Figures 11.37 and 11.38) and, following sterilization exposure, is discarded directly into the drain and rinsed away with water as part of the overall process. Despite this, it is always good practice to use gloves and eye protection, as PAA will burn the skin at concentrations of ~3% and can cause eye damage at even lower concentrations (~0.3%). The cup is vented, to prevent pressurization during the degradation of PAA over time, and should be stored in a well-ventilated area. PAA itself, even at lower concentrations when diluted for use (the final, mixed formulation in water), has a strong, acrid, vinegar-like odor that is irritating to the eyes and mucous membrane. At the time of writing, there is no defined safety (permissible) level/limit for PAA, but it is recommended that it is handled and used in well-ventilated areas to minimize any risks. In all cases, it is recommended as a precaution to use PPE when handling PAA or using PAA-based sterilization processes, to include safety glasses and gloves. Safety training should always be given according to a written procedure in relation to the correct emergency procedures in the case of an accidental spill of PAA-based sterilants and/or sterilizer malfunction within a given area.

Typical sterilizer design

An example of a PAA-based sterilization system is shown in Figure 11.38; the most widely used systems to date are the STERIS SYSTEM 1 and SYSTEM 1 E, which are similar in essential design but are also different processes.

The sterilizer load is placed within the chamber, according to the manufacturer's instructions; note that there is no packaging system for the devices being placed directly into the chamber for sterilization. Different types of insert tray systems are designed to support the various types of loads, ranging from general instrument trays to those specifically designed to accommodate larger flexible endoscope designs (Figure 11.37). Devices that contain internal lumens (rigid and flexible endoscopes) are connected to the sterilizer flow system using a series of connectors specifically designed and validated for each type/series of devices. The sterilizer is sealed by closing the lid and the sterilization process initiated. Hot potable water (typically in the 42–55°C/108–131°F range) is taken into the system through a series of pre-filters (which can vary depending on the water quality), but ultimately through a sterile water filter. In some designs this will be a designated, final 0.2 μm sterile water filter, while in others this will include pre-treatment with a UV system and then followed by a final dual 0.1 μm sterile water filter. The water is heated to the desired sterilization temperature, while

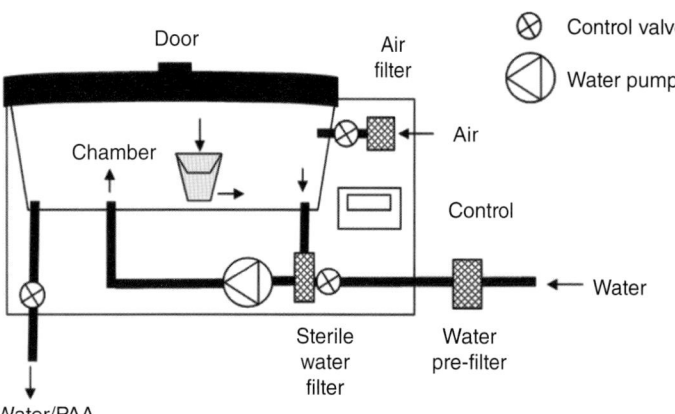

Figure 11.38 A typical design of a peracetic acid–based sterilization system. Such systems are designed to be top loading and have a single door (see also Figure 11.37).

the two-component sterilant is dissolved and mixed to give the final use dilution for sterilization (at ~2000 mg/L PAA). The sterilization phase is controlled at the defined temperature range and time (50–55°C/122–131°F for 12 minutes or 46–55°C/115–131°F for 6 minutes). All parts of the load and internal sterilizer design are exposed to the sterilant, to include the sterile water filter, followed by a drain. The final rinsing stage will include two or four sterile water rinses (fill, rinse time, and drain), depending on the defined process. The full cycle is controlled by a microprocessor and associated sensors for process control. In addition, these systems have programmed diagnostic cycles to be conducted every 24 hours that perform a series of self-tests to confirm proper functioning. The total process time is <30 minutes, but varies depending on the process and installation (e.g. water pressure requirements).

Standards and guidelines

Table 11.14 provides a list of standards and guidelines associated with the use of liquid PAA sterilizers.

Other processes

The most widely used chemical sterilization processes used worldwide have been described already, but new types of chemical sterilization processes are frequently being developed. These may or may not become available at various locations around the world, depending on local regulations and their commercial success. They can be based on any chemical that has the ability to demonstrate broad-spectrum (including sporicidal) antimicrobial activity, is developed for use as part of a sterilization process (e.g. providing an SAL of 10^{-6}), and meets healthcare requirements for safety and device compatibility. Note that the use of the term "sterilization" and how any such sterilization processes are regulated in a particular region can vary. For example, the use of a sporicidal disinfectant or sterilant does not necessarily ensure that sterilization is achieved and/or maintained during a given process. At a minimum such processes should be required to meet the requirements of various international standards, with particular emphasis on the essential requirements defined in ISO 14937 *Sterilization of health care*

Table 11.14 Standards and guidelines applicable to liquid peracetic acid sterilization processes or sterilants.

Guidelines/standards	Title	Description
ISO 14937: 2009	Sterilization of health care products. General requirements for characterization of a sterilizing agent and the development, validation, and routine control of a sterilization process for medical devices	Specifies general requirements for the characterization of any sterilizing agent and for the development, validation, and routine monitoring and control of a sterilization process for devices
ISO 11138:1 2017	Sterilization of health care products – Biological indicators. General requirements	General requirements for production, labeling, test methods, and performance requirements for the manufacture of biological indicators
ISO 15882: 2009	Sterilization of health care products – Chemical indicators. Guidance for selection, use and interpretation of results	Provides guidance for the selection, use, and interpretation of results of chemical indicators used in process definition, validation, routine monitoring, and overall control of sterilization processes
WHO: 2016	Decontamination and reprocessing of medical devices for health-care facilities	Guidance on processing, to include low-temperature sterilization
ANSI/AAMI ST58: 2013	Chemical sterilization and high-level disinfection in health care facilities	Provides guidelines for the selection and use of liquid chemical sterilants/high-level disinfectants and gaseous chemical sterilizers that have been cleared for marketing by the US Food and Drug Administration for use in hospitals and other healthcare facilities
CDC/HICPAC: 2008	Guideline for disinfection and sterilization in healthcare facilities	Recommendations on methods for cleaning, disinfection, and sterilization of patient-care medical devices in the United States
AS5369: 2023	Reprocessing of reusable medical devices in health and non-health related facilities	Guidance on processing, including low-temperature sterilization in Australia

products – General requirements for characterization of a sterilizing agent and the development, validation, and routine control of a sterilization process for medical devices. A number of existing or developing sterilization technologies are briefly discussed in this section.

There are many new hydrogen peroxide gas (particular gas plasma) sterilization systems. The essential components of such sterilization processes and sterilizer designs have been discussed earlier in this chapter. The individual sterilization processes provided in these sterilizer designs will vary widely and close attention should be given to the exact process conditions, the claims made with each individual design, and any required regulatory approvals to allow a sterilizer to be legally sold within a given country/region. Processes can range in hydrogen peroxide gas concentration, saturated or unsaturated gas conditions (i.e. liquid/gas or just gas peroxide exposure), exposure temperatures, pressures (vacuum levels), and the presence/absence and specific use of a plasma phase at various parts of the cycle. Each system should be considered unique, even though they may have similar trade names or claim equivalency to other existing systems.

Ozone, similar to other oxidizing agents such as hydrogen peroxide and PAA, is a potent antimicrobial chemical. It is a gas at room temperature and atmospheric pressure, being easily formed from oxygen (e.g. present in air at ~21% or provided as oxygen gas within an area) by applying energy in the form of a UV light or electricity (e.g. by creating a corona discharge). Also, it is a very unstable biocide that quickly breaks down to oxygen again, particularly on contact with various surfaces. It is used as a deodorizer/disinfectant (in air and water) and has often been investigated as a method of sterilization due to its potent antimicrobial activity at relatively low concentrations. For sterilization activity, optimum antimicrobial activity requires humidified ozone at a typical concentration of 50–100 mg/L. The most resistant organism to ozone-based sterilization processes is *Geobacillus stearothermophilus* spores, which are used in the development and routine testing of such sterilizer designs. Examples of ozone-containing sterilization processes that have been developed in the past include systems such as the STERIZONE® 125 L sterilization system and the OPTREOZ™ 125-Z system. The first used humidified ozone alone, while the second utilized a mixture of hydrogen peroxide and ozone gas. Unfortunately, neither of these systems has been widely used, but they are briefly described here.

Ozone-based sterilizer designs and sterilization processes, in particular the STERIZONE 125 L, are similar in many respects to those described for hydrogen peroxide gas systems, with the exception that very high humidity control is also required. The sterilizer consisted of a chamber (to hold the load), an ozone generator, a humidifier, and a piping system incorporating a vacuum pump. The process was conducted under vacuum (low pressure), within the temperature range of 30–36 °C/86–97 °F, and consisted of three phases: conditioning, sterilization, and ventilation. During conditioning a vacuum was drawn in the chamber to remove air and the load humidified by the introduction of water through a humidifier. Ozone, similar to EO and formaldehyde, requires high levels of humidity (optimally just below saturation at 90–95%) for antimicrobial activity. Following conditioning, low pressure was redrawn (at 0.01 kPa, approximately equivalent to 0.0001 bar, 0.001 psi, and 0.075 Torr), humidity controlled within the 85–100% range, and ozone introduced into the chamber at an initial concentration of 85 mg/L. Ozone was generated from medical-grade oxygen (which can be provided from a facility supply or directly from an oxygen gas tank) through a corona discharge-based generator and allowed to diffuse within the chamber for a given exposure time. Similar to hydrogen peroxide gas, the concentration of ozone could be reduced within the chamber during the exposure time (depending on the load). A vacuum could then be redrawn in the chamber and this exposure phase (vacuum, humidity, and ozone introduction) repeated. Therefore, a total of two ozone exposure pulses were conducted for each cycle. During sterilization, the ozone was degraded when removed from the chamber by passing it through a catalytic converter. The final phase was ventilation, when a vacuum was reapplied to the load to remove ozone residuals, also broken down through the converter and then returned to atmospheric pressure to release the load. The total cycle time was ~4.5 hours, and may have been longer depending on the load. No additional aeration was required due to the instability of ozone. Ozone is a respiratory irritant at low concentrations (e.g. at 0.01 ppm) and can have more serious health consequences at higher levels. A typical safety level that is recommended with ozone use is 0.1 ppm over a typical eight-hour working day (weighted average) and a short-term exposure limit of no more than 0.3 ppm over 15 minutes. Ozone detectors, including personal monitors and hand-held and room/area-mounted sensors, are available for safety monitoring. Ozone sterilizers were recommended to be installed in well-ventilated areas (e.g. with 10 or more air volume changes per hour). These designs of ozone sterilizers claimed to have low running/maintenance costs but required an intermediate cycle time (shorter than EO but longer than hydrogen peroxide gas systems). There were some significant limitations on material compatibility (to include aluminum, brass, and polyurethane), as well as their not being used to sterilize liquids, textiles, and cellulose-based materials (including paper packaging systems).

Another version of an ozone sterilizer was known as the STERIZONE 125 L+ system (or also as OPTREOZ 125-Z). These sterilizers provided a completely different sterilization process based on hydrogen peroxide gas and ozone gas together. They were vacuum-based processes, but at higher temperatures of 40–42°C/104–108°F and of similar sterilizer design to the ozone sterilizer. Hydrogen peroxide gas was generated from a hydrogen peroxide solution (at 50%) during the process and mixed with ozone during the sterilization cycle. Three types of cycles were available (ranging from 46 to 100 minutes long) that were chosen depending on the sterilizer load (e.g. lumen or non-lumen devices within the load). In comparison to the other ozone sterilizers, the cycles had shorter conditioning phases, consisting of drawing a deep vacuum (at a pressure of 0.13 kPa, equivalent to 0.001 bar, 0.019 psi, and 1 Torr) only, and then entering the sterilization phase consisting of a number of hydrogen peroxide/ozone gas exposure pulses (2–4 depending on the cycle). During each pulse the peroxide gas was introduced first into the chamber under vacuum and then ozone gas added, followed by an exposure time and then redrawing of the vacuum. A similar catalytic converter system was used to break down any ozone/peroxide gas residuals before venting into the room. In this system design, ozone was present at a much lower concentration (depending on the cycle, within a range of 2–10 mg/L) and the claimed antimicrobial effects were due to the combined action of peroxide/ozone gas. Finally, the ventilation stage consisted of two pulses of drawing a vacuum and using oxygen gas to purge any remaining ozone/peroxide gas from the load. The claimed benefits of these sterilizers, in comparison to the ozone design, were having a shorter cycle time and greater lumen penetration capability.

There are other types of gases that have been or are being investigated for use in sterilization processes. These include the use of PAA gas, chlorine dioxide (not to be mistaken for chlorine gas, which is a separate type of chemical), and nitrogen dioxide. These could include single or multiple biocide-based processes. A plasma–PAA sterilization process (similar to the hydrogen peroxide gas–plasma systems described earlier in this chapter) was developed but is no longer commercially available. Other gas plasma systems remain under investigation. As outlined in Chapter 6, a plasma can be made by applying energy to any gas. Gas plasma processes based on the generation of plasma within oxygen, nitrogen, helium, and argon or combinations of these gases (as examples) have shown potent antimicrobial activity. In all these cases, it is expected that sterilizer and sterilization process designs will be similar to the other low-temperature gas processes discussed earlier in this section. For example, PAA, chlorine dioxide, and nitrogen dioxide are all found to have optimal antimicrobial activity at higher humidity levels. Equally, such processes will need to ensure the correct balance of antimicrobial efficacy, safety, and device compatibility for routine clinical use.

There is a similar range of liquid chemicals that could be further developed as true sterilization processes. These are based on many processes already in use as disinfectants such as liquid PAA formulations, oxidized water, chlorine, liquid hydrogen peroxide, and liquid applications of chlorine dioxide and ozone (see Chapter 9 on chemical disinfection). An example is the use of various chlorine-generation systems (also known as "activated," "electrolyzed," or "super-oxidized" water applications). These operate by passing electricity through water, generally containing a low concentration of salt (NaCl, sodium chloride), to produce active chlorine species (primarily HOCl but also Cl_2 and OCl^-). Such processes can produce liquid preparations with powerful antimicrobial activity, including sporicidal activity. While their use to date has been as sporicidal disinfectants, future developments could include their optimization as part of sterilization processes in compliance with the applicable standards. Further examples include the use of various gases (or even gas plasmas) that are introduced into water or liquid chemical preparations for antimicrobial applications, such as with chlorine dioxide, water, and different types of gas plasmas.

Process monitoring

Process monitoring of low-temperature sterilization processes will include a similar series of tests as previously described for steam sterilization, such as parametric monitoring, BIs, CIs, and PCDs (see the section on the basic principles of sterilization earlier in this chapter). These quality control indicator systems are used in combination with recommended practice guidelines and standards. They will specifically include:

- Parametric monitoring, which should cover the key process conditions required for sterilization, such as cycle or sterilant exposure time, temperature, pressure, and even the concentration of the sterilant (if applicable). Printout reports from the sterilizer are commonly used and can provide useful information about each sterilizer cycle performance. In some sterilizer designs independent control systems may also be available (as an option) or installed to verify the calibration of key controlling sensors (e.g. temperature and pressure).
- Biological monitoring (using BIs), which can also be used to verify the efficacy of a sterilization process. Examples of the types of bacterial spores used to monitor chemical sterilization efficacy are given in Table 11.15. BIs can be provided in a variety of designs but are most widely used as self-contained designs and may include an additional CI.
- CIs, which are widely used to assess whether critical physical parameters of the given chemical sterilization process have been met. It is important to note that these indicators can vary in their classification and therefore their ability to indicate a successful sterilization process (Table 11.3). Similar to steam sterilization, some CIs are used as external indicators that

Table 11.15 Types of bacterial spores used for testing and monitoring of chemical sterilization methods.

Sterilization process	Test bacterial spores
Ethylene oxide	*Bacillus atrophaeus*
Hydrogen peroxide gas (including gas plasma)	*Geobacillus stearothermophilus*
Low temperature steam-formaldehyde gas	*Geobacillus stearothermophilus*
Liquid peracetic acid	*Geobacillus stearothermophilus*
Ozone	*Geobacillus stearothermophilus*

give an immediate result after the sterilization cycle and may provide an early indication of a problem in the process. Examples include various types of sterilization tapes or indicators integrated into packaging materials (similar to steam sterilization tapes). Such indicators do not show that sterilization has been achieved but rather that the item has been exposed to a given sterilization process. Internal CIs are designed to be used inside packages as a pack control to assist in confirming that the chemical sterilization process has been efficient within the load; these indicators will also vary in their specificity and sensitivity, depending on their classification and labeling. These are most commonly multi-parameter indicators that monitor at least two of the critical parameters of the sterilization process.

- PCDs, which are used in low-temperature sterilization as challenging or worst-case tests for sterilant penetration within the sterilizer. These generally consist of a barrier system (e.g. an absorbent pack or a lumened device), inside which a BI and/or CI is placed as a penetration challenge. PCDs can be used to test empty or full sterilizer loads.

Parametric release of the load is also possible with low-temperature sterilizers, depending on their design and the manufacturer's claims (see the basic principles of sterilization). Similar to steam, a low-temperature chemical sterilization process requires evidence that the sterilizer has performed the necessary cycle parameters to achieve sterilization. Parametric release for chemical sterilization will therefore require an in-depth knowledge and control of the sterilization parameters. These variables require continuous (and preferably independent) measurements and documentation, to include time, temperatures, pressures, relative humidity, chemical concentrations, and so on (dependent on the defined sterilization process). Like other sterilization processes (including steam), parametric release of loads may depend on final verification of an internal CI (in specific packs) prior to patient use.

In addition to quality control monitoring of low-temperature sterilization, personnel monitoring is often recommended or even required (according to local regulations) with some chemical sterilization methods. This is due to the staff health and safety risks associated with working with even low concentrations of chemical sterilants during work. While low-temperature sterilization processes can be used effectively to kill a wide range of microorganisms, these same sterilants may pose a serious health risk to personnel working in and around the process, if they are not closely monitored to ensure that permissible or safety exposure limits are not exceeded. Even with standard compliant equipment, ventilation systems, and well-established work practices, accidental leaks of toxic sterilant gases can and do happen and personnel working in these areas must be protected. In some cases strict guidelines and recommendations are given regarding safe levels of chemical sterilants, while in others these may not be as well defined. In some countries "immediately dangerous to life or health" (IDLH) exposure limits have been defined for airborne contaminants such as gases (Table 11.16). It is important to note that the concentration at which some chemicals can become a significant health risk can be much lower than those sensed by humans (e.g. smelled, tasted, or giving signs of irritation). The IDLH is defined as the concentration at which a chemical in a given area is likely to cause death or immediate/delayed permanent adverse health effects or prevent escape from such an area. For example, the IDLH value currently set for ethylene oxide is ~800 ppm, hydrogen peroxide 75 ppm, and ozone 5 ppm. A further important exposure limit that is often referenced is the 8-hour TWA. TWA or PEL values are based on the cumulative average concentration over a typical 8-hour day, 40-hour week to which a worker can be safely exposed (in this case, as defined by the American Conference of Government and Industrial Hygienists, ACGIH). They are intended to provide an exposure rate that most employees can safely and continuously be exposed to without significant adverse effects on their

Table 11.16 Examples of acceptable immediately dangerous to life or health (IDLH) and time-weight average–permissible exposure limit (TWA-PEL) limits for chemical sterilant gases.

Sterilant	IDLH (ppm)	8-hour TWA-PEL (ppm)	15-minute TWA-PEL (ppm)
Ethylene oxide	800	1.0	5
Formaldehyde	20	0.75	2
Hydrogen peroxide gas plasma	75	1.0	n/a
Ozone	5	0.1	n/a

health. As an example, the PEL limit of EO is 1 ppm (but a 15-minute exposure limit of 5 ppm is also given as the maximum level to which an employee may be exposed). The eight-hour PEL thus represents an exposure limit that should provide a safe work environment based on chemical toxicity and injury as well as longer-term risks from cancer and so on. The PEL for EO and hydrogen peroxide is similar, 1 ppm for both gases. The eight-hour PELs for formaldehyde (0.75 ppm) and ozone (0.1 ppm) are lower. Exposure to extremely low concentrations of ozone, for example, can cause an inflammatory response (include cough, shortness of breath, tightness of the chest, a feeling of an inability to breathe or dyspnea, dry throat, wheezing, headache, and nausea) in the respiratory tissue that can persist for up to 18 hours. Note that these safety levels can vary depending on regional requirements and are subject to change over time.

Various personnel and environmental monitoring systems are available that give an immediate indication of concentration in the work area so that workers can be protected from acute and chronic exposures.

Troubleshooting

Given the range of chemical sterilization processes and sterilizer designs, troubleshooting problems specific to each individual type are considered as outside of the scope of this chapter. Readers should ensure that they are familiar with the IFU and troubleshooting guidelines provided by the sterilizer manufacturer. Despite this, many of the typical problems (in particular process failure indicators) described in the troubleshooting of steam sterilization are applicable to chemical sterilization processes. Process indicators specific for the chemical sterilization process include CIs, BIs, PCDs, and parametric indicators that indicate failed results, which can often result from procedural issues such as:

- Devices correctly prepared and placed into the sterilizer. A typical example is with some vacuum-gas processes that require devices to be dry prior to placing them into the sterilizer.
- Whether the correct indicator or process challenge device was used with the load.
- Overloading or incorrect loading of a chamber.
- Wrong cycle chosen for a particular application in a sterilizer design.

Various indicators can also detect mechanical or other sterilizer faults and are designed to show:

- Loss of pressure (high or low), indicating a leak in the sterilizer (e.g. a failed door gasket or loose fitting in the associated pipework).
- No sterilant present within the cycle.
- Temperature not achieved within the sterilizer chamber.

As discussed for troubleshooting steam sterilization process failures, a well-planned, systematic, written procedure should be in place at the facility to address any of these potential situations as they may occur at any time. This procedure should be developed with the assistance of the sterilizer manufacturer and/or as recommended in its IFU or any associated training provided.

Some common failures or problems associated with chemical sterilization processes are:

- Failed sterilization indicators: ensure that the correct indicators (CIs, BIs, and those associated with PCDs) have been used, are within their label claims (including expiration dates), and that the correct procedures have been used concerning the use of the sterilizer (e.g. packaging, loading, etc.). In the absence of any specific procedural fault identified, the load should be considered non-sterile, the sterilizer removed from use, and investigated according to the manufacturer's instructions. Independent parametric control sensors/systems may be available in the sterilizer design and where a fault is identified, similarly the sterilizer should be removed from use and investigated according to the manufacturer's instructions.
- Self-diagnostic tests: many chemical sterilizers have self-diagnostic cycles/tests that are recommended to be performed periodically. Examples include sterilizer leak tests and filter integrity tests. Failure of such tests indicates an error in the operation of the sterilizer and should be investigated according to the manufacturer's instructions.
- Gas detection: various types of sensors are available to detect concentrations of gases above safety levels. Gas concentrations above safety levels indicate significant health risks to staff and inadequate control of the sterilization process (e.g. failed door gaskets, leaking gas tanks/feed-line systems). The sterilizer should immediately be removed from use and then investigated by trained staff/service providers. An excessive gas level can also indicate inadequate aeration of a load during or following a sterilization cycle. These should be immediately investigated as significant safety risks to staff and patients. Typical causes can include overloading of the sterilizer, insufficient aeration for certain types of devices/loads, and the use of the wrong packaging materials. Gas detection can pose a serious safety risk and will vary depending on the type of gas used for chemical sterilization.
- Moisture detection: the presence of significant levels of water on device surfaces prior to chemical sterilization may be detected or not by the sterilizer design. Failure to dry devices before processing can lead to inadequate sterilization or, in sterilizers with detection systems, delays in reprocessing of loads. Remember that the presence of moisture following use of many types of low-temperature (in particular gas) sterilizers will often indicate a significant fault or safety concern. An example is with hydrogen peroxide sterilizers, where it may

indicate the presence of concentrated hydrogen peroxide in the chamber.

- Incompatibility or device damage: damage to devices can occur for various reasons during the processing cycle, including the use of chemical sterilants. It is good practice to ensure that all devices are compatible with low-temperature sterilizer processes and examined to be fit for use following sterilization, directly prior to their use on patients (see Chapter 12). Suspected damage to a device following chemical sterilization should be reported to the sterilizer and device manufacturer for further investigation. It may be necessary in such cases to discontinue use of the sterilizer for these devices until the investigation is completed to ensure that the device(s) are compatible with the process.

12 Storage and distribution

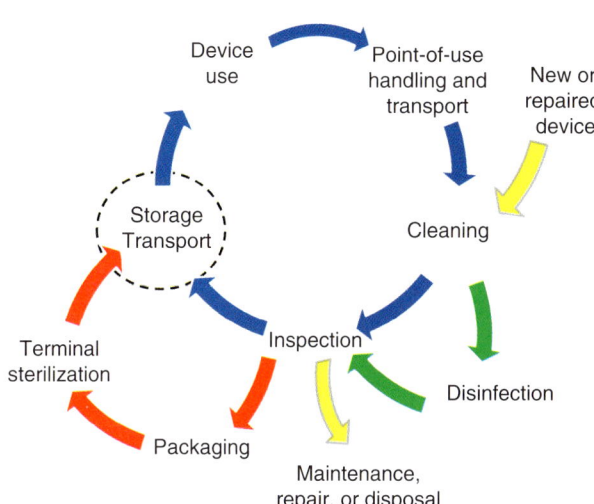

Despite the various stages of device processing and efforts to render a device clean and disinfected/sterilized, this can all be compromised through inadequate handling and storage of the devices prior to patient use. Therefore, the storage (if applicable) and distribution of reusable devices is an essential step to complete the processing cycle. In cases of non-critical and even semi-critical devices that are cleaned and/or disinfected, it is recommended that these are immediately used for their intended patient application. These devices are not generally packaged and are considered in more detail in this chapter. Similarly, in the case of immediate use steam sterilization (IUSS), previously referred to as "flash" sterilization, or liquid chemical sterilization processes (which are designed for just-in-time availability of a sterile device), the device(s) should be delivered directly for immediate use. These devices are not protected from recontamination and should not be stored before patient use, unless subjected to resterilization.

In this chapter special consideration is given to the storage and distribution of reusable devices that have been packaged and sterilized. These devices are ready either to be used on a patient or to be stored in the correct manner and made available for a patient procedure at a future date. Various types of rigid and flexible sterile barrier systems/materials have been designed for such purposes (Chapter 10); however, these systems can become compromised during storing and handling. Best practice for maintaining sterile packs is to minimize handling and to store and transport as appropriate. Other considerations include storing within clinical areas such as wards that are not typically under direct oversight of processing personnel. Restricting access to storage areas to authorized personnel is essential, in addition to adequate storage and distribution procedures that should be specified for each facility. Risk assessment of the storage areas considering co-location of processed devices with bulk consumables, mobile patient equipment/other goods, fluids, refrigerators, or warming devices (as examples) should also be considered.

Handling of non-packaged or non-sterilized devices

Non-packaged and non-sterilized devices can include:
- Non-critical and semi-critical devices that have been disinfected (high-, intermediate-, or low-level disinfection; see Chapter 9); these may have been processed by thermal or chemical disinfection methods. They are non-packaged (not processed within a sterile barrier system designed for storage/transport following the processing cycle). As a result, the surfaces of these devices can easily become contaminated when handled, transported, or exposed to the environment.
- Critical devices that have been sterilized but not contained within a sterile barrier system. Examples include the sterilization of devices in an IUSS cycle or within a liquid chemical sterilization process that is labeled as a "just-in-time" process. Such devices may be sterilized at that time, but can also become contaminated, with greater patient consequences due to their criticality.

Decontamination and Device Processing in Healthcare, Second Edition. Gerald McDonnell and Georgia Alevizopoulou.
© 2025 John Wiley & Sons Ltd. Published 2025 by John Wiley & Sons Ltd.

In these cases, at the point of disinfection or sterilization completion (if applied correctly) the device(s) should be used immediately. It is important that such devices are aseptically handled and presented for patient use to minimize any risks of contamination. Several guidelines recommend a minimum time from when they have been processed before they are able to be used on patients. For example, some European guidelines recommend the use of flexible endoscopes on patients following high-level disinfection for up to three hours after the device has been processed. However, there is of yet no universal rule. Such recommendations are based on the correct handling and storage of the device prior to use. Inappropriate handling and/or storage could allow the device to be contaminated during any interim time. Therefore, it is more prudent to consider a risk-based and event-related policy rather than focusing on a specific time period alone.

Overall, a facility policy should be in place that describes the safe handling of any non-packaged or non-sterilized devices prior to patient use. This will include:
- Disinfection/sterilization methods to be used and under what circumstances.
- Handling and/or storage procedures following processing, including any minimum or maximum times within which the device can be used.
- Handling of devices that have been compromised (even if only suspected) or that have been held/stored for greater than the allowable time.
- Return of processed devices that have definitely not been used. This situation could be governed by a blanket rule to process all devices that have left the processing department, and/or a process and criteria for restocking unused devices.

For heat-disinfected or steam-sterilized devices, it is important to ensure that the devices are allowed to cool to room temperature before handling or patient use, to prevent condensation that may affect sterility of the pack; this may require up to an hour or more to be sure, depending on the device/set and as dictated in the manufacturer's instructions. Low-temperature chemical disinfected/sterilized devices can be used immediately, ensuring that any residual chemicals have been correctly detoxified and removed in accordance with manufacturer's instructions. A common cause of patient-associated toxicity reactions is residual disinfectant remaining in or on devices when clinically used. Similarly, contaminated rinse water can lead to toxic reactions (due to the presence of chemical contaminants) and patient infections (due to the presence of microorganisms). A typical example is with flexible endoscopes, which are often processed as semi-critical devices by being cleaned and high-level disinfected (see Chapter 15 on endoscopy). Flexible endoscopes are manufactured with various types of plastic (often porous) materials and can have one or more internal lumens. It is difficult to ensure that these materials and lumens are safely reprocessed.

Common problems include inadequate cleaning, disinfection, recontamination (following disinfection, such as with contaminated rinse water), and insufficient rinsing. Residuals can therefore include cleaning chemistries, disinfectants, and chemical/microbial contaminants from the rinse water. Bacteria present in rinse water and remaining in/on the endoscope following disinfection can pose a risk to patients. These risks increase significantly when bacteria are allowed to grow within the lumens of these devices if they are stored wet (even with a low level of moisture remaining within the endoscope lumens). Residual water can remain within these channels, even if processing was conducted within a washer-disinfector or automated endoscope reprocessor (AER) that may have lumen purging/drying claims.

In some areas specific drying cabinets, referred to as controlled environment storage cabinets, are employed to assist in the drying and storing of flexible endoscopes following processing (Figure 12.1). Such cabinets should comply with European norm EN16442 and are generally designed to flow high-efficiency particulate air (HEPA)-filtered air through the various device lumens for the purpose of drying. When stored in such a manner, the manufacturer may recommend that the devices are safely maintained to prevent contamination and bacterial/fungal growth in or on the device. Such storage cabinets and any associated testing data should be carefully examined with the manufacturer to ensure they are safe for use in accordance with any facility policies. Staff training is important to make sure that these storage cabinets are correctly used and maintained.

Note that some transport systems for flexible endoscopes are designed as rigid containers with covers, to prevent contamination of the device during transport to a site of patient use (Figure 12.1); these are not sterile packaging systems and do not imply that the device can be safely stored prior to patient use. Care should be taken to read and understand any manufacturer's instructions provided with these systems. Finally, extra caution should be given to prevent storing disinfected devices in their transport cases, a common poor practice typically seen with flexible endoscopes and ultrasound probes. Such cases are often lined with foam or porous material to protect the device in transit, which increases the risk of contamination. Storage containers should be washable, non-porous, sealed, and robust, and transport cases do not achieve this.

Sterile storage environment and layout

A dedicated area should be defined for the storage of packaged, sterilized items. Ideally there should be a physical separation between the storage area and the rest of the processing area to reduce any risks of mixing sterile and non-sterile items, as well as cross-contamination. If this is not possible, care is needed to ensure that air and traffic always flow from clean to dirty areas of the facility. Access to the area should be clearly defined, with traffic controlled to minimize the movement of airborne contaminants. No through traffic should be allowed, with only staff allocated to the "clean side" being allowed access to the storage area.

The storage area should be well lit, easy to clean, and arranged in a way that will make it easy to identify packs with minimal handling. The maintenance (cleaning and disinfection) of work surfaces, floors, shelving, and transport equipment is essential. Light fittings, pipes, and air-conditioning ducts, which can collect and shed dust, should not be overlooked when cleaning. Monolithic ceilings (e.g. plasterboard versus tiles) and fixtures (e.g. lighting to be flush mounted) as well as use of bulkheads to reduce high-dusting surfaces should be encouraged. Surfaces in contact with sterile goods should be as clean as possible to minimize contamination. Care should be taken to use cleaning/disinfection chemistries that will not damage packaging materials. It is not necessary to keep surfaces disinfected, but they should be visually clean. Cleaning of the sterile storage area should be planned in such a way as to minimize handling of sterile packs, as excess handling can increase the risk of damaging the packaging materials.

The storage system should be designed to meet the specific needs of the facility. As long as the system conforms to the facility policy, hygiene, infection prevention/control, and security requirements, a manager should be free to lay out and maintain the storage area in the best way possible to meet the needs of the facility. Sterile packs should be arranged to allow them to be easily identified for their intended use. Shelving systems and sterilization baskets are most often used (Figure 12.2). The type of shelving used for sterile storage should protect the sterile packs, allow for easy stock rotation, and be easy to clean, as well as allowing air to circulate around packs. Sharp edges or parts can pose a staff safety risk as well as causing packaging materials to rip.

The environmental conditions of storage can also affect the integrity of a sterile pack. Bear the following in mind:
- Reduce exposure to environmental factors such as direct sunlight, air, temperature, humidity, and sources of water.
- Minimize handling within the storage area.
- Ensure controlled transportation to the place of intended use.

Water and air can be major sources of contamination. Examples include an overly humid environment, direct exposure to sunlight, and high temperatures over time, which may degrade the packaging material and increase the risk of contamination. High humidity may also cause condensation to form on packaging and enhance the capability of microorganisms to multiply and enter sterile packs. Likewise, very dry conditions may cause packaging materials to dry out, become brittle, and lose their barrier function. Ideal environmental

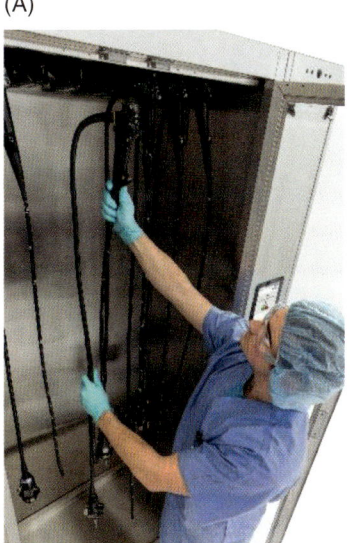

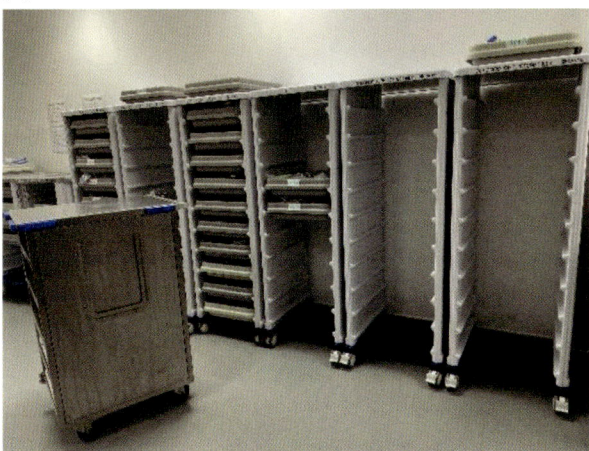

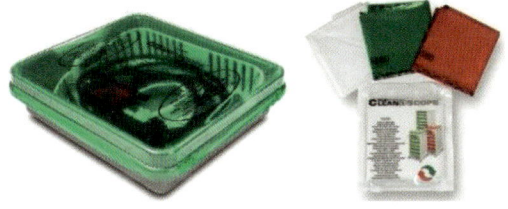

Figure 12.1 Examples of temporary storage methods used for flexible endoscopes. (A) A controlled environment storage cabinet, designed to flow HEPA-filtered air through the endoscope lumens to aid in drying. (B) A transport system comprising covered trays and carts used to transfer contaminated/processed endoscopes from one area to another using different-colored systems for contaminated and processed scopes.

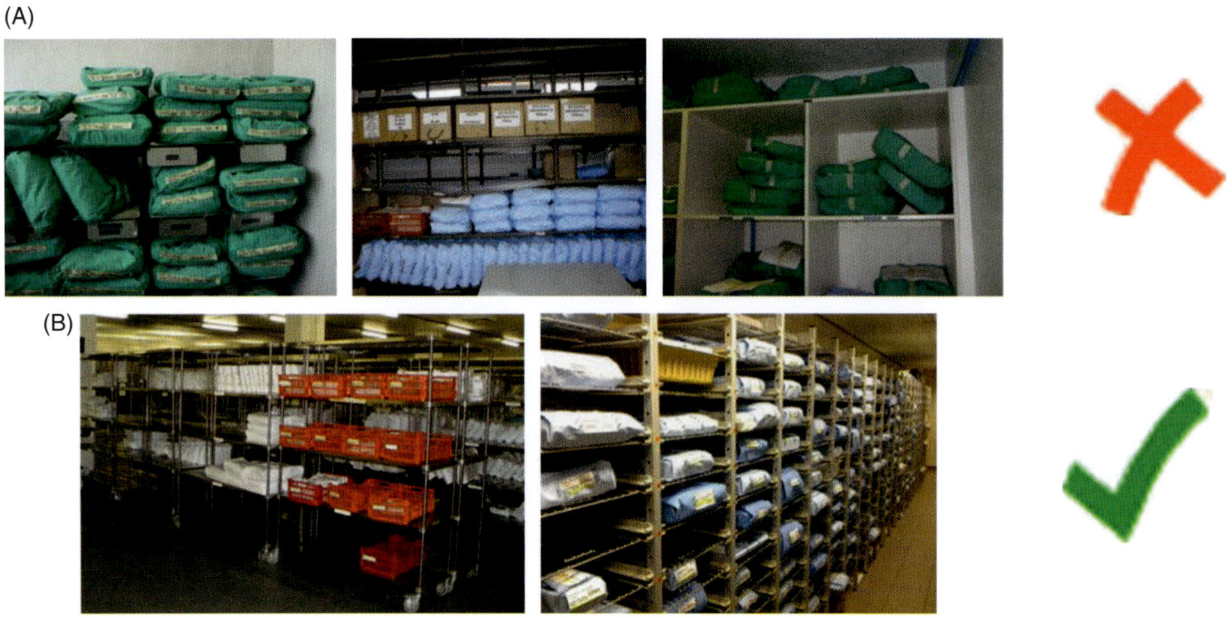

Figure 12.2 Shelving systems used for sterile pack storage. (A) Some storage conditions that may cause damage to device loads. (B) Examples of adequate storage conditions.

temperatures should be controlled at 18–22°C (65–72°F) and relative humidity (RH) should be 35–50%, although various national standards and guidelines may allow for other temperature and humidity ranges. Air supply to the storage areas should be clean and dust free, and may require (HEPA) filtration. Ideally, the sterile storage area should be maintained under a positive pressure with ~13 air exchanges per hour or positive pressure to surrounding areas, in order to reduce the possibility of airborne contamination from air outside the storage area.

Ideally all environmental conditions should be monitored. The duration and severity of excursions in temperature and RH should be set out and actions specified for facility management. Records should be kept at least daily, but in some instances automated building management systems or the use of continual data readers may be required to observe temperature and RH in real time or at defined intervals.

Sterility maintenance should be viewed as a quality management process. Several events may compromise sterility. Each processing facility should have policies and procedures in place for the labeling, storage, handling, and rotating of sterile packaged materials in the storage area. This can include other facility sterile supplies that are also used for patient surgical/medical procedures.

Sterility maintenance shelf-life refers to the period of time during which a sterilized item is considered safe to be used. Guidelines regarding sterility shelf-life can vary from country to country, and particular attention should be paid to instructions for use that are given by the packaging system/material manufacturer. Traditionally, packaged reusable devices were considered to be sterile for a given storage time (e.g. up to four weeks), after which if the pack was unused it would be recalled for processing. Internationally this is no longer considered to be valid or warranted. An alternate system, known as "event-related sterility," is more practical, reduces unnecessary waste, and is widely used. This system defines the sterility of a pack as being dependent on events that may occur during the handling, transporting, and storage of the item. As an example, if the pack has remained intact and has been stored correctly, the devices within it should be expected to remain sterile, unless otherwise specified by the packaging manufacturer. Sterile packaged devices can become compromised depending on the quality of packaging material used, the storage conditions, the conditions during transport, and the amount of handling. The greatest risk to a sterilized pack is damage to the packaging materials. Events that can compromise sterility include:

- Holes or torn wrappers.
- Broken or incomplete seals on laminated pouches.
- Securing tapes or locks that have been tampered with or removed.
- Exposure to blood, bodily fluids, or any type of moisture.

- Being dropped on a dirty surface.
- Being moved.
- Elastic bands or tapes used to bundle items and causing tearing.
- Excessive temperature or humidity conditions, for example through exposure to sun.
- External chemical indicators having faded – this may also be considered a reject, even though it may not materially have been a sterility compromise.

Sterile items should be arranged so that handling is reduced and they are easy to locate. They can be organized to suit the facility, for example alphabetically, by procedure, by discipline, or numerically using stock codes. Efficient labeling of shelves and sterile packs facilitates easier location and identification of the sterile packs, making access easier and more efficient. A good tracking system (see Chapter 14) will also make identification and location of packs easier. Packs should be stored away from direct sunlight and water and should not be stored next to or under sinks, on the floor, or on windowsills where they are likely to get wet or damaged. Common sense dictates that storing sterile items on the floor or too close to the floor, in a moist area, or not covering shelves to protect packs from dust will compromise sterility. Sterile packs should be stored at least 25 cm/8–13 inches above the floor, 45 cm/18 inches below the ceiling or sprinkler heads, and at least 5 cm/2 inches from outside walls to allow for air circulation in the room and to prevent contamination during cleaning.

There should be enough shelving and cupboard space available to store all sterile goods without having to stack them tightly or on top of one another. Shelving should be designed in a way that makes it easy to see the number of packs in storage. Shelving should be slatted, easily cleaned, and allow air to circulate around stored packs. Spacing of shelving and packs must also be planned to prevent packs from being touched, bumped, or leaned on by housekeeping staff or when packs are retrieved for distribution. Packs should not overhang the shelving. Shelving should be made of an easy-to-clean material; laminate may be acceptable, but the outer surface needs to be non-porous, non-shedding, and resistant to frequent cleaning. Wood is not adequate. Freestanding or mobile shelving provides a practical solution for handling the flow of products in and out of storage and cleaning. It allows staff to access all sides of the storage area for rotation of sterile packs. Open shelf units are more commonly used as they are convenient and less expensive than closed shelving units. Open shelves (wire mesh or bars) allow dust to pass through, making them easier to clean than solid shelves. If open shelving units are used, special attention should be on traffic control, housekeeping, and environmental ventilation. A barrier should be created between the floor and the bottom shelf. The disadvantage of open shelving units is that sterile packs are more vulnerable to accidental physical and environmental hazards. Closed shelving units or covered cabinets are often preferred for seldom-used items. Closed cabinets should have doors, preferably with a lock. When items are stored in closed cabinets, dust is limited, handling is discouraged, and inadvertent contact with sterile items is minimized.

Packs should be stored in a way that allows for easy handling to prevent injury. Personnel should avoid compromising the sterility of the item by not dragging, crushing, bending, compressing, or puncturing the package. Larger, heavier packs may be stored in transport trays to prevent tears in the wrappers during handling. Heavier packs should be placed on lower and middle shelves, with lighter, easier-to-handle packs on higher shelves. Shelf liners may be used on shelves if tears on the bottom of packs are a problem. Tears usually occur as a result of heavy packs, especially trays, being "dragged" off the shelf. The edges of the metal trays and weight of the devices increase the negative effects of friction, causing packaging to catch and tear. Burrs or sharp edges on the shelves may also damage sterile packs. When removing sterile packs from the shelf, both hands should be placed underneath the pack and the pack lifted to avoid dragging and tearing or snagging the wrapper.

When packing shelves do not squeeze packs into tight spaces, bend, stack, compress, or fold them, as this can tear the packaging and potentially rupture closures and seams if the air inside the pack is forced out. When a pack is compressed, air is forced out of the pack creating a void; when the source of compression is released – that is, the weight on top of the pack is removed – a suction is created that may potentially "suck in" contaminated air.

Rigid sterilization container systems should only be stored on shelves or racks designed to hold the weight and configuration of the containers. If containers need to be stacked due to space constraints, it is important that the manufacturer's stacking guidelines are adhered to and that the containers are firmly seated on top of each other and can be easily removed. Staff should be instructed not to hold rigid containers by only one handle, as this can lead to injury, damage to instruments, and increased risk of dropping.

Cardboard boxes should not be used as storage containers because they can release paper fibers into the environment, cannot be easily cleaned, and sometimes have rough edges that can make holes in packaging and may contain mold. It is recommended that any shipping cartons are not brought directly into the sterile storage area because they serve as reservoirs for contamination during transport. A dedicated deboxing area is recommended for the clean removal of stock for immediate storage, and disposal of boxes to recycling waste. Deboxing should ideally not occur in the sterile store.

If sterilized packages are likely to be exposed to excessive environmental challenges (e.g. transport to another location) or multiple handlings before use, dust covers or containers may be used to protect the packs. These covers/containers are designed to protect the pack against outside elements. Dust covers should be applied and sealed immediately after the cooled pack is removed from the sterilizer cart and prior to storage/shipping.

Inventory control

An inventory control and stock rotation system is important to ensure the efficient use of devices within a facility (also see Chapter 14 on inventory management). A number of stock control systems are available and should be chosen to meet the requirements of the facility. It is good practice to ensure that devices do not stay in a sterile storage area for extended periods of time and that similar device sets are equally used. This requires close coordination between staff in the processing area, storage area, those involved with transport, and at the site of patient use (e.g. in the operating room).

The longer a sterile pack has been exposed to the environment and been handled, the more likely it is to be compromised. Therefore, a common stock rotation system works on a "first in, first out" (FIFO) principle. Rotation of stock is important to ensure that "older" sterilized supplies are used before "newer" supplies. It also helps with maintain appropriate stock levels and not overstocking. Examples of such systems are:
- From left to right: older sterilized supplies are kept to the left of the storage area/rack. New supplies are added to the right side, moving older supplies to the left. Staff should be instructed only to take supplies from the left for distribution.
- From top to bottom: old supplies are removed and distributed from the top of the stock area. New supplies are added to the bottom shelves and moved up as supplies are distributed.
- From front to back: older supplies are placed at the front of the shelf and should be first to be distributed. Newer supplies are added to the back of the shelf, pushing older supplies forward.

Transport of sterile packaged items

Various methods can be used in the transport of sterile packaged items to their point of use. This can range from hand carriage (e.g. where a storage area is located close or adjacent to a point of use) to the use of trolleys and other transport systems for taking items to a remote location (within a facility or at a different facility). Similar considerations to those discussed for the storing of sterile packaged devices (see the section on storage and handling of sterile packaged devices) should be given to any immediate or remote transportation in order to reduce any risks of contamination.

Hand transport

Appropriate hand transportation of sterile packs will generally include supporting with both hands under the pack. Avoid cradling packs or carrying them under the arms. When carrying sterile packages containing devices, the package should be kept away from the body and parallel with the floor in order to avoid shifting of the instruments. Good body mechanics should be used when transporting any items to prevent injury (e.g. lifting from the knees rather straining the back; see Chapter 13 on physical and emotional health).

Trolley systems

When devices are to be taken from one area to another, trolley systems should be considered (Figure 12.3). Contaminated and sterile supplies should be transported separately in dedicated covered or enclosed trolleys with a solid bottom shelf (see Chapter 7 on transportation post procedure). The solid bottom shelf prevents contamination on the floor being picked up by the wheels of the trolley and deposited onto sterile packs. Unintentional contact with staff and other sources of contamination along the transportation route can be avoided if covered or enclosed carts are used for transportation of such items. All transport vehicles (motorized or manual) should be constructed of materials that allow for a proper decontamination (cleaning and disinfection) process; this is particularly important if the same vehicle will transport alternating sterile and soiled items. If reusable covers for carts or other transport vehicles are used, they should have a resealable opening and should be cleaned after each use. Trolleys should be cleaned and dried after each use, because even though they are used with sterile items, contamination can be picked up during transport. It is important to wash the outside tops and bottoms of shelves on trolleys used to transport sterile packages. Loaded transport vehicles should never be left unattended or in an unsecured location. If plastic or paper bags or plastic tote boxes are used to contain and transport items, the devices should be placed in such a way that would prevent them from being crushed, damaged or contaminated. Tote boxes should also be sealable for both clean and dirty distribution to prevent tampering with contents.

Packages should be placed securely in a flat position (or for individually packed items may be transported side to side), not placed on top of each other, and should not extend beyond the edge of the cart shelf or table surface, to prevent accidents.

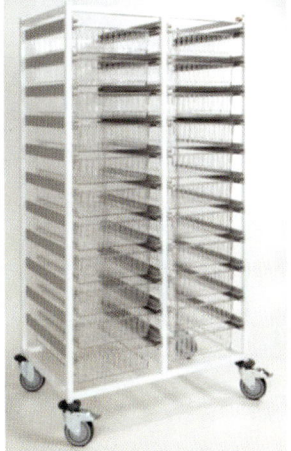
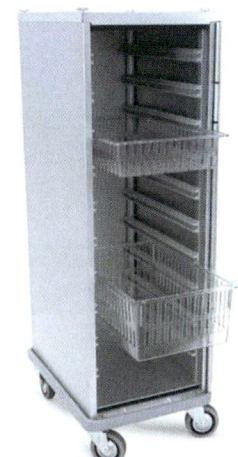
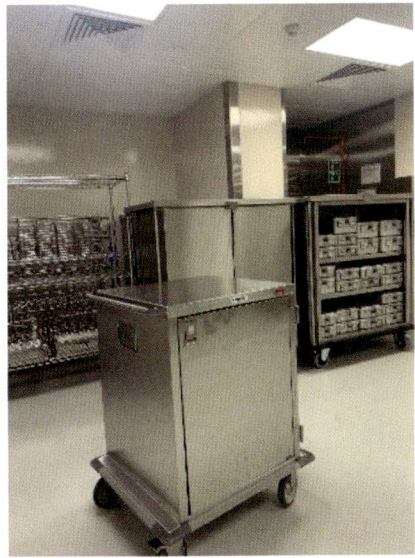
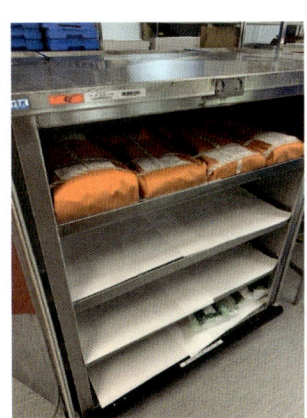
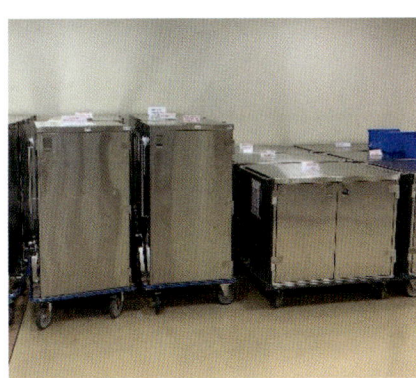

Figure 12.3 Examples of closed and open trolleys for sterile goods transport.

Dedicated lifts (elevators)

Where appropriate, separate, dedicated "clean" and "dirty" lifts (elevators) should be used to transport sterile items directly from the processing dispatch area to a point of use (e.g. operating room suite) or from the point of use back to the dirty receiving area of the processing area (Figure 12.4). Such systems can provide fast, direct transport system between the two areas, with minimal handling. This can only be done if there is a direct vertical link between the area where the devices are used and the processing area on two separate floors. Preferably the lift should lead directly into the storage/dispatch area of the processing department or to an access corridor in close proximity to this area.

The main advantage of a dedicated lift (elevator) is to increase transport operational efficiencies and lower device turnover time when the two areas are on separate levels. A dedicated dirty lift (elevator) may also assist in reducing the potential for cross-contamination of items being transported in a common patient/visitor/staff/service lift (elevator), but may not prevent airborne transmission of pathogenic microorganisms. A dedicated clean lift (elevator) will only remain clean if proper cleaning procedures of the cab, floor, ceiling, and walls are performed on a regular basis, something that is not generally done in most facilities. Poor lift (elevator) maintenance and housekeeping of the hoistways and pit can lead to an accumulation of waste, water, oil, dirt, and dust there, creating an ideal breeding ground for mold and other potentially infectious microorganisms.

If a dedicated "clean" lift is used to transport clean or sterile items from the reprocessing dispatch area, the lift should be

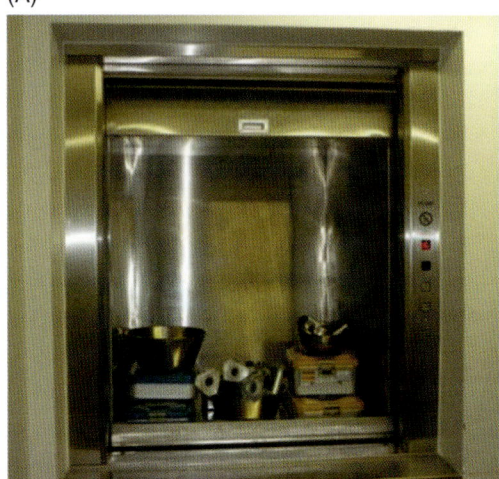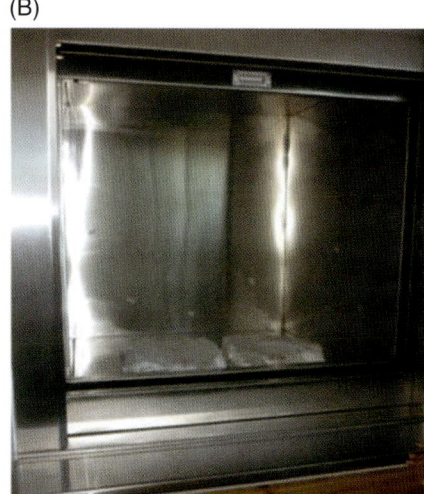

Figure 12.4 Examples of lifts used to transport items to and from a processing area. Dedicated lifts for (A) soiled items and (B) sterile items.

located in a designated "clean area" of dispatch and the point of use. The same lift should not be used for transporting contaminated and sterile items. A dedicated "soiled" lift should be available to transport soiled items from the point of use to the "dirty" receiving area and a dedicated "clean" lift should be used to transport sterile items separately. A possible disadvantage of dedicated lifts may be that longer queue times are experienced as a result of waiting for the respective dedicated soiled or clean lift (elevator). In the case of sterile items there is also the potential for condensate to occur on plastic or metal surfaces that are moved from air-conditioned areas such as theaters and the reprocessing area to non-air-conditioned environments such as lifts (elevators) and then back to another environment.

Transport to another facility

In some cases processed (including sterile) goods will need to be transported to a different off-site facility for further storage and/or patient use. In these cases it is recommended that transport vehicles are completely enclosed, with all items (clean and/or dirty) securely packed and separated in order to protect them from damage and contamination during transport. The vehicles used for transport should be able to safely separate clean and processed/sterile items from contaminated items (Chapter 7; see Figure 12.5). Processed items being transported by road should preferably have a dedicated drop-off unloading area and procedures in place for separation from any loading area for dirty items. Ideally the delivery area should lead directly to a dedicated receiving area to minimize handling. Routes and schedules should be planned to minimize transit time.

External transport vehicles should have a routine cleaning and maintenance program. If applicable, carts should be secured during transportation within the vehicle to prevent damage or cross-contamination. Vehicles should be designed in such a way as to allow for ease of loading and unloading. Many vehicles carrying high volumes of devices have a tail lift fitted to facilitate the loading of trolleys. Environmental conditions should be regularly assessed for significant changes in temperature and humidity, which may affect the load during transport; best practice is that vehicles have temperature and humidity control.

Guidance at the point of use

Sterile packaged or otherwise processed items should be inspected at the point of use. First, the external condition of any packaging should be inspected (Figure 12.6). Circumstances in which a product may be considered unsterile or otherwise compromised include:
- Incorrectly wrapped.
- Damaged or opened.
- Punctures, holes, or tears.
- Signs of moisture or stains, including if still wet after a sterilization cycle or indications that it may have come into contact with water during storage.
- Obvious signs of external contamination where packs might have been placed or dropped on a dirty surface.
- No indication of having been through a sterilizing process (e.g. an external chemical indicator not present or not changed to a defined color).
- Broken seals, including tamper-proof locks on rigid containers that are broken/missing.
- Excessive dust.
- Evidence of crushing.
- No labeling or no production and/or expiration date.

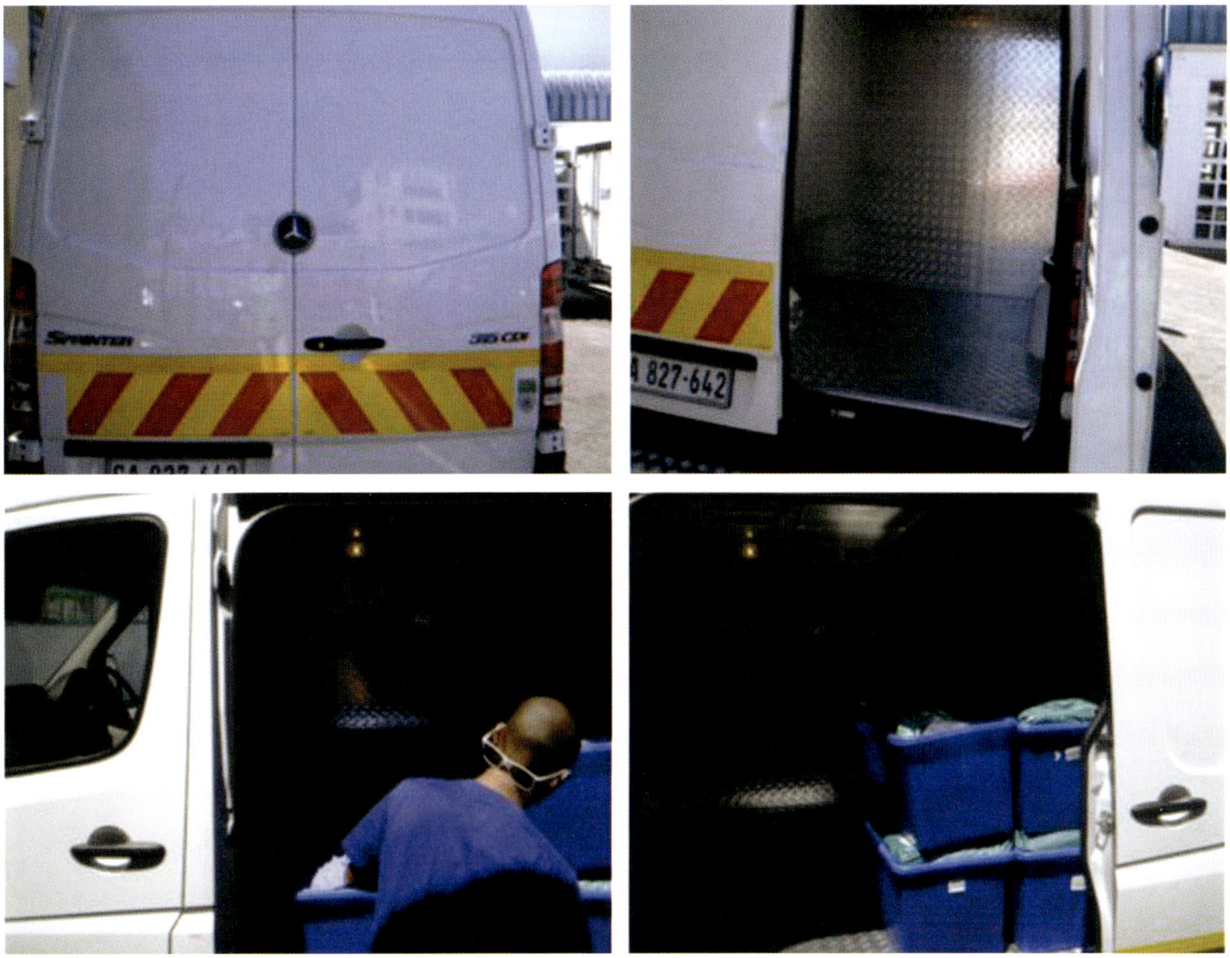

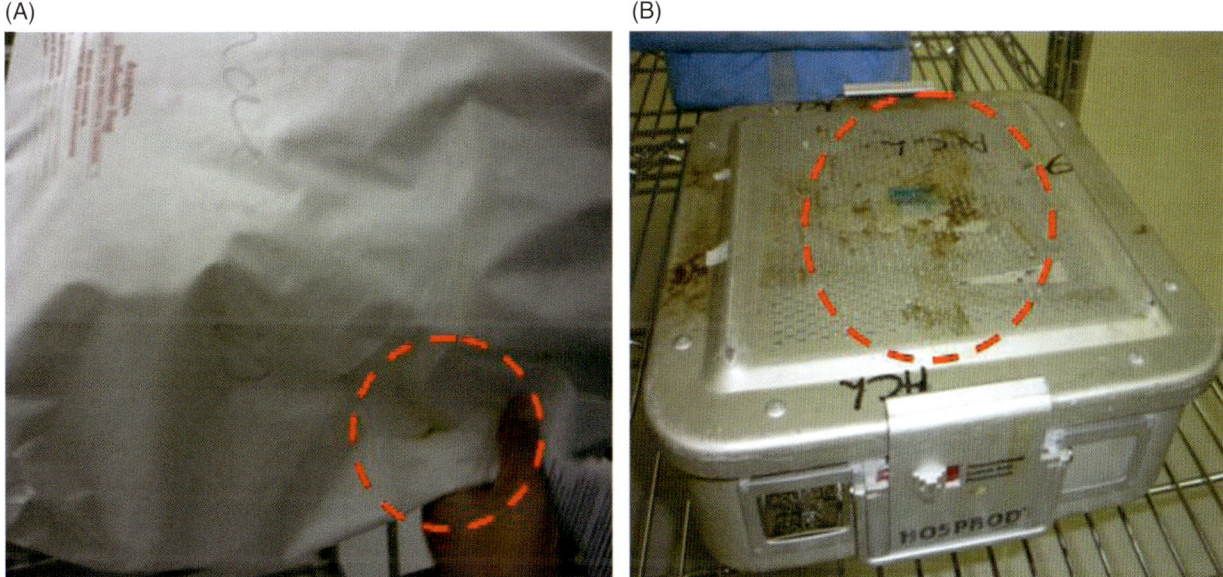

Figure 12.5 Example of a dedicated transport vehicle separating clean and dirty items. The sterile items go into the back of the vehicle (top panel), which is separated from the front by a metal divider. The dirty items (in bins) go into the front of the transport vehicle through a sliding side door.

(A)   (B)

Figure 12.6 Examples of damaged, sterile packaged goods that may be compromised. (A) Torn packaging, (B) dirty rigid container, (C) inadequate transport/storage (compressed) packs, and (D) inadequate packaging.

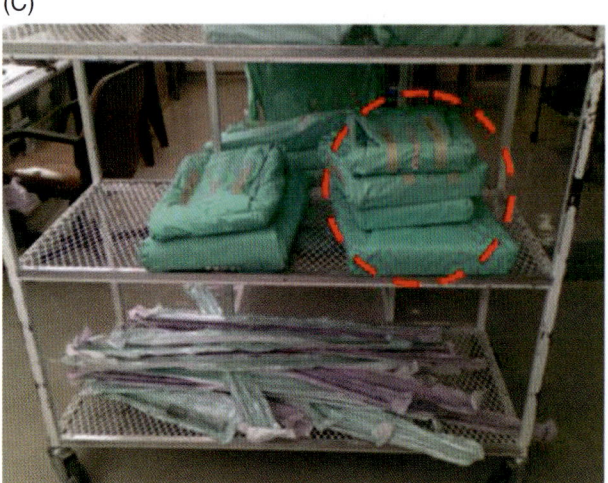 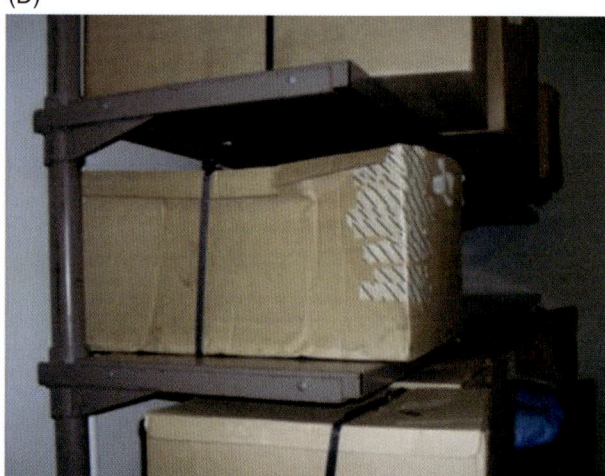

Figure 12.6 (Continued)

Table 12.1 Standards and guidelines for the storage and distribution of devices prior to patient use.

Guidelines/standards	Title	Description
AS 5369	Processing of reusable medical devices in health and non-health related facilities	Section 9 and Appendix A provide guidelines for the storage and handling of processed items
ANSI/AAMI ST79	Comprehensive guide to steam sterilization and sterility assurance in healthcare facilities	Section 11 covers storage facilities and transport requirements for steam-sterilized items
Association of periOperative Registered Nurses (AORN)	Perioperative standards and recommended practices	Standards and recommendations for peri-operative practice including decontamination and storage
CDC (Centers for Disease Control) HICPAC (Healthcare Infection Control Practices Advisory Committee) Guidelines	Guideline for disinfection and sterilization in healthcare facilities (2008)	Provides guidance on storage and handling of disinfected and sterilized goods
AAMI ST58	Chemical sterilization and high-level disinfection in healthcare facilities	Includes guidelines for device storage and transport following disinfection/sterilization
EN16442:2015	Controlled environment storage cabinets for processed thermolabile endoscopes	Specifies performance requirements for cabinets intended to be used for storage of processed endoscopes
World Health Organization	Decontamination and reprocessing of medical devices for health-care facilities	Guidance on the storage of processed devices following sterilization or high-level disinfection (endoscopes), including maintenance

Finally, when the packaging is opened at the site of use (see Chapter 3 on the operating room/procedure room) by the medical/surgical staff, they must check that the device/set is fit for use, to include verifying that:

• Any associated internal chemical indicators (where these are used) have changed to the defined color, as described by the manufacturer (see Chapter 14 on quality management).

• All devices in a set are present and operational for the procedure. The staff may check for any signs of damage at this stage. For example, rusting may have occurred during storage due to the effects of sterilization (e.g. presence of chlorine or other chemicals in steam; see Chapter 11, in the section on troubleshooting steam sterilization problems) or if devices have been stored wet. Another example is damage due to inadequate handling during storage/transport of the device/device set.

- All devices are present in a set and in accordance with a checklist.
- No recalls have been requested by the processing department (see Chapter 14 on recall).

It is essential that the devices are handled correctly and aseptically during procedure set-up and immediately prior to use to ensure that they are safe for patient use (see Chapter 3 on the operating room/procedure room). Inadequate handling at this stage can compromise the entire quality of the processing cycle and patient safety.

Standards and guidelines

Correct storage and distribution of devices and materials are important to maintain the safety of processed devices, including sterile packaged devices, throughout storage and transportation. Table 12.1 provides a list of standards and guidelines that are used worldwide.

13 Safety

Safety may be defined as the condition of being protected from danger, harm, or injury. Everything we do, privately and professionally in our work, has potential to cause harm either directly or indirectly. Safe work practices are designed to reduce these risks to a minimum while at work. Processing facilities can pose numerous safety issues, including physical activity (lifting, pushing, pulling), use of chemicals (including liquids, gases, and even radioactivity), handling of contaminated waste/devices, handling of sharp instruments, and so on. Safety in processing facilities is therefore an important aspect to consider. It is impossible to eliminate all safety risks, but these can be reduced by understanding the hazards, establishing facility policies to reduce them, providing regular training to staff, and by the dedication of staff/management to maintain safe working practices. Safety is therefore the responsibility of everyone, staff and management alike. The goal of safety management should be to reduce the risks of danger and injury where possible and to be prepared to cope with emergencies. Essential precautions such as safety policies, training, emergency procedures, waste policy, and even possible evacuation procedures are an integral part of safety management. Although it is possible to reduce healthcare workers' exposure to hazards, doing so is largely dependent on training and staff compliance with procedures. Most accidents are avoidable with correct staff training and compliance.

Types of workplace hazards

Healthcare facility staff can face a wide range of hazards on the job. These include:
- Microbiological risks, in particular the risks of being directly exposed to various different types of pathogenic microorganism (Chapter 5).
- Chemical risks, from the various types of chemicals used for cleaning, disinfection, and sterilization. Chemicals are a significant safety concern, be they in solid, liquid, or gas form (Chapter 6). The health effects can range from short to long term.
- Device risks. Many surgical and medical devices are sharp (Chapter 4) and can damage the skin, eyes, and mucous membranes. Sharps injuries are particularly common during device processing and are an even greater concern when pathogenic microorganisms may be present. Other device risks can include electrical shock, injury due to device weight or complexity (see physical health below), or exposure to chemicals used in or with the device.
- Equipment risks. These may include the risks of burns (e.g. from the internal surface of a steam sterilizer or accidental release of steam into a working area) or injury to the hands (e.g. crushing) or feet (from dropping). Any moving part of a piece of equipment is a particular safety hazard. Equipment risks can often unintentionally become a greater concern with automated equipment.
- Physical health, including ergonomics (or human factors). Included in this subject is posture on sitting or standing while working, correct design/use of loading carts, minimizing risks from bending/moving articles, and overall well-being while working in a processing environment.
- Emotional health. Although often underestimated in comparison to other safety risks, emotional health issues such as stress should also be considered. Device processing areas can often be stressful environments.

Health and safety must be at the forefront of all decisions and policies within a processing facility. The overall safety of employees and patients is the ultimate responsibility of the facility management team. But equally, all healthcare workers must be made aware of potential hazards associated with their day-to-day activities, be trained in practices that will prevent injury and accidents, and act responsibly to ensure that they follow best practices. Safety is a team effort.

Decontamination and Device Processing in Healthcare, Second Edition. Gerald McDonnell and Georgia Alevizopoulou.
© 2025 John Wiley & Sons Ltd. Published 2025 by John Wiley & Sons Ltd.

Microbiological hazards

Microbiological safety hazards are concerned with the potential exposure to pathogenic (or disease-causing) microorganisms. These have already been introduced in Chapter 5, with examples including:

• Viruses, such as hepatitis B (which can cause liver disease), human immunodeficiency virus (HIV, the virus that causes acquired immune deficiency syndrome (AIDS), a disease of the immune system), and norovirus (which causes gastroenteritis).

• Bacteria, such as *Staphylococcus aureus* (wound, skin, and other infections), *Escherichia coli* (gastrointestinal and other diseases), and *Mycobacterium tuberculosis* (causing a respiratory disease known as tuberculosis).

The problem with microorganisms is that they cannot be seen but are often deadly. Although individuals who are infected may be diagnosed (or known) to have a particular microbial disease, many more will be carriers. Carriers may not know that they have an infection (not showing signs of disease) or may be immune to or protected from the microorganism, yet are a hidden source of pathogenic microorganisms. Similarly, many microorganisms may be relatively harmful to healthy individuals but can be a particular concern to sick (in particular immunocompromised) individuals. Microorganisms can also be picked up in a variety of ways, including through the air and surface contacts such as the hands, environmental surfaces, and reusable devices (Chapter 4).

An important concept to understand is the principle of "standard (or universal) precautions." The concept assumes that all blood and bodily substances are potential sources of infection, independent of any known or perceived risk with a patient. Typical examples of precautions used throughout the facility will include wearing of personal protective equipment (PPE), hand hygiene, safe injection practices, and safe handling of any sharp materials (such as needles; Figure 13.1).

Blood-borne pathogens are an important part of this concern. They are defined as disease-producing microorganisms spread by contact with blood or other bodily fluids contaminated with blood from an infected person. Notable examples of blood-borne pathogens are the viruses HIV and hepatitis B. There is no need to know whether the patient is infected with a particular microorganism, as it is automatically assumed that he or she and any associated bodily fluids pose a risk. Devices used for surgical and medical procedures should therefore always be considered contaminated and handled appropriately. It is good practice to ensure that the same precautions are used whether blood is obviously present or not. Standard precautions are ultimately about the safety of healthcare workers, but apply equally to the patient, and should ensure that a standard processing cycle is conducted on all devices. A system of barrier techniques and safety procedures is routinely used by healthcare workers to prevent cross-contamination and the spread of infectious diseases when caring for patients, processed devices, and dealing with healthcare waste. In some cases, extra precautions may need to be considered due to the risks of the particularly high levels of microorganisms being

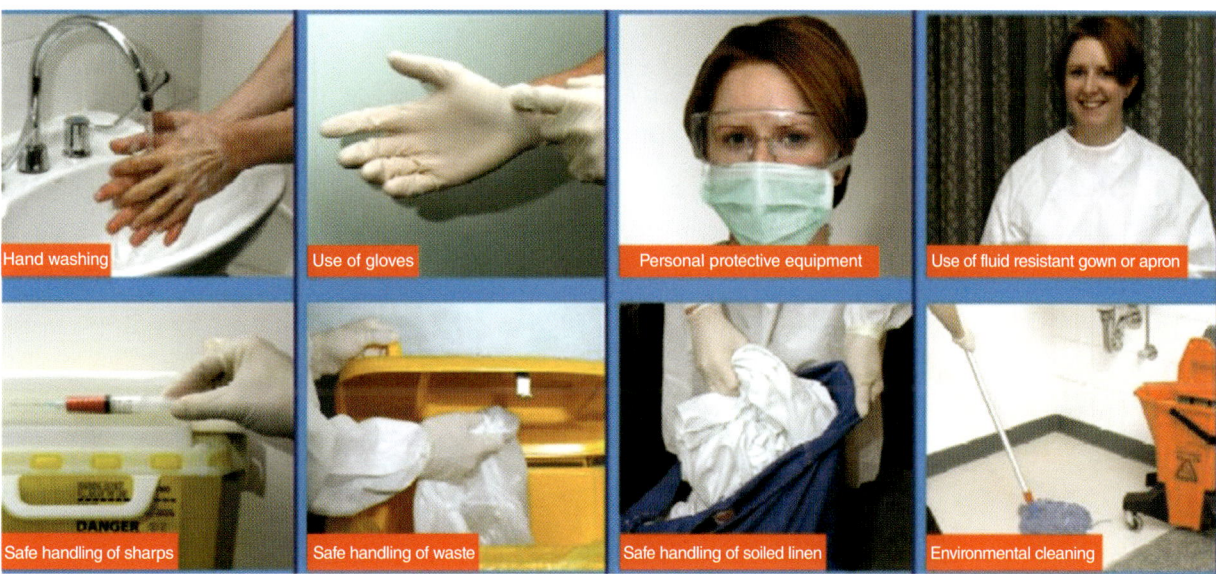

Figure 13.1 An example of a healthcare facility's standard precaution recommendations.

handled or present. Examples include precautions in the handling of wastes from patients with active Ebola virus disease or norovirus infections, which in both causes produce high viral loads in blood and diarrhea, respectively.

The role of infection prevention and control in healthcare facilities has already been introduced as procedures and practices to reduce the risks of microbial, especially pathogen, transmission (Chapter 5). These are standard precautions that are equally important in processing areas as they are in working directly with patients. Examples include:

- Use of PPE, such as gloves, masks, and eye protection.
- Frequent hand washing, in particular immediately on leaving a processing area.
- Covering cuts and abrasions when coming into contact with patients or handling contaminated materials.
- Routine surface disinfection in the immediate vicinity of patients (high-risk touch surfaces in particular) and in manual cleaning or soiled device sorting areas.
- Cleaning up known spills of blood and other bodily fluids.
- Reducing accidental cross-contamination such as by rubbing the eyes and touching the nose/mouth.
- Safe handling and decontamination of reusable devices. Clearly the greatest risk will be during the transport of soiled devices and the sorting and cleaning of devices. Devices that have been adequately disinfected (preferably to a high level; Chapter 9) can be considered safe for further handling (e.g. packaging for sterilization or transfer to a patient for use).
- Use of sterile disposable materials on patients.
- Safe handling of contaminated waste. The safe collection and disposal of needles (hypodermic and suture) and sharps (scalpel blades, lancets, razors, and scissors) is an important example (see the section on device and equipment risks). The risk of infection following a needle-stick injury with a needle from an infected patient is estimated to be 0.3% for HIV, 3% for hepatitis C, and 6–30% for hepatitis B. But this is an estimate and will depend on the precautions taken after the injury. Those precautions will include safe hospital waste management and disposal, which is discussed in more detail in the section on waste management.
- Immunization of staff against known risks (for example against hepatitis B and other viruses).

Strictly speaking, once standard precautions are in place, there should be no need to designate a set of instruments or other materials as being of greater or lesser risk, as long as the process remains consistent. Despite this, facilities may decide to have certain warnings or handling procedures in place when devices are known to be used on patients with certain diseases. Such policies should be avoided, but if not are carefully considered and kept to a minimum, as it may often be the case that diseases or associated pathogens are present but undiagnosed in a patient. Therefore, it is inappropriate to label and require special handling of devices when applying standard precautions and particularly for device processing. A current exception is the handling and processing of devices and materials used on patients with known (or highly suspected to have) prion diseases (see Chapter 5 on prions and other infectious proteins). Due to the unusual nature of these agents and particularly their unique resistance to cleaning, disinfection, and sterilization, special precautions and procedures are recommended at this time (these are considered in further detail in Chapter 15 under devices known or suspected to be contaminated with prion materials).

Microbiological safety will not only apply to patients and staff, as there may also be risks to facility visitors and to the general public. Visitor safety will be a consideration in infection prevention and control, to include various precautions depending on where the visitors will be and what they will do during their visit. Hand hygiene is always good practice (before and after visiting a hospital or clinic) and risks can also be reduced by the routine disinfection of various high-touch surfaces (such as bedrails, telephones, light switches, etc.). Visitors to a processing facility should be restricted and, when they are allowed to have access, they need to be aware of any risks and follow facility policies just like any staff (such as the use of PPE). This is particularly important for any person visiting the department for work, to include engineering or biomedical personnel (either facility staff or external contractors).

An effective facility policy should be in place to reduce microbiological risks, including in high-risk areas such as when dealing with patients, occupational exposure to blood or other bodily fluids, processing of devices/materials, and waste disposal. In addition to the specified standard precautions and procedures, guidelines should also be given to staff regarding what to do when things go wrong. Examples include a spillage of blood or bodily fluid, needle-stick or sharps injury with a contaminated device, and accidental swallowing or eye contact with soiled materials. This should include the immediate first aid required, reporting mechanisms, procedures to be followed (e.g. these may include post-exposure anti-infective prophylaxis such as taking antibiotics under care of their physician), and follow-up testing, provision of support, and counseling (if applicable).

Chemical hazards

The principles of chemistry and chemicals have been introduced in Chapter 6. A variety of chemicals in solid, liquid, and gas forms can be used in a healthcare facility, and particularly in a processing area for cleaning, disinfection, and sterilization. Chemicals are a significant safety concern and their health effects can range from short to intermediate and long term. It is estimated that nearly one-third of all occupational injuries or illnesses are linked to chemical exposure in the workplace. For example, toxic chemicals can cause health effects if they are swallowed, have contact with the skin or other parts of the body (in particular the eyes), and if harmful vapors are inhaled.

As a general statement, all chemicals can do you harm under the right conditions. Some of these are obvious, such as that strong acids and alkalis can give an immediate and even serious burn or damage when placed on the skin or eye. Others will be more subtle, with some extreme cases leading to increased allergic reactions (sensitization), toxic effects or damage over time, and carcinogenicity ("cancer-causing," where a carcinogen is a cancer-causing agent/chemical). Any chemical used during processing should be respected and the necessary precautions taken to limit exposure.

For chemical safety there are at least three considerations:
- Personal safety.
- Patient safety, which can be associated with chemicals remaining on a device surface (e.g. not being rinsed away) that subsequently contact a patient, or chemicals that could damage the device leading to other patient risks.
- Environmental safety.

Personal safety is the responsibility of each employee or worker in the area to ensure that any chemicals are correctly handled. It is the responsibility of supervisors/managers to ensure that staff are aware of any safety risks and have been given the correct training and equipment to minimize those risks. This will also apply to visitors to the processing area, as chemical accidents can happen to those in the vicinity of someone using a chemical.

In establishing and maintaining good personal safety practices when using chemicals (as for other risks), it is recommended to conduct a risk analysis (see the section later in this chapter on reducing safety risks and risk analysis). This would include identifying chemical risks in a work area, deciding and introducing measures to reduce risk (including staff training), and ensuring that these measures are maintained.

For each chemical product, it is good practice (if not also a legal requirement in most countries) for safety information to be provided by the manufacturer. This is usually provided with the product, including the product label and associated safety data sheets (SDSs). All hazardous chemicals used in the workplace (even if you are familiar with working with them at home or at work) should have an accompanying SDS specifying the risks and precautions that need to be taken when dealing with these substances. The information on an SDS will typically include:
- Product and chemical identification.
- All active constituents as well as hazardous ingredients.
- Specific health hazards.
- Precautions for use at application strength, including any exposure limits.
- Potential reactions with other chemicals/environmental conditions (e.g. temperature).
- Safe storage and handling information.
- Emergency procedures.
- Disposal methods.

Examples of SDSs are shown in Figure 13.2. It is the worker's responsibility to be aware of possible risks and the PPE that should be used.

Staff should be aware of and be able to recognize a variety of standardized warning symbols that can be used to recognize certain health risks associated with a product (Figure 13.3).

In general, the most effective ways to reduce the risks associated with any chemical hazard are to provide training, use PPE, and periodically audit that safety practices are being followed in a department. Training is the first step, to allow any chemical user to understand their risks, so that they can appreciate how PPE or other safety precautions can reduce those risks. PPE includes equipment such as gloves, safety glasses or goggles, face shields, disposable aprons/gowns, and safety shoes/covers (Figure 13.4). For example, safety glasses are usually designed to protect the eyes from splashes from the front as well as from the sides.

The final consideration is chemical safety auditing. Auditing can be defined as an evaluation or review of practices based on established procedures. When safety policies and procedures are put in place it is important to review over time that they are being followed. Audits can be defined at intervals, in cases where they are expected, or, more beneficially, they may be unexpected. They help establish that safety is important in each area, that staff/management are committed to it, and to verify that safe practices are periodically reviewed. The outcome of audits also assists in maintaining a continuous improvement culture.

Some chemicals are considered of higher risk than others and may require even tighter controls. Examples include the use of various types of gases such as ethylene oxide (see Chapter 11 on chemical sterilization) or aldehyde-based liquid disinfectants like glutaraldehyde (see Chapter 9 on chemical disinfection). Ethylene oxide gas, for example, is flammable/explosive at concentrations of ~3% gas in air, can be lethal at 800 ppm, and is considered a carcinogen (cancer causing) over time. For this reason, reasonably tight controls and monitoring systems are strongly encouraged to be employed in areas using the gas for sterilization. Special facility design or handling equipment (e.g. dedicated ventilation) may be required based on manufacturer's guidelines and local health and safety requirements.

In addition to personal safety, there are chemical hazards to patients and to the environment. Patients' exposure to chemical hazards should be minimized by correct use and removal of chemicals used for processing or for maintaining a device. Patient risks will include direct or indirect safety concerns.

MATERIAL SAFETY DATA SHEET

Supersedes: 2/1/00

Issue Date: 6/01
Issue Date: N/A

SECTION I - CHEMICAL PRODUCT

Identity: Disinfectant Powder Cleanser

Brands: COMET Disinfectant Cleanser with Chlorinol (Professional Line)

Hazard Rating: 1	Health: 1	4=EXTREME
	Flammability:	3=HIGH
	Reactivity:	2= MODERATE
		1=SLIGHT

Emergency Telephone Number: - 1-800-332-7787 or call Local Poison Control Center

SECTION II - COMPOSITION AND INGREDIENTS

Ingredients/Chemical Name: Bleach, cleaning agents (calcium carbonate, sodium carbonate, anionic surfactants), quality control agents, perfume, color. Comet Disinfectant Cleanser with Chlorinol contains no phosphorus.

Hazardous Ingredients as defined by OSHA, 29 CFR 1910.1200.

Chemical Name	Common Name	CAS No.	Recommended Limits	Composition Range	LD50/LC50
Calcium carbonate	Limestone	1317-65-3	ACGIH TWA: 10mg/m³ (total dust) / 5 mg/m³ (respirable dust) OSHA PEL: 15 mg/m³	60-100%	NA/NA
Silica, quartz	Quartz (naturally occurring component of limestone)	14808-60-7	ACGIH TWA: 0.1mg/m³ (respirable dust) OSHA TWA: 0.1 mg/m³	0.1-1%	9 g/kg/NA

SECTION III - HAZARDS IDENTIFICATION

Health Hazards (Acute and Chronic):

Ingestion: Mild mucous membrane irritant. May result in gastrointestinal irritation with nausea, vomiting and diarrhea.

Eye Contact: Mild eye irritant. Direct contact with eye may result in superficial, temporary irritation similar to those produced by other household detergents.

Skin: Mild skin irritant. Prolonged skin contact or direct contact with eye may result in superficial, temporary irritation similar to those produced by other household detergents.

Inhalation: Mild respiratory irritant. Unusually high exposures may cause coughing or irritation of nose and throat.

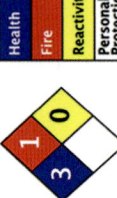

Material Safety Data Sheet
Carbamide peroxide MSDS

Section 1: Chemical Product and Company Identification

Product Name: Carbamide peroxide

Catalog Codes: SLU1123

CAS#: 124-43-6

RTECS: Not available.

TSCA: TSCA 8(b) inventory: Urea peroxide

CI#: Not available.

Synonym: Oxygel; Peroxigel; Urea peroxide; Urea Hydrogen Peroxide; Carbamide Peroxide, USP

Chemical Name: Carbamide Peroxide

Chemical Formula: CH4N2O.H2O2

Contact Information:

Sciencelab.com, Inc.
14025 Smith Rd.
Houston, Texas 77396

US Sales: **1-800-901-7247**
International Sales: **1-281-441-4400**

Order Online: **ScienceLab.com**

CHEMTREC (24HR Emergency Telephone), call: 1-800-424-9300

International CHEMTREC, call: 1-703-527-3887

For non-emergency assistance, call: 1-281-441-4400

Section 2: Composition and Information on Ingredients

Composition:

Name	CAS #	% by Weight
Urea peroxide	124-43-6	100

Toxicological Data on Ingredients: Urea peroxide LD50: Not available. LC50: Not available.

Section 3: Hazards Identification

Potential Acute Health Effects: Very hazardous in case of skin contact (irritant), of eye contact (irritant), of ingestion, of inhalation. Hazardous in case of skin contact (corrosive), of eye contact (corrosive). The amount of tissue damage depends on length of contact. Eye contact can result in corneal damage or blindness. Skin contact can produce inflammation and blistering. Inhalation of dust will produce irritation to gastro-intestinal or respiratory tract, characterized by burning, sneezing and coughing. Severe over-exposure can produce lung damage, choking, unconsciousness or death. Prolonged exposure may result in skin burns and ulcerations. Over-exposure by inhalation may cause respiratory irritation. Inflammation of the eye is characterized by redness, watering, and itching. Skin inflammation is characterized by itching, scaling, reddening, or, occasionally, blistering.

Potential Chronic Health Effects: CARCINOGENIC EFFECTS: Not available. MUTAGENIC EFFECTS: Not available. TERATOGENIC EFFECTS: Not available. DEVELOPMENTAL TOXICITY: Not available. Repeated exposure of the eyes to a low level of dust can produce eye irritation. Repeated skin exposure can produce local skin destruction, or dermatitis. Repeated inhalation of dust can produce varying degree of respiratory irritation or lung damage.

Figure 13.2 Examples of the front pages of two safety data sheets (SDSs). Note: an SDS can be a number of pages long.

A direct concern is where a chemical is mistakenly used and left on a device (residues) prior to its use in/on a patient; in these cases, toxic effects can be observed in the patient leading to health consequences. Examples can include overuse of the chemical (e.g. not diluted correctly) and inadequate rinsing (to remove the chemistry after use). Many chemical disinfectants, for example, require multiple cycles of water rinsing (sometimes up to five to six rinses in fresh water each time) to adequately remove toxic residues of the chemistry. Indirect effects are due to damage by the chemical to the device; this damage over time can lead to problems in the safe use of the instrument on a patient.

Environmental safety with the use of chemicals is a growing concern, with many countries putting restrictions on the types of chemicals that can be used or how they are handled/disposed of in a facility. The main concerns are those regarding chemicals that are not easily broken down in the environment and can therefore lead to accumulation in environmental sources (such as in water, the air, and plants/animals). It is the responsibility of the manufacturer to ensure it complies with any local or regional regulations, as well of as the healthcare facility to follow local regulations such as those on the disposal of certain types of chemicals down public drains or sewer systems.

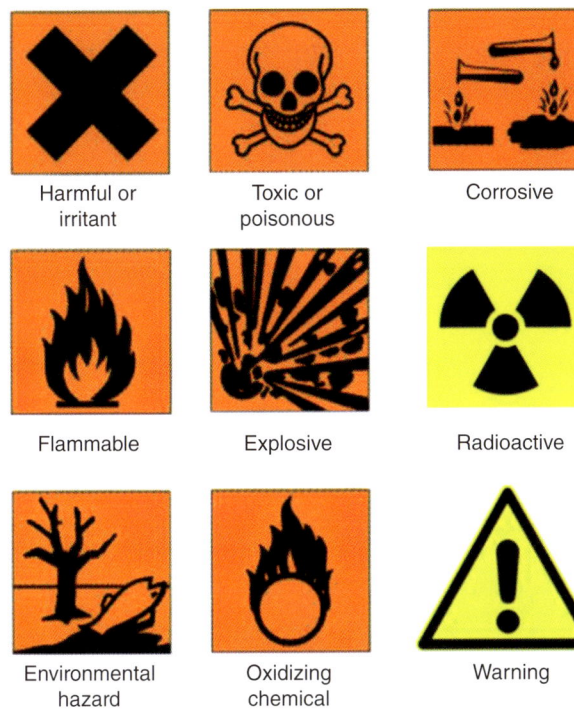

Figure 13.3 Examples of widely used internationally standardized chemical safety warning symbols.

Device and equipment hazards

Devices and associated equipment can present a range of safety risks to staff and patients alike. These include:
- General device/equipment hazards. Examples include sharp devices or needle-sticks, as well as hot surfaces (e.g. the internal chamber of a steam sterilizer or thermal washer-disinfector). Many surgical and medical devices are sharp (see Chapter 4) and can damage on contact the skin, eyes, and mucous membranes. Examples include various types of forceps, needles, scalpel blades, and scissors routinely used in surgical/medical procedures. Sharps (or "percutaneous") injuries are particularly common during device processing and are an even greater concern when pathogenic microorganisms may be present, such as during sorting and cleaning of soiled devices or other materials (see Chapter 7 on post-procedure sorting) and during waste disposal (discussed later in this chapter). An effective sharps injury program should concentrate on prevention and should include training on preventing such injuries. It should also advise on measures to take in the event of a sharps injury, such as for smaller wounds to include immediate washing, encouraging free bleeding of puncture wounds, and reporting of the incident to management. A further risk to the skin/eyes is from burns, both from heat (e.g. from the internal surface of a steam sterilizer or accidental release of steam into a working area) and from chemicals (e.g. on accidental release

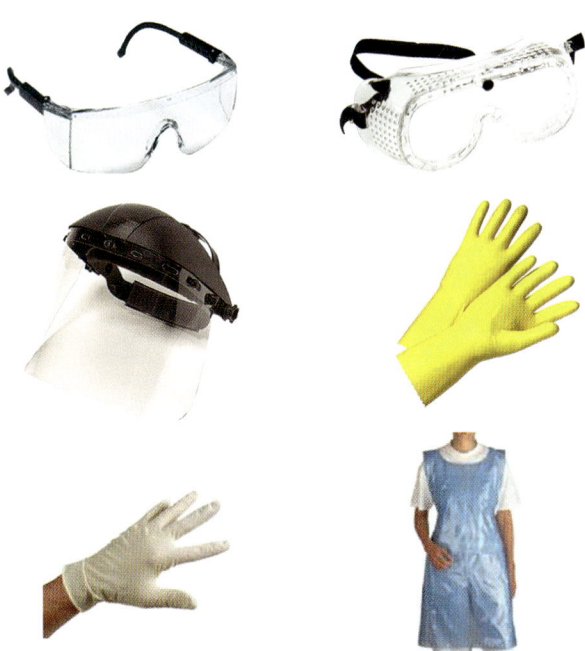

Figure 13.4 Various types of personal protective equipment.

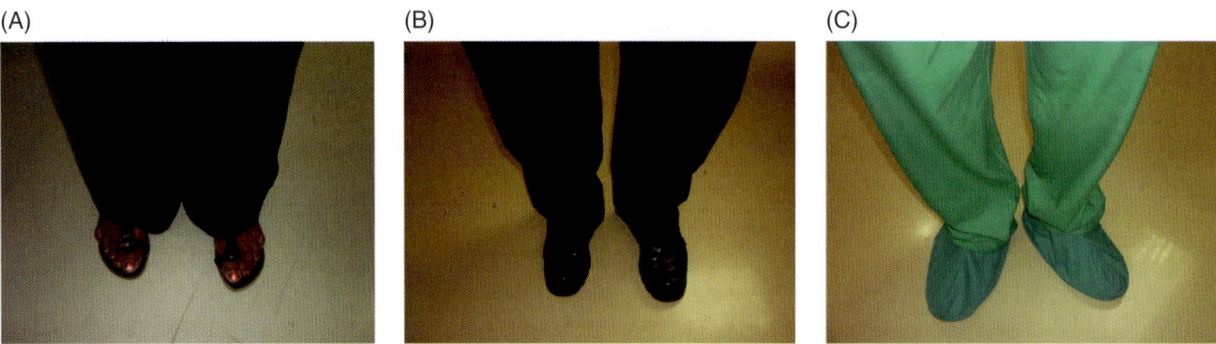

Figure 13.5 Protective footwear. (A) *Inappropriate* (although comfortable) footwear; (B, C) more protective footwear considering the risks of chemical, infectious, or weight-associated risks in a processing area.

of chemicals during an automated chemical disinfection process; chemical risks are further considered in Chapter 6).
• Mechanical hazards. Examples will include injury to the hands (e.g. crushing) or feet (from dropping). Any moving part of a piece of equipment is a particular safety hazard (e.g. washer-disinfector and sterilizer doors, as well as automated loading–unloading equipment). This will not only impact staff/visitors but may also affect device safety when damage occurs due to inadequate equipment maintenance or use. Consideration may need to be given to the use of correct footwear (in particular to protect from mechanical and spill risks; Figure 13.5).
• Electrical hazards. Many devices and processing equipment are driven by electrical power. The combination of water and electricity is a particular safety hazard, as is lack of correct maintenance of equipment/devices. Any such risks should be clearly identified by the device/equipment manufacturer in their instructions for use. Electrical risks can also be caused inadvertently by staff or be due to poor equipment installation (Figure 13.6).
• Environmental considerations. These continue to be a developing but important topic and can include the utility consumption (water, electricity, etc.) of devices/equipment, but more particularly the handling of devices/equipment on decommissioning. Regulations are developing on the safe disposal of such items, including electronic and material handling requirements.

It is important to ensure that these hazards are considered during a risk assessment and policies/procedures put in place to ensure that any risks are reduced to a minimum. Staff training is important in these cases. That will include clear designation of responsibilities and how to troubleshoot equipment malfunctions. Untrained staff should not be allowed to investigate the mechanical/electrical components of equipment; this should be the responsibility of designated internal or external engineering, biomedical specialists, or healthcare

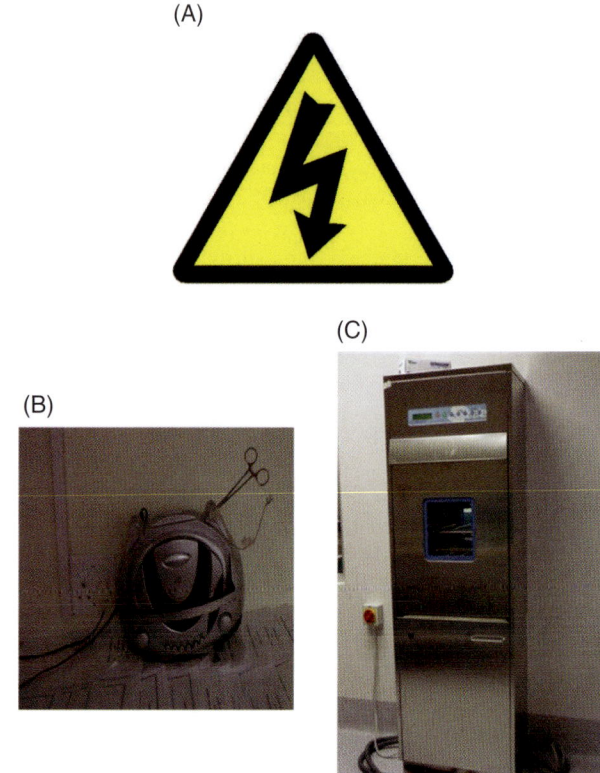

Figure 13.6 Electrical hazards. (A) A typical electrical hazard sign and (B, C) examples of potential electrical hazards. Note that (C) is a washer-disinfector that is not in use (feedwater lines shown at the front) but plugged into an electrical source; the free lines would also pose a tripping hazard to staff.

technology management professionals. Regarding mechanical, electrical, and environmental safety, any risks should be clearly identified by the device/equipment manufacturer in the instructions for use. It is the manufacturer's responsibility to reduce any such safety hazards during the design and routine testing of any device/equipment. It is equally the user's responsibility to ensure that any designated safety hazards are understood, and that devices and equipment are operated and handled correctly. The maintenance of older equipment is a particularly high risk, as the older the equipment the more likely it is that things can go wrong (and the less likely that the equipment will comply with the latest guidelines and regulations). Such equipment should be closely monitored and maintained to ensure optimal and safe use.

Physical and emotional hazards

Physical health is an important consideration in any work environment, to reduce any unnecessary physical stress or risk of injury on the body (short or long term) from any repetitive and/or periodic actions such as lifting, pulling, pushing, and so on. Ergonomics (also known as human factors) is a broad subject that considers the understanding of human–equipment interaction and design to minimize any safety risks and the optimum use of equipment. Safety risks here include:
- Posture on sitting or standing while working, including while using computers or electronic management systems (Figure 13.7).
- Minimizing risks from bending, or picking up or moving articles from one area to another (Figure 13.8).
- Correct design/use of loading carts (pulling/pushing; Figure 13.8).
- Repeated lifting and loading positions, which, if not performed safely, can impose an increased risk.
- Overstretching into, up to, or down to a particular area.
- Safe operation of equipment and accessories according to instructions for use.
- Minimizing risks with any mechanical moving parts.
- Overall well-being while working in a processing environment (e.g. stress, fatigue, shift work).

Back and neck injuries account for nearly 50% of workplace compensation claims in healthcare facilities. The most common causes of back injury are heavy lifting, over-stretching, postural stress (on sitting/standing), and repetitive job performance. The primary approach to reducing back injury should be training and reducing manual lifting and load-bearing tasks.

Examples of practices to reduce ergonomic risks will include:
- Training on safe lifting, moving, pulling, and pushing techniques. When high risks are identified, these should be reduced, such as by reducing the allowable weights of loads/packs/sets, by providing tools to aid in reaching into equipment/areas to retrieve items, or the introduction of motorized transport carts. The allowable weight of an instrument set should be based on whether personnel can comfortably carry the set in the recommended lifting and carrying posture; some guidelines recommend set weights of no more than 12 kg (~25 lb), but even this may be considered too heavy for some individuals. In some national codes of practice a risk assessment must be carried out on weights and force hazards. Considerations when conducting such a risk assessment include:
  ○ Frequency and duration.
  ○ Position of the load relative to the body.
  ○ Distance moved.
  ○ Characteristics of the load (e.g. weight and size).

Remember that the introduction of a method to reduce one risk may itself lead to another risk.
- Height-adjustable workbenches and chairs, which allow a person to adjust to the right posture position when sitting or standing (Figure 13.9). The same will apply to height-adjustable sinks or ensuring that the sink design is not too deep to allow for manual cleaning.
- Correct organization of workbench materials. All materials in a packaging area, to include packaging materials, indicators, and so on, should be located within easy reach. A similar concept should apply to device-sorting or manual cleaning areas. This will allow for not only good ergonomics but also efficient work practices (see Chapter 14).
- Wrist supports at every computer location.

Although often underestimated in comparison to other safety risks, emotional health issues such as stress should be considered. Stress can be defined as a state or worry or the feeling of being under too much pressure. It is not always a bad thing, as pressure can be motivating, improves performance, and even increases productivity; however, excessive or prolonged pressure on an individual or group of employees can lead to unhealthy stress. Stress symptoms can depend on the person and situation, but can include difficulty in sleeping, irritation, and increased mistakes. These situations should be closely monitored in staff before they become serious. Suggestions to improve emotional health include:
- Adequate facility design, including good lighting (preferably natural light), adequate ventilation, and comfortable humidity/temperature conditions.
- Sufficient staff to cope with the demands on the processing department.
- Introducing policies and procedures to protect staff from difficult situations. Examples include a policy regarding being asked to process a device and not provided with processing instructions, or being requested to skip stages of a defined decontamination cycle due to surgical/medical needs. A simple suggestion in both cases is to have a form that needs to be signed by an authorized person (which may be a senior member of surgical/medical staff or infection prevention/control) that assumes any legal risk for such a breach of policy.
- Fair and legal working practices, such as intolerance of abuse (verbal and physical), frequent breaks, reasonable

374 Decontamination and Device Processing in Healthcare

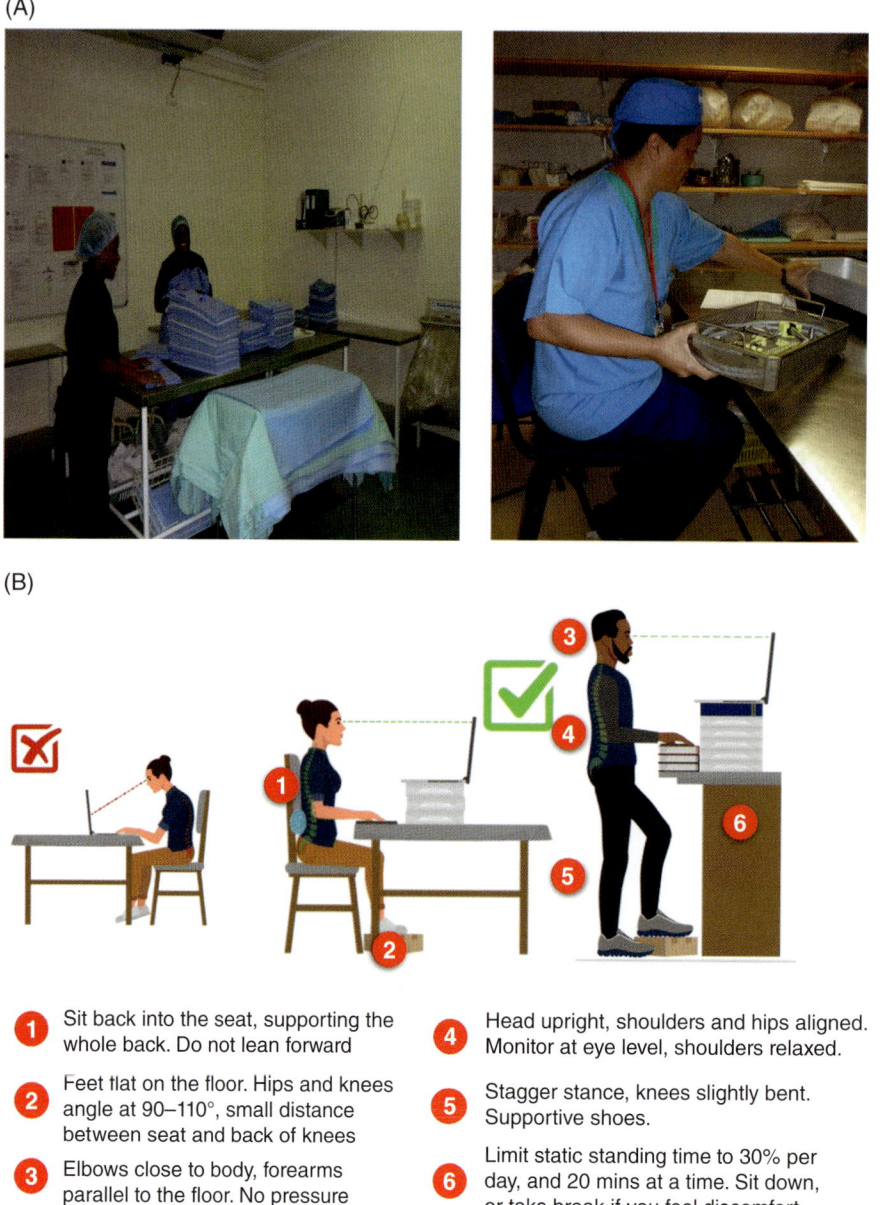

Figure 13.7 (A, B) Standing or sitting close to a work surface at the right height and with a straight back can help reduce the risks of injury.

working hours, and allowable vacations. Investment in staff, both financially and emotionally, helps to retain good-quality and trained staff.
- Including staff in department decisions and quality improvement exercises (see Chapter 14 on personnel management).
- Being a good personnel manager and encouraging teamwork (see Chapter 14).

Reducing safety hazards and risk analysis

It is important to understand the hazards within any working environment and especially when things can go wrong. Risk analysis can therefore be an important tool to identify and reduce any safety concerns. Risk analysis in reducing risks during the processing cycle is considered further in Chapter 14.

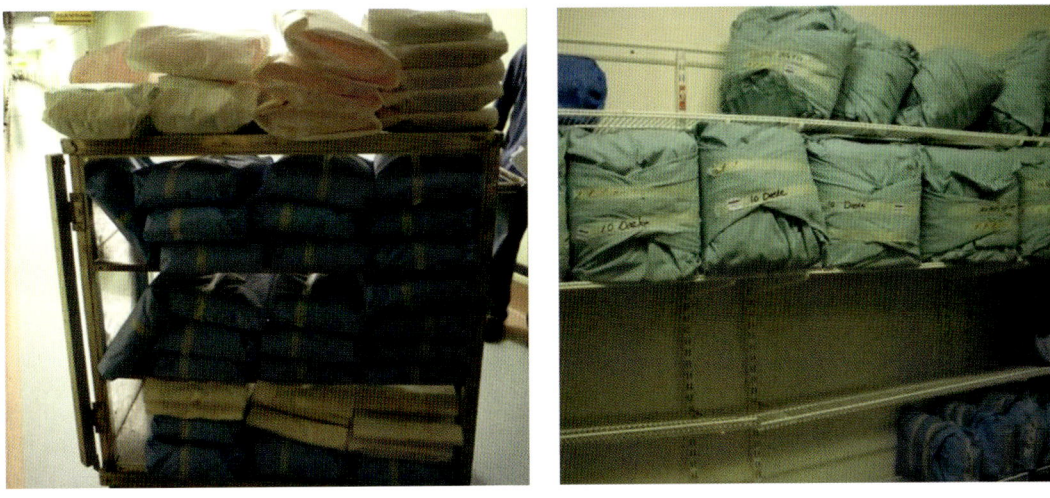

Figure 13.8 Pushing or pulling overloaded or heavy transport carts or lifting heavy loads (in the case of storage) can be safety concerns.

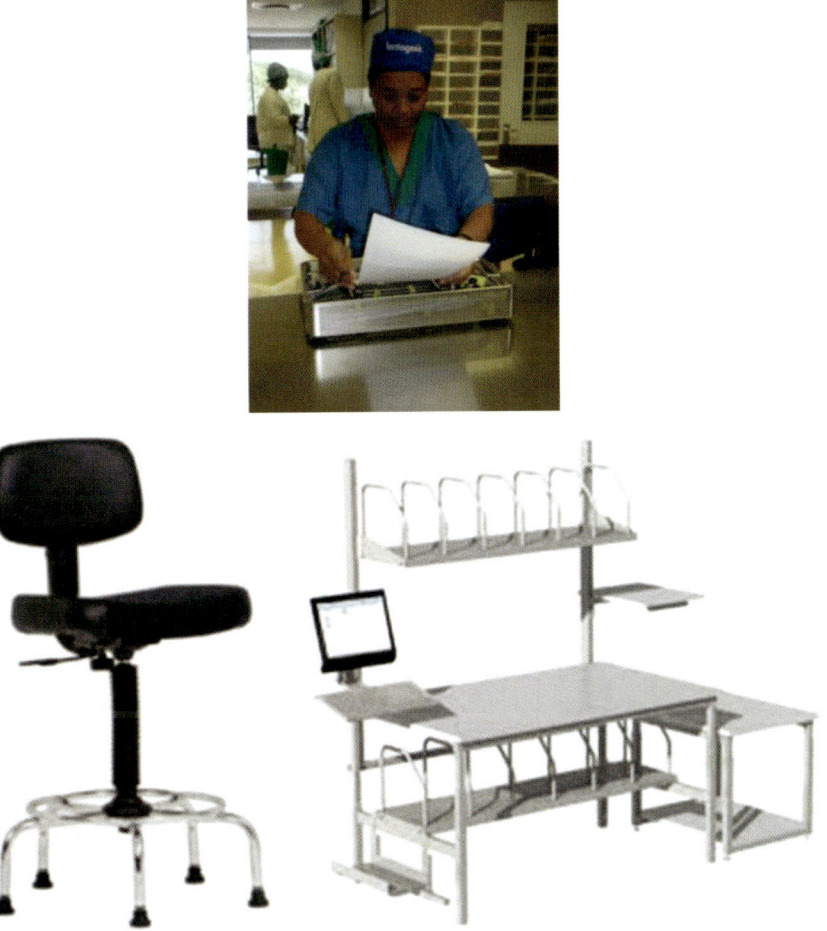

Figure 13.9 Height-adjustable chairs and workbenches.

The same concepts are applicable to safety and are further considered in this section.

A common approach is known as hazard analysis and risk assessment (or Hazard Analysis Critical Control Point, HACCP). This is widely used in industrial situations, such as in food production, but the concepts apply equally to device processing areas. There are four essential steps to consider in establishing and maintaining good and safe practices:

- Identify and understand any hazards (microbiological, chemical, device, equipment, physical, and emotional) in a given area.
- Decide what are the highest risks and what precautions are necessary to reduce these risks.
- Introduce and train staff on any procedures or control mechanisms to prevent or control the risks.
- Ensure that procedures/measures are used, are maintained (e.g. by auditing), and are optimized over time.

This systematic approach should be conducted with a team of people from many facets including but not limited to infection control, biomedical engineering, technicians, manufacturers, medical staff, and finance and legal representatives (see Chapter 14). Safe work practices are designed to reduce the risks caused by hazards and ensure that they are kept at a minimum while at work, not only for personnel but also for patients.

The first two steps are assisted by completing a safety risk analysis within the processing area, as in Chapter 14 in the section on process risk analysis. This allows for a structured teamwork exercise to consider any risks and their priority. The introduction of any control measure may include training, new or existing PPE, new equipment or tools, and so on. Many of these may require investment, either minimal or significant, therefore management should be involved in understanding any safety risks and recommendations from a risk analysis; where a specific investment cannot be made, alternative measures should be identified and introduced. The final step is equally important, as safety procedures are only as good as the people who use them. It is therefore essential to ensure that staff (and visitors) follow all safety rules and instructions within an area. Managers should lead by example. They should carefully follow the rules themselves and should have zero tolerance of any staff/visitor (despite their job description) not following safety standards within an area. It is also recommended that a periodic audit of safety measures should be conducted within the area. Audits can be expected (e.g. scheduled every month) or unexpected, but either way staff should be aware that they will occur. The audit may be conducted by a manager, designated member of staff, or an external person (e.g. an infection prevention nurse or facility safety officer). Be careful to investigate any reasons for lack of compliance with specific safety measures. For example, certain types of PPE may be uncomfortable to wear, so alternatives may be identified with the help of staff to improve compliance. As in all cases, frequent, deliberate, and/or repeated refusal to follow rules and policies, including safety measures, within a department or area may require disciplinary action.

Reducing safety risks in a work environment should be a constant goal. Continuous improvement should be encouraged. This will include full investigations of any near-misses or actual incidents, with a re-evaluation of any applicable or associated safety measures. The initial risk analysis can be periodically reviewed to ensure it is up to date (e.g. if new chemicals or equipment have been introduced) or if any further improvements can be made.

Overall, risk analysis and management can help to create a safety culture within any processing area or facility. For example, research has shown that frequent management visits to work areas and regular "safety rounds" convey a message to employees that safety is important. Another safety strategy is publishing results in the work area that highlight how many accidents have occurred or even been avoided. These are simple, yet effective methods to encourage safe working practices in any area.

Specific safety considerations

Waste management

Waste management is an important societal problem, but particular attention is paid in this section to the safe handling and disposal of healthcare waste. This can include a wide range of materials and contaminants such as:

- General paper, plastics, or other used packaging wastes.
- Patient materials, including blood, other bodily fluids/wastes, and even body parts.
- Various chemicals (used or expired).
- Damaged, old, or expired devices or equipment.
- Used single-use devices (needles, catheters, sharps, etc.).
- Pharmaceuticals.
- Radioactive materials.

Healthcare facilities are encouraged to dispose of waste (hazardous or non-hazardous) in a responsible and legal manner to avoid risks to individuals and the environment. It is therefore essential that each facility has a waste disposal policy in place for the segregation and handling of medical waste from the point of generation to any treatment and safe disposal. An audit of what waste is generated by a facility is necessary to understand the types and volumes of waste generated so that an appropriate waste management policy can be put into place.

Most countries will have legislation regarding waste management and ways of enforcing it. The legislation may stand alone or be part of a more comprehensive document (e.g. total healthcare management). Such laws are usually complemented by policy documents and technical guidelines. These should specify the requirements for the treatment of different waste categories; segregation, collection, storage, handling, disposal, and transport of waste; responsibilities; and training requirements. They will also consider any resources and facilities (e.g. incinerators) available in a particular area and any cultural aspects that may apply.

Management and treatment options should be aimed at protecting the healthcare worker, patients, and the general population while at the same time minimizing environmental exposures. Individuals who may be put at risk and potentially exposed to infection, pollution, toxic hazards, and injury by incorrectly managing waste include:

- Medical staff: doctors, nurses, technicians, etc.
- Patients receiving treatment in healthcare facilities as well as their visitors.
- Support services staff: laundries, waste handling and transportation services, sanitary staff, hospital maintenance personnel.
- Workers in any waste disposal facilities
- The general public, through contact with items found in waste outside the healthcare facilities when it is directly accessible to them (e.g. syringes).

Waste segregation and types of waste

Waste management is a specialized activity requiring well-equipped and adequately trained staff. The greatest impact of a waste management system is at the point of use. Healthcare waste is approximately 80% general (non-hazardous) waste and 20% hazardous waste that may be infectious, toxic, or radioactive. Most hazardous waste (75%) can be considered as being potentially infectious (e.g. soiled materials, used devices, or body parts), while the remainder may include various chemicals, pharmaceuticals, genotoxic waste, and radioactive matter.

The key to effective management of healthcare waste is segregation at the point of use (Figure 13.10 and Table 13.1). For example, infectious materials should be separated from non-infectious materials as they will be handled differently during disposal. Segregation and clear identification of wastes reduce disposal costs and assist in protecting the environment. The World Health Organization divides hazardous healthcare waste into the following eight categories:

- General: this includes wastes that do not pose any particular biological, chemical, radioactive, or physical hazard. They may need to be separated into recyclable or non-recyclable depending on the facility recommendations. This will also include some types of liquids and chemicals that can be safely discarded to drain, in accordance with facility, regional, and manufacturer's requirements.
- Sharps: any medical equipment that could puncture the skin, e.g. needles, infusion sets, scalpels, knives, blades, and broken glass.

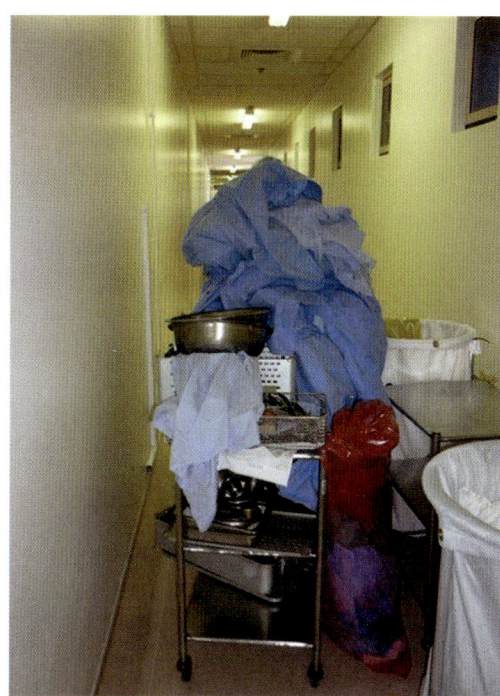

Figure 13.10 A typical example of surgical waste requiring segregation at the point of use/processing as part of facility waste management.

- Infectious: potentially containing or known to contain pathogens. Examples include discarded medical materials or equipment that has been in contact with bodily fluids such as feces, urine, blood, sputum, or other body fluids. Special consideration may need to be given to the handling of certain types of infectious wastes, such as materials with known or suspected contamination with prions (see Chapter 15).
- Pathological: human tissues or fluids, e.g. body parts; blood and other bodily fluids. Such waste will also be considered infectious but may need to be handled separately.
- Pharmaceutical: unused pharmaceuticals, such as vaccines and drugs, that have been opened, spilt, or have expired.
- Chemical: potentially hazardous chemicals discarded during the decontamination process, laboratory reagents, unused concentrated expired disinfectants, solvents, cleaning solutions, etc. This can also include materials such as batteries and heavy metals that may require special disposal procedures.
- Cytotoxic (or genotoxic): highly hazardous, mutagenic, teratogenic, or carcinogenic chemical waste, such as cytotoxic drugs used in cancer treatment. Cytotoxic/genotoxic drugs have the ability to reduce/stop the growth of fast-growing cells and are used in chemotherapy for cancer treatment. Feces, vomit, or urine from patients treated with these drugs should also be treated as cytotoxic.

Table 13.1 Examples of segregated healthcare wastes based on type. Note that color coding is not standardized and can vary depending on the supplier and facility requirements.

Waste type	Examples	Disposal	Notes
General	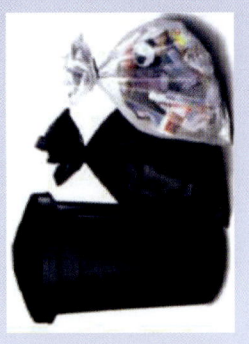	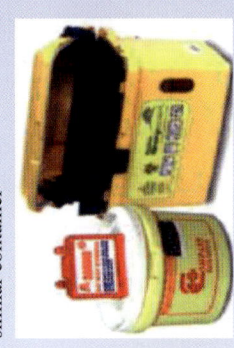 Black or clear plastic bags.	Normal, household-type waste Paper and glass segregated for recycling Normal disposal and general landfill site or similar
Sharps	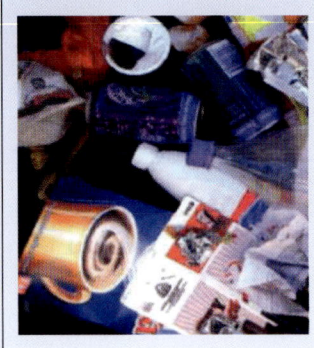	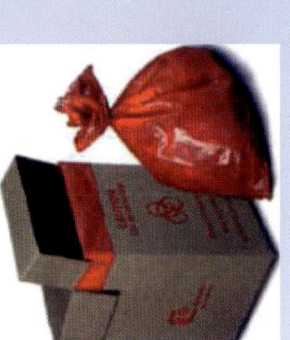 Yellow (blue or orange) locked lid or similar container	Needles, syringes, scalpels, blades, and vials Specialized collection, treatment, and disposal
Infectious		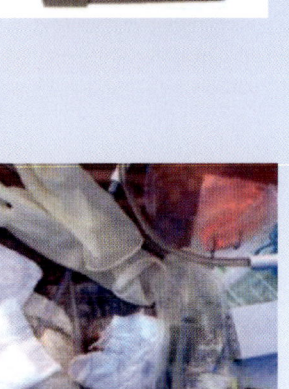 Red (yellow or orange) bags or containerized systems	Known contaminated items such as bandages, swabs, gloves Specialized collection, treatment, and disposal

Pathological

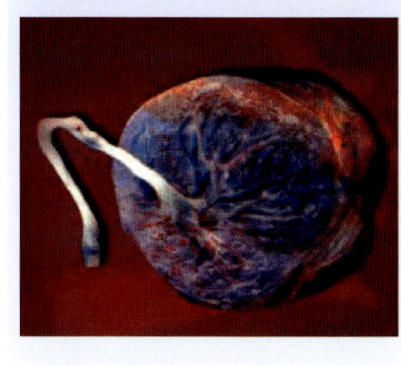

Red (or orange) bags, containers, and liquid-handling systems (e.g. with solidifiers)

Human tissues (e.g. amputated limbs) and liquids
Specialized collection (often including refrigeration), treatment, and disposal

Pharmaceutical

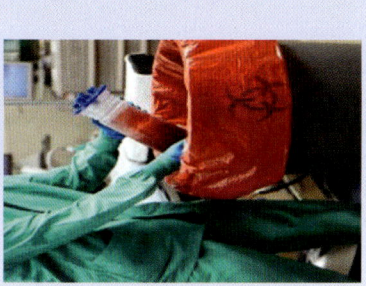

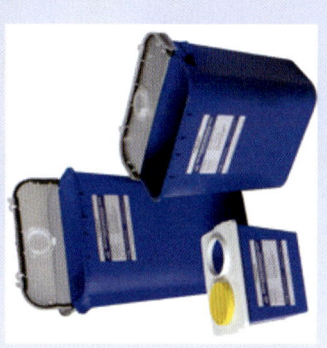

Blue containers or bags

Expired or waste medication
Specialized collection, treatment, and disposal

Chemical

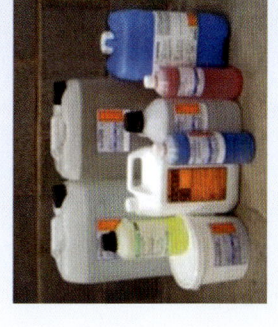

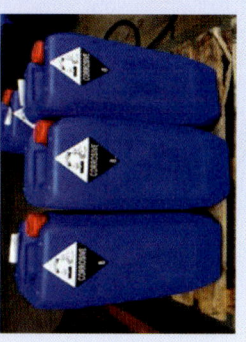

Various types of containers

Expired or waste chemicals
Some may be directly discarded in the drain but others require specialized collection, treatment, and disposal

(*continued*)

Table 13.1 (cont'd).

Waste type	Examples	Disposal	Notes
Cytotoxic		Purple containers or bags	Cytotoxic or cytostatic products Specialized collection, treatment, and disposal
Radioactive		Sealed, lead containers or disposal bags, as applicable	Waste generated by nuclear medicine or oncology Specialized collection, treatment, and disposal

- Radioactive: from the use of radiation (Chapter 6) in medical applications, such as for cancer therapy and imaging. This is typically low-level radioactive waste, including radioactive forms of chemicals such as cobalt, technetium, iodine, and iridium.

Segregation should always be at point of use and is the responsibility of the waste producer. The easiest and most effective way of identifying the categories of waste is by sorting into color-coded and correctly identified plastic bags or containers (Table 13.1). But it is important to note that color coding of waste can vary depending on the facility and provider of the various types of disposal systems. In addition to color coding the following practices are recommended:

- General, non-hazardous healthcare waste should be disposed of as regular, domestic (household) waste. It can be collected in washable containers or cardboard containers lined with black or clear plastic bags. Other types of wastes can include used containers, including pressurized containers such as aerosol cans with pressurized liquids, gas, or powdered materials, and electronic equipment, which may require special disposal in accordance with manufacturer's instructions. Care may need to be taken with certain types of materials, for instance aerosol containers or batteries should not be mixed with general waste destined for incineration due to explosion risks.
- Infectious waste should be marked with the international infectious substance symbol (Figure 13.11). Bags and containers

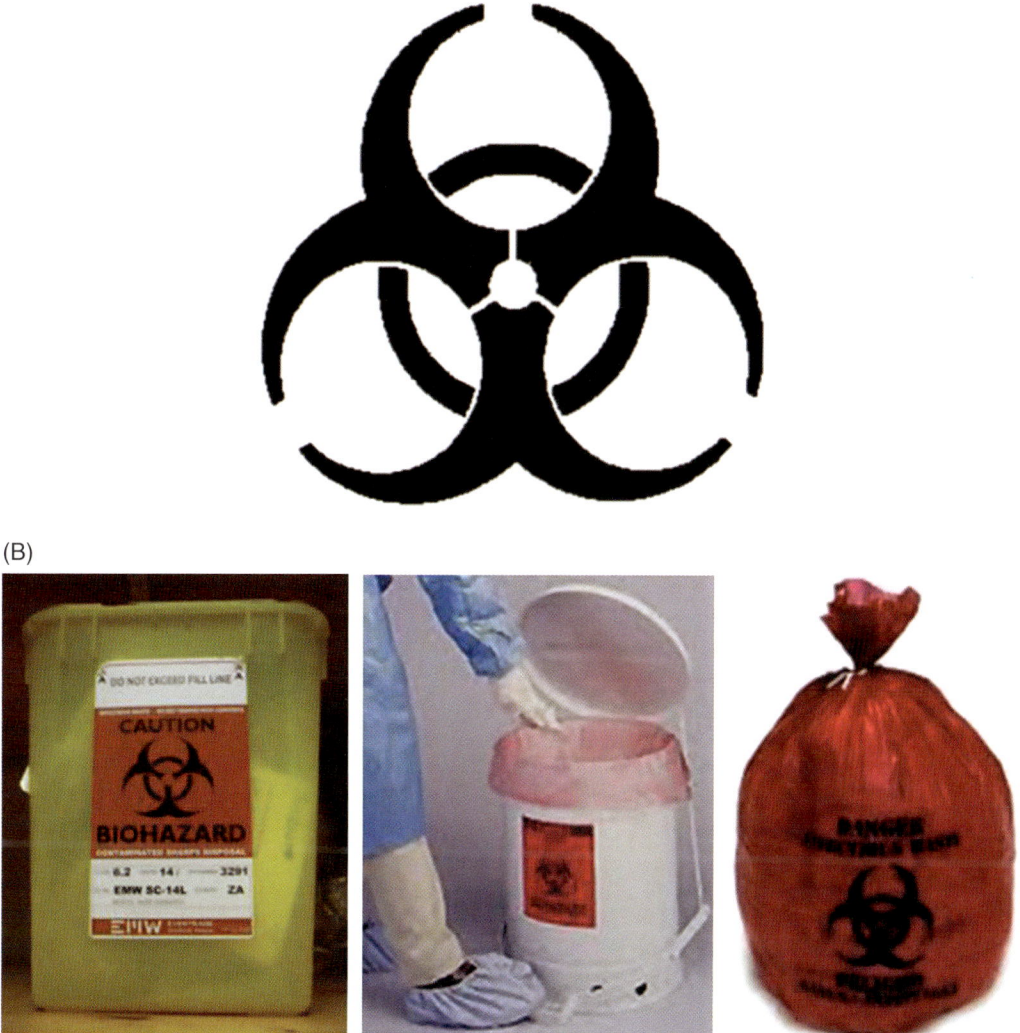

Figure 13.11 (A) The international symbol for an infectious substance and (B) examples of its use on waste containers/bags.

for this waste are generally colored red, yellow, or orange. Colored bags should be supported in washable containers or cardboard containers lined with a red or yellow plastic bag. Small amounts of chemical or pharmaceutical waste may be collected together with infectious waste. It is recommended that infectious waste should, whenever feasible, be sterilized as soon as possible by steam (autoclaving) or by incineration. Special handling may be required for waste materials considered to be "highly infectious," in particular large volumes or high concentrations of infectious waste.
• Cytotoxic waste should be collected in strong, leak-proof containers clearly labeled as cytotoxic (Figure 13.12). Containers/bags for cytotoxic waste are often colored purple.
• Sharps wastes are generally collected together, regardless of whether or not they are known to be contaminated/infectious. Containers (Figure 13.13; usually designated as biohazardous) should be rigid, impermeable, tamper proof, and covered so that they safely retain the sharps and any residual liquids that may be present (e.g. from syringes).
• Chemical (non-cytotoxic) and pharmaceutical solid wastes are typically collected in brown or blue plastic bags or containers. Large quantities of liquid/solid/gas chemical waste should be packed in chemical-resistant containers with the identity of the chemicals clearly marked on the outside and sent to specialized treatment facilities. Hazardous chemical wastes of different types should never be mixed, with reference to their respective SDSs (see the earlier section on chemical risks and Figure 13.2). Some wastes that are known to contain a high content of heavy metals (e.g. cadmium or mercury) may need to be collected and treated separately. These heavy metals can be found in broken mercury-containing thermometers and blood-pressure gauges.
• Large quantities of obsolete or expired pharmaceuticals stored in hospital wards or departments should be returned to the facility pharmacy for safe disposal.
• Radioactive waste, where applicable, should be collected in a lead box labeled with the symbol for radioactivity (Figure 13.14). Bags or containers for radioactive waste are usually colored yellow. Low-level radioactive infectious waste (e.g. swabs, syringes for diagnostic or therapeutic use) may be collected in bags or containers for infectious waste, but may require special handling in compliance with local/regional requirements.

Staff should refrain from correcting segregation mistakes by removing items from a bag or container after disposal. If general and hazardous wastes are accidentally mixed, the mixture should be treated as hazardous.

Waste transport and storage

Accumulation of waste is a significant health risk in any facility. Waste should be collected and removed according to the facility's policy on a regular basis. It is recommended that waste containers/bags should not be overfilled. For example, when bags are three-quarters full they should be closed with

(A)

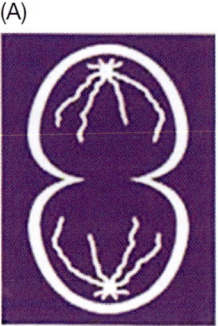

(B)

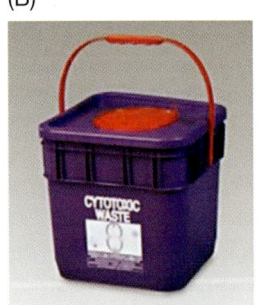 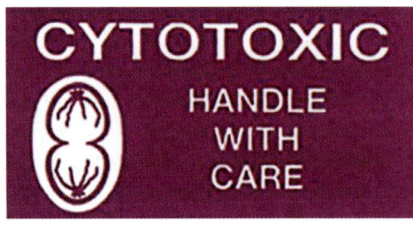 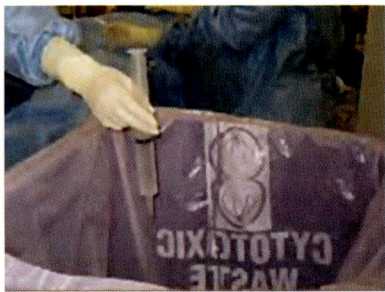

Figure 13.12 (A) The international symbol for a cytotoxic hazard and (B) examples of its use on waste containers/bags.

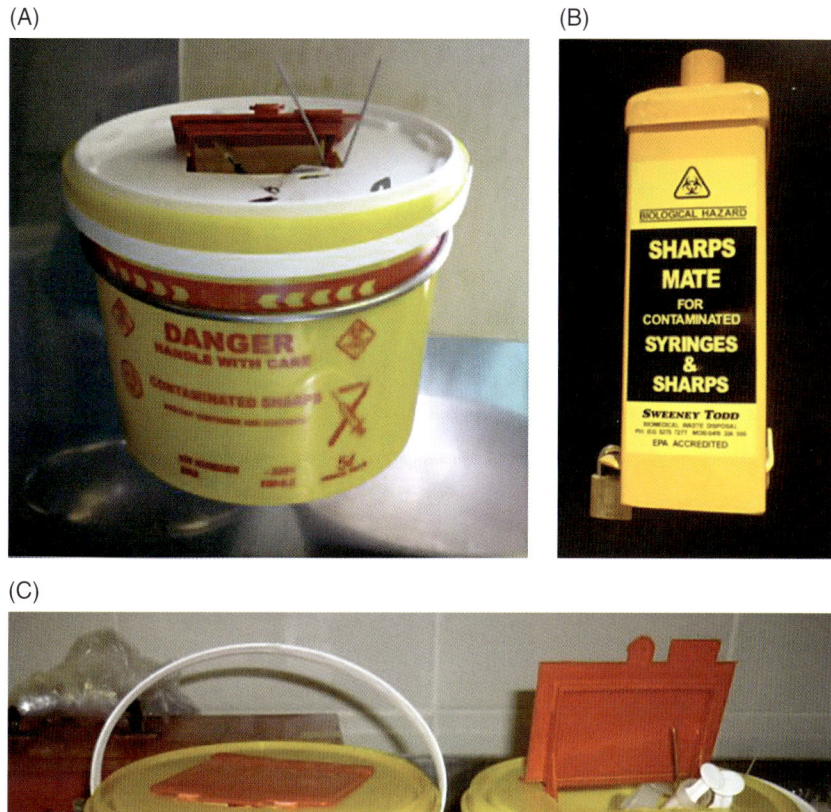

Figure 13.13 (A–C) Examples of sharps disposal containers. Note that in (A) and (C) there is inappropriate use of the container with items protruding from the lid.

plastic cable ties or other methods and placed into larger containers or liners in designated intermediate storage areas (if applicable; Figure 13.15).

Such storage areas should be close to the wards/departments, not accessible to unauthorized persons (such as patients and visitors), and be correctly labeled/signed as being a storage area (Figure 13.16).

An optimum storage area should have an impermeable, hard-standing floor with good drainage; it should be easy to clean and disinfect, with an accessible water supply for cleaning purposes. The area should be protected from outside elements, inaccessible to animals/insects/birds, and not situated near certain areas (e.g. fresh food stores, food preparation areas, or patient waiting areas).

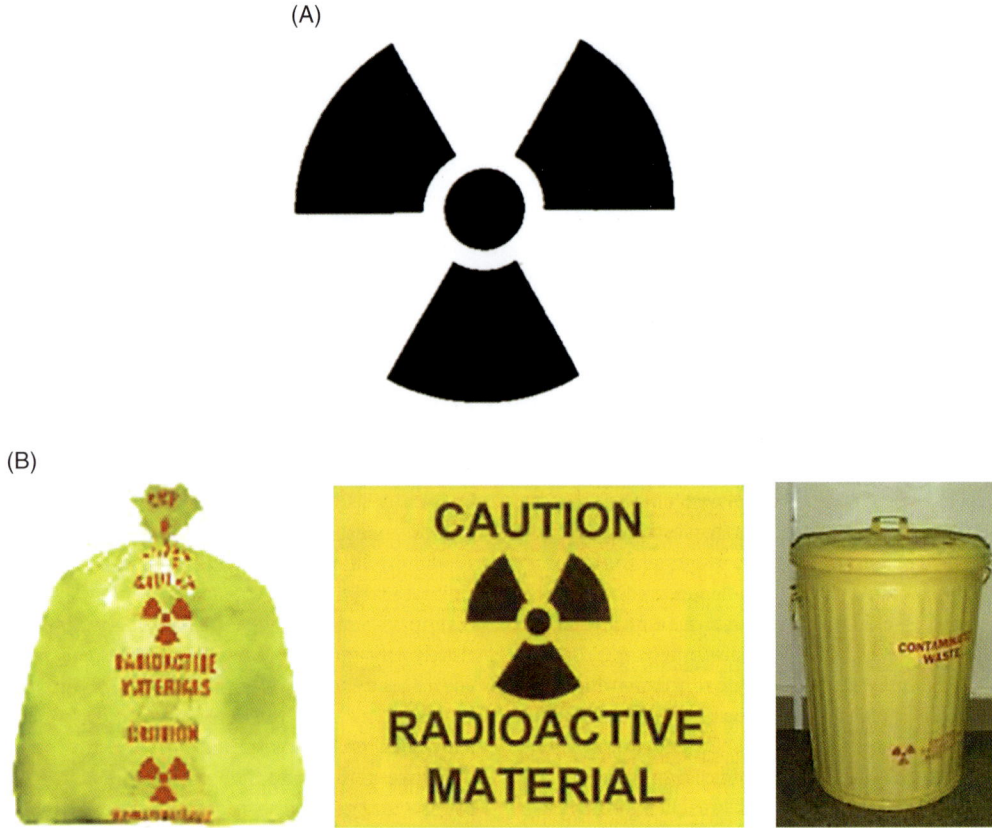

Figure 13.14 (A) The international symbol for radioactivity and (B) examples of its use on waste containers/bags.

Transport of waste to a designated central storage area should be performed using a wheelie bin or trolley that is easy to load and unload, has no sharp edges that could damage waste bags or containers, and is easy to clean/disinfect. Ideally, transport bins should be the same color as the corresponding bags and be covered. General waste should be transported separately from other hazardous wastes to avoid potential cross-contamination or mixing. Waste should be transported along designated routes avoiding patient care, visitor, and clean areas where possible.

The central storage area should follow the same guidelines as for any intermediate storage area. It should be sized according to the volume of waste generated by the facility as well as the frequency of collection. As a general rule, storage time should be minimized and not exceed 24–48 hours, especially in countries that have a warm and humid climate. Further external transport (e.g. for incineration) should be done using dedicated vehicles. The transportation should always be properly documented and all vehicles should carry a consignment note from the point of collection to the treatment facility.

Terminal waste disposal and the environment

Waste has a huge impact on the environment, potentially leading to pollution and even contributing to climate change (e.g. from greenhouse gas emissions). The amount of waste materials is increasing and their nature is becoming more complex, in particular with technological advances. For instance complex mixtures of materials, including plastics, precious metals, electronics, and hazardous materials, can be difficult to safely dispose of. Each year in the European Union alone it is estimated that 3 billion tonnes of waste is generated, with 90 million tonnes of it hazardous. This amounts to about 6 tonnes of solid waste for every person every year. Healthcare is a significant contributor to this problem. Most healthcare waste is either incinerated or dumped into landfill sites, with both these options creating environmental concerns. Landfill not only takes up more and more valuable land space, but also causes air, water, and soil pollution, discharging carbon dioxide (CO_2) and methane (CH_4) into the atmosphere and chemicals and pesticides into the earth and groundwater. This, in turn, is itself harmful to human health, as well as to plants and animals.

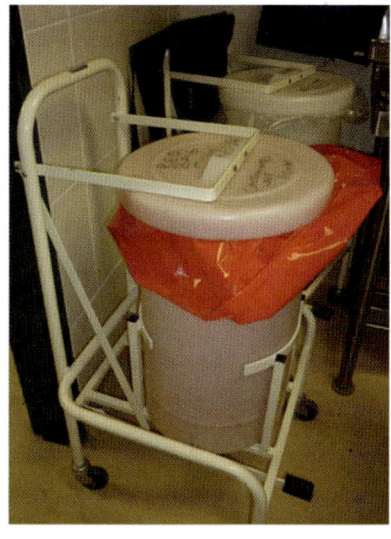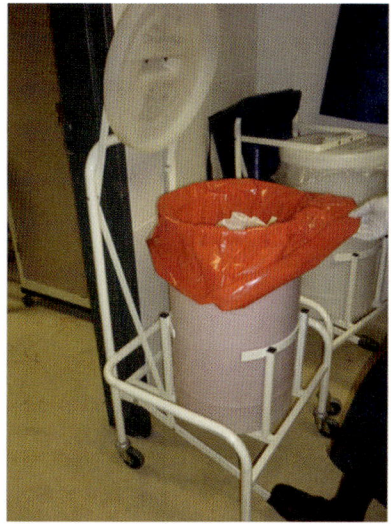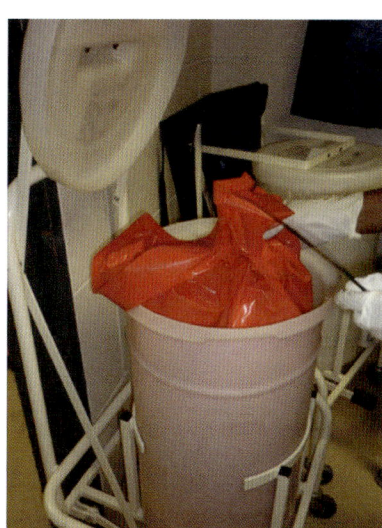
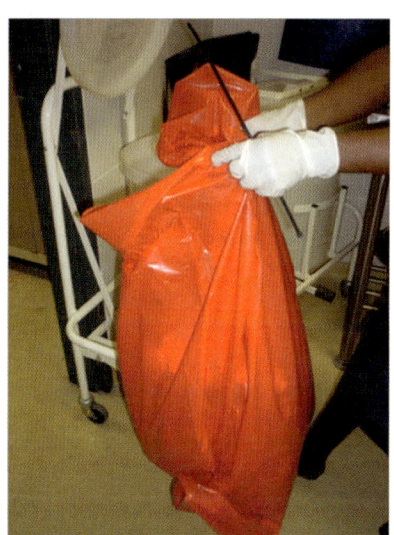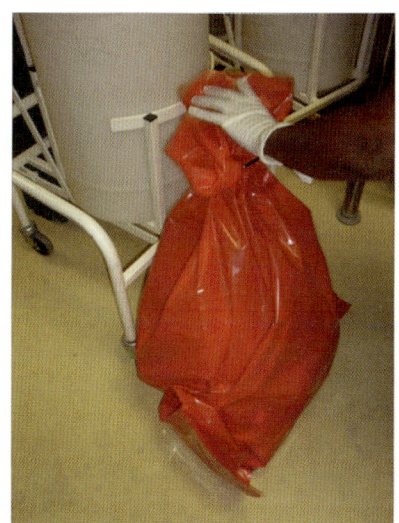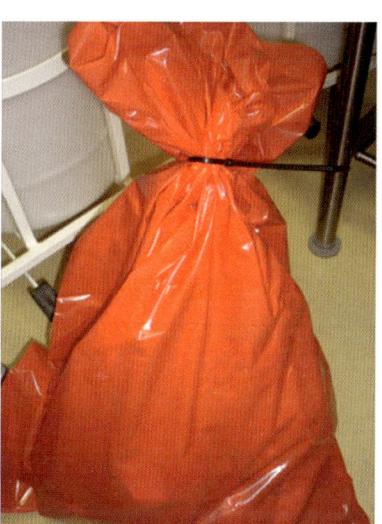

Figure 13.15 Disposal of a waste bag.

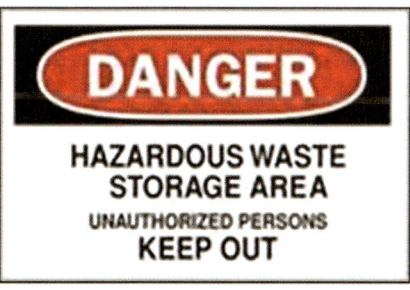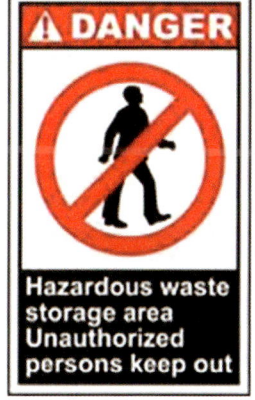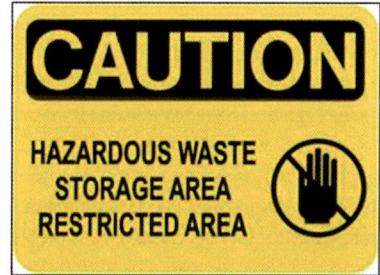

Figure 13.16 Examples of hazardous waste storage area signs.

It is therefore important to highlight that the most important step in waste disposal is the separation of waste at the source of generation. This will help to minimize the various types of wastes that are designated for disposal in accordance with facility and local policies.

The public can be affected either directly or indirectly through the dumping of waste in uncontrolled areas, for instance by its contaminating soil and underground water supplies. Controlled areas for the disposal of solid waste on land are generally known as landfill and this is both one of the most widely used methods of terminal waste handling and the least desirable option. Landfill sites are specially engineered and constructed to reduce hazards to public health and safety. They usually consist of a large hole in the ground, such as an old quarry or mine, but may also be an area where rubbish is piled above ground, creating a hill, which is then naturally covered (such as with grass) in a process known as land raising. Such waste is generally compacted to the smallest practical volume and covered with soil to minimize any risks (including to public health and safety). Landfill sites are generally used for the disposal of non-hazardous solid wastes. However, there can be significant complications relating to their use, including the production and release of methane and other greenhouse gases into the air. Landfill gas is produced from the breakdown of organic material in waste. It can consist of 50–60% methane (CH_4), 30–40% carbon dioxide (CO_2), and 10% nitrogen (N_2). If not controlled, it can also build up in the landfill mass and cause explosions. A further complication is the leaching of hazardous materials into natural water sources.

Incineration (burning to ash; see Chapter 11, Figure 11.18) of wastes has been widely practiced for many years (see Chapter 11 on dry heat sterilization) and has many advantages. For example, it reduces waste volume to a minimum of ash and is also considered safe for the terminal treatment (sterilization) of infectious, hazardous waste. Historically all hazardous/infectious healthcare waste was incinerated, but alternative methods are now being encouraged. This is partly due to the increasing volume of plastic wastes such as polyvinyl chloride (PVC, widely used in many disposable items) that releases toxic substances such as dioxin (a bio-accumulative toxin) on incineration. There is also ongoing controversy over the incineration of healthcare waste, particularly in high-population areas. The incineration of materials containing chlorine can generate dioxins and furans, which are classified as possible human carcinogens and have been associated with a range of other adverse health effects. Dioxins and furans are persistent substances that do not readily break down in the environment and that can bio-accumulate (providing a risk to our food chain). The risks of dioxin/furan release is higher at lower incineration temperatures (<800°C; 1472°F). Modern incinerators are recommended to be used that work at 800–1000°C (1472–1832°F) and include special emission-cleaning (chemical-filtering) equipment that can ensure that no significant amounts of dioxins and furans are produced. More environmentally friendly alternatives to incineration include separation and autoclaving of infectious waste, chemical treatment, and microwaving. These may be preferable under certain circumstances.

Overall, healthcare waste should be disposed of in accordance with all relevant national legislation, including regulations related to waste in general, environmental protection and air quality, and prevention/control of infectious disease. Environmentally friendly waste management is based on three principles:

- Waste prevention. If the amount of waste generated is reduced, this reduces any hazards by reducing the presence of dangerous substances in products, automatically simplifying disposal.
- Recycling and reuse. If waste cannot be prevented, as much as possible should be recovered, preferably by recycling.
- Improving final disposal and monitoring. Where possible, waste that cannot be recycled or reused should be safely incinerated, with landfill used only as a last resort.

Examples of international agreements that include these principles are:

- The Basel Convention, a global agreement ratified by over 190 member countries to deal with the problems and challenges posed by hazardous waste. The key principles of the convention are environmental health and safety protection. They include the reduction of hazardous waste, disposal of hazardous waste as close to the point of generation as possible, and minimizing the movement of waste.
- Stockholm Convention on Persistent Organic Pollutants, a global treaty that protects human health and the environment from persistent organic pollutants (POPs), defined as chemicals that remain intact in the environment for long periods. The key principle of this convention is that it is the duty of any organization that generates waste to dispose of the waste safely.

Accidental spillages/leakages

It is recommended that all healthcare facilities have an emergency spillage procedure in place stating what precautions must be taken and what procedures followed in the case of an accidental spillage of hazardous waste (chemical, infectious, etc.). The procedure will depend on the physical characteristics and volume of materials being handled, their potential toxicity, and the potential for releases to the environment. A major consideration for processing areas should be in the handling of accidental spillages, considering the use of various types of chemicals (solids, liquids, gases) and/or materials in these areas.

Before drafting a policy for accidental spillages, it is strongly recommended to review what chemicals are present and their associated SDSs, as well as other references/guidance for recommended spill cleanup methods and materials (including PPE such as respirators, gloves, protective clothing, etc.). Spill control procedures and control materials/kits should be readily available for any reasonably anticipated chemical spill. Place spill control materials and protective equipment in a readily accessible location within or immediately adjacent to the area where the chemicals are used. Chemical spill procedure guidelines will vary depending on the chemical risk, but in general the following should be considered:

- Management notification and who will be responsible for determining the nature of the spill and coordinating the necessary clean-up actions.
- Evacuation procedure of the contaminated area, if applicable.
- Immediate first aid and decontamination procedure for the eyes and skin of exposed personnel.
- Protective clothing/equipment that should be worn by personnel involved in the clean-up.
- Measures to be considered to limit the impact of the spill. Examples include protecting floor drains or other means of environmental release. Spill "socks" and other absorbent materials may be placed around drains as needed.
- Methods to neutralize or disinfect the spilled or contaminated material if indicated.
- Methods to collect all spilled and contaminated material. For example, sharps should never be picked up by hand; brushes and pans or other suitable tools should be used. Spilled materials and any disposable, contaminated items used for clean-up should be placed in the appropriate waste bags or containers.

Fire

Healthcare facility fires are especially dangerous, as they not only require staff to evacuate themselves, there is also the need to evacuate patients (many of whom may be bedridden/immobile). A fire emergency is defined as an uncontrolled fire or imminent fire hazard, the presence of smoke or the odor of burning, the uncontrolled release of a flammable or combustible substance, or a fire alarm sounding.

The most common fire hazards in hospital settings include patients/staff smoking, compressed gas cylinders, solvents, and faulty equipment. The widespread use of combustible liquids presents a major problem. Many liquids or gases used, including in processing areas, may be flammable or combustible and can be ignited by a spark or static electricity. A liquid may be classified as flammable or combustible depending on its flash point (the temperature at which it gives off enough gas to form an ignitable mixture with air). A flash point can be at or above 37.8°C (100°F). Examples of flammable liquids include most alcohols, benzene, acetone, and "combustible" liquids such as some lubricating oils, ethylene glycol, and carbolic acid. Their flammability can also depend on their concentration, such as with alcohols that are dramatically less flammable when mixed with water (e.g. 70% alcohol).

For a fire to ignite, oxygen (in the air), fuel (the liquid or gas), and an ignition source (e.g. spark) are needed. To prevent fires caused by liquid chemicals, consider the following guidelines:

- Restrict the amount of flammable liquids in the working area.
- Carefully read manufacturer's instructions and SDSs.
- Store large amounts of flammable liquids in a metal cabinet.

Many types of gases are used in healthcare settings, for example oxygen, anesthetic gases, and sterilizing gases (e.g. ethylene oxide and hydrogen peroxide). Although oxygen is labeled as non-flammable it is an oxidizing gas that will aid combustion. Most gas cylinders are flammable as they are all under pressure and can present a fire risk. Such cylinders must be handled with care. They should be secured and stored in a well-ventilated fireproof, dry area at a temperature not exceeding the gas supplier's recommendations. Cylinders should be handled carefully (never drop or bump them) and stored away from boilers/hot water pipes/flammable solvents, open flames, and so on.

Electrical equipment malfunctions are a further major cause of fires. Equipment that is not maintained or is incorrectly grounded (electrically) is often the root cause. Because processing facilities have many damp or potentially damp areas, electrical maintenance and safety are important.

Where evacuation from an area or facility is needed due to a fire, general regulations require that a fire alarm signal is given continuously and for fire safety signage to be in place to assist with evacuation and/or firefighting. All staff must be familiar with an emergency exit plan. Signs (Figure 13.17) are needed to:

- Warn of hazards.
- Identify safe routes for escape.
- Indicate the location of fire equipment.
- Give consistent instructions.

If a fire is initiated or discovered, the following is recommended:

- Alert people in the area of the need to evacuate.
- Activate the nearest fire alarm.
- Call for assistance and leave the area immediately, if you are not a trained firefighter. Do not try to retrieve personal items.
- Close doors behind you.
- Do not attempt to use elevators.
- Assemble at the area designated in your emergency action plan and remain there until instructed that it is safe to re-enter the building.

Overall, a policy should be in place that describes the necessary preventative and action procedures in the case of a fire. It is important that area managers keep an accessible record of any particular safety risks (chemical, infectious, or equipment) for the information of emergency personnel (e.g. fire officer). Staff should be trained on this policy and periodic drills should be held of the evacuation procedure.

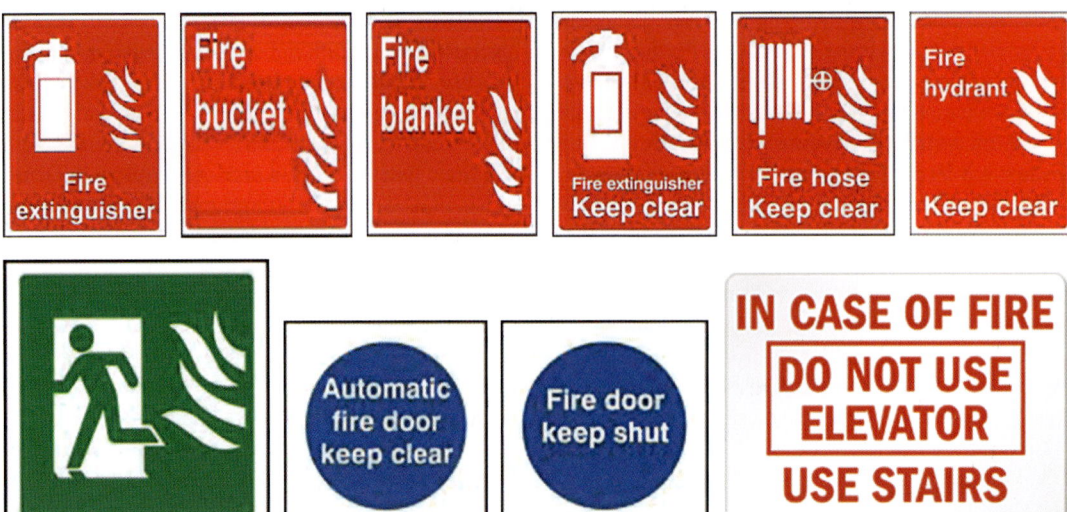

Figure 13.17 Examples of fire-associated signs.

Disaster planning and management

A disaster is defined as a sudden and usually massive accident, mishap, or natural occurrence. Examples include nuclear accidents, facility fires, terrorist attacks, wars, transportation accidents, bomb blasts, riots, and industrial explosions, as well as natural disasters such as floods, tsunamis, epidemics, droughts, and tornados. In such situations healthcare facilities are immediately affected, with significant demands being placed on personnel, resources, and facilities. Facility disaster management plans are designed to best deal with such situations, which should include any processing areas (both existing and temporary based on the facility's needs).

The aim of a disaster plan is to provide maximum benefit to the maximum number of affected people with the available staff and resources. This involves coordinated planning of all departments within a healthcare facility as well as coordinated outside community assistance. During a disaster, healthcare systems will be confronted with increased demands and decreased availability of resources. Local or regional healthcare systems best understand their own needs and resources and are therefore recommended to develop specific disaster medical capacity and capability plans, including for processing areas.

Disaster planning should reflect any local or country-specific regulations and guidance. Every healthcare facility should have a collaborative and coordinated crisis plan, including protocols, checklists, and signs to facilitate efficient hospital management and minimize chaos during emergencies. This applies equally to processing areas, where increased needs for medical equipment and supplies will be necessary. Protocols within the processing area during disasters should be as simple as possible, concise, realistic, workable, and located in an easily accessible place to all staff. Contingency plans may be necessary, such as alternative methods of cleaning, disinfection, and sterilization that may not be optimal but will be sufficient to reduce any cross-contamination risks under a disaster situation.

14 Management and quality

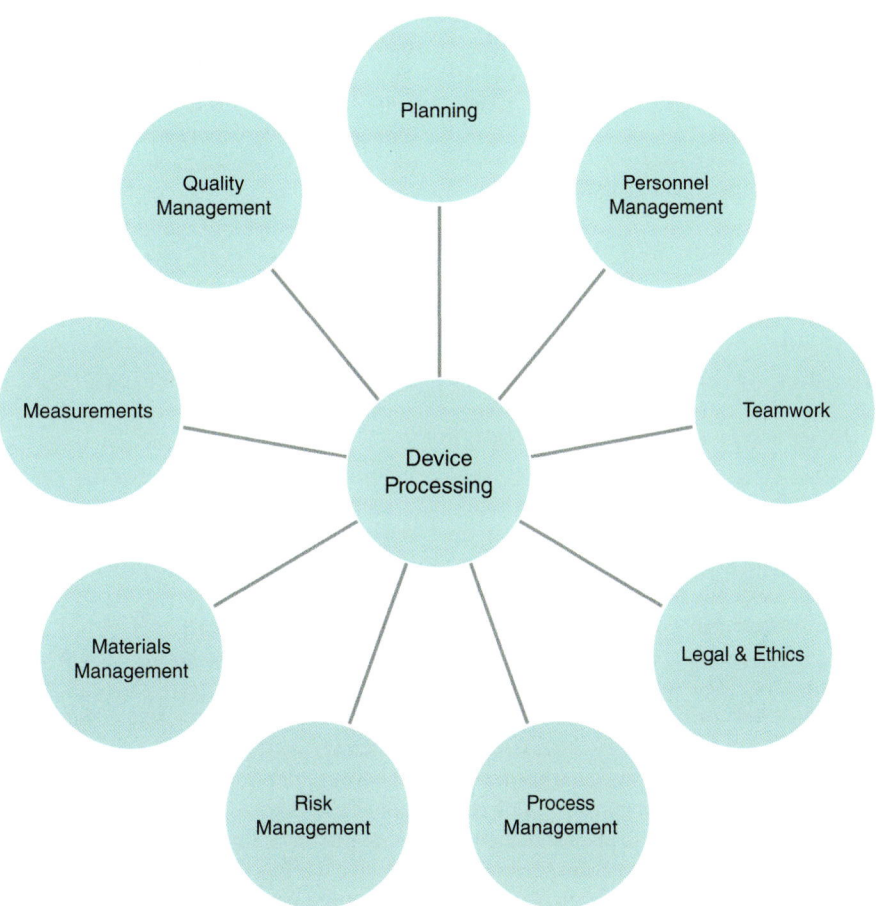

The term "management" refers to actions taken to ensure that processes and people are performing to plan. The four common management principles are planning, organizing, leading, and controlling. While it sounds simple, management can be quite complex and requires a well-organized approach to be successful. To help translate these principles into applicable processing area activities, the principles and how they apply to processing areas can be expanded to consider:

- Planning
- Personnel management
- Teamwork
- Legal and ethical responsibilities

Decontamination and Device Processing in Healthcare, Second Edition. Gerald McDonnell and Georgia Alevizopoulou.
© 2025 John Wiley & Sons Ltd. Published 2025 by John Wiley & Sons Ltd.

- Process (including risk) management
- Materials management
- Measurements
- Quality management

These areas are all supported by measurements, risk management, and quality. Managing is about being organized and proactive, being able to anticipate and adapt to an ever-changing and increasingly diverse environment with numerous challenges. Effective managers and management systems are proactive and make things happen, as opposed to ineffective managers and systems that may only react to problems (i.e. crisis management) and can lead to problems. Management is therefore not only the responsibility of an individual head of department or area manager but takes a team effort to ensure that the overall process is efficient.

It is the responsibility of a manager to create and maintain an internal environment that enables others to work efficiently and effectively. Basic management skills include problem solving and decision making, planning, meeting management, delegation, collaboration, and most importantly effective communication.

Managers cannot be effective without having the dedication of their co-workers (both within and outside a department under their leadership) and efficient management processes in place. The processing area is a dynamic area, often with increasing demands, and is therefore dependent on a team environment with staff cooperation at all levels. Processing area personnel need to work collaboratively with surgical and medical staff to ensure that the demands for sterile or otherwise processed devices are consistently met. For the area to keep up with changing technology, regulations, and demands, individual staff members must excel at their specific jobs and work together as a team. Teamwork is particularly important because without it processing can be inefficient and even increase the risks of mistakes being made. With the right teamwork, efficient management processes can be put in place and optimized over time. These will include management of people, process, materials and device supplies, and quality to ensure compliance with local and international regulations and standards.

Planning

Having the right plan is the first step in managing a successful processing department. To do so, managers should complete the following four steps of strategic planning:
- Customer requirements. Understand what your customers require from the processing department. A "customer" can be defined as the recipient of a product or process result, in this situation a processed device, device set, or piece of equipment.
- Resource requirements. Based on the customer requirements (including timelines), determine what resources are needed to fulfill those requirements, including labor, equipment, space, and supplies.
- Create a workflow. Design a workflow or value stream that supports meeting the customer requirements with the resources available.
- Standard work instructions. Document and standardize the workflow and individual tasks required to complete the work.

Whether you are opening a new department or managing a current department, the planning process can and should be reviewed annually for budgeting purposes and whenever activities or scope of work change for the department.

Customer requirements

Processing departments may have several customers within or outside the healthcare facility that they provide services to. It is imperative to understand each customer's requirements. The primary customer for most departments is the operating rooms (ORs) at the facility. It is very common, though, for a processing department to serve multiple customers, including facility or off-site clinics, physicians' offices, endoscopy departments, nursing floors, labor and delivery, and the emergency department. Every customer may have different requirements and perceptions of what the processing department can and should provide and deliver.

It is critical to establish a relationship based on mutual respect, trust, and strong communication. The customer's requirements must be clearly and succinctly expressed in such a manner that the processing department can successfully meet them and measure their performance against them. Avoid vague or general terms that can led to misunderstandings.

Defining expectations will require a face-to-face meeting between the processing leadership and the customer. Do not underestimate the importance of such meetings in building a positive relationship and clarifying mutually agreeable expectations and requirements. This will also be the start of ongoing conversations that are vital to a positive long-term relationship.

When meeting with a customer, consider these best practices:
- Keep the conversation focused on the customer's needs.
- Openly state the purpose for asking any questions about requirements/expectations.
- Do more listening than talking.
- Ask what is most important to the customer and what specifically they value.
- Ask open-ended questions.
- Do not be defensive. Take criticism graciously.
- Ensure you understand why the customer has their particular requirements.
- Ask clarifying questions to ensure mutual understanding.

Sometimes it takes more than one meeting to come to agreeable expectations to meet the customer's requirements. If they state that they expect instrument trays to be 100% complete with no quality issues, that expectation may be agreeable as a goal but not an immediate reality. To meet the customer's expectation the processing department may need to state its expectations in how the customer returns instruments to the processing department, the inventory on hand, and realistic turnaround times.

A healthy relationship between a processing department and its customers requires both parties to understand each other's processes, business objectives, and potential roadblocks to ensure their common goal of positive patient outcomes. If a customer expects to carry a low inventory of instruments and requires the processing department to process instruments between surgical cases within one hour, the expectation is unrealistic and must be addressed in an honest and factual manner. When agreeing to achievable and sustainable customer requirements or expectations, three key factors are helpful:

1. Capability of the processing department:
   - Adequate technical proficiency.
   - Adequate workforce skills.
   - Sufficient processing capacity.
   - Demonstrated ability.
2. Commitment from both parties:
   - Concern for each other's success.
   - Common and mutual goals.
   - Honesty and integrity.
   - Courtesy and respect.
   - Cooperation and flexibility.
   - Explaining actions that may impact others.
   - Becoming familiar with one another's processes.
   - Promoting open, two-way communication.
3. Consistency in performance:
   - Honoring commitments.
   - Delivering expected performance.
   - Timely responses.
   - Open exchange.
   - Effort to understand as well as be understood.
   - Periodic assessment or survey.

Having developed mutually agreed requirements, it is important to communicate these expectations to processing staff and engrain them into the operational culture and belief system. Having staff focused on meeting the customer requirements creates a customer first culture and ensures that their daily decisions are driving the correct actions. This has a direct correlation to the patient experience and a positive healthcare outcome.

In addition to clarifying and documenting all their customers' requirements, processing leadership should take the time to review their own requirements within their processes as well as realizing their relationships with other departments within their healthcare organization.

Requirements within a processing department include how the instruments are cleaned and disinfected and presented to the clean prep and pack staff. For instance, there should be documented and measurable expectations that instruments should be pre-cleaned appropriately, positioned correctly for automated cleaning–disinfection, and sharps clearly identified and discarded as appropriate. In fact, every step in the processing process can be viewed as a requirement with expectations.

Other requirements for a processing department include its relationship with human resources, biomedical, environmental services, and facilities staff. Each of these internal departments provides services to the processing department that should be mutually agreed, documented, and measured.

Resource requirements

Having agreed on customer expectations, it is important to determine the resource requirements to fulfill those expectations. This is where a detailed operational plan should be developed to ensure what should happen, when it should happen, how long it should take, and what the results should be. In determining resource requirements, a plan can be defined against which the processing department can be measured. The steps taken to determine resource requirements will also directly impact budget allocation and available capacity to process the workload forecasted, and identify any limitations or changes in demand.

The first step is to accurately *forecast* the workload that each customer is anticipating sending to the processing department. Reusable instrument trays, single items, case carts, and clinic trays are common high-level workload indicators that are utilized in the initial forecast. Customers such as the OR staff may provide workload forecasts that are not readily applicable to forecasting processing volumes. An example is an OR forecasting the number of surgical procedures but unable to explain how many instrument trays will be used. Most processing departments utilize some type of electronic tracking system so the availability of historical data can be utilized to forecast future volumes in these cases.

Since most processing departments do more than clean, disinfect, prepare, pack, and sterilize instruments, it is important to document all tasks performed by the department and the forecasted associated volume. Training, education, meetings and huddles, clinic pick-ups and deliveries, and any other tasks should be documented, and volumes forecasted. Clarifying the volume of work by complexity can be important to consider. Showing the loaner set (vendor) tray volume separately from the clinic tray volume will allow different time standards to be assigned and resource requirements to be more accurately forecast. Other options include categorizing trays by sterilization modality, container versus wrap, large versus small, complex versus simple, and surgical versus clinic. The size of the processing department may also dictate how detailed a forecast is required. Small departments may find a simple forecast works well while large, multi-location departments require detailed analyses.

By collecting detailed information on all tasks performed, labor and equipment requirements can be accurately determined based on verified data. Facilities with actual data examples also have a better chance of receiving the resources needed versus those estimating what they need. An example of a workload is given in Table 14.1. Using weekly estimates as the frequency for forecasting workloads is recommended for its ease and accuracy. Daily tasks usually vary between midweek and weekends and thus weekly frequencies can remove the variations.

Labor requirements

Labor requirements typically represent the largest variable cost to processing departments and are reviewed with greater scrutiny by executives and finance teams. Having verified data to justify the labor need for the department is critical. Data also allows the processing leadership to measure actual performance to a plan while driving continuous improvement initiatives.

Labor requirements can utilize a simple software-based (e.g. Microsoft Excel) staffing model utilizing the data previously collected from the department workload. The spreadsheet should list every activity the department performs, the frequency with which it is performed, the volume per frequency, and the time standard required to perform the activity. Using the previous forecasting workload example, an additional column can be added to the table for a reasonable time estimate (Table 14.2).

As shown in Table 14.2, some activities have been duplicated to represent multiple process steps. OR tray processing can be broken into various steps such as decontamination and assembly (prep and pack) to better reflect the different activities, different time requirements, standard work instructions, and physically different locations.

Table 14.1 An example of forecasting workload.

Activity	Unit	Frequency	Volume
OR trays	Tray	Weekly	1300
OR quick turn trays	Tray	Weekly	22
OR loaner trays	Tray	Weekly	78
OR peel packs	Peel packs	Weekly	500
Clinic trays	Tray	Weekly	70
Case carts	Carts	Weekly	250
Steam sterilizer loads	Load	Weekly	96
Low-temp sterile loads	Load	Weekly	65
Medical equipment	Items	Daily	10
OR supply restocking	Occurrence	Daily	1
Crash cart restocking	Cart	Monthly	5
Sterilizer testing	Occurrence	Daily	1
Washer testing	Occurrence	Daily	1
Daily staff huddle	Huddle	Daily	1

OR, operating room.

Table 14.2 An example of labor requirements.

Activity	Unit	Frequency	Volume	Time (min)
OR trays decontamination	Tray	Weekly	1300	6
OR trays assembly	Tray	Weekly	1300	15
OR quick turn trays	Tray	Weekly	22	20
OR loaner trays decontamination	Tray	Weekly	78	6
OR loaner trays assembly	Tray	Weekly	78	10
OR peel packs decontamination	Peel packs	Weekly	500	–
OR peel packs assembly	Peel packs	Weekly	500	2
Clinic trays decontamination	Occurrence	Weekly	5	30
Clinic trays assembly	Tray	Weekly	70	6
Case carts picking	Carts	Weekly	250	15
Steam sterilizer loads	Load	Weekly	96	15
Low-temp sterilizer loads	Load	Weekly	65	8
Medical equipment	Items	Daily	10	3
OR supply restocking	Occurrence	Daily	1	60
Crash cart restocking	Cart	Monthly	5	25
Sterilizer testing	Occurrence	Daily	1	35
Washer testing	Occurrence	Daily	1	10
Daily staff huddle (20 people)	Huddle	Daily	1	200

OR, operating room.

Once all activities have been listed in a manner that makes sense for determining labor requirements, the next step is determining the time standard to use. The objective in setting time standards is multi-faceted. Setting a time standard based on the fastest possible time will result in a goal for individuals to achieve but not a reality situation for planning, as not everyone will constantly be able to perform at that level. Setting a time standard based on current averages may set a realistic staffing requirement as it reflects current performance. The best practice is to identify what the best time would be for an experienced staff member following standard work practices without interruptions and then compare that to the current average department performance. Setting current labor requirements to the average performance and then agreeing to find opportunities to improve performance allows for constant improvement opportunities. Remember that the objective is to find ways to work smarter and remove waste from the process as opposed to making people work faster.

In addition to calculating the number of staff required to process the forecasted workloads, it is critical to understand the type of staff and leadership required to effectively manage the department (see the section on personnel management).

Equipment requirements

Processing equipment needs can be determined by combining the forecasted workloads with the capacity of each piece of equipment within the process. It is worth noting the difference between capacity and throughput. Capacity refers to the potential amount of work that a process or piece of equipment can produce. Throughput refers to the actual amount of work that is being produced. For example, an instrument washer-disinfector may have the capacity to process 9 trays every 30 minutes, 18 trays in 1 hour, or 432 trays in 24 hours. But this does not mean that a department forecasting a workload of 430 trays will only need one washer-disinfector. Equipment requirements will be based on arrival times of instruments, staffing availability, requirements to begin the cleaning process as soon as possible, manufacturer's instructions for use (IFU), and other variables (including the provision of time for equipment maintenance). For small departments equipment requirements may be easier to determine, while larger departments may require workload and equipment calculations that specialists or equipment vendors can assist with. The following section considers a large department and some concepts that can be utilized.

The first step is to determine the volume to plan for, which may include estimates for an average day, busy day, peak volume day, or some other volume indicator. Additionally, in planning a new department consider future growth in forecasted volumes to ensure planning for the capacity to support future volumes in 5, 10, or even 15 years' time. This will include the need for shift work and new equipment over time, including washer-disinfectors and sterilizers.

The second step is agreeing to the acceptable amount of backlog at each step of the process. Accepting or not accepting backlogs has a direct impact on equipment requirements. The cleaning process should have minimal backlogs, as IFU and best practices state that soil should be removed as soon as possible after use. Other steps in the process where soil is not an issue, such as in inspection, packaging, or sterilization, may allow for acceptable backlogs without degradation to the instruments. But such backlogs must not negatively impact achievement of the customer's expectations.

For example, a hospital processing department processes on average 310 instrument trays per day, with a busy day reaching 396 and a record day being 480 trays. Using data from the department's experience (e.g. a tracking software system), its managers created a graph showing the number of times they processed trays on an average day on and what they considered to be a busy day that occurred more often than planned. The graph in Figure 14.1 provides a visual depiction of the tray volumes and assists managers to make decisions on what volumes can be planned for their equipment requirements. Using the average day would provide enough capacity for any day that was less busy than average, but create backlogs on any day that was busier than average. In this example it can be assumed that managers agreed they wanted the capacity to handle a 90th percentile workload, or 396 trays per day with minimal backlogs.

The next step in this theoretical example is to break down the 396 trays into an hourly workflow to understand when the trays will arrive at the department:
- The surgery department starts sending used trays to the processing department around 9 am and finishes most of its day's work by 7 pm, equaling a 10-hour window.
- 396 trays divided by 10 hours = 40 trays per hour on average with an average of 6 trays per case cart, equaling about 7 dirty case carts per hour.

Therefore, equipment requirements in this example would include:
- Cart washers: based on 8 carts per hour capacity, one cart washer would be required to handle 7 case carts.
- Pre-cleaning sinks: based on 10 trays per hour being processed through a sink (assuming it is staffed), 4 sinks would be required to handle the 40 trays. Remember, some situations where more detailed manual cleaning is required may be a source of backlog in the sinks.
- Ultrasonic washers: consultation of IFU for ultrasonic equipment shows that 50% of the trays require sonic washing with a typical 15-minute cycle. Based on 4 trays per hour (single-tray sonic washer), 5 sonic washers are required to handle the 20 trays.
- Instrument washer-disinfectors: based on 18 trays per hour capacity, 2.2 washer-disinfectors would be required. Rounding down to 2 washers would mean an increased backlog or

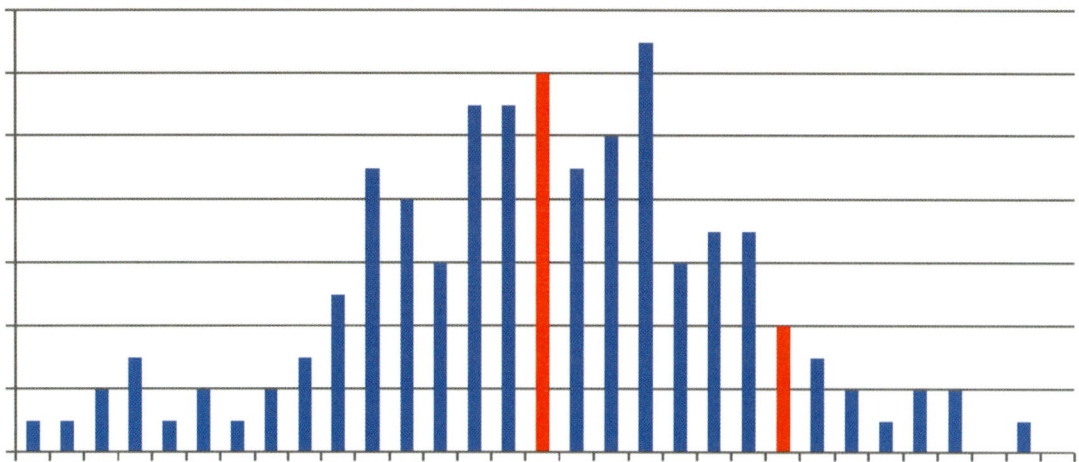

Figure 14.1 Graph (histogram) showing the theoretical number of trays processed per day, with an average (red, at ~310 trays/day) and a 90% percentile (red, at ~396 trays/day) representing a typical busy day.

rounding up to 3 would ensure that backlogs are minimized. A large number of devices requiring detailed hand cleaning in advance should be removed from this calculation as they will take longer to process.
- Preparation and packaging tables: based on 4 trays per hour (agreed throughput based on staffing performance), 10 tables are required to maintain workflow. Here is where reasonable backlogs could be planned to ensure staff remain productive and to take advantage of additional hours of the day if the department is comfortable with trays sitting in the processing department. Be careful, though, as the trays may be needed for the following day's surgical cases.
- Sterilizers: depending on the size of the sterilizer(s) at the facility, the required number of sterilizers can be calculated based on the workload. Steam and low temperature would need be broken out separately, depending on equipment capabilities.

Once the capacity for each step in the process has been determined, a balanced process can be predicted to help eliminate potential backlogs within the department. Figures 14.2(A) and 14.2(B) show examples an out-of-balanced process and an in-balance process. The intent is to create a balanced flow of work through the department where no one area represents a significant capacity restraint or overabundance of capacity.

Materials requirements

Planning for materials has a direct connection to daily material management routines. For planning purposes, the goal is to identify the amount of materials needed to maintain operational workflows and meet customer requirements. Materials include the various consumable supplies used in device processing, as well as the customer instrument inventory. This step will also help identify space requirements for the department.

Examples of consumable supplies used regularly by a processing department will include the following categories:
- Environmental: towels, mops, cleaning–disinfection chemistries.
- Instrument cleaning: automated and manual chemistries, brushes.
- Instrument maintenance: lubricants, spare parts, inspection equipment.
- Quality tests: cleaning indicators, biological indicators (BIs), and chemical indicators (CIs) for sterilization, air removal, or other periodic tests.
- Low-temperature sterilization sterilant and other accessories.
- Sterilization packaging: peel pouches, wrap, plastic covers, corner protectors, tray liners, locks, filters.
- Personal protective equipment (PPE): decontamination PPE, various types of gloves, scrubs, shoe and hair covers, safety monitors.
- Miscellaneous: paper, pens, printer cartridges, labels, etc.

The amount of supplies required is determined by the clinical requirements including manufacturer IFU, regulations, customer-identified requirements for use, and the volume of work being processed.

Customer instrument inventory is often stored within the processing department, but even if it is not the processing department is typically responsible for the maintenance of inventory, including sterile product storage. Determining instrument requirements is 100% based on the customer's usage schedule or surgery schedule. Determining instrumentation requirements will require collaboration with facility-specific customers to understand current and/or future requirements. For departments already utilizing a computerized trace-and-track system, especially if tracking case cart

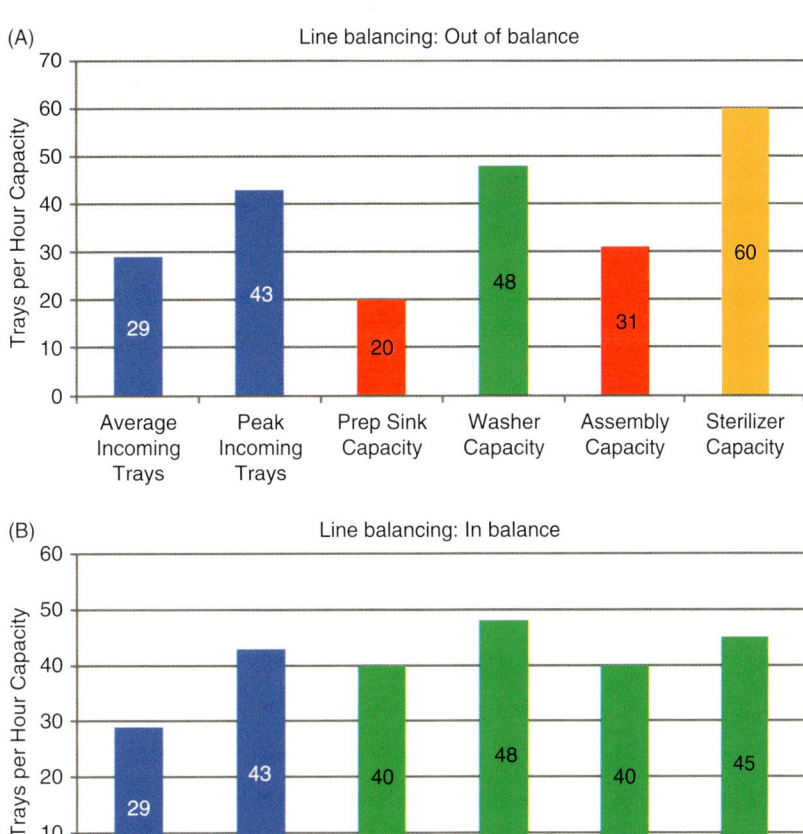

Figure 14.2 Examples of (A) out-of-balance and (B) in-balance processing capacities based on various steps of the processing cycle. The red/yellow bars show opportunities in the workflow to balance capacity.

selection, run reports can show the usage of instrumentation by day to understand the daily variances. It is important to note that using averages for instrumentation usage is not typically recommended, as surgery schedules may perform similar types of surgeries on specific days of the week. This results in higher than average demand for instrumentation on one day of the week that should be planned for.

Once the potential maximum daily requirements for each instrumentation tray or item are understood, the current inventory should be reviewed to determine whether additional purchases are required. It is important to consider whether the processing department is going to be tasked with same-day quick turnaround of the same sets of instrumentation twice or more times in a single day due to lack of inventory. Overall, inventory usually requires negotiation and budgetary planning to achieve an optimum balance between having enough devices/sets to meet the schedule but not too many that result in low utilization and thus wasted financial investments.

Space requirements

The next resource requirement to determine is space to work. While many processing departments are already built and can no longer change or adjust their space, space is a critical element when planning for a new department or renovation. A first consideration will be any local, regional, or international regulatory or standard requirements. These continue to develop internationally and can be mandated in certain countries. Space requirements are then a culmination of the previous three resource requirements – labor, equipment, and materials. Each step of the process should be understood to determine the required space to fit the equipment, have space for staging of work, be conducive to efficient workflows, meet the regulatory and IFU requirements for processing, and provide room to grow in the future. Taking time to design a future department with all the details required, such as management of waste bins, PPE changing locations, eye-wash stations, storage and staging space, incubation or testing equipment for quality monitoring, and other specific items required in the department is time well spent. Sometimes the reorganization of an existing processing facility can facilitate greater throughput and efficiency.

Workflow

An evaluation of the previous requirements can allow for the development of a practical workflow for the department with the resources available. Workflow refers to the series of necessary activities to complete a task, such a device processing. To best explain this, it is important to note the differences between a value stream map (VSM) and a process flow diagram (PFD). A VSM depicts the overall process while identifying process steps in three categories: those that add value, those that are non-value but with required waste, and non-value waste. VSMs commonly view the workflow at the process step level instead of the individual activity or task level. For example, the cleaning and disinfection steps within decontamination might be a single step in a VSM versus detailing out each activity that occurs in decontamination. VSMs should then add additional information in workflows such as wait times, backlogs, staffing, resources required, and opportunities to reduce waste and improve value. These are important in a process concept known as "lean," which is the concept of maximizing productivity while continuously minimizing waste.

A PFD is designed to detail the specific activities and tasks that occur within each process to understand the details and complexities of the workflow. A PFD may cover one process area such as preparation and packaging or sterilization, or combine the entire process throughout the processing department. Combining elements of a value stream into a PFD is often the most useful approach (Figure 14.3).

Creating a PFD allows for a visual representation of the process and each activity identified as value-added or non-value-added. PFDs are best used to accomplish the following:
- Engaging staff in identifying improvement opportunities in specific activities.
- Understanding the detail of how a process works, variances in practice, and lack of standardization.
- Identifying better ways to get the work done.
- Understanding what really happens versus what is supposed to happen.
- Identifying specific improvement opportunities.

Fortunately, completing a PFD is a simple process, using materials such as paper/pen but optimally a large blank wall, with sticky notes and markers. Start by defining the boundaries of the process from start to finish. It is recommended to engage with staff in documenting the current processes and let them provide the details of what really happens. Ask questions to ensure you understand every possible action staff take in doing their work and encourage them to be honest in their feedback. Document variances between what staff do and the required work processes as these will indicate opportunities for improvements. Discuss points of waste (e.g. time or resources) and break down the issues the staff face in accomplishing their tasks. Once the PFD is completed, improvement activities can be planned as well as standardizing the work.

Standard work instructions

A final consideration in planning is to document and standardize the workflow and individual tasks required to complete the work. Standard work instructions are a powerful and simple concept that is fundamental to every successful process. The use of standard work helps reduce waste and errors by consistently applying best practices and eliminate variance in work.

Standard work instructions document exactly how an activity or task should be completed. This includes the sequence of steps and desired method to complete the activity, quantities of work in process, and the pace at which the process must be completed. When followed, standard work should help staff complete activities the same way and processes should be consistent and repeatable without variation. Standard work is utilized in training and education and becomes the foundation for continuous improvement. Optimal training should be threefold to include verbal, demonstration, and written/signed and dated methods.

Policies, procedures, and standard work instructions can provide various levels of description. For example, a policy may state the hospital's desire to reduce the risk of surgical site infection or other surgical complications. A supporting procedure may state that the processing department will follow manufacturers' IFU to support the infection risk policy. The standard work instructions describe how to perform step-by-step activities including inspection of the IFU and following the essential steps to ensure correct processing to standardized department requirements. It is this level of detail that provides the means to achieve process repeatability, discipline, and predictability of outcomes.

Creating standard work instructions will also allow the designation of an amount of time to complete the activity. Standard work can help reduce time variances between staff as they all begin to perform tasks the same way according to the standard work.

Personnel management

Skilled and dedicated staff should be considered the most valuable resource for any processing area. Safe processing in a busy department can be labor intensive and relies heavily

Management and quality 397

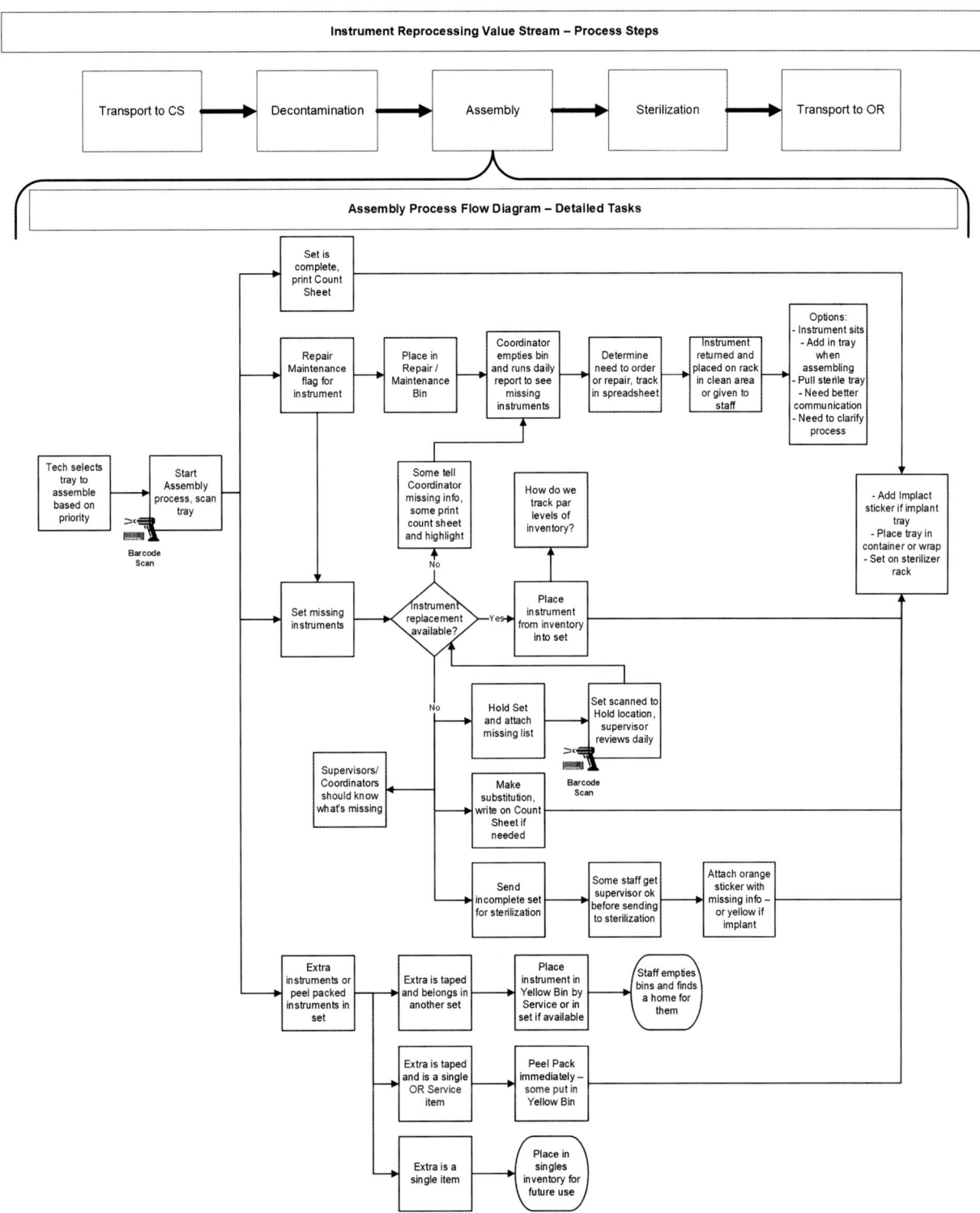

Figure 14.3 An example of a simple value stream with a process flow diagram for one area of a central sterilization (CS) cycle.

on having the right people. Staffing resources should be decided by considering customer (medical/surgical) demands (as discussed in the earlier section on planning), but consideration may also be given to other variables such as available processing equipment and the flexibility of the available staff who may have other clinical roles (junior and senior, often specialized staff). This can range from existing medical/surgical staff as part of their job description to a fully dedicated processing team. Device processing is important for staff and patient safety, therefore these tasks should not be underestimated or designated to existing staff who are already focused on or overwhelmed by other responsibilities. Processing area staff can be dedicated to this specific role or may be responsible for many different tasks, depending on the size and needs of a facility. If the department has employees who do not have adequate skills or training, quality will be compromised and this can impact patient safety. Targeted recruitment and training of the workforce should be identified to ensure quality and consistent processes. Designating the right time and staff to the process can have many benefits in patient safety, the care of equipment/devices, and job satisfaction.

Organization

Most processing roles or specific jobs are part of larger organizations that can vary from a few to thousands of people. Examples include a small dental facility with one or two dentists and dental nurse assistants, or a large hospital system with dedicated departments. All will have some kind of personnel organization, ranging from various managers, heads of departments, and business owners to supporting staff, including technicians. Whatever the size of the organization, each level should have clearly designated roles and responsibilities. Examples of this case in a processing facility will include:
- Department manager: this position requires a highly skilled individual manager who should understand processing services, management principles, and leadership. This person will be responsible for managing staff, the department processes, budgets, and the overall functioning of the processing area. The department may include multiple areas, such as operating areas, endoscopy departments, infection control/prevention, and supplies.
- Section manager: generally qualified in the field of processing services and responsible for the day-to-day management of staff/service, as well as staff training and ensuring standards are maintained.
- Team leader/supervisor: supervisors are an important part of the management team since they are the representatives of management in closest contact with the people who produce the work. They are very much first-line managers and should be regarded as such by both senior management and employees. Each part of the processing area (e.g. dirty or clean areas) may have a team leader who is skilled in the functions of that area and is responsible for overseeing training and the running of the area.
- Technician/operator/assistant operator/entry-level operator: depending on how long they have been working in the area these staff can have different levels of expertise, but should all be trained to ensure the same level of knowledge. They may have specific roles (e.g. packaging or cleaning) or be capable of moving from role to role. They work together as a team in carrying out the actual processing work. The key responsibilities of a technician's job can include:
  ○ Following department policies and procedures.
  ○ Collecting and transporting soiled items from wards and theaters.
  ○ Manual and/or mechanical cleaning of devices.
  ○ Device inspection and packaging.
  ○ Safely operating all types of equipment, such as washer-disinfectors, ultrasonic cleaners, and sterilizers.
  ○ Ensuring sufficient supply of consumables are available.
  ○ Cleaning and maintaining all equipment according to manufacturer's recommendations.
  ○ Monitoring and maintaining accurate records of the decontamination process.
  ○ Interpreting and maintaining accurate records of quality test results, such as Bowie–Dick (B–D) tests, BIs, physical tests, etc.
  ○ Maintaining tracking and traceability records.
  ○ Overseeing sterile storage and dispatch procedures.
  ○ Transportation to the site of use such as the OR or a ward.

In a larger organization, career development and growth are important considerations. Career growth can be defined as progressing through different stages of a job, where as you grow and become more competent you are introduced to new challenges, activities, and responsibilities, as well as learning new processes, ultimately leading to a job that has more duties and receives more compensation. Career growth and personal development also encompass acquiring educational and practical qualifications. For in-house training to be successful it must generate commitment from the participants and this can be achieved by linking to personal and career development.

Skills and knowledge requirements

Device processing has become a specialized profession and should be recognized as a specialty in its own right. Processing departments play a specific and important part in the running of any healthcare facility, requiring highly qualified personnel, highly technical equipment, and quality requirements. Working in such departments can be challenging, demanding, and varied. Historically, processing responsibilities used to fall within existing nursing structures and responsibilities; this is no longer always the case and processing is more often managed by a specific, independent, and highly skilled manager, trained specifically in processing medical devices and ensuring the availability of safe medical supplies. Depending on the country, there are many structured training programs that consider processing as a unique discipline and allow for career development.

It is the responsibility of the top management of any healthcare facility to make sure that staff education and training are appropriate to their specific functions, and this includes decontamination and processing. It is the processing area manager's responsibility to identify specific developmental and training needs of all staff in the department to ensure patient safety, quality, and an effective and efficient process. Considering the range of chemical, microbiological, and equipment risks to staff and patients, it is essential that all personnel involved with device/material reprocessing have an in-depth knowledge of the full decontamination process and are adequately trained. Initial and regular (refresher) training is of equal importance. This will not only reduce any safety risk but can be an important cost saving to a facility by improving efficiencies and reducing accidents.

It is recommended that those working in a processing area have a good general education, including numeracy and literacy skills, to ensure compliance with area procedures and processes including use of equipment, tools, and chemicals. An ability to follow detailed instructions and work quickly and precisely is an advantage. Good communication and teamwork skills are also highly regarded in this area of work. A mandatory training program should be aimed at improving the skills and abilities of the technician. All new technicians should be required to undergo routine induction training in hospital policies and procedures related to safe work practice. Regular additional or refresher training should also be considered and is often mandated in different countries to ensure staff are kept up to date on facility policies, procedures, and standards. Senior management maintaining their current knowledge on or even participating in the development of regional or international best practices and standards is always a benefit.

Training for staff in processing areas can be broad and may include:
- Basic microbiology, including infection prevention/control, chemistry, and anatomy.
- Essentials of device types and designs.
- Environmental monitoring and controls (when applicable).
- Department policies, procedures, and standards.
- Risk assessments and analysis.
- Awareness of legal and ethical requirements.
- Health and safety issues, such as safe work procedures.
- Personal hygiene, PPE, and dress codes in order to protect the individual, colleagues, and patients from harm.
- The various steps in the decontamination process.
- Specific procedures applicable to their area of work (e.g. disassembly, cleaning, disinfection, packaging, use of equipment, etc.).
- Safe operation of chemicals and equipment.
- Accidents, incident reporting, and emergency procedures.

The most important measure of competence is that an individual understands why they are doing what they are doing. Examinations can be a useful tool to check the success of any staff training, skill, or knowledge.

Managing people

Managing people is a skill and often does not come easily. Some managers or shift leaders have a natural ability to manage people and situations, while others only gain this ability over time and with experience. In all cases, training and mentoring (or advice from others) will help to develop strong management skills over time. These skills not only apply to the management of individuals who may be under direct supervision, but also to individuals in other departments/areas and even to senior managers/superiors.

There are many management styles, approaches, and recommendations. Some simple guidelines for managing people include:
- Focus on your common goal: staff/patient safety and ensuring efficient medical/surgical equipment supplies. Consider setting targets, including departmental, group, and/or individual goals/objectives. These will encourage ownership and continuous improvement.
- Build relationships: working environments are all about people and individuals. Individuals make things happen and deserve respect. Building relationships does not mean making friends but does mean building mutual respect. It is helpful for managers to understand what motivates their staff. This can be different for each person, and may include monetary compensation, formal recognition, benefits, promotion, extra time off, etc.
- Develop effective communication skills.
- Be prepared to listen to your staff, co-workers, suppliers, and senior management: they can have different perspectives and needs, but by listening you can help develop mutual understanding, trust, and respect. Patience often helps too.
- Be sensitive to the diversity of your staff and co-workers: take into consideration age, gender, language, and cultural differences. These factors influence how you should communicate and manage various individuals.
- Managing people and processes does not mean doing all the work yourself: learn to delegate responsibility and encourage responsibility in others. Staff should be responsible for their actions; admit your own mistakes and encourage staff to do the same. Everyone makes mistakes, but everyone should also learn from them. Discuss and rectify mistakes quickly and with respect.
- Build a team spirit: encourage staff to work as a team, including having team goals and responsibilities. This is equally important in and outside the processing area.

- Develop your staff: encourage leadership and ensure training is adequate to meet current and future demands. Set goals and then praise and celebrate success.
- Conflict management: deal effectively with staff within and outside of the department, including customers, suppliers, and management.
- Set standards and lead by example: encourage staff to be part of setting these standards and optimize existing processes within a department. The more you involve staff, the more ownership and pride they will have in their roles.
- Be honest, ethical, and fair: enjoy your work and others will enjoy it with you.

Shift leaders and managers will have their own unique style of managing people, but here we can consider three basic management styles. An autocratic leader can be considered very controlling, makes all the decisions, and gives all the instructions. A participative leader allows the staff to be involved in decision making, can delegate to others some responsibilities, but may still make the final decision and take responsibility. A casual leader leaves all the decision making to the staff and is generally a hands-off manager. Each style can have advantages and disadvantages, and managers may need to consider adjusting their style to the circumstances and the individuals they are dealing with. In an emergency, for example, the leader may need to be more autocratic. Overall, an effective leader will make use of all management styles depending on the situation.

Decision making is an important part of everyday life and an important skill in management. There is only one thing worse than making a decision and that is not making a decision. In making important decisions try to follow a series of steps, including:
- Gathering information (including listening to others).
- Understanding the problem.
- Looking at alternatives.
- Choosing an alternative and implementing it.
- Evaluating the results or outcome of that decision.

In addition to utilizing the appropriate management style, leaders should implement formal staff performance systems and build a positive employee engagement culture.

Staff performance

Staff performance is simple to say but often difficult to execute, depending on the leader's ability to have critical conversations. The first step is to ensure that clear expectations are set for each employee. These often include quality, productivity, teamwork, work ethic, and other attributes associated with that staff position's objectives. Expectations should follow the "SMART" goals approach by being **S**pecific, **M**easurable, **A**chievable, **R**elevant, and **T**ime bound.

Once expectations are set and agreed to, leaders should frequently review employee performance and promote employees reviewing their own performance. Positive performance and skills should be reinforced and recognized. Opportunities for improvement must be discussed, with action plans and required support agreed to, including resources and timelines. These critical conversations are not only beneficial to departmental performance, but also beneficial in showing employees fair treatment, support when needed, and a focus on qualitative performance metrics versus emotion.

Managing staff performance is also a part of building a positive employee culture along with employee engagement. It allows for the opportunity to build and appreciate leadership roles within the team that will be a benefit in the future, including supporting training budgets to develop staff.

Employee engagement

A common measurement of effective personnel management is employee engagement scores. A short and simple definition of positive employee engagement is a culture in which employees happily participate in helping achieve the department's goals and objectives. Employee engagement includes the following elements:
- Cultivating alignment of individual goals and values with those of the organization.
- Providing motivation for employees to contribute to the organization's success.
- Encouraging active employee involvement in continuous improvement processes.
- Providing employees with a sense of well-being, belonging, and satisfaction.
- Conducting periodic satisfaction surveys (e.g. yearly).

A point often missed by well-intentioned leaders is that employee engagement does not come from simply being open to listening to ideas from your employees. Numerous departments have reached out to their employees for improvement suggestions only to never follow through on them. This lack of follow-through results in employees withdrawing from actively engaging, with the attitude that management never listens to them anyway.

Employee engagement is the result of a positive and engaging culture that is developed by numerous factors. Most prominent is the leadership's ability to motivate staff by developing positivity, inclusion, physical and emotional safety, and a caring environment. Staff will be engaged when they feel safe, treated fairly, listened to, and respected.

An easy sign to determine the level of staff engagement is how often they try to help make the department better and continuously improve. This also assumes that department goals and objectives have been communicated, and that the team understands their performance expectations. From this point, the following five components can help to build engagement and continuous improvement from staff:
- Have a process to capture ideas or suggestions: whether in writing or verbal, staff need to have a safe outlet to voice their

improvement ideas. Set guidelines, such as that improvements must be focused on the department's objectives. Then determine how to capture ideas and suggestions, such as suggestion boxes, team huddles, or meetings. The main point is to build trust among staff that they are safe to voice their ideas.
- Provide a venue to encourage discussion within the team: a successful employee engagement program should be visible throughout the process, from suggestion to approval to implementation, and become a standard part of periodic discussions. Use these times to show the department's metrics and expectations for improvements. Discussion should also include progress on implementation of past suggestions and results from suggestions already implemented.
- Devise a system of timely review and approval: employees will engage when they believe their engagement makes a difference and is not ignored. Leaders should provide timely feedback on employees' suggestions and involvement. To do so, first set a limit on how many suggestions can be worked on. Let the staff know how many suggestions can be adequately accepted based on the time required to review and provide feedback. Long delays in receiving feedback or implementation can seriously degrade a process improvement program/ employee engagement effort and lead employees to believe that leadership is not serious about listening to their ideas. Early in the process, the leader should resist the temptation to over-analyze and reject suggestions. Instead, take the opportunity to coach and improve the development and presentation of ideas. Facilitate idea creation and implementation to ensure that a continuous improvement culture develops. Remember that not every suggestion or implementation will be successful or improve performance. The point is to not expect perfection, to allow people to learn from their mistakes, and to continue to work at improving processes without undue fear of failure. Encourage a culture of finding solutions to problems.
- Formally document the suggestion: even the smallest of changes should be documented because this encourages review and idea sharing. Remember that every change must be standardized, trained to, and added to the routine training and competency programs. Documentation provides the structure to ensure that the change is understood, the risks have been considered, it has been implemented correctly, and all employees involved have been consistently trained.
- Organize visual sharing and recognition: the last step is to visually share and recognize the improvements and suggestions. Be sure to promote these both internally in the processing department but also to the department's customers.

One more common employee engagement measurement is to periodically survey employees and use the information they provide. Most healthcare organizations already have internal employee engagement surveys that highlight opportunities to improve culture and employee satisfaction.

Teamwork

Teamwork is about a group of interdependent individuals, often with different abilities, talents, experiences, and backgrounds, working together to achieve a common goal. Teams can be specific to certain processing areas or contain a wider range of skilled workers from different departments and possibly different organizations. It should be remembered that the processing department can depend on others within the healthcare facility and likewise other departments depend on the efficiency of the processing cycle. Consider, for example, the dependence of a modern processing area on support from engineering or biomedical staff to ensure the efficient operation and maintenance of equipment, but with surgical and medical staff demanding the immediate availability of processed devices for a patient procedure. Device and material processing is one of the cornerstones of infection prevention and control within a facility, requiring close cooperation. Less obvious, yet important, staff members who may be involved can include finance, legal, and quality representatives to understand budgets (today and future) and risks that could affect the performance and even reputation of the facility.

The goal of a team approach to processing is to ensure optimal and efficient device processing for all concerned, including the patient. Any such team needs a leader, whose challenge is to gain the trust and cooperation of all involved and encourage them to work together. A smart leader, which may or may not be the manager of the processing area, will use all available resources to get the job done.

Effective communication is generally the key to these collaborative teams succeeding. If team members do not communicate effectively among themselves the task will not be accomplished. Communication can be achieved in many ways, but open discussion and agreement as part of a team should be considered the most beneficial. Consider regular meetings, speaking face to face, or using the telephone rather than writing emails that may not convey the message properly or may be misconstrued. Irrespective of how smart or educated any one individual is in the team, the combined talents, expertise, experience, and ideas of the group will always be more effective. Great team members should consider themselves part of the whole process and goal, with positive attitudes, willingness to listen to others, and belief in themselves to play their role. A team must have operating ground rules, policies, procedures, principles, and values to function efficiently.

Team leadership

To enable team success, a leader should be nominated who is able to lead effectively through experience, example, motivation, and delegation. Unfortunately, not all managers are considered effective leaders. The behavior of leaders and management will generally be similar throughout the organization; therefore, focusing on providing an efficient service within a processing area can have greater effects throughout the facility. If team members are treated as valued members of the team and with respect, no matter what position the team member occupies, they will be motivated to do the same to others. If team members feel that their efforts are not recognized, they become demotivated and less inclined to do a good job. Effective personnel management skills equally apply to managing a team under direct supervision and to a wider multidisciplinary team. Consider the following guidelines in managing any team:

- Define what the team is trying to achieve and make sure the team agrees.
- Make sure that all team members are aware of and understand the team rules (policies, procedures, ethics, etc.).
- Know what skills each member of the team has to offer.
- Ensure that all team members are capable and trained to do their specific job.
- Manage the team fairly.
- Delegate responsibilities (see next paragraph).
- Give recognition and praise where it is due; it motivates people.
- Deal directly with any conflict and differences of opinion.
- Enforce agreed policies and positively discipline team members who break these rules.
- Represent and support the team.

Delegation is one of the most important team management skills – and one of the easiest to get wrong. It is defined as empowering individuals or groups to take responsibility for certain tasks or goals. Delegation can help individuals and teams to be more effective and efficient, but also motivates and develops staff, including new leaders. Poor delegation can cause frustration, demotivation, and failure to get the task done. Delegation is not about telling someone what to do, but rather about empowering and enabling others to take control of tasks/goals and holding them accountable for the outcome. This can be particularly effective if team members understand, are involved with, and agree with the goal. If team members are required to think about the task/goal, consider alternatives, and make choices, the work becomes more challenging, with the added advantage of motivating team members to succeed. For effective delegation consider the following points:

- Define what must be achieved, particularly with the team member you are delegating to, and even better if it is their idea.
- Ensure the chosen person is trained and able to perform the activity.
- Explain what is expected and agree on a timeline.
- Make resources available, if required. Consider people, location, premises, equipment, money, materials, and other related activities and services.
- Offer support and encouragement, but do not interfere, unless the outcome is critical.
- Periodically review to let the person know how they are doing.
- Congratulate when they are doing well and offer advice when not.

Do not always try to fix their problem. It may appear quicker or easier for you, but it often does not help either of you in the long term. You must be willing to absorb the consequences of failure and pass on the credit for success.

Team communication

Effective communication is at the core of any successful team and organization. One of the first signs that a team is not working together is a lack of communication. Effective communication should concentrate on the basics; that is, listening, speaking, questioning, sharing information, and mutual respect. When successful, communication improves morale and overall performance, reducing the opportunity for confusion and conflict. Communication moves in many directions: downward, across to your peers, and upward. Downward communication is the way management communicates with employees. Every employee needs to know how the organization functions and what the organization's mission statement, values, and goals are. Employees should be aware of all the up-to-date personnel policies and procedures. Managers should have regular face-to-face meetings with employees to recognize and celebrate major achievements. This helps employees perceive what is important, gives them a sense of direction and fulfillment, and lets them know that management is aware of their contributions. All employees should receive at least an annual review (if not more frequent) from their managers, regarding their performance, their goals for the future, accomplishments, needs for improvement, and management plans to assist the employee to accomplish the improvements. Across communication will be important in ensuring teamwork, understanding, and support from other departments. The manager of a processing area will depend on their management partners in many other departments, including ORs, biomedical engineering, engineering support and/or maintenance, suppliers and supplier management, and others areas that depend on the processing department. Upward communication can be equally important, from employees to various levels of management. Examples can include assistance with budget management, headcount resources, and conflict management. This can be done informally or formally at an individual level or at team meetings; it is important to use these opportunities to discuss any current concerns and ideas from employees, including managers.

The processing area often deals with an interdisciplinary team that includes representatives from various departments. Communication outside the department can therefore be as important as inside it. The processing area should develop communication patterns between the individuals involved and their respective departments; these should be meaningful, direct, open, and honest. Be clear and precise about the direction of the department, its intentions, expectations, and values. It is recommended to focus on one issue at a time, using facts rather than judgments. Effective communication is only possible in an atmosphere of trust and openness. As for internal teams, if other team members do not understand or agree to your goals then you can expect that the message will be lost.

It may appear simple, but there are three components to effective communication:
- Sender
- Message
- Recipient

Before communicating with others, the sender needs to be aware of what they want to communicate; that is, what message must be understood by the recipient. Communication is a two-way process and to communicate effectively both parties need to take turns at listening. When communicating with staff members, ask them to explain what you have just told them, to make sure that you conveyed the correct message and that they understood the message clearly. The sender sets the tone of the communication. If the sender is aggressive the recipient will more than likely ignore the message and even respond aggressively. The expectations that you communicate will shape the response that you get; if the recipient does not understand the meaning of the message that the sender has tried to impart, the communication has failed. Remember that face-to-face or phone conversations are better to resolve issues quickly and effectively. Other methods, such as emails, can also be effective in providing information to a larger group of interested team members. Within any organization, an email should be considered as an official document within or provided outside a facility and can have even legal implications; it will reflect on the sender, their department, and even the organization. Care should also be taken to ensure that what is written is necessary, accurate, concise, professional, and inoffensive.

Change management

Change is a fact of life. We may not be able to control change, but we can choose how we respond to change. Change should be embraced and seen as an opportunity to do things differently, to grow, and to develop new strengths. If change is to be effective the team should be involved in planning the changes and decision making from the beginning; if the team is involved, they are less likely to resist change. Change can be disruptive but forces the group to make choices. A good team leader will anticipate change and prepare the team to face the challenges. It is their role to challenge, motivate, and empower the team through the change(s), while maintaining the dynamics of the team. Sharing the group, department, or facility vision of the future with employees, defining their role and what they need to achieve, as well as the benefits of change to them, will encourage them to embrace the change.

Having a process in mind to consider the change is important. Remember that the change may range in its impact, such as the introduction of a new set of devices, change in IFU, new equipment for processing, new regulatory requirements, or expanding the design of a process or processing area. In all of these cases, having a standard way of considering and implementing the change as a team leads to a greater opportunity to succeed. This can take time, but the time you spend on this up front will benefit the success of the desired change.

Conflict management

Disagreements and conflicts, both personal and professional, are a normal occurrence, but how we deal with them can be successfully managed. The basic principle of conflict management is about understanding that not all conflict can be resolved, but it can be managed in a way that will decrease the impact on the team. The most common reasons for conflict among members of a team are:
- Ambiguous expectations and role clarification.
- Lack of time or resources, which can either be perceived by a team member or be real.
- Feelings of unfair treatment.
- Gender- and generation-based differences.
- Cultural differences.
- Personality differences.
- Lack of clear communication to team members.
- Ineffective leadership.

Conflict is natural and inevitable, but is often a symptom of problems and the need for change. But conflict itself is not the problem; unresolved, destructive conflict that is not dealt with and erodes the team is the real problem. This is a responsibility of a team leader and should be taken seriously. An effective "conflict manager" must be aware of some conflict management skills and be able to use communication effectively to resolve or minimize the conflict. These include:
- Do not ignore conflict: manage it.
- Set team and individual goals, ensuring that adequate resources (staff, equipment, etc.) are available. Getting staff to work together and depend on each other can be helpful to diffuse disagreements.
- Hold regular staff or team meetings to discuss goals and problems.
- Build a team spirit and good working relationships.
- Set team rules, including mutual respect. These may include already defined facility expectations, such as gender, social, and racial equality. When rules are broken, be quick and firm to reprimand.
- Consider having a means for anonymous feedback.

Resolution of conflict is dependent on effective communication and compromise when possible between the two "warring parties." Underlying issues need to be openly expressed and addressed, with the goal of gaining a mutual agreement. The outcome should be mutually satisfactory, but often with neither party feeling that they have been completely satisfied. Sometimes an excellent compromise is when neither party feels completely fulfilled. By discussing issues related to conflict management, teams can establish an expected protocol to be followed by team members when in conflict.

Effective teamwork

As an example of an effective team, let us look at a professional soccer or football team. The aim is not only to win a game but also to win the league. To win the league, you must be the best. To be the best, you must have the best team, not just the best players. A great team works together as one unit, producing fast, creative, wise, decisive, and consistent results. All team members must be aware of what they are trying to achieve and of what rules need to be adhered to. These rules give the team a sense of stability in knowing what to expect. A team needs rules on how to manage itself and play the game. These rules are usually defined by the football authorities and tradition (e.g. if the goalkeeper is hurt the ball is kicked out of play). The team will also have its own rules regarding how many practices a player can miss, how many red or yellow cards are acceptable, and so on. To score goals against the opposing side all members of the team must work together and contribute; it is difficult for 10 players to win against 11. The team is only as strong as its weakest link. If players are injured or suspended the entire team is affected. If one person forgets their role or does not perform adequately, the opposing team could score a goal. Team members need to monitor each other and be accountable to each other.

A team that wants to be great (world class) needs to stop every once in a while and look at how it is doing. Losing should not shut the team down. The team must learn from failures, refocus, and move forward. If a team loses, they should look for mistakes, identify weaknesses, and work on those weaknesses. Improvements can only be made if problems are identified. It is not a good sign if players start skipping practice, arriving late or unprepared for games, or are being sent off. These are signs of the team starting to break down. To prevent this, the team will need to be reassessed regularly. The team manager is crucial in developing a winning strategy. For optimum production the manager will need to constantly observe the team and look at ways of working together more effectively by:
- Identifying differences and problem areas.
- Identifying and recording all process non-conformances.
- Setting immediate/corrective/preventative actions and reviewing the effectiveness of the actions.
- Deciding if it is time to do things differently.
- Helping the team develop through training.
- Bringing in new players or even coaches.

Finally, when the team goal is achieved, there is a payoff for all team members. In soccer this may include end-of-season bonuses, but also the sense of achieving the best, which all depends on how the team is playing. If the team is playing well and winning, then the stadiums will be full and supporters will be happy. They will continue to support and invest in the team. The supporters will expect the team to maintain a certain high standard, to change with the times, and to meet their expectations. The better the team the more supporters there will be (everyone loves a winner), and the more investors the club will attract. If a team is doing badly, players and supporters tend to look for more exciting clubs.

Legal and ethical responsibilities

All processing area workers have a legal and ethical responsibility to safely prepare devices and materials for patient use. The patient, their family and friends, and the healthcare facility depend on this and each employee should clearly understand their role and responsibility. The responsibility overall lies with management and staff to ensure they understand and apply the applicable laws, regulations, standards, and best practices that apply in the country they live in and the facility they work in. Knowledge and an understanding of these requirements are important, and should not be underestimated.

The word "ethics" is derived from the Greek word *ethos*, which means "the sum of good values of a character." Socrates, a Greek philosopher, is often considered to be the father of ethics. A person is said to be ethical when they respect others, follow the rules, and value life and the community. Being ethical is essentially being fair or doing the right thing. This means understanding a situation from another person's perspective – not just your own. An important concept here is to embrace diversity, equity, and inclusion in the work environment as best principles.

Legal responsibility refers to understanding and following the laws of any region, state, country, or area to which you belong. This can often be complicated, changing and differing from region to region. Legal responsibilities can include civil and criminal laws.

Civil laws deal with relationships between people and protecting their rights. Examples are:
- Negligence (malpractice): this can lead to injury, including infection, to you, other workers, and patients. Examples include not reporting a defective piece of equipment or device or intentionally providing a non-sterile device for a critical procedure.
- Defamation: providing false or inaccurate statements about a person that could damage their reputation. Included under

defamation are statements that are spoken ("slander") and/or written ("libel").
• Assault and abuse: physical, verbal, or mental abuse can include hitting, swearing, and gender, sexual, and racial abuse.
• Invasion of privacy: this includes revealing personal or private information about a person without their consent, which could include employee or patient information.
• Occupational health and safety: most countries have strict regulations regarding employers providing safe working environments and employees following safe working practices/procedures. This includes the correct provision and use of PPE (see Chapters 5 and 13).

Criminal laws deal with actions against a person, property, or society with intent. Many of the examples given under civil laws may also be considered as criminal, depending on the nature of the act. These may include:
• Health laws, specifically directing facility leadership to provide safe care to patients. Facility management and/or an individual may be directly responsible for negligence in the care of patients, an example being infection transmission or action leading to a staff accident, which could have serious civil and criminal legal consequences.
• Stealing equipment and materials.
• Illegal disposal of chemicals or wastes.
• Deliberate damage to persons or property.
• Accepting bribes, directly or indirectly, including money or a gift that alters the behavior of the recipient (e.g. using a new product or influencing the acquisition of equipment/supplies).

Employees should be aware of the facility's and their personal legal responsibilities and understand the long-term consequences of negligence, omissions, and unlawful and unethical behavior. The facility's legal responsibilities should be based on current regulations and laws applicable to their region, state, country, and/or region. Employees must also be knowledgeable about the law, as in certain situations they may be involved in writing or modifying facility guidelines. For example, various regions, states, and countries may periodically introduce or adopt various regulations, standards, and guidelines that directly affect the processing area:
• A regulation is a rule or order issued by a country, community, or administrative agency, generally under legal authority, and has the force of law.
• A standard is a document that specifies the minimum acceptable characteristics of a product or material, issued by a standards organization. Examples include the International Organization for Standardization (ISO) and the European Committee for Standardization (CEN). Standards may or may not have legal stature within a given country.
• A guideline is a document used to communicate recommended procedures, processes, or usage of certain practices. In general guidelines do not have legal stature, but are often considered best practice at the time of writing.

In some cases the correct adoption of the various regulations, standards, and guidelines within a facility or department will be periodically audited by independent bodies and can have significant consequences including closure, legal penalties, or loss of reputation. Examples include the US Joint Commission (www.jointcommission.org), the Council of the European Union Medical Devices Directive (Directive 93/42/EEC), and the UK Quality Care Commission (www.cqc.org.uk).

Process management

As discussed earlier in this chapter, device processing requires up-front planning to ensure that the department has the appropriate space, equipment, labor, materials, workflow, and leadership to meet customer requirements. These resources must be effectively managed together to provide an efficient, effective, and quality process.

Process hazard analysis and risk management

It is important to understand potential hazards associated with processing devices and the risks they impose on the process. Performing a hazard analysis and risk management can be important tools in identifying and reducing risks in any process, but also in identifying opportunities for process improvement. A typical risk analysis will consist of two steps:
• Review current processes and procedures to identify key hazards in each area. Examples include devices not available for a patient procedure, insufficient cleaning, failed disinfection or sterilization conditions, and damage to packaged goods during transport to the location of use.
• Evaluate the hazards and determine their level of risks, their significance, and any action items for risk reduction. Discuss how to control and monitor hazards.

Teamwork is the best approach in performing a risk assessment. Depending on the process or area being evaluated, risk assessment teams may include processing staff, nursing and or other surgical/medical staff ("the customer"), equipment and device manufacturers, consumables manufacturers, infection prevention, health and safety, equipment maintenance, and engineering and facility management staff. It is recommended to focus on one area or process at a time to allow individual team members to provide their perspectives on items relevant to their expertise. Risk analysis should be a continuous effort that develops over time and maybe periodically updated. The team should consider rating the level of risk on an agreed scale such as the one provided in Figure 14.4. Such analysis allows for any risks to be graded from high to low, enabling the team to identify the more significant risks and consider action to reduce them. Start simply and continue to build on this over time. You may want to initially focus on risk analysis in areas that have had complaints or known quality issues in the past.

			Hazard scale				
			5 Death or total systems loss	4 Major injury or illness	3 Lost time, injury or illness	2 First aid incident	1 Very minor, little consequence
			Catastrophic	Critical	Serious	Marginal	Negligible
Likelihood scale	5	Likely to occur frequently	Frequent	25 = Rethink	20 = Rethink	15 = Rethink	10 = Reduce	5 = Inform
	4	Likely to occur several times	Probable	20 = Rethink	16 = Rethink	12 = Reduce	8 = Reduce	4 = Inform
	3	Sometimes	Occasional	15 = Rethink	12 = Reduce	9 = Reduce	6 = Inform	3 = Inform
	2	Unlikely but possible	Remote	10 = Reduce	8 = Reduce	6 = Inform	4 = Inform	2 = No action
	1	Very unlikely assumption that it will never occur	Improbable	5 = Inform	4 = Inform	3 = Inform	2 = No action	1 = No action

Figure 14.4 An example of a matrix that can be used to grade risks identified in a process. Each identified risk is scored from 1 to 5 on its likelihood of occurring (on the left) and the severity of the hazard (on the top). Overall, the risk is scored by multiplying the numbers on each scale (likelihood × hazard). The final score dictates if the risk is low (e.g. <2) or high (>15), therefore requiring action or not (in this example four different levels or grades are defined).

There are many different methods, guidelines, and standards that can be used in conducting risk analysis. An example is ISO 14971, *Medical devices – Application of risk management to medical devices*.

Pre-cleaning, cleaning, and disinfection

Managing the process of decontamination, the cleaning (and disinfection, when appropriate) of dirty devices, focuses on maintaining a continuous flow to remove soil (including bioburden) as soon as possible before it dries. This requires proper staffing at the point of use and the area of arrival at a designated processing area, and an understanding of the time requirement to properly clean and disinfect the items. Adherence to manufacturers' IFU is critical to ensure proper steps are taken to remove soil and render the items safe for handling on the clean side. Compliance with IFU is often most difficult during the cleaning process and use of technology is recommended to ensure that staff are not relying on memory alone to know what and how to clean different types of devices.

During planning, the required equipment, supplies, and workflows should have been determined for effective cleaning and disinfection for the planned volume of instruments or other devices. During work in this area, process management becomes focused on ensuring that adequate staff are available, a system for identifying priorities is in place based on customer requirements, tools and technology are in place to assist with regulatory and IFU compliance, staff are trained for the tasks they are performing, adequate PPE is available, and department leaders are monitoring performance.

In many cases, depending on the department, cleaning and disinfection may be a fully manual process and/or an automated process. It may also be a terminal process (as in the case of non-critical equipment) or steps prior to further processing (as is the case for critical devices). Planning the handling of non-critical and critical device processing should be considered in the area. Some non-critical equipment will be directly returned to clinical use from this area, with the requirement for separate handling/flow of product to ensure that dirty and clean/disinfected equipment are not mixed. Other equipment may be used together with critical devices for transportation to a storage area or for clinical use, as in the case of carts or trollies. They will typically require some form of routine cleaning–disinfection that can be manual or automated (e.g. cart washers or washer-disinfectors). For transportation equipment, the process flow in and out of these areas will be important to consider and the risks need to be evaluated. Provisions for moving equipment, instruments, and devices between this and other processing areas will be important (e.g. pass-through hatches between areas and how/why they are used).

Preparation and packaging

Process management in preparation (including maintenance and inspection) and packaging (when appropriate) continues to focus on continuous flow to ensure that devices are processed in a timely manner and provided for sterilization and sterile storage. Customer priorities, requirements, and, in particular, missing (or damaged) devices become important factors in this area. Most often at this stage devices are safe for handling, but special provision may need to be made for a process to accommodate devices that remain biohazardous due to lack of standard processing (e.g. contaminated cables or other devices that may not be able to be exposed to water immersion or heat decontamination processes, or devices found to still have residual soil present). The department can focus on processing devices that have been prioritized based on the customer or surgery schedule and available inventory. Technological advancements provide integration between OR or other area scheduling and instrument tracking systems to assist in prioritizing processing based on customer requirements, available inventory, and the real-time status of devices/trays in process. This type of augmented intelligence can assist in performing and prioritizing workload to ensure that customer requirements are met.

Another aspect in preparation/packaging that requires process management is the handling of missing or extra instruments found in a tray during the reassembly process. Depending on how well the surgical or clinical teams returned the instrumentation to the correct tray, the processing staff may find trays with missing items or with extra items in the tray. Standard work for handling these situations must be developed, trained to, and adhered to in order to provide complete trays. This will include provisions for waiting for feedback from users, as well as options for repair, replacement, and so on.

Consideration in terms of time and process needs to be given to the requirements for inspection (e.g. of cleanliness or damage) and often maintenance (e.g. lubrication) that will have to be conducted at this stage, as well as the associated record keeping of the results from such actions (see under quality requirements later in this chapter).

Sterilization and sterile storage

Process management within the sterilization process focuses on maintaining workflow, ensuring compliance to manufacturer's sterilization parameters or IFU, and ensuring that all documentation is properly captured. Instrument tracking system technology is widely used in this area to ensure proper documentation and even provide built-in quality checks that the proper cycle selection is made that matches each instrument's requirements.

Processing departments typically have two modalities of sterilization: steam sterilization and some form of low-temperature sterilization. Steam sterilization handles items that can withstand high temperatures and pressure as it utilizes pressurized steam to sterilize items. Low-temperature sterilization can be provided by different means and chemicals, with the most common worldwide being the use of hydrogen peroxide gas systems. The lower-temperature gas processes are commonly used for items with plastics, rubber, or other material that would melt at high temperatures. Both steam and low-temperature sterilization have required documentation as well as testing and monitoring requirements that will be discussed in the quality management section.

Understanding customer needs

No matter how well you plan, measure, work as a team, and manage your people and processes, if you do not deliver what your customer needs daily, you are not going to be successful. Meeting your customer's daily needs is the top priority within process management. Although the requirements and approach will vary from location to location, some of the basic considerations will include:

- Review expectations with your customer 24–72 hours in advance. Are there significant changes in the surgical cases that were unexpected? Ensure that the customer confirms their requirements and the vendor trays needed, and reviews any surgeon preferences. In some cases this may be possible, but in others it may be more difficult (e.g. in cases of trauma surgery). Communication with the customer can establish shared expectations.
- Develop plans for inventory shortages or customer requests to quickly process items for a second or multiple use on the same day. Ensure that there is a documented process for handling these priority situations, and what is considered acceptable or not.
- Develop a process within the preparation and packaging team to prioritize the reassembly of trays based on customer requirements. This process can be utilized for same-day needs but also for next-day needs in advance of any surgical case requirements.
- Some health systems utilize surgical case carts to deliver all instrumentation and supplies for a surgical case. The processing department may be responsible for picking the items for such carts prior to the case. If so, utilize the process to develop a needs list of items that are missing or not available for surgical requirements.
- Develop a system to audit the devices, sets, or other items supplied to the location of use such as the OR prior to the customer receiving the items. This will help ensure that all items required are provided.
- Continuous improvement. Follow up with your customers to identify issues and root causes if items were not provided properly and work to implement solutions to avoid future mistakes.

Leadership routines

Process management depends on leadership routines to follow up, monitor, support, and improve operations. These are regularly scheduled actions that team leaders, supervisors, managers, and directors can take to ensure that processes and people are working to plan and in compliance with standard work and regulatory requirements.

Leadership routines can be simple checklists guiding the leader through specific actions to capture current state performance and opportunities for continuous improvement. As with any process and especially processes dependent on people, regular follow-up is recommended to ensure that the potential for process drift is managed and controlled. Being present to observe and verify practices is important and should be expected by staff members. Regular follow-up allows leaders the opportunity to reinforce positive behaviors and high performance, address opportunities in real time, engage with staff, and see what is really happening versus what should be happening. Leadership routines are core to the opportunity for process improvement as well.

Process improvement

Managing a process includes the opportunity to understand how it can be improved and the implementation of change to make improvements. Improvements can focus on performance to plan and quality issues, or on finding ways to improve performance to exceed the plan. Process measurements (considered later in this chapter) can provide the data and information that identify process improvement initiatives. Failed outcomes or quality measures that are below customer expectations should drive immediate process improvement efforts, while process or waste measurements may drive ongoing incremental change. Either way, measurements of where you are starting from (and associated reasonable goals for where you would like to be) are required for process improvement to be successful and meaningful.

Improving processes can be done through many established and proven standardized methods, a few of which are:
- 5 Whys. This is a simple but systematic method to identify the root causes of a problem. It refers to the practice of asking the question "why" five times to understand the real reason a defect or failure occurred in a process. Each successive question allows a deeper understanding of the cause of the issue being investigated. Five is a relative number that forces you to analyze and continue asking questions until there are no more whys to answer. You may need to ask why more or less than five times to get to the real reason. In theory, the root cause is eventually identified and then can be acted on. The technique is used to ensure that the real cause of the problem is addressed and not just a symptom.
- Structured problem solving. There are many methods described by various steps (often as acronyms) that follow a similar approach to problem solving and process improvements. They help ensure that root causes are identified and addressed instead of simply treating the symptoms. The goal is that problems are clearly recognized and measured against clear objectives and standard processes. Examples include PDCA (Plan, Do, Check, and Act) and DMAIC (Define, Measure, Analyze, Improve, and Control). PDCA starts with taking time to "plan" what you are trying to do and ensure that you understand the real problem and root cause being addressed. You should use this time to gather information on the current state and conditions, then plan your action items for correcting the problem and establish a clear goal for what the outcome should be. Then "do," implementing your planned changes and how you will measure success in the goal. "Check" to follow up and measure the new process performance and determine whether the changes are meeting expectations. Finally, "act": if the new changes are successful, ensure that they are standardized and methods implemented to sustain the improvements. If the outcomes are not successful, then return to plan and start over, incorporating the newly learned lessons and what did not work. DMAIC has a similar outline. "Define," by taking time to identify the problems, current conditions, the improvement opportunity desired, and a clear goal for the expected outcome. "Measure," by gathering data on the current process or operational performance you wish to improve. "Analyze" the data to identify the root causes of the issue. "Improve," by developing and implementing new processes and operational improvements to eliminate or reduce the root causes and improving performance. And finally, "control," to measure the new operational performance to determine whether the changes were successful and then manage and sustain the improvements.
- Lean principles. The core principles of lean can be described as people working together and continuously improving to create customer value and meet requirements without generating waste. It is therefore a never-ending philosophy that continually looks to meet changing customer requirements while finding ways to be more efficient and eliminate waste from operational processes. The core concepts were initially developed in automobile manufacturing but have been embraced worldwide by all industries.

Let us consider lean principles further. The earlier discussions in this chapter on management incorporated lean principles without even mentioning lean. Creating an operational plan to achieve continuous flow and balanced line processing are lean concepts. Standard work and employee engagement also encompass lean concepts. As with all other process improvement approaches, lean requires measurements to be in place to measure opportunity and improvement against. The different improvement methods described earlier are considered lean tools. Perhaps some of the most

famous lean principles are known as the seven wastes of lean and are:
- Overproduction: producing more than your customer requires.
- Waiting: delays, backlogs, no value being added.
- Transportation: movement of material without adding value.
- Inventory: material beyond what is needed based on customer demand.
- Motion: excessive motion.
- Overprocessing: doing more work than the customer requires.
- Defects: items not meeting customer specifications requiring rework.

Embracing lean principles is therefore best accomplished by embracing the culture of continuous improvement, employee engagement, and a team effort to measure and quantify opportunities while always looking for ways to eliminate waste. But no matter what approach you take to process improvement, you will find similar concepts. The most important points are:
- Establish a cross-functional team that is involved in and dependent on the process.
- Understand the customer's needs and build your processes and workflows to meet those needs while identifying potential limitations.
- Use quantitative methods to monitor and measure performance. Examples include customer-facing defect rates, internal process defects such as bioburden reaching the prep and pack area, turnaround times, and employee productivity.
- Identify and prioritize improvement opportunities, involve the team in finding ways to improve, and collectively make changes while documenting and training to standard work.

Recall

A recall situation is important to consider as part of processing management. Recall is the notification and retrieval of items deemed unsafe, potentially unsafe, or non-sterile that have been placed in sterile storage, provided to a customer, or used on a patient. All processing facilities should have a written recall policy in place stating when and how items will be recalled. Examples of such situations could include failed BI or CI tests, washer or sterilizer malfunctions, or if sterile packs are known to have been compromised. In the event of such process failures, items known or suspected to have been affected must immediately be recalled for correct processing or discarded. In addition, any equipment or processes will need to be evaluated and if applicable taken out of service.

It is recommended when a recall is required that the details are documented, to include any known causes, affected items, retrieved and processed items, and if any items have already been used on patients. As it becomes apparent that items need to be recalled, processing personnel will immediately notify users and retrieve the supplies from storage or directly from users as soon as possible. A recall is usually authorized by the most senior staff member on the shift, or according to the facility's policy. The processing failure may be due to problems identified in the processing area, site of device use, or even from patient information (e.g. infection, toxic reaction, or complication).

Affected departments should be advised verbally as soon as possible, with a follow-up, written confirmation stipulating which items from a particular batch are suspect and should be returned. Departments should be requested to check their stocks, used and unused, for any suspect items. Recalled items should be labeled "under quarantine" while in transit back to the processing area, where they can be safely handled and/or discarded; this will depend on the cause of the recall and should be in accordance with the facility's policy.

A recall should be conducted by an authorized team. This will at least include processing staff, surgical staff, and particularly any facility infection prevention representative. Infection prevention should assess any risks to patients who may be affected by suspect items. Team members may include other staff, such as hospital management, legal, and engineering biomedical representatives, as well as external suppliers or manufacturers, depending on the risks to patients and in order to resolve any identified problems. As a final note, the cause of the recall should be fully investigated, a report written, and every effort made to reduce the risk of reoccurrence.

Materials management

Materials management refers to the purchasing and managing of supplies and equipment to enable the processing department to operate effectively. Departments may manage this directly with suppliers or with assistance from other departments such as supply chain, purchasing, or finance. It may include supplies specific to processing, such as cleaning and disinfection chemicals, indicators, equipment, or packaging materials, but also the various devices required for surgical use in the facility. Two aspects of materials management are particularly important to processing departments: inventory management for both processing supplies and device/instrument inventory, and tracking/traceability systems.

Inventory management

Inventory management applies to every item used during processing, including supplies used in processing and finished goods such as instrument trays. Effectively forecasting, procuring, and maintaining inventory needs will ensure that the processing area has the correct amount of stock in the correct place at the correct time to meet the needs of the facility.

Inventory management includes the monitoring and recording of inventory at each site of use, including how much to keep on hand, when to purchase, how much to purchase,

controlling loss due to damage or waste, and managing shortages and back orders. There are many methods for controlling inventory, all designed to provide an efficient system for deciding what, when, and how much to have or order. Effective inventory management to maintain the right level of stock is particularly important in the supply of consumables (materials used during processing) and devices both new and processed. The levels of inventory will depend on a number of factors unique to the facility, such as the reliability of supply and how steady the demand/use is. When deciding on what level of stock to hold the following questions can be considered:
- How reliable is the supply, what is the lead time, and are alternative sources available?
- Can demand for processed items be accurately predicted?
- What are the cost implications of holding or not holding essential inventory?
- What is the impact of any expiry dates (typically with single-use items) and implementing a first-in–first out policy?
- What is the minimal functional stock level – can we identify a minimum stock level and reorder when stock reaches that level? This is known as the reorder level.
- Is there an alternative, back-up, and equivalent supplier?

There are advantages and disadvantages to holding too little and too much inventory or stock, which are outlined in Table 14.3.

Effective inventory management will enable the department to accurately track all materials and processed items in order to meet or exceed facility expectations. It can ensure consistency of supply and better understanding and control of costs.

Of particular importance to customers will be managing surgical instrument inventories, which include instruments processed and kept sterile, both peel packs and instrument trays, plus back-up single instrument inventories kept non-sterile and available to replace missing or broken instruments. To forecast required inventories of sterile items, the processing department leadership and surgical or customer leadership must jointly evaluate usage and forecasted demand against current inventories to determine what an adequate inventory level would be. This will also take into account the facility's ability to rapidly process items, while maintaining compliance with regulatory requirements and IFU, for multiple uses in the same day. It should be noted that allowing multiple uses of an item in the same day requires the processing department to prioritize that item before all other items and creates a parallel processing workstream that must be managed separately and accurately.

Surgical scheduling will be important, as surgical procedures are often grouped together in blocks to meet a surgeon's or service line's schedule of procedures on one day, which will also drive the instrument inventory requirements. A block schedule that drives four similar surgical cases back to back will require four similar instrument inventories to support the procedures. If those same four cases were booked one per day for four days, only one set of instruments would be required. Processing leadership must continually work with the surgical teams to evaluate the scheduling and instrumentation needs that can be effectively processed.

Tracking and traceability

Inventory management is best optimized using an instrument tracking system, which is an important topic to consider for modern processing departments and healthcare facilities. The original intent of instrument tracking systems was to provide a means to track instruments and monitor their progress through the processing cycle, commonly referred to as "track and trace." But modern tracking systems can offer much more and provide a wide variety of benefits.

Tracking inventory is still a core part of every tracking system, which rely on barcodes or other electronic readable codes to quickly scan the item to a location or process. With inventories that can often include thousands of instrument

Table 14.3 Advantages and disadvantages of holding too little or too much consumable/device inventory.

Too little stock	Too much stock
Just-in-time (JIT) systems reduce costs by storing minimal inventory Items are ordered when needed and used	Easy to manage – there will always be enough inventory
Stock does not expire	Stock may expire – first in, first out (FIFO) system will need to be in place to ensure that inventory is used before expiry
Less storage space is needed	Larger storage area is needed
Makes it difficult to deal with emergencies	Easy to deal with emergencies
Risk of running out of stock if there is a supplier issue	Little risk of running out of stock
Generally costs the facility less	Generally costs the facility more

trays spread across multiple storage locations and used in multiple locations, it is valuable to understand inventory location and availability. Understanding the complete instrument inventory assists in controlling costs, scheduling patient procedures, and determining processing priorities. An efficient tracking system assists in inventory monitoring, control, and associated replacement costs.

Modern instrument tracking systems offer a wide variety of workflow management tools and applications that can be invaluable to the processing manager's ability to manage and improve the department's performance. A few of these capabilities include:

- Surgery schedule integration: integration allows the surgical schedule and associated required instrumentation to be exported into the tracking system. This allows the tracking system to compare surgical requirements to instrument inventory, prioritize processing efforts, and highlight inventory shortages and conflicts in advance of the surgery.
- Loaned (or vendor) tray management: tracking systems can offer the ability to manage the flow of and communication with vendors about loan trays when preparing for surgical procedures with surgical teams and the processing department. They can provide communication and visibility to the trays being provided for the surgery, current status, arrival date and times, and processing status. Automated emails and texts are available to improve communication.
- Quality tracking: tracking systems can allow users to enter quality events and link them to the instruments/sets and their processing history. This can include parametric data/controls (e.g. temperature and pressure) and results from indicators.
- Education and competency: education modules can be included that allow processing departments to track their employees' competencies and even control which tasks employees are allowed to perform based on their competency.
- Performance dashboards: since tracking systems can collect vast amounts of processing data, it is possible to provide performance dashboards for departmental performance.
- Productivity: most tracking systems allow for some type of individual and group productivity tracking based on labor standards and time spent working on specific tasks.
- Endoscopy: endoscopy and flexible scope processing can be included in tracking systems with their own unique workflows, when appropriate. This can also include links to drying cabinets and maintenance requirements.
- IFU compliance: tracking systems can offer modules and functionality that assist in complying with IFU and regulatory requirements. Capabilities range from manual input of instructions in the form of pop-up windows as the employee is using the system to full guided workflows that the employee follows step by step.
- Surgical or clinical case cart preparation: many tracking systems, especially those integrated with surgical scheduling systems, provide functionality that scans and tracks case cart contents, providing further visibility to the operational performance and status of customer case carts.
- Patient tracking: another benefit of tracking systems is their ability to link instruments to patients and cases for complete traceability. An example of this is tracking a set of devices that may have been used on a patient known or suspected to have Creutzfeldt-Jakob disease or a similar disease (see Chapter 15 on devices known or suspected to be contaminated with prion material).
- Process documentation: besides scanning for location of inventory, tracking system scanning points and functionality can provide process documentation from processing equipment (e.g. sterilizer) cycle information to confirm that process steps have been completed.

Overall, tracking systems have evolved into total workflow and departmental management tools. Important to any such tracking system is the ability to be able to identify instruments, loaned kits/equipment, equipment, and/or sets of devices, using unique device identification (UDI) tracking numbers, also known as barcodes (see Figure 14.5).

Unique identification codes

For instrument trays where multiple individual instruments are placed together in a basket or container, a traditional 1D (or linear) barcode is commonly used (Figure 14.5). 1D barcodes are commonly used on consumer goods and use a series of variable-width black lines and spaces to encode data. These require the simplest barcode readers to read them and are used worldwide. Many manufacturers and processing facilities are now using 2D barcodes such as data matrix or QR codes for their trays. 2D barcodes use patterns of squares, dots, and other shapes to encode data and can hold more data than a 1D barcode. The data is encoded based on both the vertical and horizontal arrangement of the pattern and thus it is read in two dimensions, which is why it is called 2D.

Figure 14.5 Examples of 1D and 2D barcodes used for device/set identification.

Since instrument trays are unique to each facility and can be customized to contain instruments specific to the surgeon's preferences, there is no global harmonizing effort to standardize trays or sets of instruments. But many types of trays or sets are designed by the manufacturer to meet surgeons' requirements. Processing departments can therefore create or use barcodes for their trays as they wish. The labeling of individual instruments is part of a worldwide effort to create standardized UDI numbers. While government and non-government regulatory organizations create and enforce standards, GS1 is an international standards organization that assists in harmonizing and bringing together countries and industries to standardize the use of barcodes and commercial data labels. With members from over 100 countries, GS1 has become the worldwide standard in creating international standards, including how surgical instruments' UDI numbers are created and standardized.

The GS1 device identification system is intended to provide a global identification of devices through manufacturing, distribution, and subsequent use or reuse. The UDI, conveyed by using automatic identification and data capture (AIDC) and, if applicable, a human readable interpretation) is based on a standard UDI-D (device identifier) and linked to a public UDI database. In simple terms, instruments should have a unique identifier that can be looked up in a public database to allow everyone to be able to understand what the instrument is and its unique information. At the time of writing this book the implementation of this system was ongoing, including provision for marking existing instruments in clinical practice or new instruments with marking applied during the manufacturing process.

GS1 standards use a unique set of identification numbers for products, manufacturers/companies, locations, services, and even customers. These identification numbers are further sub-classified into groups, with the two applicable to processing being:

- GTIN: global trade item number. This is used to uniquely identify each product or item; that is, products and services that are sold and delivered at any point in their supply.
- GIAI: global individual asset identifier. This is used to identify any fixed asset, which includes all property that will not be consumed through immediate use (e.g. equipment and reusable devices).

GS1 identification numbers include identification of the company, a unique number assigned to the asset manufacturer or owner. No matter where a business is based or what language is used, GSI codes are unique and can be easily understood. The GIAI is the part of the GS1 system of standards typically used for the identification of reusable devices. It provides both the GS1 company prefix and the individual device number or serial identifier. Figure 14.6 shows an example of a

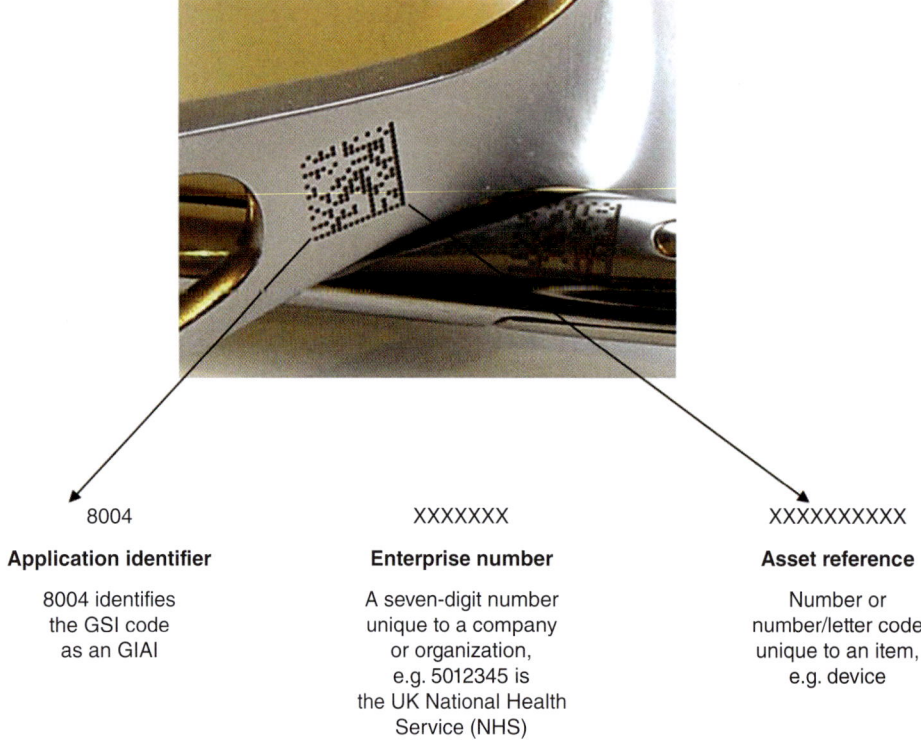

8004	XXXXXXX	XXXXXXXXXX
Application identifier	**Enterprise number**	**Asset reference**
8004 identifies the GSI code as an GIAI	A seven-digit number unique to a company or organization, e.g. 5012345 is the UK National Health Service (NHS)	Number or number/letter code unique to an item, e.g. device

Figure 14.6 Example of a GS1 unique identification code for a reusable device. GIAI, global individual asset identifier.

GS1 UDI in a 2D data matrix code. The combined GS1/GIAI reference cannot exceed 30 digits. The benefit is that it is unique and allows tracking from the manufacturer to its repeated use on patients.

Coding and marking methods

For devices that require processing, how the UDI is attached or marked on the instrument is important. Markings should not interfere with the safe use or processing of the device. For example, laser etching that cuts into the instrument's protective passivation layer should not be used as it creates small scratches that can collect soil and hide microorganisms. Three options currently being utilized to place unique 2D barcodes on instruments include electrochemical marking (ECM), laser marking, and marking dots. ECM uses an electrical current and electrolyte fluid to place the mark on the instrument with a stencil. The mark does not alter the surface, thus preserving its passivation. Laser marking uses a laser to heat the mark into the instrument. Marking dots are sometimes used on instruments that due to shape or size are difficult to laser mark. The dots have adhesive and stick to the instrument, with the 2D barcode printed on the dot.

Scanning/identification

AIDC is the use of machine-readable codes to identify, quickly and accurately, an item or process. Once the trays and or instruments have been marked, they can be read with the use of a barcode or other type of scanning device. The most common types of scanners are handheld devices as shown in Figure 14.7.

Another method to track instruments and trays is by radio-frequency identification (RFID). This technology provides passive identification, meaning that the RFID tags are

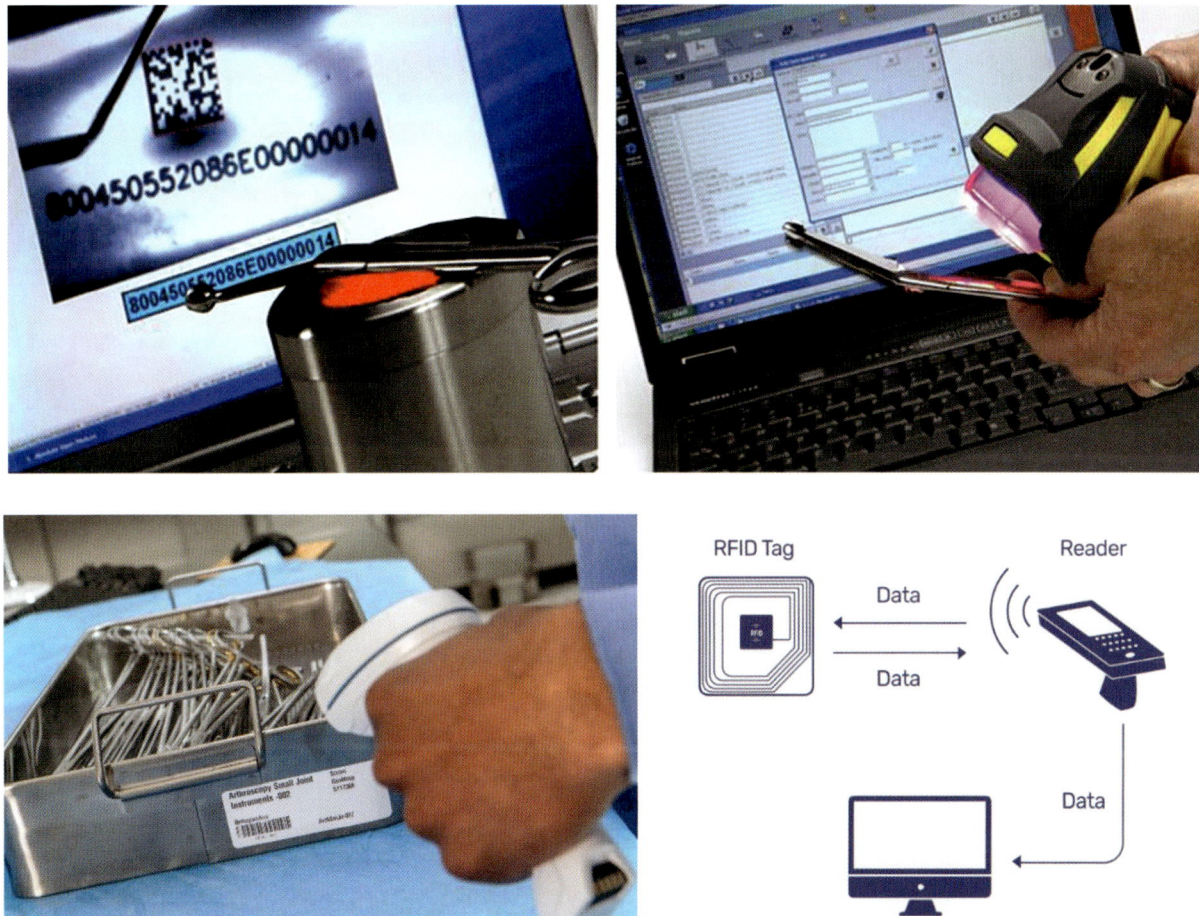

Figure 14.7 Examples of scanning systems for surgical instruments and tray identification using fixed, handheld, or remote scanners/readers.

automatically read by physical receivers without human intervention. While RFID technology is widely used in other industries, the use of it within processing departments is limited to date. The easiest RFID application is at the tray level, where an RFID tag is attached to the tray and can be automatically read by either handheld readers or fixed antennas. RFID tags for trays are available that have been tested to withstand steam sterilization. The cost of installing antennas and placing tags on all the trays should be considered as well as the limited ability to track the tray location depending on distance from the tracking system. RFID on individual instruments is also available, but has had limited application due to the financial cost of attaching the small transmitters to individual instruments. Individual instrument RFID applications have been shown to provide benefits in the tray assembly task as readers can identify a tray of 60 instruments in less than five seconds.

Measurements

An important consideration in management is the efficient use of measurements. The previous sections on planning, personnel, process, and material management measurements highlighted the importance of difference measurements for processing, as well as why measurements may be helpful to identify process limitations and improvements (e.g. lean concepts, discussed earlier in this chapter). Data can help managers measure and manage how well a department is performing, identify opportunities for improvement, create a practical operational plan, and request resources.

Most processing departments will measure how well they meet customer requirements in terms of quality and inspections, and this is discussed in detail later in this chapter (as well as in earlier chapters on cleaning, disinfection, inspection, and sterilization). If the customer experiences a defect, a missing instrument, the presence of unexpected soil, device damage, and so on, it can be reported and investigated. This is a typical outcome measurement that focuses on the customer's experience or how the product or service provided met the requirements. Outcome measurements are critical, required by associated guidelines/standards, and should be included in device processing measurements. There are two other types of measurements that can be considered: process measurements and waste measurements. Process measurements are used to identify if the process is working to plan and provide opportunities to find defects before they reach a customer. Waste measurements identify process waste and help guide improvement opportunities to become more efficient.

Measuring operational performance and sharing the information with employees can be a powerful cultural change agent. Given the right leadership and environment, measurements can motivate staff and leadership to continuously improve, ensure customer satisfaction, and improve operational efficiencies. As individuals and organizations, we have a natural tendency to be motivated and perform according to how we are measured. Therefore, having the right measurements in place can be important. Timely reviews of these measurements is equally important. A manager or employee who is aware of poor performance early can make appropriate corrections and affect the results quickly. Timely, consistent review of performance measurements is necessary for success.

Performance measurements can also help establish the difference between perception and reality. A customer may have a perception that your quality is poor because they continue to remember the incident last month, but measurements can clarify their perception with facts that the quality is indeed very good. Performance measurements provide baselines to which improvements can be compared. They should also be presented in such a way that drives the processing team to act. The three types of measurements are considered further next.

Outcome measurements

Outcome measurements are the most common and represent the final product or service quality, customer experience, and culmination of effort. They are frequently used to set organizational goals, determine rewards, compare to benchmarks, and are the final reflection of the department's work and the measurement of success or failure.

While outcome measurements are important, they are only a reflection of an underlying process and do not provide details of where or why the process broke down when a defect is identified. They do provide data that drives organizations to act and motivate individuals to find ways to improve. Outcome measurements are valuable, but should be combined with process and waste measurements to create a balanced scorecard.

While every processing department may have differences, including the need to serve different customers, the following outcome measurements are commonly shared among most sterile processing departments:
- Instrument tray quality (defects).
- Complete instrument trays.
- Complete case carts.
- On-time delivery.
- Customer experience.
- Customer satisfaction.
- Staff satisfaction.

For all measurements, it is important to agree on the definition of the measurement (what a tray quality defect is), how it will be identified and communicated (who and how the surgical team notifies the processing department of a defect), and how the measurement will be reported.

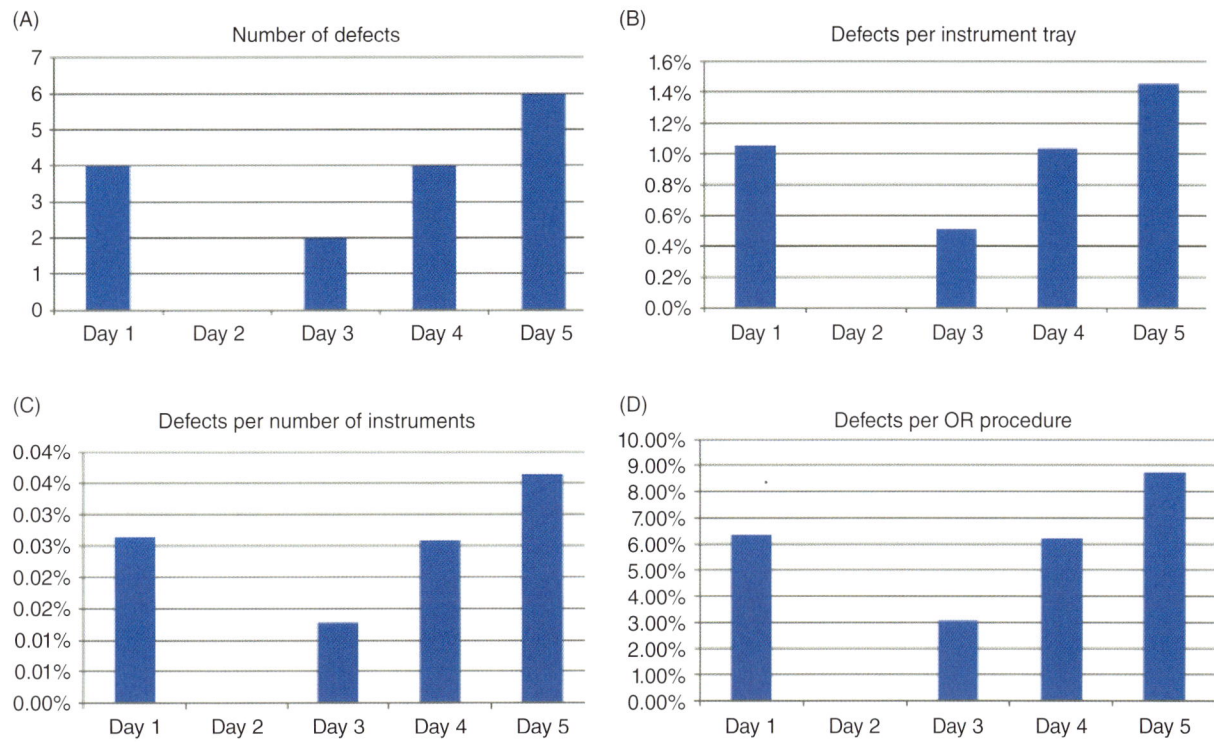

Figure 14.8 (A–D) Different ways of presenting quality defects in processing. Note the differences in how the same data is reported (defects) depending on how it is presented (differences in the Y or vertical axis in each graph). OR, operating room.

Take the example of quality defects. Measuring defects can be completed in different ways and presented in formats that have very different visual impacts. Figure 14.8 depicts the same number of defects but presented in different ways and thus seeming to tell a different story. Figure 14.8(A) shows that it is good to focus on the raw numbers, review the root cause of each, and strive for zero. But if there are too many defects to address each one individually, a Pareto analysis of the most common types may be utilized to narrow down the focus. Figure 14.8(B) shows the same defects as a percentage of all trays processed and allows for comparison to other quality indicators (since it shows the raw data as a defect percentage). Figure 14.8(C) makes the processing department's quality look even better by changing the data to show the total number of individual instruments processed versus the number of trays. The number of defects is still the same and this level of reporting is often associated with departments demonstrating the overall success of their processing quality by simply changing how it is reported. Finally, Figure 14.8(D) converts the same defect data but using OR procedures to show what percentage of procedures are impacted. In this case the OR finds a quality defect over 5% of all cases and thus their perception of quality will be very different that the percentage defect of trays or instruments shown in the other graphs. This graph directly speaks to the customer's perception of the processing department's quality.

Process measurements

For departments focused on ensuring quality and building this into their processes in advance of reports of defects, process measurements are an important focus. Process measurements are not as easy to measure as outcome measurements and require additional effort, but provide the best opportunity and information to improve operational performance.

To understand process measurements, remember the importance of process handoffs. Every process is made up of individual tasks and at some point a task hands off the product to the next process or task. Standard work instructions explain how to perform the tasks, but they should also detail the requirements that task should fulfill when handing off that work to the next step. In other words, step #1 provides a product to step #2 and then step #2 provides a product to step #3, and each handoff should be measured against an agreed expectation.

Within a processing department these handoffs can be measured for quality and timeliness to determine if the process is working to the planned standard. This is where quality is built into the process and measured before the product reaches the final customer. Process measurements can also include compliance with standard work, often confirmed through observations or audits, but also workflow backlogs measuring how well the work is flowing or not flowing through a process, as well as productivity. Potential process measurements for a sterile processing department may include:
- Compliance of procedures within the OR when sending dirty devices or case carts to the processing department.
- Transport to the department and handoff procedures.
- Instrument backlog in decontamination.
- Adherence to decontamination standard work.
- Decontamination handoff compliance in inspection and packaging areas.
- Dirty instruments identified during inspection.
- Instrument backlog in inspection and packaging areas.
- Total trays received or delivered to the OR.
- Handoff to sterilization.
- Compliance with sterilization standard work.
- Sterilization handoff to sterile storage.
- Delivery of devices to a point of use and compliance with standard work.
- Productivity.
- Task completion.

It is recommended to make process measurements a focused objective and choose only a few where improvement opportunities have been prioritized. Remember the two main concepts of process measurements: the need to implement and measure compliance with standard work instructions; and creating and measuring compliance with handoff expectations. Examples of process measurement graphs are shown in Figure 14.9.

Waste measurements

Waste measurements are the most difficult to measure and the least utilized. They are helpful in identifying opportunities to eliminate waste by clearly measuring a specific data point. Waste can be defined as any activity that is not adding value to the product or service. Another way to define waste is any activity that your customer is not willing to pay for. Sterile processing customers depend on the minimum requirements for cleaning, preparation and packaging, sterilization, and delivery of the instruments. Everything else could be considered waste. This will also include redundancy of equipment/devices

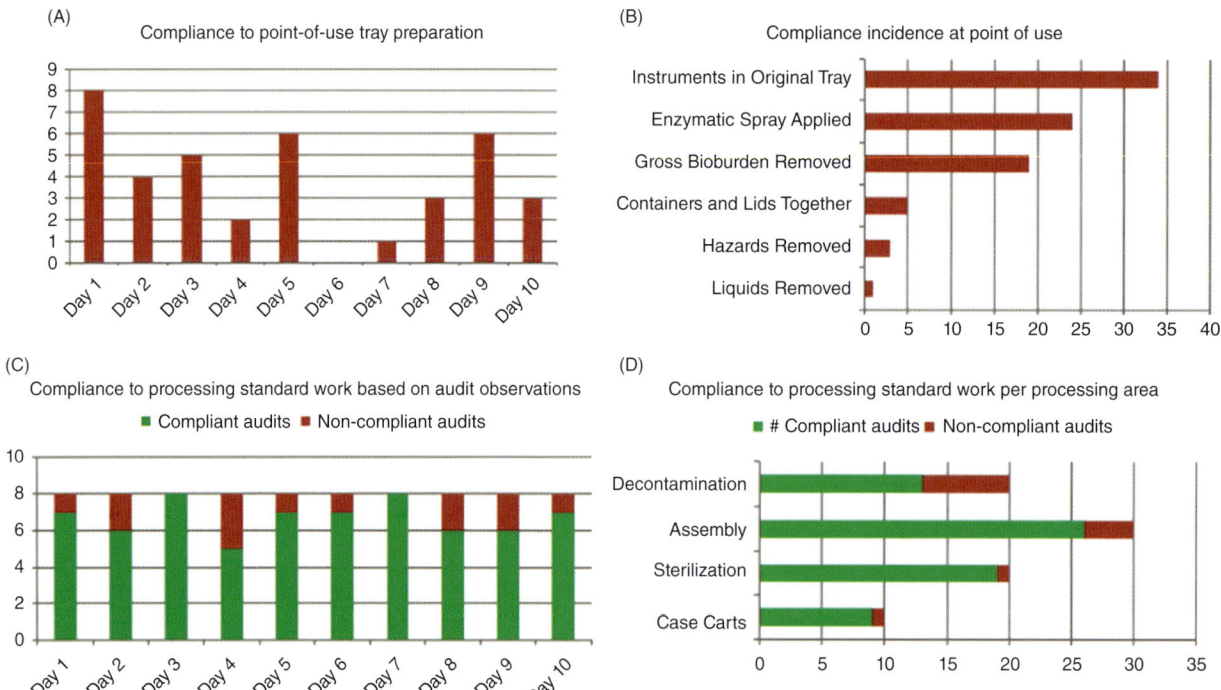

Figure 14.9 (A–D) Examples of process measurements during device processing.

that are not used, and overall waste of supplies such as devices, packaging, and so on during operating room or clinical use. Overall, reduction of waste is not only good environmental practice but also makes economic sense.

An example of waste is when an instrument tray was found to be defective at the point of use, causing the tray to be returned for processing again, using a second instrument tray in the interim, and even delaying the surgical procedure. All these activities are considered waste caused by the original defect. To narrow down the waste to a specific measurement, the department could track and measure the number of special deliveries to the OR that could have been avoided if the proper items had been provided in advance.

Departments can also identify waste and implement process improvement initiatives without first measuring the waste. If the waste is obvious to identify, then it is best practice to eliminate it. Some forms of waste are so common that they are often overlooked or assumed to be a necessary step in the process. An example is simply the walking required between stakeholders, as it rarely adds value. Remember that the processing definition of value-added activities is cleaning, prepping, packaging, sterilizing, and delivering. Keeping this strict definition in mind can help identify waste throughout the process and opportunities to improve.

An important topic to consider is sustainability. This can be defined as avoidance of depleting natural resources in order to maintain an ecological balance. It has become a major objective for many countries and individual healthcare facilities, as it makes good social and economic sense. Although overall it is outside the scope of this book, some important considerations for sustainability within a modern device processing facility will include:
- Planning with operating rooms or other clinical areas the minimum requirements for the provision of devices and equipment. Monitoring waste in this analysis will be important.
- Ensuring the conservative use of water during the processing cycle, and if possible the reuse of water (e.g. critical water for rinsing can be used for earlier steps in cleaning or disinfection processes).
- Choosing chemicals that are more environmentally friendly or naturally degrade in the environment. Also ensure the minimal use of chemicals for specific uses during processing.
- Reducing the use and increasing the recycling of packaging materials.
- Choosing equipment for processing that uses less water and/or chemicals to achieve the desired cleaning, disinfection, or sterilization requirements.
- Reducing energy consumption, in particular when equipment or facilities are not in use (e.g. at night). This can also include the reuse of energy, such as heat exchangers for water heating during washer-disinfector or steam sterilizer use.
- Sharing or consolidating resources within or across facilities.
- Considering the reuse of single-use devices or at least recycling. Note that the energy requirements to reprocess single-use devices may not always improve sustainability goals (e.g. energy, chemicals, and other requirements to reprocess devices can be high and also require greater controls than those associated with reusable devices due to device labeling and safety).

All these examples create opportunities to be more sustainable, reduce waste, and overall reduce costs to facilities. But care should be taken to consider and document the risks associated with these objectives to ensure that they do not compromise patient or staff safety (see the earlier section on process risk analysis).

Quality management

Quality can be defined in many ways, but is essentially a measure of meeting an expectation or a standard. The previous section on measurements defined three measurement categories (outcome, process, and waste measurements). Outcome measurements are often directly associated with quality, since they measure how well the product or service met the customer's requirements. But process measurements can also be associated with internal quality between one processing area and another when considering internal handoffs. From a processing point of view, quality can be defined as providing devices and materials that are safe and effective for patient use, on time, and compliant with any essential regulatory requirements.

Quality is best defined by the customer's (external or internal) point of view and expectations. While general definitions can be applied industry wide, each facility and customer should define their expectations so that they are clear, documented, and measurable. Once expectations are defined, processing departments can work to ensure that their systems and processes can meet those requirements as well as measuring their performance.

A healthcare organization or department can establish, document, and implement a quality management system (QMS). The system describes the organizational structure, procedures, processes, and resources needed to implement quality management in any facility. To assist organizations, systems and best practices are defined by international standards such as ISO 9001 *Quality management systems* and ISO 9004 *Quality management – Quality of an organisation – Guidance to achieve success*. These are used by many different types of companies worldwide to demonstrate their ability to consistently provide products and services that meet customer and regulatory requirements and to demonstrate continuous improvement. For medical device situations, the ISO 13485 standard *Medical devices – Quality management systems – Requirements for regulatory purposes* is used to demonstrate the ability to manufacture and provide products and services to meet those requirements. Although this standard is applicable to device manufacturers, it may also be considered in some countries as necessary or as best practice for device processing departments, as they are providing a process of consistently supplying safe devices for patient use. An example of a specific QMS for device processing is ANSI/AAMI ST90: *Processing of health care products – Quality management systems for processing in health care facilities*.

QMSs have the following core components:
- Purpose of the work (why).
- Applicable procedures and regulations to follow (what).
- Responsibility for the work (who).
- Timing of the work (when).
- Location of the work (where).
- How to do the work (how).
- Monitoring and/or measuring the outcome of the work. Monitoring refers to the indication of measured values in comparison with pre-determined specifications (e.g. temperature, time, pressure, etc.).
- Management responsibilities and review meetings/requirements. This will include risk management, internal audits or reviews, and training/education.
- Management of non-conformance and continuous improvement.

Quality management has two main components. The first is quality assurance (QA). This includes *proactive* activities that create an assurance that quality will be achieved. At the top level this includes writing a quality policy (a brief statement that aligns with an organization's purpose and mission) and a quality manual (typically written with upper management). The quality manual is a document that defines the scope of the system, any exclusions, and a list of associated documented procedures (e.g. for cleaning, disinfection, and sterilization). This includes standardizing processes and documenting standard work, training employees, calibrating and testing equipment used in the process, creating leadership routines, and measuring performance. The second is quality control (QC). These are *reactive* activities that measure, audit, and test current products and processes to ensure they are currently conforming to the essential and pre-defined quality requirements. QC is focused on determining whether the process is functioning and the quality assurance activities implemented proactively are successfully producing quality products and services.

An example of the differences between QA and QC can be found in cleaning soil from instrumentation. QA includes standard work being implemented in the decontamination area to ensure that staff follow the procedures and manufacturer's IFU when cleaning an instrument or equipment, that staff are properly trained, that appropriate equipment and supplies are available, and that any associated equipment being used (e.g. an automated washing or washing-disinfecting machine) is routinely maintained, tested, and operating appropriately. QA tells us that the processes are in place to produce a quality, clean product. QC in this example is the instrument/equipment inspection performed by staff to ensure that the device is visibly clean and/or using other clean indicators. QC confirms that the QA process was performed as required or identifies a defect (e.g. during inspection that soil is still visibly present on the device). The frequency of QC inspection is up to the facility to determine based on its risk analysis and compliance with any regulatory requirements. Frequently, cleanliness and functionality (including damage) inspection following cleaning is considered vital to the quality of instrumentation with the potential for a high-risk patient impact and thus it is performed 100% of the time. Other inspection criteria or audits of the cleaning process that may not score high in a risk analysis may be performed less than 100% of the time.

QA activities should be applied to every process and activity that may impact product or service quality. In other words, almost every task an employee performs in a processing department should have standard work, training requirements, and the appropriate supplies and equipment made available to ensure quality. QC activities are then utilized as needed based on the risk involved and the level of confidence a facility desires in inspecting, auditing, or testing the processes or devices being processed.

A core requirement to fulfill any QMS and to help satisfy these components is to document standard work for all processes and tasks performed in the department. Documentation and control of records are essential to any QMS, to provide evidence of conformity to defined processes, requirements, and established QC procedures. Quality records need to be legible and retrievable and to meet any organizational requirements for retention of such records as defined by any legal requirements (e.g. as defined by the organization or local regulations).

A final, general consideration is continuous improvement in any quality management program. This was considered briefly in the section on measurements, where monitoring of performance criteria and other quality measurements can be used to measure and identify improvement opportunities. Common terms in continuous improvement include corrections, corrective actions (CAs), and preventative actions (PAs). A correction is an action to fix a mistake (often referred to as a non-conformity or NC). Examples include repeating a procedure correctly or resterilizing a product when the packaging material was inspected and found to be damaged. A CA can go further to eliminate the cause of the situation, such as ensuring that all staff are trained on that process. Another is investigating why the packaged material was damaged (e.g. torn due to sharp surfaces in storage or handling procedures). PAs go even further and can be proactive (where risks have been identified in advance of even seeing a problem). They eliminate the cause of a potential problem or undesirable situation. An example may be periodically observing staff performing the process in compliance with a procedure (auditing performance), introducing new equipment that reduces the risk of not following procedures correctly, or putting new systems in place for storage or handling of sterilized product to prevent damage or ensuring close inspection by staff. It is important to consider in these cases that staff performing such duties daily may often identify good opportunities to reduce risk proactively.

The remainder of this chapter will focus on the QC or monitoring activities that are performed by processing departments. Due to the risk of patient infection from nonprocessed or incorrectly processed devices, many of these monitoring activities can be performed 100% of the time to provide confidence that the items are safe for use. Monitoring is a series of routine observations, providing evidence that the correct conditions were present in every item processed. Specific monitoring methods are carried out to show the extent of compliance with a formulated policy and/or standard (Table 14.4).

It is impossible to ensure that every device is clean, disinfected, inspected, sterile (as applicable), and delivered correctly to its point of use. Quality is therefore a series of procedures and monitoring approaches that can be combined to ensure an overall quality process. For this, concepts such as the identification of worst-case products (for cleaning, sterilization, etc.), product families (grouping products based on similar designs or attributes that can be considered the "same" or equivalent to each other), and master products (a device, set of devices, or equipment that represents a worst-case situation for cleaning, sterilization, etc.) can be useful to identify and include during facility monitoring processes.

Monitoring cleaning

The most important and practical method to monitor the effectiveness of any cleaning process is by carefully inspecting the cleanliness of instruments and materials. Visual inspection relies on the individual's eyesight and can be enhanced by inspecting in a well-lit area and by use of a magnifying lens.

Care should be taken, where possible, to inspect areas of the device where soil may become lodged or that are difficult to clean, such as a box joint on hinged instruments (e.g. forceps; see Chapter 4, in the section on instruments for cutting and dissecting). Although visual inspection has the advantage of being relatively quick and easy to perform, it is known to be variable, non-quantitative, and dependent on the vigilance of the staff inspecting the devices. Also, certain types and levels of soil may not be easily detected by the naked eye. Despite these disadvantages, visual evaluation of device cleanliness is currently considered best practice and is required during processing. Visual inspection can be enhanced by using magnification, lighting, and equipment such as boroscopes (see Chapter 8 on inspection).

There are recommendations in some countries that visual examination should be complemented by other detection methods to confirm cleaning efficacy. It is proposed that over time such methods will be more widely used as they become more practical for routine use in a reprocessing department. Many are already in use, particularly for laboratory investigations. These include microbiological and biochemical tests.

Microbiological tests are rarely, if ever, used for monitoring cleaning and are based on the detection of microorganisms, directly or indirectly, on a surface. A direct method is taking a microbiological sample by swabbing or extraction from the device surface and sending the sample to a microbiology laboratory to determine the number of bacteria present. Such methods are limited, in that they can only be used to determine certain types of live bacteria and potentially fungi, and require specifically trained staff using strict aseptic technique and microbiology methods. Further, the results may or may not correlate with a defined level of cleanliness on a device (e.g. to include alive or dead, organic and inorganic materials; see Chapter 5). Overall, such methods are not considered practical for the routine testing of cleaning efficacy in a processing department.

An indirect method of microbiological testing may include the use of a chemical marker that is found in microorganisms. An example is in the detection of adenosine triphosphate (ATP), a chemical found in most living cells such as bacteria, fungi, and human cells where it is used for chemical transfer of energy in cells that respire, which is the process of converting nutrients into cell energy. The presence of ATP can therefore be used as an indirect marker for the presence of bacteria or fungi. In addition, as ATP is present in human cells (which make up various types of human tissues, including blood), it may also be used as a biochemical marker for cleaning efficacy.

Biochemical tests (Figure 14.10) can essentially use any molecule that is present in human cells to indicate the presence or absence of human and microbial soil. This will include proteins, carbohydrates, lipids, nucleic acids, and other molecules that make up cellular structure and function (see Chapter 2). Other such indicators could be the presence of certain types of chemicals in specific soils, such as in blood, or more generally the presence or level of carbon present, since all organic molecules, including proteins

Table 14.4 Examples of various monitoring methods used in a processing area. This should not be taken as an exhaustive list.

Reprocessing area	Monitoring

Cleaning	Manual:
	    Volume of water and cleaning chemistry
	    Water temperature
	    Frequency of water and chemistry changes
	    Inspection of accessories, e.g. cleaning brushes
	    Rinsing
	    Visual or biochemical cleanliness
	Automated:
	    Ultrasonic efficacy
	    Spray arm movement and non-blocked jets
	    Chemistry delivery
	    Process variables such as temperature, pressure, flows rate, etc.
	    Soiling and cleaning indicator tests
	    Visual or biochemical cleanliness
	    Presence and use of personal protective equipment (PPE)

Disinfection	Process variables such as temperature, pressures, chemistry delivery, etc. Acceptable levels of process controls (e.g. A_0 for thermal disinfection) Equipment independent monitoring/process data collection Chemical indicator pass/fail Number and method of rinses (chemical disinfection) Sensor calibration Presence and use of PPE
Packaging	Visual check for cleanliness, residues, and damage Rejection policy (presence and compliance) Check all instrument sets against a list to identify missing items Presence of in-pack chemical indicators Heat sealer efficiency and operation Visual damage to packaging such as staining or wetness
Sterilization	Process variables such as time, temperature, pressures, chemistry delivery, etc. Sterilizer printout and/or data collected Sterilizer sensor calibration and equipment maintenance Pressure leak tests Biological and chemical indicators both internal and external Process control device testing, including Bowie–Dick tests for pre-vacuum steam sterilizers Gas sensors and calibration Gas or liquid storage conditions both internal and external; check that all packs have external chemical indicators before loading into autoclave Items removed are intact, dry, and undamaged Failed indicator policy Water or steam quality/purity
Storage	Stock rotation Damage of packaging materials Area humidity/temperature
Handling	Check all instrument sets against a list to identify missing items Cleaning and disinfection frequency of carts
Site of patient use	Check all instrument sets against a list to identify missing items Visual examination of device cleanliness and damage Aseptic technique Check in-pack chemical indicators

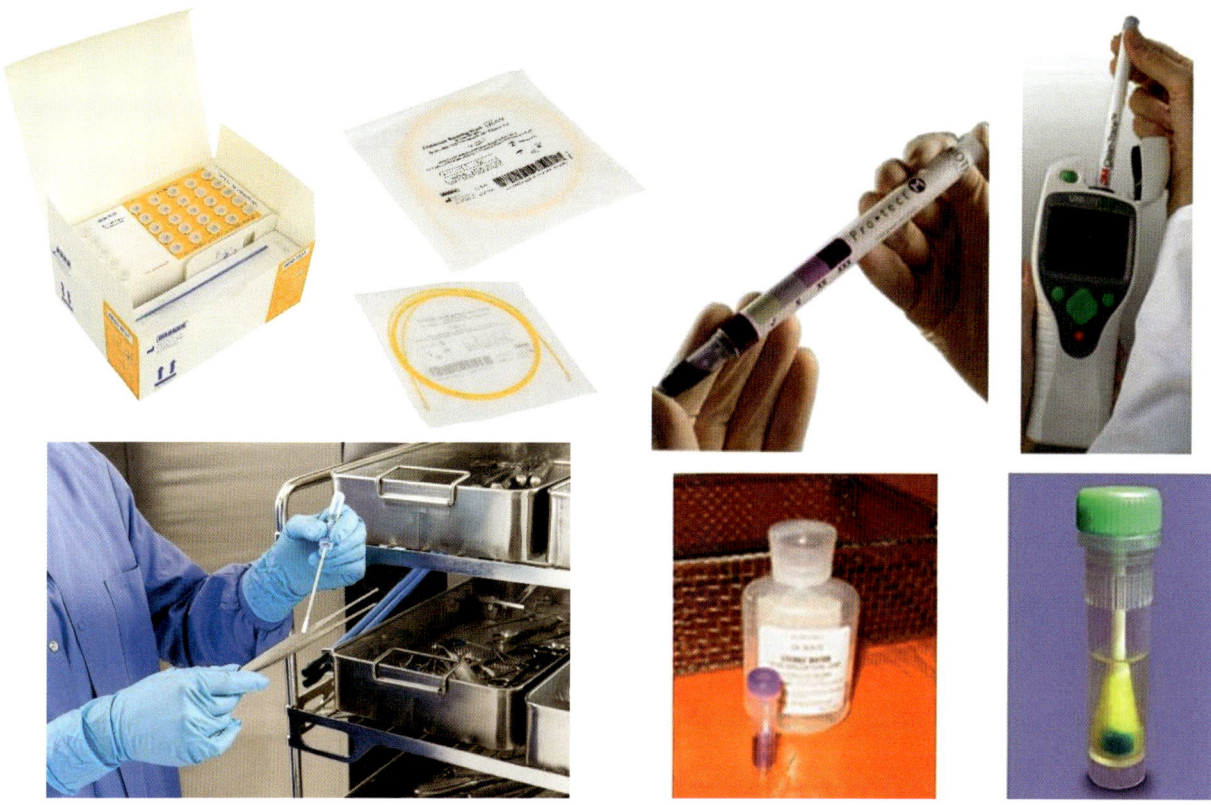

Figure 14.10 Various types of soil-detection kits. On the left and center are various types of protein-detection kits (including swab-based tests). On the far top right is an adenosine triphosphate (ATP)-based test (with detector) and bottom right a qualitative residual blood test.

and lipids, include carbon (see Chapter 2). To date, the most widely used biochemical indicators are protein, blood, and ATP.

Protein is one of the most important molecules in the structure and function of cells (microbiological, human, plant, etc.) and viruses (Chapter 2). Protein-detection methods have therefore been widely used to test for residual soil, significantly below the levels that can be directly seen by the eye. A variety of chemical reaction–based methods (such as those based on biuret or ninhydrin reactions) are used to detect protein and/or peptides (smaller protein structures). Easy-to-use protein-detection kits have become widely used for testing cleaning efficacy in processing departments (examples are shown in Figure 14.10). As an example, a swab is used to sample the device surface and then treated with the chemical protein reagent that reacts with a broad spectrum of proteins and peptides to give a blue to purple color; blue or purple indicates the presence of protein above a detection level (usually defined by the kit manufacturer). The acceptable levels of detectable protein to claim that a critical or semi-critical device is clean have been harmonized to two levels, an alert level of $\geq 3\,\mu g/cm^2$ and an action level of $\geq 6.4\,\mu g/cm^2$ protein. Overall, the action level is the most important to achieve, but levels between the alert and action levels may warrant further investigation to ensure that the device will be consistently cleaned over multiple processing cycles (not allowing for soil accumulation over time). It is important to remember that the most challenging area for device cleanliness (based on various device features that may be less accessible to cleaning) should be chosen for testing, as they are considered worst case (see Chapter 8).

A traditional method to detect blood uses hydrogen peroxide (at low concentrations such as 3–6% in water), due to the action of enzymes found in blood cells that break down peroxide to release oxygen, shown as bubbling. Similar but more sensitive tests are based on a swab test that turns green/blue in color in the presence of blood/hemoglobin (Figure 14.10). Unlike protein, blood may not always be present on a soiled device, but is a very common soil component in the use of many surgical/medical instruments. The final method uses ATP, a molecule found in actively respiring cells as described earlier, which has also been used as an indirect indicator of the presence of contamination on a surface. It includes test swab or strip-based tests that give a color change on reaction with ATP at a certain level of detection ("qualitative") or a fluorescent (light-generating) reaction that is read using a handheld sensor/detector to give a quantitative level of ATP (Figure 14.10).

Care should be taken to read and understand the IFU provided with residual soil-detection kits to ensure their correct application and interpretation. It should also be remembered that cleaning tests do not guarantee that a device, set, or load is clean, only that the surface tested passes or fails a cleaning indicator test.

Manual cleaning processes can be considered variable, depending on the operator, cleaning method, attention to detail, and so on. Despite this, some quality controls can be used to reduce risks. Examples include standardizing the volume of water used in a sink by measuring and indicating the amount of water to a defined level, and an automated pump to ensure that the volume of chemistry used is in compliance with the manufacturer's instructions. Modern washer-disinfectors can provide greater control and cleaning assurance. Monitoring tests used in automated systems can include parametric tests, cleaning indicators, and cleaning test soils.

Parametric tests monitor key parameters that have been specified as required for the automated cleaning process. This will include the cleaning phases (pre-cleaning, cleaning, rinsing), time, temperature, pressure, draining, chemistry dosing volume, and so on. Some washer-disinfectors (in particular those compliant with ISO 15883-1 *Washer-disinfectors: general requirements, terms and definitions and tests*) have independent sensors and separate process control sensors to confirm many of these important parameters. The data from these systems may need to be manually or automatically checked by the washer control/computer system to verify the correct process conditions. In addition to automated tests, various manual QA tests can be specified, including checking drains, spray arm and nozzle circulation, and lack of blockages (Chapter 8).

Cleaning indicators are designed to provide a standardized challenge to a cleaning process (Figure 14.11). They are ready-to-use indicators with soil dried onto representative surfaces. Cleaning indicators can be used to test for the efficacy and reproducibility of cleaning in a washer and washer-disinfector. They may be used during installation and/or periodic testing of a washing process, but can also provide a routine test daily or on every load to confirm cycle performance. There are currently no standards that define the design of such indicators, but they do specify their performance.

Cleaning test soils are designed to represent patient soils that may be present on device surfaces following surgical or medical use. There are many types of test soils that are used for the development or routine testing of cleaning processes. Many were traditionally developed for specific country use, and more recently examples of internationally recognized test soils and requirements for test soils have been published in ISO 15883-5:2021 *Washer-disinfectors: Performance requirements and test method criteria for demonstrating cleaning efficacy*. These can be prepared with basic laboratory equipment. In addition, some commercially available test soils are available (Figure 14.12). Soils are composed of many materials, such as defined proteins, starch, and egg yolk, and some contain pigments so that they can be detected more easily during visual inspection. The test soils are applied manually, usually by brushing onto the instruments, washer chamber walls, and any associated racks, and then dried for a specified time prior to testing. The instruments are then examined for traces of this soil following a cleaning cycle.

Additional monitoring tests may be recommended, depending on the washer technology. These will be specified by the manufacturer and/or in local/regional guidelines. For example, ultrasonic washer tests can include some tests of cavitation energy. Ultrasonic cleaning uses ultrasonic (sound) waves, generally in combination with a cleaning chemistry,

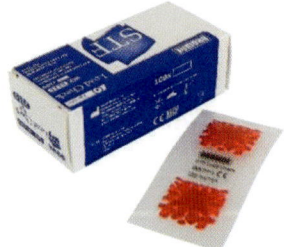
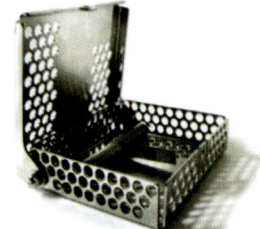
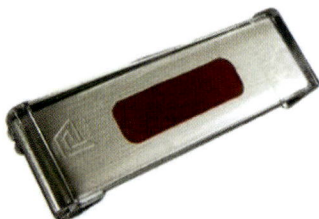

Figure 14.11 Examples of cleaning indicators.

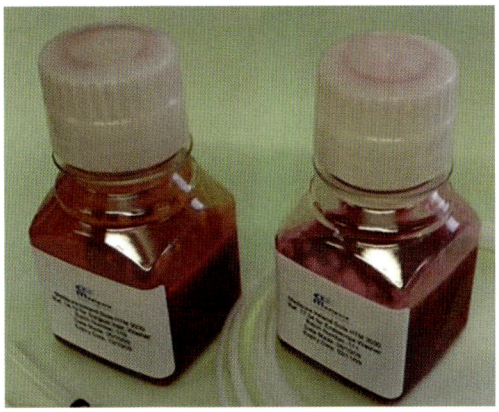 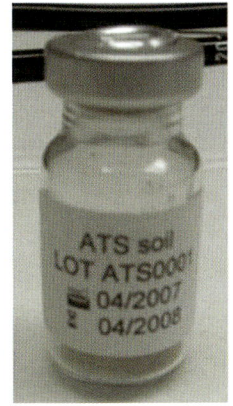 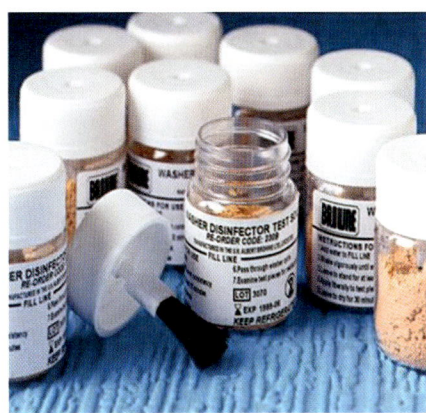

Figure 14.12 Examples of cleaning test soils.

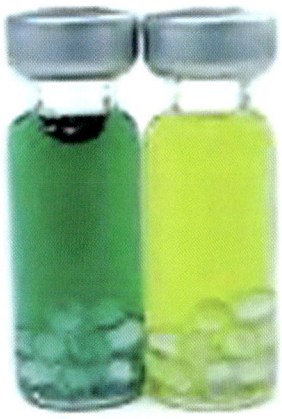

Figure 14.13 An example of an ultrasonic cavitation test. The indicator is provided as a green liquid (left) and changes color to yellow (right) on exposure to defined ultrasonic conditions.

to cause the disruption and removal of soil from surfaces. When ultrasonic waves are applied within a liquid it causes "cavitation," the production and collapse of small bubbles along the surface of the device. This process can be confirmed using a color-change indicator that is designed to indicate the correct energy and other conditions (Figure 14.13). An older test that is still used sporadically is the aluminum foil test (Figure 14.14). This is used to test the ultrasonic efficiency in various locations in the washer. Strips of aluminum foil (e.g. 10 cm × 20 cm) are suspended at various locations within the ultrasonic bath. The ultrasonic bath is then turned on for a typical cleaning cycle and the foil removed and inspected. All foil samples should be perforated and eroded to about

the same degree if the system is operating correctly. Other methods use cavitation meters to directly measure the ultrasonic energy within the bath, as well as other indicators (e.g. ultrasonic pencil tests).

Monitoring disinfection

The main method of monitoring thermal (heat) disinfection is by measuring and/or confirming the temperature and exposure time. This may be conducted manually or in automated systems (washer-disinfectors, pasteurizers, etc.). Similar to cleaning processes (see the section on monitoring cleaning), modern washer-disinfectors will include independent monitoring systems to verify the correct disinfection conditions, in accordance with ISO 15883-1 *Washer-disinfectors: general requirements, terms and definitions and tests* and other parts (see Chapter 9). Process monitoring sensors will require periodic calibration (to verify that they are operating correctly, usually with reference to specific standards or manufacturer's claims). Periodic testing may also include the use of temperature monitoring equipment to verify the temperature distribution in the disinfection chamber over time.

Chemical disinfection can be more challenging. This is often best controlled in automated systems. ISO 15883-compliant washer-chemical disinfectors will include various parametric measures of the process, in compliance with Part 1, Part 4 (*Requirements and tests for washer-disinfectors employing chemical disinfection for thermolabile endoscopes*), and Part 7 (*Requirements and tests for washer-disinfectors employing chemical disinfection for non-invasive, non-critical thermolabile medical devices and healthcare equipment*). This will include systems to confirm the correct chemical dosing, temperatures, pressures, flow rates, and so on during the process. Some systems may also include chemical disinfectant sensors that

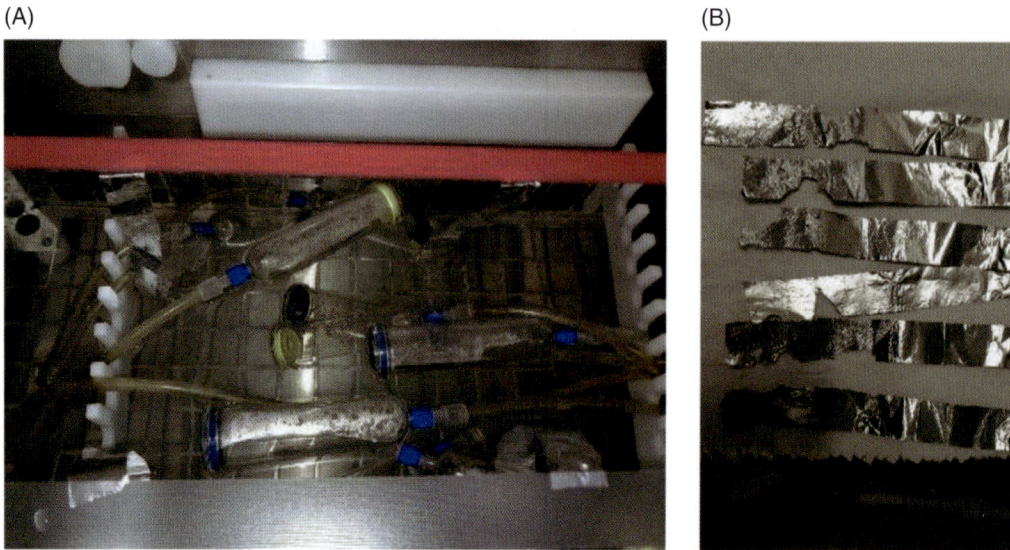

Figure 14.14 Ultrasonic bath aluminum foil test. (A) Test strips of foil are shown suspended at several locations within the bath and (B) a close-up of the strip after exposure, showing perforations.

monitor the concentration directly or indirectly during the process. Manual chemical disinfection is also widely used, and it can be more difficult to ensure a quality process due to the inability to validate a manual process. Suggestions will include the use of timers, recording sheets on the use of the disinfectant, in particular with reusable chemical disinfectants, and verifying the number of and times for each rinse for rinsing methods.

In both automated and manual chemical disinfection processes, it is recommended (and often required) that CIs are used that are specific to the type of disinfectant, usually specified by the disinfectant manufacturer (Figure 14.15). The overall use of CIs (and other types of quality indicators) is discussed in further detail in the next section.

Monitoring sterilization

The requirements for monitoring the various physical and chemical sterilization methods can vary from country to country. There is no practical method that can confirm a sterile device, but various methods can be used to verify that a defined sterilization process has been achieved within a device set or load. These will include a variety of parametric and indicator-based tests, usually specified by guidelines and standards and/or the sterilizer manufacturer. An example is in steam sterilization, where process monitoring within a sterilizer is based on the concept of "parametric release"; that is, a declaration that the product is sterile, based on records demonstrating that the process parameters were delivered within specified tolerances. The critical parameters here are

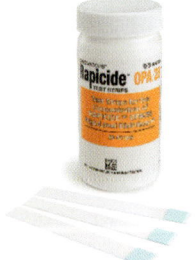 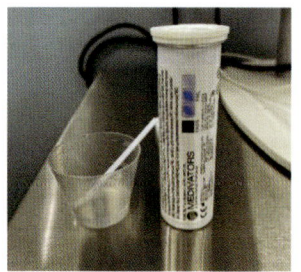 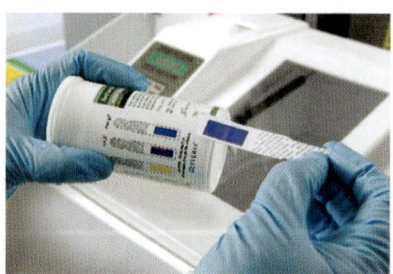 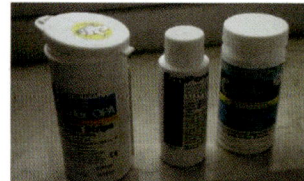

Figure 14.15 Examples of disinfectant chemical indicators.

attainment of minimum values of time, temperature, and presence of moisture, but of course other variables can affect the efficacy of the process (such as air removal, pressure, water/steam quality, and so on; see Chapter 11, the section on steam (moist heat) sterilization). Therefore, a combination of steam sterilization monitoring and validation methods is employed, to include:
- Parametric monitoring of time, temperature, and pressure.
- CIs and/or BIs.
- Process challenge devices (PCDs), such as the B–D test and hollow load test (to test air removal/steam penetration)

Many of these monitoring methods (for physical and chemical sterilization) have already been introduced in Chapter 11, in the section on the basic principles of sterilization, and are further considered here. These are given as a guide; local guidelines and standards and manufacturers' guidelines should be consulted to determine the minimum requirements for the routine monitoring of any sterilization process.

Parametric monitoring

This refers to the monitoring of the important parameters that have been specified as required for sterilization to be achieved. Steam is a useful example, as its successful application for sterilization is dependent on reaching the correct temperature (that can only be achieved by steam under pressure; see Chapter 11). Therefore, physical monitoring of the temperature and time of the process is a good indicator that the process has been correctly applied. Other parameters will include various types of air-detector systems, as effective air removal and steam penetration are important considerations for steam sterilization. For a chemical sterilization process this may include the concentration (directly or indirectly) of the sterilizing agent(s), humidity levels, temperature, pressure, and other process variables, depending on the sterilization process. Overall, these various types of sensors can be used for monitoring the effectiveness of the process and can provide this information immediately for inspection and control.

Sterilizers have various gauges, sensors, timers, recorders, and/or other devices that monitor their function. These are all required to be periodically maintained and/or calibrated in accordance with the manufacturer's instructions. Some will have independent monitoring systems separate to their control sensors and may have various alarm systems that are activated if the sterilizer fails to operate correctly. Monitoring records for each cycle should be inspected and maintained, as dictated by local guidelines or regulations. The details of sterilizer designs can vary considerably; therefore close inspection of the operator manuals is recommended.

Typically, at the end of a cycle, and before the items are removed from the sterilizer, the sterilizer records (printouts,

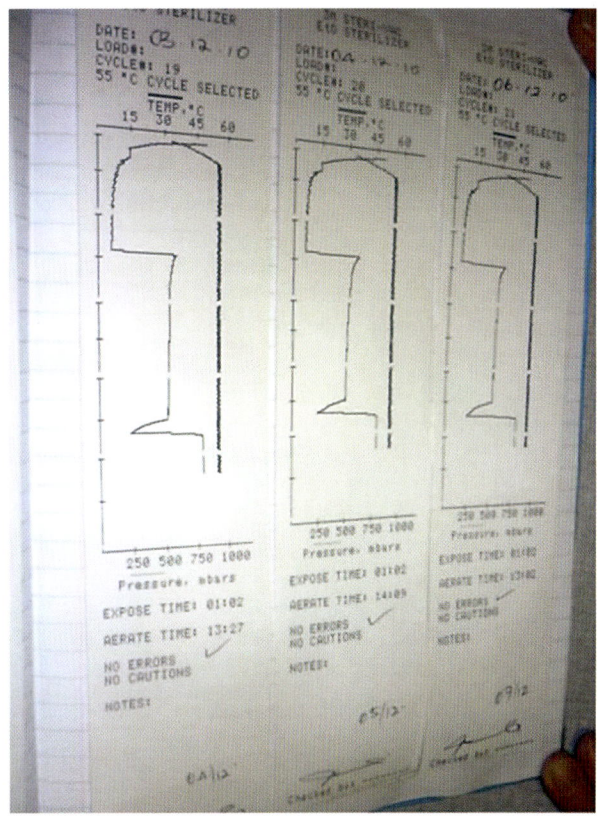

Figure 14.16 Examples of the inspection of sterilizer-recorded data (printouts) for verification and/or archiving.

collected data, etc.) are examined to make sure that the process conditions have been achieved, and then signed by the person inspecting the record for future confirmation before releasing the load (Figure 14.16).

Although parametric monitoring can provide assurance that the sterilization process has been applied, there are limitations associated with each sterilizer design. Therefore, parametric monitoring is most often complemented by other tests, such as those based on CIs and BIs (see later).

The term "parametric release" refers to the release of loads as being "sterile" and ready for patient use, without the specific need for inspection of other CIs or BIs. This concept originated in the pharmaceutical industry, where a very high level of product and process understanding, change control, and documentation are demanded. Parametric release has traditionally been used for many industrial sterilization processes (in particular steam, ethylene oxide, and radiation) and requires a high level of consistency and control of all steps of the process. It has been also applied to the processing of devices and materials, but has not (as yet) been accepted in all regions. An effective parametric release program requires a QMS to be in place (see the section on quality management). The system needs to be well designed and maintained, following various guidelines and standards (such as ISO 13485 *Medical devices – quality management systems – requirements for regulatory purposes*). The QMS should be documented to include policies, standard operating procedures, safe work instructions, test measurement protocols, and reference documents, as well as a quality plan applicable to all elements of the sterilization process. An important part of the system is the definition, monitoring, and maintaining of parametric release criteria with the sterilization process. These will need to be defined with the sterilizer manufacturer and may or may not be available depending on the sterilizer design. Once defined, the entire process must be tested, validated, commissioned, and documented to ensure that it will consistently yield the defined sterilization process. This will include:

- Installation qualification (IQ): the process of obtaining and documenting evidence that equipment has been provided and installed in accordance with its specifications (including requirements for water, air, etc. as required).
- Operational qualification (OQ): the process of obtaining and documenting evidence that installed equipment operates within pre-determined limits when used in accordance with its operational procedures.
- Performance qualification (PQ): the process of obtaining and documenting evidence that the equipment, as installed and operated in accordance with operational procedures, consistently performs in accordance with pre-determined criteria and thereby yields a product meeting its specification.

Chemical indicators

CIs are generally used in combination with parametric monitoring to ensure the consistency of a sterilization process. They are defined as test systems, usually in the form of test strips, that reveal a change in one or more pre-defined process variables based on a chemical and/or physical change resulting from exposure to a process. They are generally provided as color-change indicators and are widely used in monitoring sterilization processes. The ISO 11140-1 *Sterilization of healthcare products – chemical indicators* standard classifies indicators into six basic types, according to their intended use or performance criteria (Table 14.5).

The various types of CIs are considered in more detail next, with consideration for how they are typically used in a reprocessing area.

Process indicators

A process indicator is the most basic of CIs and is commonly placed on the outside of a package to verify that the package has been exposed to a sterilization process. Such an indicator should be clearly visible on the outside of the sterilized package. This helps differentiate sterilized from unsterilized items (Figure 14.17). Process indicators are available as tapes, labels, or printed onto sterile packaging materials.

Table 14.5 The classification of chemical indicators. Based on ISO 11140 *Sterilization of healthcare products – chemical indicators.*

Type	Indicator type	Description
Type 1	Process indicator	Simple indicators to demonstrate exposure to a process and to distinguish between processed and unprocessed units Generally used outside packaging to indicate it has been exposed to a sterilization cycle A common example is steam sterilizer (autoclave) tape
Type 2	Indicators for use in specific tests	Used to indicate a specific type of test, generally established in another standard Examples include the Bowie–Dick test (for confirming air removal/steam penetration into a porous load) and hollow load tests (for testing sterilant penetration into a lumen) Generally routine tests
Type 3	Single variable indicators	Designed to respond to only one critical process variable (e.g. concentration of a biocide)
Type 4	Multi-variable indicators	Designed to respond to two or more critical variables (e.g. temperature, time, and concentration of a biocide)
Type 5	Integrating indicators	Designed to respond to all critical variables of the process and generally similar in performance to a biological indicator (e.g. indicators containing bacterial spores used to test sterilization processes)
Type 6	Emulating indicators	Designed to react to all critical variables for a complete specified cycle Indicator performance matched to the critical parameters of the sterilization cycle

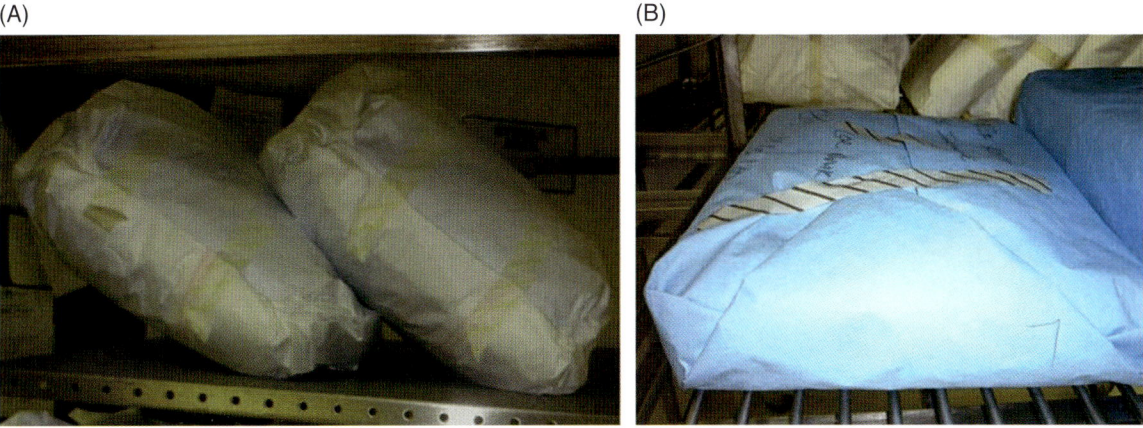

Figure 14.17 Example of the color change with a type 1 (process) chemical indicator, in this case for steam sterilization. The tape on the unsterilized packs (A) are clearly differentiated from the tape on the sterilized packs (B).

These indicators are affixed onto the outside of the package or rigid containers once they have been assembled for sterilization (Figure 14.17). They may also be provided as an integrated part of the packaging material. Following exposure, the process indicator should be checked to ensure that it has changed color according to the manufacturer's instructions and prior to release for patient use or storage.

In-pack internal chemical indicators

These are mainly supplied as test strips and are generally placed inside packs to be sterilized. Different types of CIs may be used, such as ISO 11140 types 3, 4, 5, or 6. This will depend on how many critical process variables are to be monitored and any local guideline or standard requirements. An in-pack CI can detect sterilizer malfunction or error in packaging or loading of the sterilizer. It is recommended that the CI is placed in the package, instrument tray, or rigid container in an area that is considered to be the least accessible to sterilant penetration. This may not always be in the center of the package (Figure 14.18).

In-pack CIs cannot be examined until the pack is opened at the site of use. Therefore, it is important that surgical/medical staff are trained on the correct monitoring and interpretation of the CI result. The associated pack or devices should not be used in the case of a failed indicator. Any non-responding or partially responding indicator signifies a failed sterilization process, and the contents of the package should not be used. A facility recall (see the earlier section on recall) should be initiated in such cases.

Biological indicators

BIs are defined as test systems containing viable microorganisms providing a defined resistance to a specified sterilization process. Examples are shown in Figure 14.19. For sterilization applications, BIs contain bacterial spores of various types that are considered the most resistant microorganisms to their respective sterilization processes (Table 14.6). They contain a known high population of bacterial spores (e.g. 10^5 or 10^6) and are supplied in many ways, including:

- Sealed vials or ampoules (in suspension).
- Placed onto a carrier material (e.g. paper or a stainless steel disc) and provided as:
  ○ Dry spore strips or discs in envelopes. These are required to be recovered, transferred to growth media, and incubated following exposure. Note: close attention to aseptic technique (microbiological handling methods to prevent cross-contamination) is required.
  ○ As a self-contained system incorporating a growth medium and typically a CI. These require no specific handling precautions following exposure, but ensure that the spore strip/carrier is exposed to the provided internal growth medium and then incubated as described by the BI manufacturer.
- Included in specially designed challenge packs (known as PCDs).

A BI is designed to be able to show growth (i.e. spore viability) or no growth on incubation of the BI following exposure to a sterilization process. Growth would be a fail result and no growth a pass result. Incubation time can range from 20 minutes to 24 hours or longer (based on the product being used and its associated labeling) before the final result is known. Some BI designs (known as "rapid-read" designs) include an indirect CI of this final result, such as a color change (based on a change in pH in the growth medium), the presence of enzyme activity (indicated by the production of light), or even direct detection of spore growth, all suggesting that spore growth is occurring as soon as possible and within the requirements of different standards and regulatory

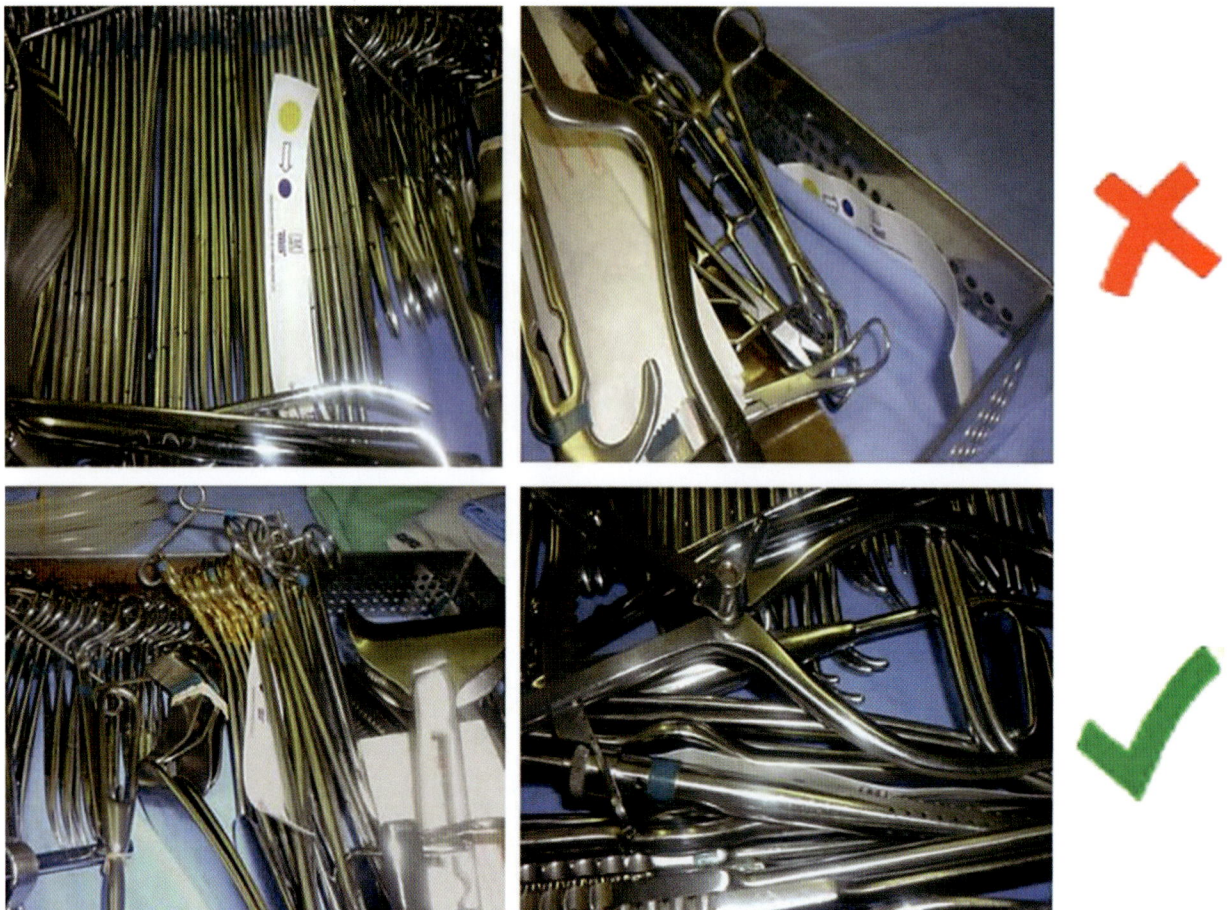

Figure 14.18 Positioning of chemical indicators within a load. The lower locations are optimal.

requirements. In some, but not all, cases these early indications of growth are considered preliminary and require verification of growth or no growth for the final result, and must be verified at a later stage according to manufacturer's guidelines. With other designs no further incubation time is required to verify the rapid result.

BIs are often recommended to be performed on a regular basis such as daily or weekly in each sterilizer. In some countries BIs are required to be tested with certain types of sterilization loads such as when including implantable devices. Similar to CIs (see the previous section), BIs should be placed in the chamber/load in the least favorable position for sterilization, which for steam sterilization is typically on the bottom shelf over the drain.

After sterilization, the BI is retrieved from the load (allowing cooling if applicable), checked with any associated CIs (if provided either within or separate to the BI design), and, if the CI passes, it should be ensured that the BI is incubated at the correct growth conditions for the indicator. These instructions will be provided by the BI manufacturer and may require specific handling to ensure aseptic technique to prevent cross-contamination. Self-contained BIs are preferred in such cases as they require minimal handling post exposure. In these cases a medium-containing vial is crushed or otherwise exposed to the spore carrier following exposure and without direct contact with the internal components of the BI. The incubation conditions will depend on the BI instructions and can vary depending on the manufacturer, types of spore, and associated sterilization method under test. For example:

- *Geobacillus stearothermophilus* spore-containing BIs (such as for steam and hydrogen peroxide gas processes) are typically incubated at 55–60°C for 20 minutes to 48 hours depending on the BI manufacturer's instructions.
- *Bacillus atrophaeus*-containing BIs (such as those used for ethylene oxide sterilization processes) are typically incubated

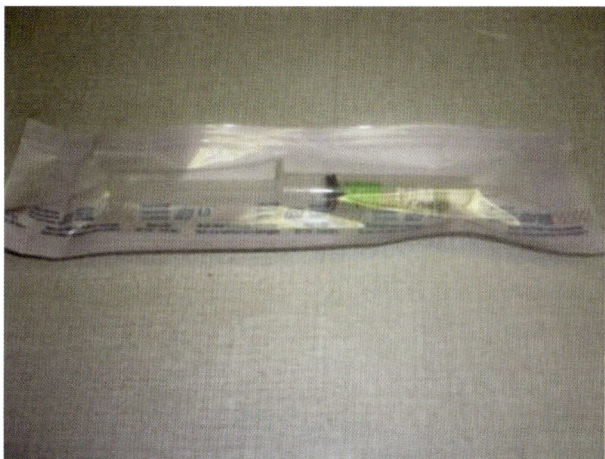
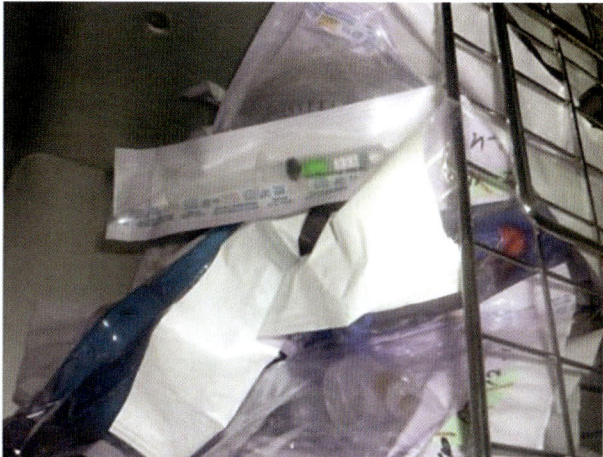

Figure 14.19 (A) Examples of biological indicators (BIs), in this case color coded according to their use in specific types of sterilization processes. Thy include blue (flash sterilization), brown (steam sterilization), and green (ethylene oxide). (B) An example of a biological indicator (BI) test. In this case a BI (self-contained) is placed into a syringe and a peel pouch as a challenge within the full load.

Table 14.6 Sterilization methods and types of bacterial spores used in biological indicators for routine monitoring. These microorganisms are widely accepted and used for the testing of their respective sterilization method.

Sterilization method	Bacterial spores
Steam under pressure	*Geobacillus stearothermophilus*
Humidified ethylene oxide	*Bacillus atropheus*[1]
Hydrogen peroxide gas (with or without plasma)	*Geobacillus stearothermophilus*
Liquid chemical peracetic acid	*Geobacillus stearothermophilus*
Humidified formaldehyde	*Geobacillus stearothermophilus*
Dry heat	*Bacillus atropheus*[1]

[1] Previously known as *Bacillus subtilis*.

at 35–39°C for 48 hours to 7 days, or the equivalent rapid-read indications depending on the manufacturer's instructions, e.g. 4 hours at $37 \pm 2°C$ ($99 \pm 3°F$).

It is important to note that bacterial spore growth requires specific temperatures and incubation time and these variables should be closely controlled. These conditions can be tested by using another BI that has not been exposed to the sterilization process as a positive control. If this BI fails to show growth then there is a problem with the method (e.g. not following manufacturer's instructions or the incubator is malfunctioning), the batch of BIs, or the incubation conditions.

As already described, a preliminary result (presence or absence of bacterial growth) may be provided depending on the BI design. Such "chemical" indicators may include the release of acid (which changes the color of the medium) or other indicators of spore germination and growth. But the final result will be determined following the full incubation conditions as defined by the manufacturer. A negative (pass) result is defined as a lack of growth following exposure to a sterilization process, while a positive (fail) result is the presence of growth.

Specific sterilization monitoring tests

A variety of specific sterilization tests may be used or required depending on the sterilization process. They are typically designed as routine tests and are therefore not often used for testing in specific product loads. Some tests are designed only to be tested in specified sterilizer cycles defined for that purpose. Many of these tests are described in various guidelines or standards, while others are developed by manufacturers specifically to test a sterilizer design. They often incorporate CIs and/or BIs under some challenging test conditions. Examples are PCDs, which were previously discussed in Chapter 11 (see Figure 11.13). These are designed to provide a specific challenge, such as a penetration challenge, for a sterilization process and used as a more robust or worst-case method to monitor the performance of that process.

An example is a hollow load (or helix) test described for testing steam sterilization. Similar tests are also described for other gas sterilization processes. The hollow load test consists of a length of tubing, with one end open and the other closed; the closed end is designed to hold a CI or BI. The test simulates a worst-case challenge for sterilant penetration through a long-lumened device. An important example of a specific test for steam sterilization is the B–D test.

The Bowie-Dick test was developed in 1963 by Dr. J. Bowie and Mr. J. Dick to detect problems with air removal and steam penetration in a pre-vacuum sterilizer, particularly within a "porous" load represented as a pack of towels.

The test works by being able to trap air within it and therefore preventing the penetration of steam. If the sterilizer's air-removal stage is working properly (see Chapter 11), the air is removed and replaced with steam. The steam then reacts with the special indicator ink on an internal test sheet and changes color evenly to show that all the air has been removed. If, on the other hand, all the air is not removed from the test pack, the air/steam mixture will not have the right temperature or moisture content to change the test sheet and a failed result will be observed. The original B–D test required a standard test pack consisting of 25–36 washed all-cotton towels. The towels were folded in half three times to provide eight thicknesses, each with an area of 300 mm × 225 mm, and stacked one above the other to form a stack approximately 270 mm high. The exact number of towels often depended on how often they had been used. The indicator was then placed on a piece of paper in the middle of the stack and the whole stack wrapped to keep it in place. In most situations, commercially made single-use test packs are now used. It is recommended that any B–D test packs are checked for compliance with established standards (e.g. ISO 11140-3 *Sterilization of healthcare products – chemical indicators – Part 3: Type 2 indicator systems for use in the Bowie and Dick type steam penetration test*). Specific manufacturers' instructions, provided for both the B–D test and the steam sterilizer, should be followed to ensure the correct use and interpretation of the test. It is important that the B–D test pack is placed *on its own* on the bottom shelf of the sterilizer over the drain and close to the door, as this is likely to be the coolest part of the sterilizer. The reason the B–D test must be run on its own is that if the sterilizer contains other packs as well, they can also trap air within them, which will decrease the sensitivity of the test. A B–D test is typically designed to be run for specific test cycle conditions, such as 3.5 minutes of steam sterilization, where other cycle conditions with longer exposure times will invalidate the results.

If the B–D test result is unsatisfactory (a fail), the sterilizer should be taken out of use and the fault investigated (this may require testing by a designated test person). It is important that the sterilizer and the associated steam supply are at full operating temperature before carrying out the test. A warm-up cycle will not only ensure that the sterilizer chamber and jacket are at the correct temperature, it will also purge the steam supply of any moisture and non-condensable gases, for example CO_2, which build up when the sterilizers are not being used or sit overnight. All water contains a certain amount of non-condensable gases, but the colder the water the higher the concentration of gases. When the steam supply is not active, the temperature of the steam drops, leading to a build-up of water in the supply system. As this water cools it absorbs non-condensable gases. The first cycle on the following day can therefore contain unusually high levels of non-condensable gases as they are flushed out of the system. It is recommended that if, after carrying out a warm-up cycle, the B–D test fails, a second B–D test should be performed. This is to ensure that the first fail was not simply further contaminants still being flushed out of the steam supply. If the second B–D test also fails, then the cause must be investigated in more detail. It is important to remember that the CIs used in B–D tests may deteriorate in storage due to contamination or unsuitable conditions; therefore, any test shelf-life and test conditions should be finally verified to ensure an accurate pass/fail result.

15 Special interest topics

During the development of this book a number of special interest topics were highlighted as requiring further consideration. This chapter considers these aspects in further detail, with cross-references to other chapters and sections of the book.

Water quality/purity

Water is an essential component during device processing, including its use for cleaning, rinsing, disinfection, and sterilization (see Chapter 6, the section on solids, liquids, gases, and plasma, for an introduction to the chemistry of water). Examples of the use of water during processing include:
• Dilution of concentrated cleaning and liquid chemical disinfectant/sterilant solutions to provide in-use dilutions for cleaning and disinfection.
• Rinsing of devices/materials to remove patient soils and chemical residues during and following cleaning and use of chemical disinfectants/sterilants.
• Thermal (hot water) disinfection.
• Thermal (steam) sterilization.
• Humidification of loads as a conditioning requirement for some low-temperature sterilization process (e.g. ethylene oxide and formaldehyde).
• Hand washing with soaps or antiseptics.

It is important to note that water, as we typically receive it for safe drinking or other purposes, is rarely "pure" but is actually found to have a range of different chemical, microbial, and other contaminants (Table 15.1). These can include various types of chemicals that are dissolved or other materials suspended/floating in the water. Most of these cannot be seen but can play an important role in device processing.

Water contaminants can vary depending on the water source (reservoir, lake, water table, etc.), any purification steps (e.g. to render it safe for drinking), how it is transported to and within a facility, and if any further treatment is done within the facility. Facility treatments can include the addition of antimicrobial chemicals (such as chlorine) or the removal of certain contaminants (such as the use of chemical/microbial filters, ultraviolet (UV) light treatment, or water "softening"). The quality or purity of the water will also vary over time, especially between seasons. For clarification, on the discussion of steam sterilization (Chapter 11, in the section on water quality and steam purity), water "quality" refers to the physical properties of steam (e.g. saturation, non-condensable gases, and dryness), while "purity" refers to the chemical (and microbiological) contaminants that may be present. Elsewhere within the book both terms are used interchangeably to refer to chemical and microbial contaminants in the water.

Examples of various negative effects of water quality include (also see examples of these effects in Figure 15.1):
• Device and equipment damage: a common example is rusting (or the development of rust, chemically known as ferric oxide, FeO_3) on stainless steel surfaces. Rust can be seen as a reddish-brown material on the surfaces of instruments (particularly on any moving parts). It will also be observed as "pitting" or the development of small pin holes on the surface of the device. Rusting is a visual sign of surface damage. One of the most common causes of premature rusting of stainless steel devices is the presence of a high concentration of chlorine in the water, particularly when the water is heated. Another is the presence of high levels of silicates. High levels of chlorine and water at unusually high ("alkaline") or low ("acidic") pH can also lead to device/instrument/equipment damage such as bleaching (loss of color) and decay of anodized aluminum.
• Chemical deposits: water hardness (scale, limescale, or calcium/magnesium carbonate) is a particular concern and is often detected by the presence of "spotting" or a white, grainy deposit on surfaces (Figure 15.1). Hardness (also known as "scale" when seen on a surface) refers to the concentration of calcium and magnesium ions in water, measured chemically as parts per million (ppm) or milligrams per liter (mg/L) $CaCO_3$. Water can have high concentrations of hardness (e.g. over 400 ppm) without being seen, but such high concentrations will precipitate out as a salt when heated. The precipitate may also be otherwise colored (e.g. appearing more green or brown

---

Decontamination and Device Processing in Healthcare, Second Edition. Gerald McDonnell and Georgia Alevizopoulou.
© 2025 John Wiley & Sons Ltd. Published 2025 by John Wiley & Sons Ltd.

Table 15.1 Examples of components that can be found in water. Some components are dissolved in (or in solution with) water, while others are suspended (floating in or on water).

Component	Examples
Water-dissolved components	
Inorganic materials	Pure water (H_2O)
Organic materials	Calcium (Ca), magnesium (Mg), chlorine (Cl_2)/chloride (Cl^-), silicates (molecules with SiO^{-4}),
Gases	Sodium (Na), nitrates (molecules with NO_3^-), iron (Fe)
Suspended components	
Inorganic materials	Calcium carbonate ($CaCO_2$), clay, silt, silica
Organic materials	Endotoxins, proteins, fats, oil
Microorganisms	Bacteria, viruses, protozoa

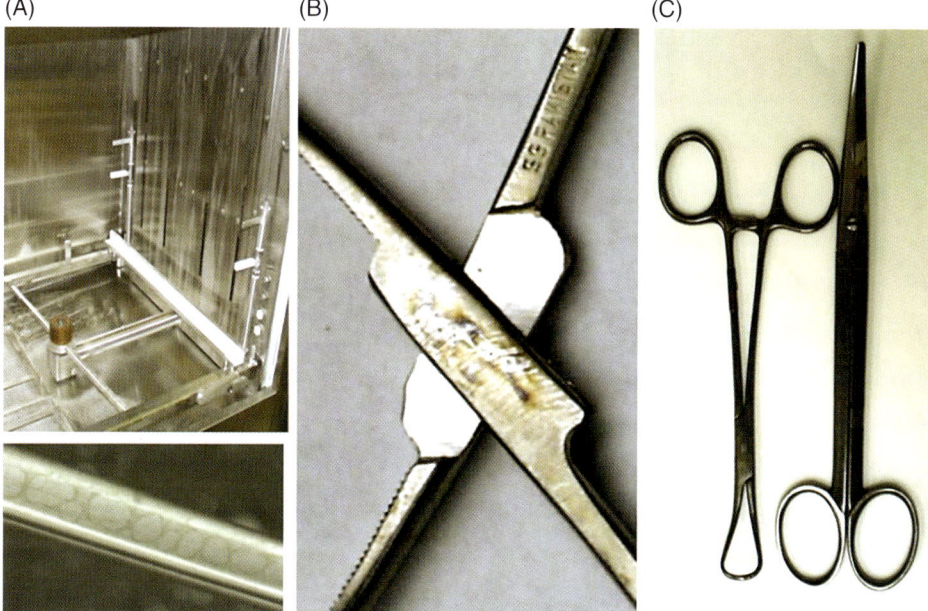

Figure 15.1 Examples of problems associated with water quality/purity. They include (A) water hardness deposition (seen as white precipitate in a washer-disinfector and "spotting" on a device surface); (B) rusting; and (C) staining (black staining on stainless steel devices).

due to the presence of other metals such as copper in the water that precipitate with the hardness). When water is dried any chemical component(s) will remain on the surface and these deposits can also have negative effects.
• Staining of devices, materials, and equipment: in addition to the rusting (red/brown) and hardness (white, grainy) stains already discussed, other examples include:
  ○ Multicolored staining (often seen as a rainbow effect, including yellow, brownish, blue, and violet) covering large areas or drop-shaped or irregular, insular shapes, which is usually due to increased content of silicates in water.
  ○ Orange-brown staining, often due to high levels of phosphates in the water.
  ○ Black staining: acidic (pH <6) water.
  ○ Gold-tinting: high chlorine levels.
  ○ Purple/blue staining: high levels of amines in water (note that many of these effects may be due to various treatments of water within a facility, e.g. amines are often added to water boilers and steam generators).

These are also discussed in Chapters 8 and 11 in the sections on troubleshooting cleaning or steam sterilization problems respectively.

- Inefficient cleaning: various chemicals can negatively impact the ability of a cleaning chemistry to work, reducing cleaning efficacy. Another example is the increased production of foam (e.g. in a washer-disinfector), which can reduce cleaning and cause damage to the equipment over time.
- Patient toxicity: this can occur with any device depending on how it is used, but the greatest risks are with critical and semi-critical devices and are often due to the lack of adequate rinsing following cleaning or high-level disinfection. Examples include complications of eye and other microsurgical techniques from various water components left on the device during processing. These can be chemical (such as the various deposits discussed earlier) or microbial/biochemical (e.g. bacterial endotoxins; see Chapter 5, in the section on bacterial contaminants).
- Patient infections: bacteria and other microorganisms present in water can remain on a surface (e.g. introduced following chemical disinfection of a semi-critical device), can multiply (in the case of bacteria), and can lead to patient infections (depending on the use of the device). A typical example is in the processing of flexible endoscopes (see the section on endoscopes and other lumened devices), where water is used to rinse away chemical residues prior to patient use. The use of poor-quality water contaminated with bacteria can lead to risks even with critical devices that are subject to sterilization, and can be a source of toxicity (e.g. endotoxins, see Chapter 5 and later in this chapter).

It is best practice to form or connect with a facility multi-disciplinary team to address water quality/purity and its impact on device processing and patient safety. This will include facility engineering and maintenance staff, water quality equipment suppliers or maintenance consultants, processing staff or management (which may include multiple locations/departments such as endoscopic areas or surgical staff), infection prevention/control, laboratory personnel, clinical engineers, and maybe others. The idea is to use the multi-disciplinary team to best define and manage the different risks associated with the clinical use of water in processing areas.

Three basic steps are recommended to reduce the risks of problems associated with water quality:
- Test and review water quality. It is important to understand the quality of water at the site of use (such as delivered to a sink, equipment, or machine). Water will enter a facility but then various treatments may occur (even periodically without prior knowledge, a particular concern in larger facilities). A typical example is the addition of chlorine (or other chemicals) to the water to be able to control bacterial levels (e.g. *Legionella*, a common bacterial contaminant in water that can lead to a lung disease). High levels of chlorine can have a significant impact on device/equipment safety, resulting in damage and increased costs. The transfer of water through a facility can also mean contamination sources, such as in older facilities that have lead or copper pipework. Also consider that there may be different sources of water, such as cold, hot, and "treated" or "purified." These can be of different quality and should be individually tested.
- Identify potential water quality problems and introduce methods to reduce their impact. A summary of typical chemical water quality problems and suggested methods of reducing their levels is given in Table 15.2. Microbial contamination can also be a concern in water used for final rinsing of chemically disinfected devices and even in water used for thermal disinfection/sterilization. This includes:
  ○ High levels of bacteria or other microorganisms. Disinfection can be compromised by rinsing with contaminated water and may lead to patient infections. The microbiological quality of water is generally tested by estimating the quantity of viable, aerobic bacteria. An example of recommended levels of bacterial contamination is:
    – <1 cfu/mL: satisfactory.
    – <1–9 cfu/mL on a regular basis: acceptable, indicates that bacterial numbers are under reasonable control.
    – 10–100 cfu/mL: unsatisfactory, investigate the potential problem and/or repeat testing.
    – >100 cfu/mL: unacceptable, out of service until quality is improved.

  These levels may or may not be acceptable depending on the use of the device or water (e.g. as discussed in Chapter 9, in the section on flexible endoscopes). Country-specific recommendations regarding the levels of microbial contamination in water may be specified for some device (e.g. flexible endoscope) reprocessing applications.

  ○ High levels of bacterial endotoxins. These may be present at high concentrations in the water due to the presence of Gram-negative bacteria (such as *Pseudomonas aeruginosa*). Endotoxins are a class of toxins present in a microorganism but released only on cell disintegration (see Chapter 5, in the section on bacteria). High levels of endotoxins can lead to toxic reactions in patients (specifically fever and more serious complications). As components of Gram-negative bacteria, the bacteria may be inactivated by disinfection and sterilization methods but the endotoxin may remain as a risk. Heat-based methods such as dry heat and moist heat sterilization have been shown to inactivate endotoxins, as well as certain types of chemical sterilization methods (such as using hydrogen peroxide gas or gas plasma processes), but these should not be depended on alone to reduce the risk of endotoxin contamination. The levels of endotoxin that may cause a toxic effect are often debated, but a conservative estimate is levels >200 EU/mL water. Despite this debate, final rinse water (or disinfection water) is recommended to be ≤20 EU/mL. In some countries levels in rinse water or in steam are recommended to be ≤10 or even 0.25 EU/mL (note: this reflects the typical levels that should be present if

Table 15.2 Examples of common chemical water quality problems and how they may be addressed. Lower specifications may be recommended for certain applications (e.g. for heat disinfection or sterilization; see Chapter 11, in the section on water quality and steam purity). Specific requirements can be given in country-specific standards or guidance documents.

Water quality indicator	Suggested warning levels[1]	Intervention
Hardness[2] mg/L ($CaCO_3$ equivalent) Generally the following terms are used: 　"Soft" water: 0–60 mg/L 　"Moderately hard" water: 60–120 mg/L 　"Hard" water: >120 mg/L	≥150 mg/L, although lower levels may be suggested for heat disinfection/sterilization methods (e.g. ≤20 mg/L)	Softening: a technique that removes hardness (calcium/magnesium) by replacing with another chemical (e.g. NaCl, common salt) May also reduce levels of other chemicals such as iron (Fe)
Chlorine mg/L	≥120 mg/L: during cleaning chloride concentrations >240 mg/L chlorine can be very damaging to surfaces Equally, at higher temperatures chlorine can be more aggressive at even lower concentrations (10–120 mg/L)	Activated carbon filtration: this can reduce chlorine (and chlorine-containing chemicals such as chloramines) as well as some organic materials
Conductivity (or resistivity) $\mu S/cm^{-1}$ Measure of the concentration of "ions" and therefore various metals and molecules in solution Will include iron, copper, chlorine, and manganese	≥100 $\mu S/cm^{-1}$ For example, a conductivity level at 40 $\mu S/cm^{-1}$ is equivalent to a chloride level of 10 mg/L, but this will also be affected by the presence of other chemicals	Specific chemical contaminants may be removed/reduced by boiling or (as an example) carbon filtration More efficient processes include deionization, distillation, or reverse osmosis
Total dissolved solids (TDS) mg/L	Generally recommended to be <100 mg/L; a similar measure to conductivity	Specific chemical contaminants may be removed/reduced by boiling or (as an example) carbon filtration Better processes include deionization, distillation, or reverse osmosis
pH: a measure of how alkaline (high pH) or acidic (low pH) the water is	Water should not be lower than pH 6.5 or higher than pH 9.5 and should generally be in the neutral (pH 6–8) range for potable water	Will involve further investigation to identify the source of the acidity/alkalinity, given the typical range of potable water
Total organic carbon (TOC) mg/L, a measure of any organic (carbon-containing) materials in the water, including microorganisms	Generally recommended at <1 mg/L during disinfection and steam sterilization processes	May be reduced with certain types of filtration methods (including activated carbon) or may require more efficient processes including deionization, distillation, or reverse osmosis

[1] Remember, "≥" means "greater or equal to," ≤ is "less than or equal to," and ≈ is "approximately equally to."
[2] The official units of measurement for hardness are mg/L ($CaCO_3$ equivalent), but others include parts per million (in this case, 1 ppm is ≈1 mg/L), German degrees (°dH, defined as 10 mg calcium oxide per liter of water and ≈17.8 mg/L $CaCO_3$), and French degrees (°f; defined as 10 mg/L $CaCO_3$).

a water purification system, such as reverse osmosis, is used to treat the water).

- Monitor the water quality over time. As highlighted previously, water quality will change periodically and sometimes dramatically. Also, uncontrolled water treatment methods can themselves cause problems if not maintained correctly. Therefore, routine monitoring is suggested. In some countries and for some applications it is often mandated. Monitoring can include a simple or more complex series of assays (tests) and can vary depending on the use of the water. For example, water used for cleaning, thermal disinfection, and steam sterilization can be monitored by periodically checking the pH, conductivity, chlorine, and hardness levels. Equally, water used for the terminal rinsing of devices may need to be periodically checked for microbial and even endotoxin levels.

Methods for the analysis of water quality have already been discussed in Chapter 6, in the section on other common chemical measurement methods. In some cases, such as monitoring of pH, conductivity, chlorine, and hardness levels, simple test kits or equipment can be used to directly monitor water quality on site. In others, specific laboratories are required for analysis, such as inductively coupled plasma–optical emission spectroscopy (ICP-OES) analysis for testing the levels of different chemicals and bacteria/endotoxin testing. The method of water collection for such analysis is important to consider. The wrong sampling method or equipment (such as water collection bottles) can be a source of contamination and provide inaccurate results. For example, specific types of water collection bottles will be required for chemical analysis. For microbial analysis, the water bottle should be sterile and those collecting the sample should be trained in aseptic technique; these samples should also be refrigerated on collection and transport to a test laboratory.

The specific recommendations for the quality/purity of water at different stages of device/material processing can vary from country to country. These requirements are becoming essentially harmonized internationally, based on international standards and guidelines such as ISO/TS 5111, *Guidance on quality of water for sterilizers, sterilization and washer-disinfectors for health care products*. Examples include the requirements for utility and critical water or steam purity as defined in ANSI/AAMI ST108 *Water for the processing of medical devices*, the English requirements for water purity for steam and water used in washer-disinfectors (HTM 01-01: *Management and decontamination of surgical instruments (medical devices) used in acute care*: Part C: *steam sterilization* and Part D: *washer-disinfectors*), and the Australian/New Zealand AS 5369 *Reprocessing of reusable medical devices and other devices in health and non-health related facilities*. A guidance on these recommended levels of contaminants is given in Table 15.3, but this list is not exhaustive and is provided as a guide.

Some of the more widely used methods of water treatment or purification (Figure 15.2) are:
- Water softening: a technique that removes hardness (calcium/magnesium) by replacing with another chemical (e.g. NaCl, common salt). This may also reduce other chemical levels such as iron (Fe).
- Filtration: filters are used to remove various water contaminants based on their size. The use of filtration as a disinfection

Table 15.3 A guideline for recommended levels of water contaminants at various stages of device processing. The focus of this guidance is for the processing of critical and semi-critical devices. Consideration should also be given to any local guidelines and standards for water quality. Note that chemical and equipment manufacturers may specify requirements for water quality greater or lesser than the ranges given in this table.

Parameter	Units	Cleaning	Disinfection	Rinsing (post chemical disinfection)	Steam	Pure water[1]
pH		6.5–9.5	6.5–9.5	5–7.5	5.0–9.2[2]	5–7.5
Conductivity	µS/cm	<500	<10	<10	<10	<10
Hardness	mg/L	<150	<150	<1	<1	<1
Total dissolved solids (TDS)	mg/L	<100	<100	<100	<50	<0.5
Total organic carbon (TOC)	mg/L	n/a	n/a	n/a	<1	<0.5
Bacteria	cfu/mL	<500	<500	<10[3]	n/a	<10[3]
Endotoxin[4]	EU/mL	n/a	n/a	<10	<10	<10
Visual inspection		Colorless, clear, no sediment	Colorless, clear, no sediment	Colorless, clear, no sediment	Colorless, clear, no sediment	Colorless, clear, no sediment

n/a, not applicable.
[1] Pure water by reverse osmosis (RO), distillation, or other water purification method. Other indicators include chloride <2 mg/L, silicates <1 mg/L, and phosphates <0.5 mg/L.
[2] The pH range for steam is wider than for critical water as some steam may not be generated locally but from a centralized/facility system. The need to add chemicals to the boiler and the steam to travel distances over black iron piping may result in higher pH requirements. A pH <7.5 in these systems should be avoided.
[3] <1 cfu/mL: satisfactory.
<1–9 cfu/mL on a regular basis: acceptable, indicates that bacterial numbers are under reasonable control.
10–100 cfu/mL: unsatisfactory, investigate the potential problem and/or repeat testing.
>100 cfu/mL: unacceptable, out of service until quality is improved.
Some guidelines recommend specific testing for certain types of microorganisms such as *Mycobacteria* and *Legionella*.
[4] In some guidelines the safe level of endotoxin is described as 0.25 EU/mL; the scientific basis for these levels is often debated, although pure water by RO or distillation should provide this level if the supply is designed and maintained correctly.

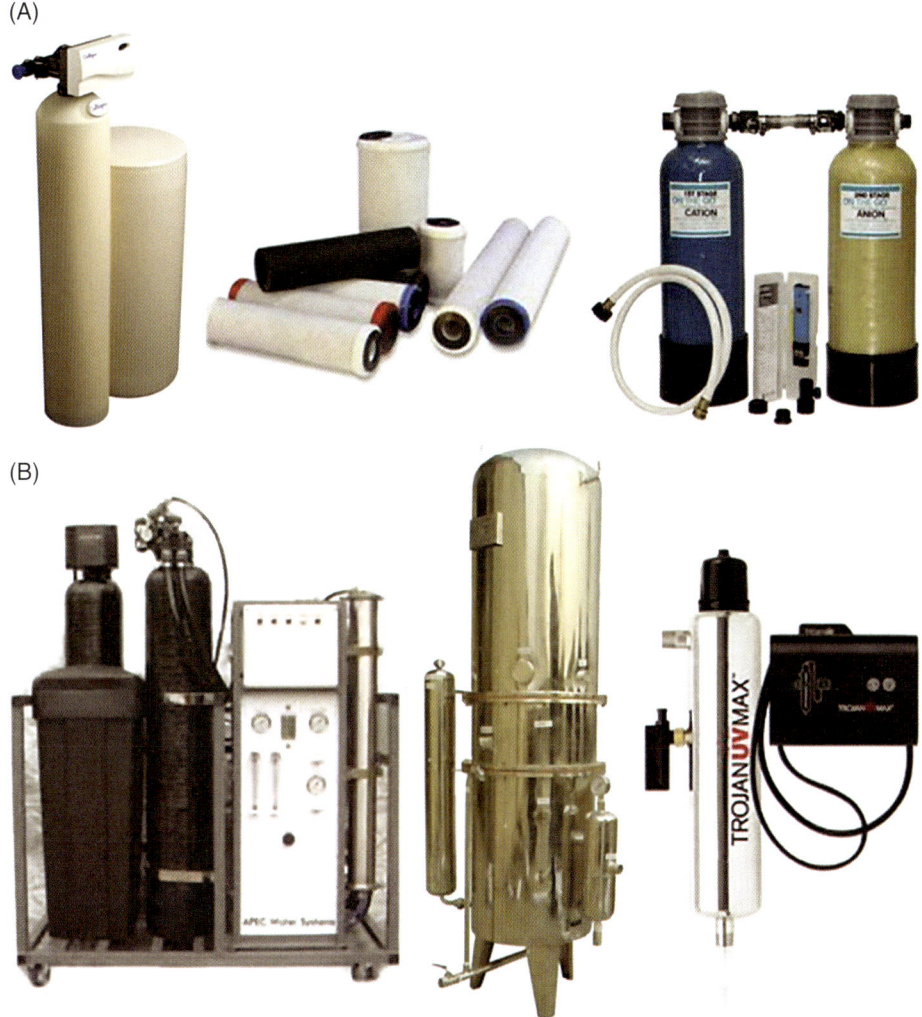

Figure 15.2 Examples of various types of water treatment or purification methods. (A) Left to right: water softener, activated carbon filters, deionizer. (B) Left to right: reverse osmosis, distillator, ultraviolet light.

method, filtration for the removal of microorganism, and the theory of filtration are discussed in further detail in Chapter 9. Filters can also remove chemicals/materials by binding or neutralizing these materials. An example is with activated carbon filtration, used to remove chlorine (and chlorine-containing chemicals such as chloramines) as well as some organic materials, or "green sand" for the removal of iron or manganese. Reverse osmosis, as a water purification method, is based on a method of filtration.

- Distillation: a process that involves the heating of water to make steam and its condensation back into water, to separate the water from its contaminants (see Chapter 6). The process needs to be controlled, as some contaminants can transfer over in the steam and be included in the condensed water.

- Deionization: a process that removes various "charged" chemicals from water by exchange (removing in exchange for other, innocuous chemicals). This is an efficacious process for any charged chemicals but not for uncharged chemicals/materials.
- Reverse osmosis: a filtration (membrane)-based method that is based on filtration and contaminant rejection. It is widely used for the generation of pure water, but requires constant maintenance and control to ensure the expected water quality output.
- UV light disinfection: UV refers to wavelengths of light that have a higher energy level just above visible light (specifically in the 10–400 nm wavelength range). These lights are commonly used to reduce microbial contamination in water

(see Chapter 9 on radiation). Other methods of microbial disinfection can include the addition of various types of chemicals such as chlorine and silver/copper (Chapter 9).
- In addition to antimicrobial chemicals added for disinfection purposes, other chemicals may be added for specific purposes to include:
  ○ Acids or bases/alkali to modify water pH.
  ○ Bisulfite (e.g. sodium bisulfite) for removal of chlorine.

The addition of one chemical for a particular reason can lead to problems elsewhere during the processing cycle, so any decisions to add or modify various chemical treatments should be considered with the processing facility.

Overall, water is an essential component of most processing steps and can affect the safety and efficacy of these processes. Control and monitoring of water quality/purity are highly recommended to ensure process effectiveness and device safety.

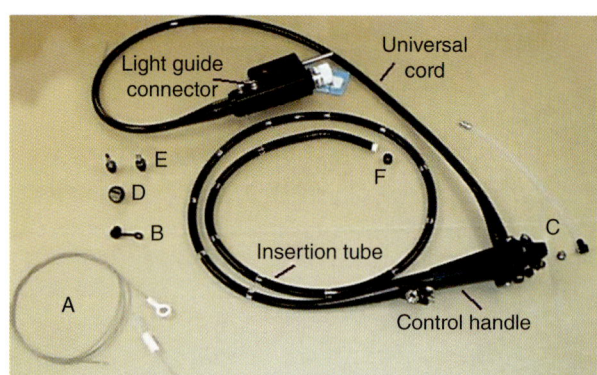

Figure 15.3 A flexible endoscope with various accessories. Included are (A) cleaning brush, (B) biopsy valve cap, (C) channel adapter, (D) port accessory, (E) valves (in this case two valves are used during the patient procedure), and (F) insertion tip (with tip cover shown).

Endoscopy

Endoscopy has been one of the fastest-growing areas of medical and surgical technology and practice for patient care. The word endoscopy is derived from the Greek *endon*, meaning "within," and *scopeo*, meaning "examine." Endoscopy therefore refers to any procedure to look inside the body, for medical, diagnostic, or surgical purposes. Endoscopic procedures comprise a significant percentage of healthcare procedures across the world. Coupled with the tremendous growth in the adoption of various cancer screening programs, the volume of endoscopic procedures is estimated to rise even further. The various different types of endoscopic procedures were introduced in Chapter 3 in the introduction to endoscopic procedures, including their use in robotic-assisted surgery. Endoscopes are dedicated medical devices to perform endoscopic procedures. They are advanced, sophisticated types of viewing devices serving both diagnostic and therapeutic roles. They can vary in design, construction, materials, and intended use. In many cases, flexible and rigid endoscopes use a variety of other devices/instruments during a procedure to access internal tissues and to operate. These include separate devices used as part of the procedure, such as light and suction source instruments, injection and aspiration needles, trocars, snares, forceps, irrigation catheters, coagulating electrodes, cytology brushes, retrieval nets, and many more; others are specific parts of the device, such as the procedural valves (Figure 15.3). Reusable endoscopic accessories, just like the endoscopes themselves, should be checked thoroughly for function and integrity before and after each use. The various designs and features of endoscopes and their accessory devices were introduced in Chapter 4 in the section on endoscopy.

In addition to being some of the more expensive devices to purchase (hence there is usually a limited inventory for specific models in service), endoscopes are extremely delicate and are often associated with expensive repairs. They are also reported as the most common types of reusable devices associated with cross-infection in patients. A good understanding of their design, function, as well as proper care and handling during clinical use and processing are essential to maintain the endoscope in optimum condition and prevent disease and infection transmission.

Special attention is required for processing flexible endoscopes, such as those used in respiratory, urinary, and gastrointestinal procedures, because it requires some unique procedures compared to those used with any other reusable medical devices. Therefore, they are often considered separately and processed in a dedicated area of a healthcare facility separate from other devices. In many countries this area would be near the endoscopy procedure rooms to facilitate the high demand and quick turnaround time. In other countries, endoscope processing is conducted in a central location such as a central services department. The specific decontamination procedures may occur either in a single processing room or in two or three rooms designed to allow for physical separation (dirty side, clean side, and storage/use side) based on the expected room bioburden levels and in accordance with the principles of the design of a decontamination area (see the introduction to Chapter 1). Regardless of the location and the layout of the dedicated processing area, endoscopes and their accessories are at minimum expected to flow through strict unidirectional processing procedures and be processed in a standardized manner to reduce the risks of cross-contamination and/or cross-infection between patients. Naturally, compliance and strict adherence to topical, local standards, processing guidelines, and manufacturers' instructions are essential. Yet despite the emphasis on this topic, at the time of writing there continues to be an increase in

endoscopically transmitted infections attributed to water-borne and multi-drug-resistant organisms. The correct processing of endoscopes remains a significant and challenging concern globally. Several discrepancies across the world include:
- Assuming that flexible endoscopes are low risk, limited device availability, and insufficient time planned for processing between patient use.
- Inadequate and/or lack of training and competency of decontamination staff in the design (particularly internal components), care, and handling of flexible endoscopes.
- Complex design of endoscopes in conjunction with inconsistent and/or poor manufacturers' instructions for use and processing.
- Lack of standardization of endoscope processing and lack of established policies.
- Failure to adhere to standards and guidelines.
- Lack of verification and quality control measures specific to endoscope processing.
- Abbreviation of processing steps, which are often demanded by the increased clinical need.
- Inadequate processing environments overlooking capacity of the facility, area layout and room size, workflow and traffic patterns, equipment and utilities required for endoscope decontamination.
- Omission or inadequate point-of-use treatment and processing/use of endoscopes that can result in biofilm development over time (see Chapter 5 on bacteria).
- Failure to clean, inspect, and disinfect/sterilize all internal channels and device parts.
- Failure to clean and disinfect/sterilize associated accessories.
- Failure to use appropriate decontamination tools, such as brushes, irrigators, automated endoscope reprocessor (AER) connectors.
- Poor selection of cleaning and disinfectant solutions that may not be compatible with the endoscopes or may not be effective against different types of soils and pathogens.
- Failure to follow the manufacturer's recommended exposure time and temperature for chemical solutions, e.g. detergents and high-level disinfectants.
- Use of poor-quality water or contaminated water while rinsing (post chemical disinfection).
- Inadequate drying and storage prior to patient use.
- Lack of scheduled preventative maintenance and failure to notice and/or report malfunctions of devices and equipment.

As a first step, it is important to consider the clinical use of the flexible endoscope. Devices used for critical procedures (contacting sterile areas of the body, including blood contact) should be cleaned and sterilized, while those used for semi-critical procedures (where the device could contact mucous membranes or non-intact skin) should at a minimum be cleaned and disinfected (see Chapter 1 on the Spaulding classification). Simple as this classification may appear, it can often be difficult to make a decision regarding the risk to a patient. In the past, many of these flexible endoscopes would only have been used for simple diagnostic purposes and would be deemed semi-critical because they are used by being passed into naturally occurring orifices of the body that are not in themselves sterile. In recent years, however, their intended use has changed and many endoscopes are frequently used surgically for advanced therapeutic procedures and required to be sterile during clinical use. In parallel, advances in the technology of modern gaseous sterilizers allow endoscopes to be readily sterilized in a reasonable time frame for practical clinical use, which relieves the common compromise of needing to perform high-level disinfection due to time constraints and clinical pressure for readiness. For example, there are various VH_2O_2 sterilization cycles available that accelerate the availability and throughput of such devices, in addition to allowing them to be stored as sterile wrapped devices in readiness for patient use. In many parts of the world many flexible endoscopes are already being recommended to be sterilized, including duodenoscopes, cystoscopes, and bronchoscopes. When consensus is not reached, it is recommended to perform a risk assessment (see Chapter 14 on management and quality) to see whether sterilization is feasible and if transitioning to sterilization will improve the quality of medical device processing as well as the level of patient care. It is important to remember in this evaluation that disinfection or sterilization is only one consideration in risk assessment. Others that are of significant concern due to unfortunate reports of endoscope-associated patient infections include lack of cleaning, rinse water quality, inadequate drying prior to storage, and contamination during clinical use (e.g. from water bottles or accessories).

Written policies and procedures should be in place that ensure the safe and efficient processing of endoscopes and their accessories. Procedures should consider processing recommendations provided by the endoscope manufacturers and any cleaning, disinfectant, and/or sterilization process/equipment/chemistry manufacturers used for processing. They should also comply with local, national, and regional standards and guidelines. Staff should be trained in these procedures and understand the significance to patient safety of any deviation, and processing areas should be periodically inspected for compliance/staff competency.

Recommended procedures should include:
- The appropriate handling of endoscopes and associated accessories, to ensure they are not physically damaged during clinical use, transportation, cleaning, disinfection/sterilization, and storage. These devices are very complex, delicate, and fragile, and are more susceptible to damage compared to any other device. The distal tip is especially complex and easy to damage in ways that may not be obvious; minor bumps can cause major problems. Endoscopes can be easily cut, cracked, punctured, or scratched, and most of these problems come

from human error, poor handling, and lack of care. It is worth mentioning that it takes about 6–8 working hours to replace the distal tip when sent out for repair. Care must be taken while carrying endoscopes in the hands, since the optics are easily damaged if left to dangle or knocked against a hard surface. Hold carefully the control head, the light guide connector, and a loop of the insertion tube in such a way that you are controlling the distal tip. The other hand can hold the tip or help support the weight of the cables (Figure 15.4). As a different example, endoscopes have a minimum bend radius (how tightly they can be coiled) that is usually defined by the device manufacturer. Over-coiling endoscopes into loops smaller than intended to fit into small transportation boxes, wash sinks, or storage containers can lead to buckling and wrinkles on the flexible endoscopes. This can eventually damage the various channels and other components critical to functionality or impact their stiffness, which can prevent certain movements with the device during clinical use. Repeated bending should be identified and corrected before it leaves a permanent effect.

• Preparation of the device prior to processing. This is specifically considered in Chapter 7 on point-of-use treatment and transport and Chapter 8 on cleaning. At the point of use endoscopes ought to receive an initial treatment in preparation for cleaning. This step requires the insertion tube to be wiped with a cloth impregnated in a cleaning solution to remove gross soil as well as aspiration through the suction channel and flushing through the remaining channels as appropriate for the endoscope (Figure 15.5). The volume of fluid used is dependent on the model and length of the channel. Always confirm with the manufacturer's instructions for use. Single-use sponges, valves, and other clinical accessories are discarded at the end of the treatment. They should not be sent to the processing area unless they are reusable (reusable valves may often be used).

• Fluid-resistant caps or "soaking caps" may need to be attached (placed over the lightguide connector end) to protect any electrical components that may be present prior to immersion in water. Newer generations of flexible endoscopes may be labeled as waterproof and will not need such an accessory.

• Leak-testing procedure. A main source of damage with flexible endoscopes is from fluid invasion. Most of an endoscope's internal components are not made to be chemical or fluid resistant. Fluid invasion (or entry into these areas) can damage these components, making the endoscope inoperable. A leak test is designed by the manufacturer to identify punctures,

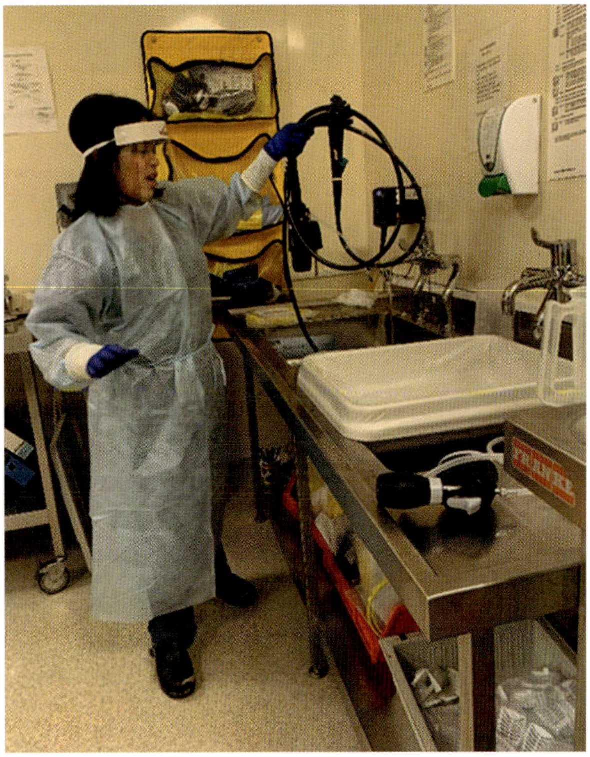

Figure 15.4 Endoscope processing technician holding the control head, the light guide connector, and a loop of the insertion tube in one hand while controlling the distal tip just before placing the endoscope into the wash sink for manual cleaning.

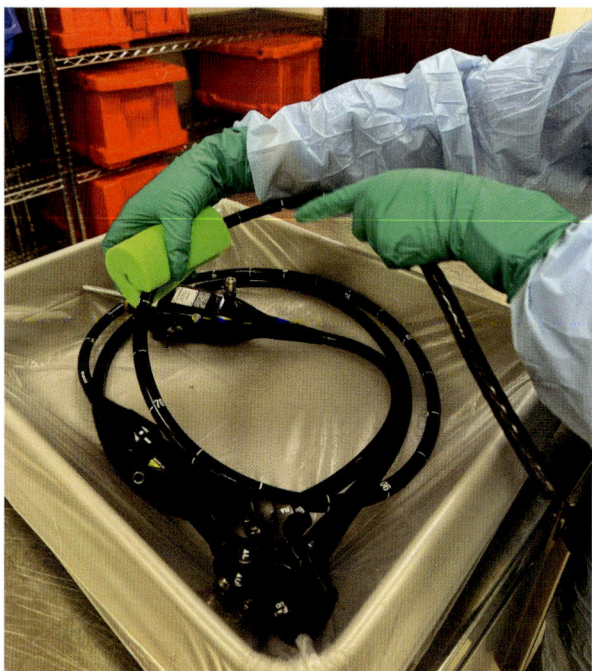

Figure 15.5 Point-of-use treatment of a flexible endoscope; a disposable sponge impregnated in cleaning solution is used to wipe gross soil down the insertion tube (flushing of internal lumens is not shown).

tears, failed seals, and other damage that could cause fluid to enter the internal space of the endoscope prior to processing. According to repair service providers' statistics, 60–70% of leaks will come from the bending rubber sections of the device, with damage to the biopsy channel and then the control body being responsible for the remaining locations of leaks. During a leak test the internal compartment of a flexible endoscope is pressurized with air. Pressurization can be either manual using a handheld air pump or automated using an electrical leak tester. Staff look for visible signs of leaks by either observing a pressure drop (dry leak test) over time or by looking for bubbles while submerging the entire endoscope in water (wet leak test; see Chapter 8 on endoscopy). The endoscope must be pressurized prior to submersion and angulated in all directions to ensure that all surfaces and seals are assessed for leaks. It is imperative that the leak test is performed for the full duration, which typically takes 90 seconds or as stated in the manufacturer's instructions. Pin-hole leaks may not identify themselves immediately.

- Cleaning of the endoscope, including external and internal (lumen) parts. Cleaning must start quickly after the point-of-use treatment is completed. The longer the time between point-of-use treatment and cleaning, the more difficult the endoscope becomes to clean. Most instructions for use do not provide a specific time. Some guidelines state that "cleaning should be initiated within one hour or as determined by the facility based on their own documented risk assessment." Manual cleaning is often recommended by the device manufacturer, even if automated cleaning systems are available or used. Manual cleaning consists of brushing and flushing the various internal lumens with a cleaning chemistry, followed by rinsing with water, in accordance with the recommendations from the chemistry manufacturer (Figure 15.6). Manual cleaning requires a proper set-up including using an ergonomically designed sink with convenient depth to allow immersion of all lengths of endoscopes. Brushing is a critical step in this phase of endoscope decontamination that unfortunately is often overlooked. Skipping or abbreviating this or any step could result in residual soil and pose a serious risk of infection or other patient adverse effects. Brushes should meet the endoscope manufacturer's specifications. They should be appropriately sized to fit the channel being cleaned, contact all surfaces of the channel and ports, and pass easily through the channel without excessive friction. If brushes are labeled for single use, use them only once and then discard. Reusable brushes need to be cleaned and disinfected between uses and replaced as they become worn. While brushing, the endoscope needs to be submerged under water to prevent aerosolization. Aerosolization is a major concern for safety and therefore current and full use of personal protective equipment (PPE) is highly recommended (see Chapter 13 on safety). Besides brushes, several other cleaning accessories may still be needed, such as adapters and channel irrigators, and they are often specific to the device being cleaned. The irrigator forces fluid through all the endoscope channels at the same time, helping to flush debris out of the device. Accessories may require special adapters. Depending on the device design, semi-automated irrigation systems may be used. It is also important to consider any accessories used as part of the device. An important example is the processing of reusable flexible endoscope valves (Figure 15.3).

- Inspection of flexible endoscopes. This is required to identify both residual soil as well as any signs of damage including surface and cosmetic issues and/or malfunctions (see Chapter 10 on flexible endoscopes). A procedure should be in place to allow for a simple, easy-to-use, standardized and consistent inspection process. Detailed visual inspection is the minimum and can be enhanced with technology using lighted magnifying glasses or electronic borescopes to view where the human eye cannot. The value of such inspections is dependent on image quality, but is also impacted by the skill and technique used by the operator of the inspection device, hence training is critical. An example of a borescope for inspection of lumens is shown in Figure 15.7. Furthermore, recent revisions of international standards advise that a cleaning verification test should be incorporated into the facility's inspection procedures prior to high-level disinfection/sterilization. The various biochemical tests that can be used for this purpose were discussed in detail in Chapter 8 on cleaning and Chapter 14 on management and quality. At the time of writing, there is no standardized global requirement for the frequency of such tests in endoscopy. Some countries require that cleaning verification testing is performed on every high-risk endoscope – that is, bronchoscope – after each use following cleaning and rinsing. Low-risk endoscopes should be tested on initial receipt

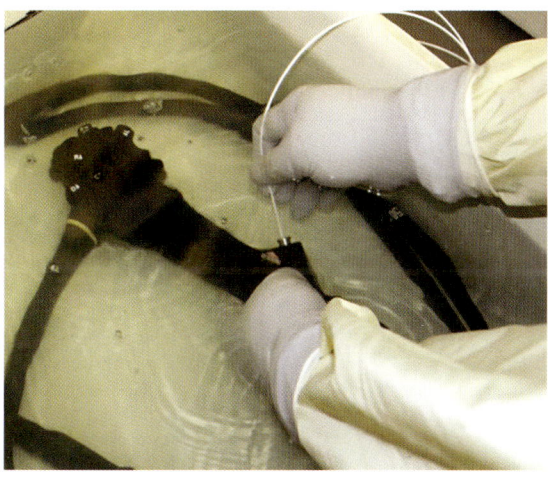

Figure 15.6 Manual cleaning of a flexible endoscope.

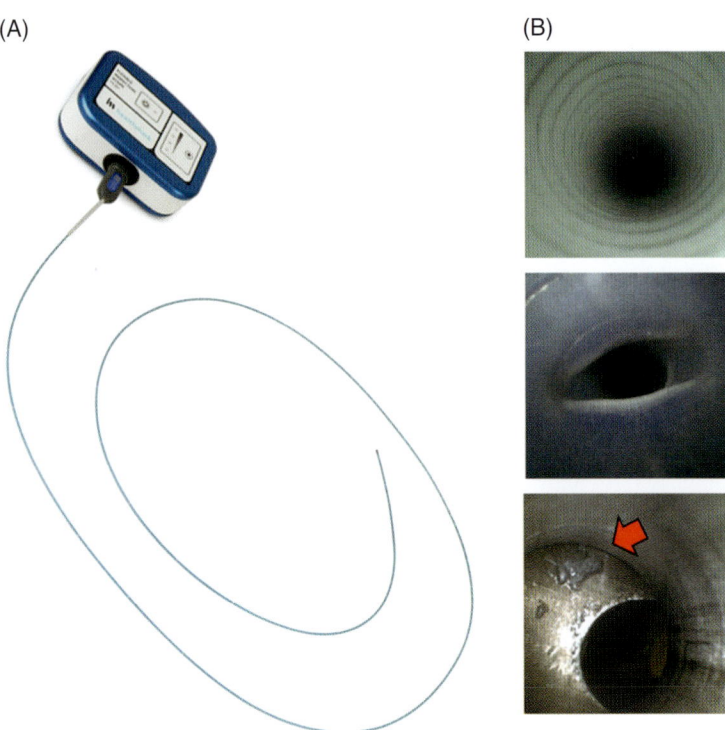

Figure 15.7 (A) Example of a borescope for inspection of lumens. (B) Examples of a new, clean lumen (top), a damaged (crushed) lumen (middle), and soil present in a lumen (arrow, bottom).

and then periodically at intervals that are defined by the facility. Some countries will also include implementation of microbial surveillance using a standardized sampling method and periodic observational audits.

- The antimicrobial process. Disinfection of temperature-sensitive endoscopes can be achieved by manual immersion or by an automated system using a variety of liquid chemical (high-level) disinfectants (these are discussed in further detail in Chapter 9 on disinfection). Liquid chemical and gaseous sterilization systems may also be used, depending on the sterilization system manufacturer's claims (see Chapter 11 on sterilization). When using aldehyde-based disinfectants or sterilization processes, consideration should be given to the possibility of the presence of certain types of bacteria that can present with higher tolerance or resistance profiles to these processes (e.g. mycobacteria). Overall, the choice of the antimicrobial process is dependent on the facility's risk assessment and standard/guidance documents applicable to the region/country. For example, a facility may choose to sterilize bronchoscopes since bronchoscopies are associated with higher infection rates, but to high-level disinfect colonoscopes due to their lower risk of infection.
- Rinsing. Following manual or automated liquid chemical disinfection, all internal and external surfaces should be safely rinsed in accordance with the disinfectant manufacturer's instructions. This is to ensure that no chemical toxic residuals remain and the device is safe for patient use. There are unfortunately frequent reports in the literature of toxic reactions in patients due to inadequate rinsing. In some cases, up to five or six rinses in fresh water of the required purity may be required. Water purity is an important consideration, as considered earlier in this chapter. In some cases, following gaseous sterilization methods (e.g. with ethylene oxide or formaldehyde) devices may require extended aeration to similarly ensure that no toxic residuals (the sterilization gas or by-products) remain on the device. In other cases, validation processes may be sufficient to ensure that safe residual levels have been achieved, but in these cases other quality checks may be required (e.g. inspection for moisture).
- Drying and any potential storage of the device. For gaseous (flexible/rigid endoscopes) or high-temperature (rigid endoscopes) sterilization methods, the devices are sterilized in sterile barrier systems and should be stored in accordance with facility policy. Devices that are not terminally packaged may require drying prior to storage and/or the use of a drying cabinet (see Chapter 12 on storage and distribution). This is particularly important with disinfected devices, as low levels of bacteria can be allowed to grow during storage, in the presence of water (e.g. in a lumen), and over time. Moreover, drying is essential to ensure effective sterilization

prior to low-temperature gaseous sterilization processes such as those based on ethylene oxide, formaldehyde, and vaporized hydrogen peroxide. There are various drying practices across the world: air drying, placing devices in an area of limited access allowing water to evaporate from the device; towel drying, using a non-linting towel to absorb water from the surfaces of the device; and mechanical drying, removing water with heat or forced air from device surfaces. When cloths are used, consider the type of cloth – cotton, reusable or not – the duration of use, and how to process it. Introducing forced air into channels is a common practice either as part of the drying phase of an AER, or employing specific-purpose air guns or simply syringes. Residual water can remain within the endoscope channels, even if processing was conducted within an AER that may have lumen purging/drying claims. Details about the type of air to use, how to apply the air, and the time required should be specified as dictated by the device manufacturer. Attention should be paid to thoroughly drying all endoscope surfaces, not just the channels; for example, drying the control crevices is often challenging and verification means of drying efficiency may be needed. In some areas specific drying cabinets, referred to as controlled-environment storage cabinets, are employed to assist in the drying and storage of flexible endoscopes following processing. Such cabinets are generally designed to flow high-efficiency particulate air (HEPA)-filtered air through the various device lumens for the purpose of drying. When stored in such a manner, the manufacturer may recommend that the devices are safely maintained to prevent contamination and bacterial/fungal growth in or on the device. Such storage cabinets and any associated testing data should be carefully examined with the manufacturer to ensure they are safe for use in accordance with any facility policies.

It is of note that some professional associations and standards recommend using alcohol to enhance dryness coupled with vertical hanging to drain residual alcohol. Alcohol flushing is somewhat controversial due to its fixative properties and the potential patient health risks, because residual alcohol could be introduced to patients' tissues during endoscopic procedures if not removed during the pre-operative inspection of endoscopes and associated accessories such as valves.

- Storage. Procedures must also be in place that will define for how long a processed endoscope can be stored before it needs processing again. An event-related policy is highly recommended based on a risk assessment (see Chapter 12 on storage and distribution). If a storage cabinet is used, a risk assessment will help determine the period over which a processed endoscope can be stored and reused. Storing endoscopes in transport bins, in their original shipping cases that are lined with foam or porous material, or in wooden cabinets should be avoided at all times.

Single-use devices

The various different types of instruments and devices were discussed in Chapter 4, including their classification (in the section on single-use and reusable instrumentation definitions). An important example was the designation of a device as being for single use or reuse. A reusable device is designed to be used many times on different patients, being provided with detailed instructions on how it can be safely reprocessed between each patient. A single-use device (SUD) has been designed by a manufacturer to be used on a single patient only and then discarded. The emphasis here is on a single patient, where a device may be used multiple times on the same patient, depending on its design and manufacturer's instructions.

The internationally recognized symbols used with SUDs are shown in Figure 15.8. As highlighted in Chapter 4, some SUDs are provided sterile and ready for use, while others are provided non-sterile and are required to be cleaned and sterilized prior to patient use (see later in this chapter on loan devices sets and implants). Examples of the labeling and types of these devices are shown in Figure 15.9.

Some are designed to be processed multiple times (or even indefinitely in accordance with the instructions for use), but once used on or with a patient are not allowed to be processed further. Examples include implantable screw or plate sets that are designed for use in trauma or orthopedic surgical procedures (Figure 15.9). The sets (or replacements for individual screws or plates) can be provided non-sterile, are processed prior to surgical use, and some of the implants are used for the surgical procedure, but all are not used during that procedure. If the remaining screws have not been soiled, damaged, or

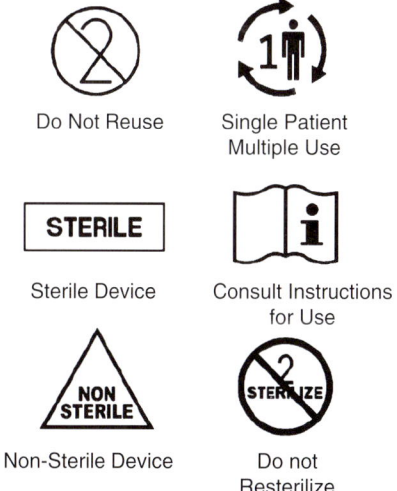

Figure 15.8 The internationally recognized symbols used with single-use devices.

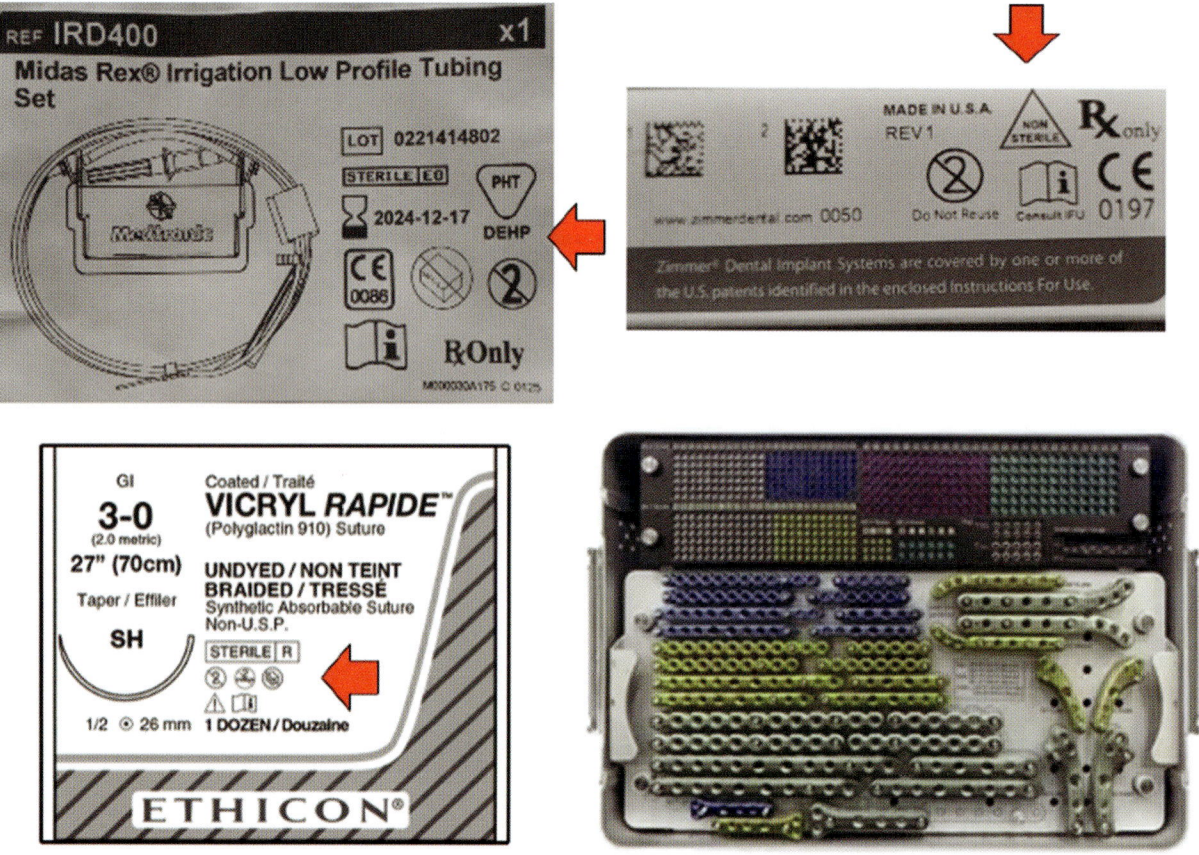

Figure 15.9 Examples of single-use devices provided sterile (left) and non-sterile (right). Note the differences in labeling. An example of a set of non-sterile orthopedic implants is shown on the lower right.

used, they can be labeled for processing in preparation for the next surgical procedure. But other types of SUDs have not been designed or labeled by the manufacturer to be processed. They can be labeled as single use and not to be resterilized (Figure 15.9).

Although many types of sterile SUDs have not been designed to be processed, in many parts of the world healthcare facilities will decide to process such devices and allow them to be used on other patients. The decision to process a used SUD should not be taken lightly. In some countries reuse of SUDs is considered illegal, while in others it is accepted if the correct procedures are used to ensure that the device is safely processed without adding any additional risk to another patient/user. Although the benefits may appear to be reducing costs and environmental considerations (less waste for incineration or other disposal method), risks will include damage (seen and unseen) to the device (which can lead to adverse patient effects), toxicity and infection concerns, how to define a new lifetime (i.e. how many processing cycles and inspection criteria), and legal considerations. Any decisions regarding the processing of SUDs should be taken at the highest level of any healthcare facility, in collaboration with infection prevention/control and with written approval by management.

Single-use/disposable items are widely used in healthcare, including for wound care, catheterization, and radio-diagnostics. They are often used for minimally invasive procedures and in accident/emergency departments as a cost-effective alternative to processing similar instruments or devices. The types of disposable instruments used most frequently include suture sets, dressing forceps, and nursing scissors. More complex examples used in neurosurgery can include disposable instruments that are routinely used for brain biopsies. By having a stock of sterile, packed items ready for use, medical or surgical staff can always have supplies in stock. Many of these can be expensive and in some cases the whole set may not be specifically used during a particular procedure (or not even used but opened), giving the concern that the device/set may appear wasteful to discard.

Legally, sterile SUDs are not designed to be processed and the manufacturer will inform the buyer that the device is for single use only by labeling it accordingly. The manufacturer is not obliged to give reasons why the item has been classified as single use. When the manufacturer attaches the symbol for one-time use only to a device, it may mean that the device concerned can only be used once, but it may also mean that the manufacturer has not identified adequate processing guidelines for the possible reuse of the device. What should be made clear is that if any harm is caused to the patient on reusing the device, the healthcare facility alone has to bear the legal consequences. Processing of SUDs is not recommended or covered by the manufacturer's legal declaration of conformity to any local/international regulations, and attempts to do so will nullify the manufacturer's warranty. While the legal assessment of such cases remains controversial, it is clear that the liability and penalty risks involved should be borne by those processing the device.

When processing an SUD, in the absence of guidelines, it is important that the processor considers all the requirement of a safe processing cycle:
- Removal and inactivation of microorganisms to the defined level of safety (e.g. on non-critical, semi-critical, or critical devices and the defined requirements for cleaning, disinfection, and/or sterilization).
- No associated toxicity, as adverse patient reactions may include chemical toxicity due to residual soil materials (e.g. due to inadequate cleaning), chemical residuals (from cleaning, disinfection, sterilization, or even water residuals), or other contaminants (e.g. on handling the device) and changes to the device during processing.
- Device compatibility, ensuring that no damage (seen or unseen) is done to the device or its intended purpose following processing.

For example, complex disposable devices are sometimes constructed in such a way that they cannot be disassembled for effective cleaning. Many single-use items are manufactured from plastics that contain plasticizer oil compounds to preserve flexibility and inhibit or prevent the "drying out" and cracking of the plastic over time in storage. Some of these plasticizers can be removed from the plastic during use and processing, which is why the device may only be guaranteed by the manufacturer for single use. Equally, the effects of steam or other sterilization techniques on a device may not be obvious (e.g. stress cracking, leaking, residual sterilization chemicals, etc.). Therefore, it must be assumed that processing SUDs constitutes a potential hazard to the patient's health, as deterioration in the quality of the product may not be known or ruled out.

When the decision to process an SUD is made in a facility, the facility is responsible for ensuring that the processed device has the same level of safety as a new device. This will require a defined reuse protocol that has been confirmed to be safe, effective, and thereby minimizes any risk to a patient. Processing staff must have enough knowledge or information on the device to show that any processing steps (including cleaning, disinfection, and sterilization, if applicable) will not damage the quality of the SUD or result in any material (mechanical, geometric, optical, electrical, and biocompatible) defects to the device that may compromise the patient's safety. Unfortunately, this information is not always readily available from the manufacturer and cannot be verified through visual inspection of the SUD alone. Overall, the points to consider will include:

- It may not be illegal but is it ethical to reuse single-use items? Does the patient need to be informed (e.g. if the procedure is being directly paid for by the patient/insurance provider)?
- What are the legal implications?
- Why is the product being reused? Is it economics or is there no alternative reusable item available? What are the cost benefits?
- Who decides if the device can be safely and effectively processed, and for how many times? Has management approved the practice?
- What are the effects of processing methods (cleaning/disinfection/sterilization) on the materials used to manufacture the device? Do the people making the decision have enough knowledge to decide if it can be safely processed?
- Can the device be safely and effectively processed?
- How many times can each individual device be safely reused, and how will this be tracked?

Items labeled for limited reuse are different, based on their manufacturer's instructions for use, and must not be confused with single-use items. Limited reuse devices are designed for reuse but the number of times they can be used/processed is limited by the manufacturer. Examples are certain types of diathermy leads (which may have a limited life cycle of 100 cycles), diathermy scissors, types of minimally invasive surgical instruments, and many robotic devices with complex designs. It is important that the use of these devices is tracked through the number of times they are used in/on patients and processed. A specific standard operating procedure should describe the limited number of uses, how these will be recorded, how the items will be processed, what checks will need to be made, and how the devices will be disposed of when their life is deemed to be over. In these cases care should be taken to review the manufacturer's instructions for use in detail, including requirements for inspection, defined reuse requirements, and processing details.

Loan devices, sets, and implants

For various reasons there are many times when healthcare facilities need to loan or rent instrumentation for specialized surgery or surgical implants from a supplier, an individual (e.g. a surgeon), or a neighboring facility. The term "loan" device/set can be defined as any device or group of devices that may be used by a healthcare facility for patient procedures this is not part of that facility's device inventory. This can include surgeons' specialized instruments, instruments and/or implants belonging to surgical manufacturers, and instruments borrowed from other healthcare facilities, all of which will eventually be returned to the supplier/owner. Typical examples include orthopedic and neurosurgical procedure sets. These may be provided as a set on a fee-per-use basis or as a mixture of reusable and single-use (implant) devices for certain surgical or medical procedures (e.g. where the facility is charged when an implant is used). In some cases, the equipment or devices may be on long-term loan to a certain facility (where devices/sets are known to be under consignment). It is important that the same processing procedures and controls, in compliance with the manufacturer's instructions for use, apply to the use of these devices/sets, irrespective of where they come from.

Standard procedures should be identified for the management of loan sets and implants for specialty procedures. There are many advantages and disadvantages to using loaned devices. Device sets are often prohibitively expensive and unaffordable to many facilities, with the convenient option being to loan items from the supplier. This is a practical way to have such sets available for patient use without the high investment costs. Unfortunately, however, the facility using such instrumentation may not have knowledge of or control over the item's history (including prior use/processing procedures). A further concern is that loan items/sets will not be available when needed for a patient procedure without previous planning and will typically require full processing before use. Load devices/sets can be provided directly from the supplier/manufacturer or from another healthcare facility, and may or may not be correctly processed (including detailed inspection) for direct patient use.

Policies and procedures must be in place to manage, control, and track any loaned instrumentation from the time it is received by a facility until it is returned to the lender. In the absence of effective procedures and controls confusion can arise, equipment can be lost, and, most importantly, patients, employees, and the facility itself can be placed at unnecessary risk. Ideally, a standardized loan agreement should be in place between the device manufacturer/lender and the facility department/borrower. The agreement should include procedures and policies, created in collaboration with both parties, to include costs, ordering, transport, receipt, pre-procedure processing/preparation, post-procedure processing, dispatch, and transport out of a facility. Instrumentation supplied from the lender should include a transport/loan list that identifies the items being delivered (including quantities, if applicable) and a copy of the device manufacturer's written handling and processing instructions. Ideally, the loaned set or equipment should be checked and processed by the facility, but this is not always necessary and should be reviewed with the provider of the loaned devices. On receipt, the facility staff intending to use, process, and otherwise handle the instrumentation must be informed of all specifics related to the loan agreement, including the number of instruments/trays and the specific surgical/medical case for which items will be used. It is best practice in accordance with blood-borne pathogen risks that the instruments or equipment have been at least cleaned and disinfected prior to transportation, but this should be verified by the receiving facility. Note: this is not only a concern to those receiving the devices but also to those transporting them from one facility or area to another. The manufacturer's processing instructions should have been provided for each loaned device and, when applicable, must be followed carefully as the item is prepared, cleaned, disinfected, inspected, and/or sterilized. Procedures for transporting instruments to and from the facility are also important; for example, sterile instruments should ideally be packed in locked, secure, tamper-proof containers to help reduce the possibility of cross-contamination and damage during transport (see Chapter 12 on transport of sterile packaged items).

Accountability should be clearly stated and agreed, to include the responsibilities of both the lender and facility staff. Facility staff members who are involved in handling any aspect of the device/set must be trained by the manufacturer or a designated member of staff. It must be remembered that accountability includes from the time of receipt and continues after the surgical procedure is completed until the loaned set is returned to the owner. This will include responsibilities for cleaning, disinfection, inspection, and/or sterilization prior to returning the loaned devices/equipment for transportation to another facility.

Recommendations on the use of loaned devices/sets include:
- A contract should be in place between the supplier and the facility.
- The facility should have a written policy regarding the receipt, handling, and use of loaned devices/sets.
- Unless otherwise agreed with the supplier, all loaned instrumentation should be considered contaminated when it is received. As contaminated, it should be handled appropriately in accordance with facility policies and subjected to processing prior to use.
- An area and responsibilities should be designated for receiving and returning all loaned items. This may include a processing area or site of patient use (e.g. operating room), where applicable.
- Instrumentation packaging should include a transport/loan list that identifies the items being delivered, which may include:
- Identification of the device/set or equipment.
  - Number and types of instruments/implants (especially to include pictures of the set with devices identified).

- ○ Signature of the individual delivering the items.
- ○ Signature of the individual receiving the items.
- ○ Signed verification that the devices/device sets have been previously processed or are provided clean, inspected, sterilized, and ready for use.
- ○ A copy of or access to the device manufacturer's processing instructions.
- If delivered ready for patient use, devices should be inspected immediately prior to use in accordance with the facility's policies (see Chapter 7).
- If the device/set requires processing, normal facility protocols for cleaning, disinfection and/or sterilization, and distribution should be followed. Loaned devices may require specific procedures, including disassembly, cleaning, sterilization, and transport to a site of use. This is often due their size, weight, and complexity. For example, device sets may need to be completely disassembled prior to cleaning/rinsing/disinfection and reassembled in preparation for sterilization. The weight of metal in larger sets is often too great to be sterilized as one tray, resulting in inadequate sterilization and wet packs (see Chapter 11, in the section on troubleshooting steam sterilization problems). Lifting and transporting of such trays can also pose a safety risk to staff.
- Procedures should be in place to allow the devices to be tracked within the facility.

In conclusion, due to the increase in technological complexity and costs, there is frequent use of loaned devices/equipment in healthcare facilities. The use and processing of loaned devices/equipment should be carefully managed. It is important to identify and understand the full loan process and all potential problems that may arise. A management program requires close collaboration between the lender and the facility using the set, to include all staff who may be required to handle these devices during their use/reuse. To ensure accountability, a written agreement between the facility and the device/set/equipment supplier should be in place to cover the entire process from receipt of the loaned items to their return.

Loaned device sets can often include implantable devices or "implants." A surgical implant is defined as a critical device that may be used to support, enhance, replace, or repair a missing, abnormal, or damaged structure within the body. It can be further defined as:

- Having a minimum use in the patient of three months.
- Penetrating living tissue.
- Having a physiologic interaction.
- Being retrievable.

This definition excludes short-term implantable devices such as most catheters (defined as a thin flexible tube that is inserted into a part of the body to inject or drain away fluid or to keep a passage open). Implants are also considered as separate to a transplant (or bio-implant), which is the introduction of foreign tissue. An implant is generally manmade and includes metal, plastic, ceramic, or other materials; in some cases it can include skin, bone, or other bodily tissues. Bio-implants made from skin, bone, or other bodily tissues are commonly used in maxillo-facial orthopedics, reconstructive prosthetics, cardiac prosthetics (artificial heart valves), and in procedures on the skin and cornea. In some cases implants contain electronics, for example artificial pacemakers and cochlear implants; these are called "active" implants and are generally powered using batteries or other energy sources. Implants can be designed to deliver medications, monitor body functions, or provide support to organs and tissues. They can be permanent (e.g. hip replacements/dental implants/stents) or they can be temporary, being removed once they are no longer needed (such as chemotherapy ports or pins/plates to repair broken bones).

Implant surgery is not always 100% successful due to a number of associated risks. These include difficulty in surgical placement or removal, infection, rejection (a reaction to the materials used in the implant), and implant failure. Implant-associated infections can occur and are often sourced from patient skin contamination at the time of surgery, but may also be due to an otherwise contaminated implant device (e.g. because of inappropriate handling or processing). Due to the nature of orthopedic surgery (see Chapter 3), this is probably the area in which the largest number of implants are used; it is also an area where implants may not always be adequately processed, due to the wide variety of pins, screws, small plates, and other small orthopedic implants that are needed. These implants are often repeatedly processed in loaned device racks or trays (Figure 15.10).

Orthopedic implants are devices that are placed over or within bones to hold a fracture or a prosthesis that would replace a piece or the whole of a joint or bone. There are many types of orthopedic implants available, including specific

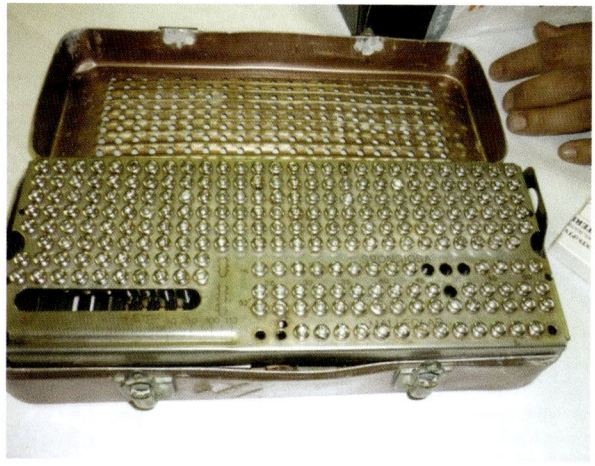

Figure 15.10 A set of loaned orthopedic screw implants.

procedures involving the hip, knee, shoulder, elbow, and other bones. Some examples are interlocking nails, screws, wires, and pins; mini, small, and large fragment implants; cannulated screws; angled blade plates; and hip/knee/shoulder prostheses. Concerns have been raised that many of these smaller implants are continually processed (e.g. pins, plates, screws) but may not be individually tracked or adequately processed, and as a result may not be safe for patient use. This can be due to poor handling and inadequate processing, especially when they are used at multiple facilities as part of loaned device sets. Implants when provided with these sets are classified as single use, which means they must not be reused following contact with or use in a patient (see the section on SUDs earlier in this chapter). They are designed for single patient use but also to be processed multiple times prior to use, if they have not been soiled (even if just accidentally) or used in surgery. Because the surgeon does not always know what size of plate or screw they will need at the time of a patient procedure, a large assortment of sizes is provided for each surgery. A good example is in trauma surgery, where the damage to a patient is unpredictable and requires flexibility during surgery. Often a surgeon may measure or start using a particular plate or screw that is then replaced in the set and a larger or smaller size used for the procedure. In some cases these pins/plates/screws may be used temporarily, may be merely rinsed (if practical), and returned to the set holder in the theater. When the holder is returned to a processing area, it is typical for only the missing screws to be replaced and the whole set processed for the next patient use. As a result, many of these sets can circulate for many years with the same screws that have been processed many times. As mentioned previously, when processing is not followed in compliance with the instructions for use, debris and residues can be present on processed implants and can potentially contribute to implant failures and other problems, such as through infection or inflammation/toxic reactions in the patient.

There is also a concern that in repeated processing (e.g. with bad water or steam quality) implants can become unexpectedly corroded or damaged. This has clear implications for increasing implant failures over time. Another example is that these implants should not be exposed to lubricants, such as in the traditional use of lubricants in washer-disinfectors. Lubricants may be expected to interfere with the intended use of the implants. Inspection and strict compliance with instructions for use are important to reduce these risks. In many cases such implants may be labeled as being for "limited reuse" (see the section on SUDs earlier in this chapter). The consequences of implant failure depend on the critical nature of the implant and its position in the body. Thus, heart valve failure is likely to threaten the life of the individual, while breast implant or hip joint failure is less likely to be life threatening.

Overall, facilities should clarify with device manufacturers the recommended number of reuse or processing cycles, or the life span of implantable screws, wires, and plates (i.e. the number of times the item can be cleaned and resterilized without compromising functionality). Care should also be taken to carefully follow device manufacturer's instructions regarding the safe processing of such sets, including their inspection following cleaning. Overall, it is optimal for facilities to consider the use of individually processed and presented sterile screws/plates or other implants when practical.

Surgical and medical laundry

Laundering of surgical/medical linens and textiles should follow the same chain of events as the processing of any other surgical/medical devices. These have been previously outlined in Chapter 8 on textiles and laundry and Chapter 9 on laundry to include (see Figure 15.11):

- Post-procedure sorting and separation of waste from materials to be reprocessed (see Chapter 7 on post-procedure sorting).
- Safe transport to a processing site (see Chapter 7 on transportation post procedure).
- Cleaning (see Chapter 8 on textiles and laundry).
- Disinfection and drying (see Chapter 9 on laundry).
- Inspection (see Chapter 8 on textiles and laundry) and packaging (if applicable).
- Sterilization (see Chapter 11) if required (e.g. if used directly or contacting critical devices used directly for patient procedures).
- Safe transport to storage and/or site of patient use.

Textiles and linens can be designed for single use or reuse. Reusable surgical textiles can be made from various grades and weaves of cotton with or without special waterproofing treatments. They can become heavily soiled during medical/surgical use and should be safely handled, cleaned, disinfected, or even sterilized prior to their use with another patient. It is therefore important to ensure that an in-house or external laundry is used that is capable of handling such materials and ensuring that an efficient cleaning and decontamination process is applied. The healthcare facility should have a medical/surgical textile reuse policy in place, as well as a tracking and monitoring system that will monitor the number of times the item passes through the laundering process. The number of processing cycles to which these materials can be subjected varies but can generally be assumed to be between 50 and 300 cycles. It is important to remember that the criteria for reuse, as for devices and equipment, will depend on how the materials are used and processed, including visual inspection, which can limit the overall lifetime.

The healthcare facility, and any external laundering facility, has a health and safety obligation to prevent the risk of infection to staff handling contaminated textiles. Only authorized

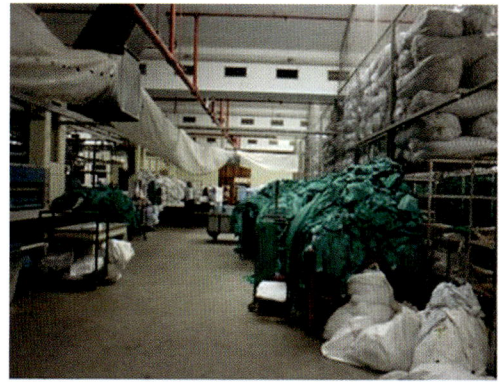 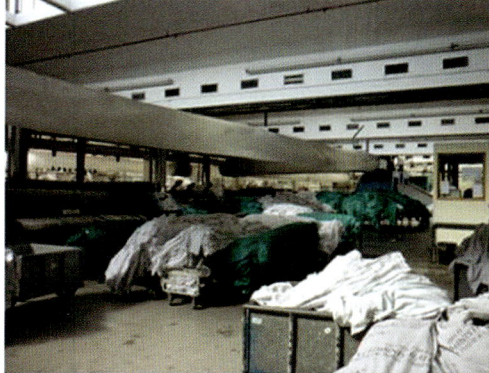

Contaminated surgical laundry is sorted and weighed.

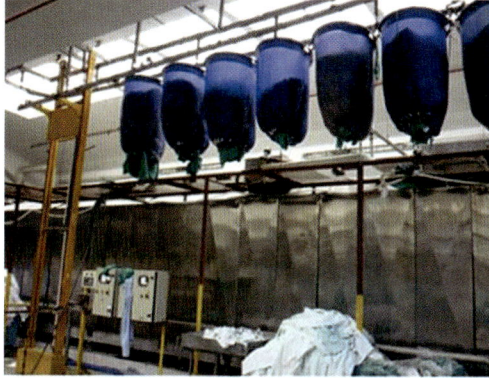 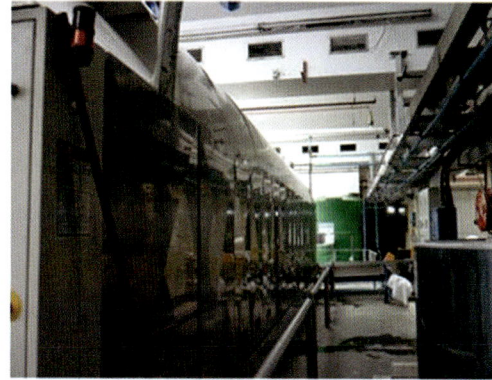

The weighed laundry is transported to the washer-disinfector.

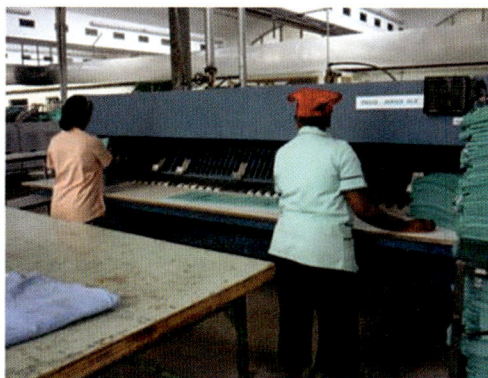 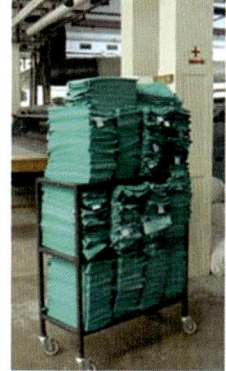

After inspection laundry is ironed, folded and ready for use or for further sterilization.

Figure 15.11 Various stages of a laundry process.

personnel should be allowed in storage, dispatch, or laundering areas. As with instruments, all textiles that have been exposed to patient use, whether they may appear to be used or not, are assumed to be soiled and therefore contaminated. When used/contaminated surgical laundry is handled, it is important that the worker is well protected and wearing the correct PPE, as they can often be at a higher risk of being exposed to contaminants than those dealing with contaminated instruments. All staff working in the receiving/sorting area must wear the appropriate PPE, for example waterproof aprons and gloves, and should be fully trained in operating any associated laundry equipment. There is also the very real risk of potential harm to laundry staff and damage to surgical textiles by a failure of the end user to separate "sharps" from dirty surgical laundry before it is placed in laundry bags. Sharps and waste segregation procedures must be in place, as well as adequate PPE to protect staff dealing with used textiles from these risks (see Chapter 13).

The laundry area should follow the same design recommendations as a device processing facility (see Chapter 1 on design of a decontamination area). For example, the receiving/sorting area should be functionally separated from the area handling cleaned/disinfected textiles. Functional separation can often be achieved by using pass-through washer-disinfectors (often referred to as washer-extractors, continuous tunnel washers, or washer-driers). It is also recommended that contaminated surgical laundry (such as drapes, gowns, and towels) is laundered and kept functionally separated from general hospital laundry.

The laundering process has many of the same essential processes as medical/surgical devices, with the addition of separate drying, ironing, and folding stages. On receipt of contaminated laundry items should be sorted, often weighed (or other method of controlling the load size), and placed into dedicated washers or washer-disinfectors. Heavily contaminated soiled textiles are often recommended to be pre-washed (sluiced) to remove as much organic material as possible prior to loading into the washer; this practice may be recommended to be more safely performed as a pre-treatment step in the washer-disinfector to reduce exposure. This will assist in stain removal. Staining is a concern not only due to difficulty in cleaning and disinfection/sterilization, but also in that visually stained textiles are not acceptable to patients/staff (even if they are disinfected/sterilized). If stains cannot be removed the items may need to be discarded according to the healthcare facility's policy. Loading the correct weight of material into a washer is important to ensure adequate cleaning/disinfection. The way the washers are loaded is a critical step; if they are not loaded according to manufacturer's guidelines (e.g. too heavy or too light a load) the laundry process will not be efficient. The washing process is generally followed by a thermal and/or chemical disinfection cycle. A typical heat disinfection process includes holding the load for a minimum of 10 minutes at 65°C (150°F) or 3 minutes at 71°C (160°F). The cleaning and disinfection cycle will depend on the equipment design, validation, and can even vary depending on the load (as defined by the equipment manufacturer). For chemical disinfection, the entire process (including washing, dilution, and disinfection) is often recommended to be capable of reducing the viable count of microorganisms by 5 $\log_{10}$. In some cases this may not be at all sufficient due to high contamination rates. As examples:

- Materials contaminated with lower intestinal soil (feces) can have more than 10^8 bacteria per cm^2 (8 $\log_{10}$ or 100,000,000 bacteria!).
- Materials contaminated with blood from some patients with active virus infection in their blood can have similar or higher levels of virus present and, depending on the virus infection, can be easier or more difficult to inactivate (e.g. Ebola virus or rotavirus; see Chapter 5).

The impacts of pre-washing, cleaning, rinsing, disinfection, drying, and ironing can all contribute to reducing these levels to ensure the laundry is safe.

Like any processing equipment, laundry washer-disinfectors will require routine testing and maintenance to ensure their safe operation (see Chapters 8 and 9).

Drying is an important step in the laundry decontamination process. The most widely used method is by using heat and extractor-based drying, with or without tumble dryers, as this process can also be efficient in further reducing microorganisms. In the absence of a mechanical dryer, air drying in full sunlight is also an option, but can also lead to cross-contamination depending on the use of the materials. Wet textiles should be dried as soon as possible following cleaning–disinfection, to prevent the growth of microorganisms. Once dried, textiles should be protected from cross-contamination during ironing, folding, transport, and storage.

Working surfaces in the clean area (e.g. table tops, trolleys, and ironing equipment) should be kept clean of visible soil, dust, and lint. Before or during ironing and folding, textiles should be visually inspected for staining and damage. Any stained textiles should be rejected and discarded for esthetic reasons according to the healthcare facility's policy. Any damaged or torn items should also be removed from service and/or sent for mending according to laundry protocol. Damage is usually repaired using heat patches; it is not recommended that tears are sewn as this only serves to increase the number of potential holes. Following inspection, textiles are ironed and folded. When ironing, care should be taken not to recontaminate items on the floor or other surfaces.

When transporting unwrapped textiles following the decontamination process, they should be placed into dedicated clean surgical laundry carts or hampers and covered; the textiles should remain covered at all times during transport. If carts do not have a solid bottom or sides, they should be lined with impervious plastic/paper or a cover. It is recommended that decontaminated textiles are stored in a clean storage area on slatted shelving 2.5–5 cm (1–2 in.) from the walls, 15–20 cm (6–8 in.) from the floor, and 30–45 cm (12–18 in.) from the ceiling to allow for circulation of air and periodic cleaning. Textiles for use in higher-risk patient procedures (such as in the operating room within or adjacent to the sterile core; see Chapter 3 on principles of aseptic (or "sterile") technique) are recommended to be packaged and sterilized by an appropriate sterilization process (see Chapter 11). Laundry sterilization processes include the use of steam and dry heat.

Devices known or suspected to be contaminated with prion material

Prions are unusual infectious agents (see Chapter 5 on prions and other infectious proteins). They are considered infectious proteins, and are strongly implicated in causing a group of rare diseases known as transmissible spongiform encephalopathies (TSEs), with the most common being Creutzfeldt-Jakob disease (CJD), but also Gerstmann–Sträussler–Scheinker syndrome (GSS) and fatal familial insomnia (FFI). Variant Creutzfeldt-Jakob disease (vCJD) is a similar yet distinct disease in humans. It is particularly notable as it was found to have been transferred to humans presumably from eating meat from animals with another prion disease, bovine spongiform encephalopathy (BSE, or more commonly known as "mad cow disease"). Overall these diseases are considered very rare, with the typical risk in a population being 1–3 cases in a million people.

TSEs are known to be transferred through contaminated tissues (particularly brain and other nervous tissues/organs) on items such as reusable devices. They are also considered to have a higher resistance to decontamination and inactivation methods, including widely used sterilization methods. For these reasons, in most countries in the world (including older recommendations by the World Health Organization published in 1999, https://iris.who.int/handle/10665/66707), additional precautions and handling procedures are recommended with patients known or suspected to have prion diseases. These are considered in this section, with cross-references to other parts of the book that consider this subject.

Prion diseases are transmissible through contaminated reusable devices; this has been confirmed clinically and experimentally in the laboratory. Due to the long incubation times associated with the development of prion diseases and the difficulty in diagnosis, it is currently unknown what the true risks of device-associated prion transmission are. Although the research into these diseases and their implications to patient safety will continue, such patient safety risks can be significantly reduced by routine decontamination practices. To date, particular care has been taken to estimate such risks, based on the knowledge that a patient is known to be or suspected of developing a prion disease. Special decontamination procedures are recommended when reusable devices are used in such cases, although in some countries the recommendation exists that any such devices should be removed from use (or destroyed). In general, most national and international recommendations include the following points:

- Develop, document, and implement a policy in advance regarding the handling of devices and materials used on patients with known or suspected prion disease.
- As part of the policy, any potential risk groups (such as patients with a family history or with clinical signs suspected to indicate a prion disease) should be identified to clinical staff and these patients should be specially tracked during their time at the facility.
- Devices used on a person known or suspected to have a prion disease risk will require special handling. This is particularly the case when devices are used for any high-risk surgical procedures. A high-risk procedure is any procedure that contacts tissues that are known to contain potentially high doses of the prion agent. These include the brain, spinal cord, and certain major nerve tissues (such as the optic nerve associated with the eye). It is recommended in such cases that:
  ○ Disposable devices should be used and, if not available, that a facility should strongly consider safe disposal (incineration) of any devices (including reusable devices) that are used.
  ○ Reusable devices should be decontaminated using specific procedures. These include rigorous cleaning (see Chapter 8 on devices known or suspected to be contaminated with prion material), chemical decontamination (e.g. with 1–2 N NaOH for 1 hour; see Chapter 9 on environmental disinfection), and/or elongated steam sterilization (e.g. 134°C for 18 minutes; see Chapter 11 on prion sterilization). Some of these methods are, however, considered damaging to devices, in particular high concentrations of NaOH.
- Devices that are considered to have a lower risk, such as those used for other surgical procedures (e.g. with blood contact and/or contacting other tissues), are sometimes recommended to be similarly discarded or processed, and in other cases to be decontaminated according to normal facility practices. Non-critical devices are not considered to present a patient risk and are also recommended to be routinely decontaminated. It should be noted that these recommendations can be expected to be periodically updated based on new research. This can include local and international requirements. A good example is precautions on biosafety requirements for handling devices known or suspected to be contaminated with prion material, where recent evidence has shown the accidental transmission of disease to laboratory workers due to needle-stick injuries. Planning is important and it is practical for a specific prion policy to be developed and applied within a facility. Consideration should be given to any country-specific guidelines or recommendations in the policy implementation.

There is much debate regarding the safety and efficacy of these general recommendations. The reasons for this debate include:

- Known (diagnosed) or suspected cases of prion diseases are only considered part of the at-risk population. For example, 80% of CJD cases alone are known to be sporadic (or not associated with any known risk factors) and the incubation time of the disease before clinical signs can be very long. Therefore, many more patients may be incubating these diseases but will not be identified for some time, if ever.
- Recent research with more sensitive detection methods detected the prion agent in various other patient tissues (not just the brain and spinal cord), depending on the stage of the disease. The levels of detection are low, again depending on the stage of the disease, but can be in blood, lymph nodes, and muscle. Although the levels of prion contamination are dramatically lower than those observed in brain tissue, the significance of such low-level contamination is uncertain.

- Some of the methods recommended (in particular immersion in NaOH, a strong alkali, or elongated steam sterilization) are not typically recommended by device manufacturers. Such treatment may damage devices and lead to other patient complications (e.g. breakage on use). Although such methods have been tested under laboratory conditions their safety/efficacy may not be tested for clinical use. At this time, prion decontamination or inactivation methods are not typically approved or cleared by regulatory authorities, although some countries do provide guidelines on prion processing recommendations.
- Prions are known to be very difficult to clean from surfaces. It is a fact that the use of some chemistries in specific cleaning processes can significantly reduce prion contamination levels, but in other cases they appear to render the material *more difficult* to decontaminate. The reasons for this are currently unknown.
- Cleaning (with some chemistries) followed by steam sterilization (e.g. at 134°C for 4 minutes or 18 minutes) can be a very effective method of prion decontamination. But, as already highlighted, this will depend on the cleaning process used. The combination of an effective cleaning process known to reduce the risk of prion contamination followed by steam sterilization can be a useful precaution against the potential of prion transmission. Similarly, some low-temperature sterilization methods have been reported to be effective in reducing the risk, based on peer-reviewed literature reports.

In consideration of various guidelines and published data at the time of writing, the following recommendations can be made:

- A facility policy should be in place that describes the handling and potential processing of devices used on patients with or suspected to have a prion disease. A cross-functional team should be responsible for developing the policy, to include clinical, infection prevention/control, surgical, and processing representatives. The team should not only consider the risk to patients, but also the risks to staff from handling devices and exposure to alternate decontamination methods (e.g. high chemical concentrations or alkali). The policy should be periodically reviewed and, if necessary, updated to ensure it is current according to country-specific guidelines and research.
- Facilities should consider the implementation of routine decontamination procedures and best practices that provide standard precautions to reduce any risks of prion decontamination. This can include specific cleaning, disinfection, inspection, and sterilization products/processes that have been shown to reduce the risks of prion contamination. Care should be taken to carefully inspect any such efficacy claims to include their associated applications (temperatures, contact conditions/times, etc.).
- Prions are regarded as being infectious proteins; however, methods that are known to inactivate or degrade proteins, such as specific enzymes (proteases) and heat, may *not* be effective against prions. Any data claims against prions should be carefully inspected to ensure they substantiate efficacy against these agents.
- Special handling and decontamination procedures may be considered with devices used on known or suspected cases of prion disease. These should be particularly considered when used in high-risk surgical procedures associated with the brain, spinal cord, or posterior eye. Consider the use of disposable devices/items where possible. Difficult-to-clean items should be discarded. Reusable items may be cleaned with a cleaning process (with a specific chemistry) shown to be effective against prions, followed by a high- or low-temperature sterilization process that has been shown to be effective (e.g. 134°C for 18 minutes).
- Do not allow devices to dry prior to decontamination. It has been shown that drying of prion-contaminated soil can render the device harder to decontaminate.
- Cleaning recommendations have been considered in detail in Chapter 8, in the section on devices known or suspected to be contaminated with prion material. Cleaning chemistries and processes used should be supported by data that shows that such products have been demonstrated to reduce the risks of prion contamination. The most effective cleaning processes reported to date are alkaline cleaning formulations, but this does not mean that all alkaline detergents are or will be effective. Remember, cleaning process conditions are important to consider, not just the chemicals used. Ensure that devices are correctly rinsed and prepared for subsequent disinfection/sterilization.
- Disinfection recommendations have been considered in detail in Chapter 9 on environmental disinfection. High concentrations of chemicals such as NaOH and NaOCl have been shown to be effective as disinfection agents against prions, but can lead to device damage; they are not recommended for use. Moist heat disinfection has been shown to have little benefit in prion decontamination. Any disinfection method that could lead to protein fixation, such as dry heat, aldehydes, and alcohols, should not be used. Any alternative disinfection methods and/or chemicals should be supported by research data.
- Device inspection is important (see Chapter 10). Cleanliness is essential, but particular attention needs to be paid to areas that are harder to clean or inspect (see Chapter 8). Methods to enhance visual detection, especially to detect the presence of protein below the visual detection level, are recommended to be used. But also consider the risk of device damage, due to some of the decontamination methods that may be used for prion decontamination.
- Steam sterilization is considered an effective method and is discussed in more detail in Chapter 11, in the section on prion sterilization. Steam cycles that are considered to be effective include pre-vacuum cycles at 134°C/274°F for 18 minutes,

gravity displacement cycles at 121°C/250°F for 1 hour, and pre-vacuum cycles at 134°C/274°F for 4 minutes (when shown to be effective in combination with an effective cleaning process). Routine steam sterilization cycles may also be effective when preceded by an effective cleaning cycle that is known to reduce the risk of prion contamination. Dry-heat sterilization should be avoided.

- Some low-temperature sterilization processes have been shown to reduce the risk. These include hydrogen peroxide gas processes (see Chapter 11 on hydrogen peroxide gas). As highlighted earlier, any low-temperature sterilization process claiming to be effective should be supported by research data. Also, any chemical used that could lead to protein fixation, such as formaldehyde and ethylene oxide, should not be used.

It is anticipated that in the coming years the understanding of prion diseases and their successful decontamination will continue to improve. This will allow for the development of more practical guidelines and standards to control the risks of prion decontamination and the introduction of standard precautions to reduce their risks in parallel with those of other infectious agents.

Sustainability

Sustainability may be defined as the avoidance of the depletion of natural resources to maintain an ecological balance for the future. The relationship between sustainability and healthcare is an important topic of interest and attention globally. Many healthcare facilities are committing to meeting country-specific and global commitments to reducing waste and making decisions that have a positive impact on sustainability as well as costs.

Until recently, use of the term sustainability has been mostly related to the impact on environmental degradation or damage. An example is the harm caused to the environment due to inefficient use of energy, inappropriate disposal of plastic wastes, and the effect of chemicals. These all can have negative effects on human, plant, and animal well-being, and they are considered major threats to environmental health in the 21st century. The healthcare industry can positively or negatively impact this harm, having a substantial and multidimensional effect on the environment through its use of resources, waste generation, and pollution. Nonetheless, it also has the potential to be a sustainable development champion, extending far beyond curing illnesses and ensuring equitable access to healthcare services for all in the future.

The significance of sustainability has evolved over recent years. According to the definition in the ISO Guide 82:2019, *Guidelines for addressing sustainability in standards*, sustainability is the overall state or health of our global systems, including environmental, social, and economic aspects. It is important to consider how the needs of the present can be met without compromising the needs of future generations. The environmental, social, and economic aspects are often referred to as the three pillars of sustainability. A fourth pillar, the human element, is also considered, offering an alternative viewpoint for achieving sustainable development by focusing on human factors/behaviors.

International healthcare facilities will continue to define sustainability strategies or goals considering each of these pillars. Examples include staff and patient safety, water and energy conservation, and ethical practices. Prevention of environmental risk factors and long-term thinking are instrumental to the success of these strategies. Emphasis can be placed on ensuring that resources are used efficiently and responsibly. Circular economic principles (a model of production and consumption that involves sharing, leasing, reusing, repairing, refurbishing, and recycling existing materials and products for as long as possible) are used to mitigate the impact on the overall carbon footprint of a healthcare facility. The carbon footprint refers to the overall emission volume of greenhouse gasses, those that can trap and release heat and contribute to climate change.

Best practices in device processing can include removing unused items, streamlining single-use device/sets/personal PPE, and switching from single-use to reusable equipment where appropriate. When "reduce and reuse" strategies are not feasible, the life span of items can be renewed and extended through routine maintenance, repair, and remanufacture and the recycling of waste. This approach, in turn, can help promote economic development and reduce the overall burden on healthcare systems.

Integration of innovation and emerging technologies, for example the use of telemedicine, wearable devices, digital/remote patient monitoring, or centralized lean electronic records, provides high-quality services to patients and caregivers while reducing carbon impacts. Equally, investment in medical research, technology, and healthcare professionals' training and competency raises the opportunity of a high standard of service while creating jobs and even improving prosperity. Sustainability can also be an important component of the facility's quality management system (QMS), and may be used to mitigate the negative impacts of a service and reduce variation (see Chapter 14 on management).

Embracing a transformative, sustainable approach to healthcare requires the work of many stakeholders who can balance collaboration, adaptability, inclusion, and exchange. These are all important in the management of a device processing service. Examples of considerations in device processing that can impact sustainability include:

- Choosing chemicals, materials, and services that are aligned with the healthcare facility's sustainability plans or regional regulations.

- Management of materials and devices, working with surgical and medical staff who are needed for specific procedures, thereby reducing waste and the need for surplus product processing.
- The reuse of specific types of SUDs and materials. As highlighted earlier in this chapter, the reuse of SUDs may appear to reduce costs and environmental impacts, but remember to consider the overall impact of the costs of processing time, energy, detergents, processing materials, risk, etc.
- Separation of contaminated and non-contaminated materials for waste handling and safe disposal. Contaminated items are required to be decontaminated and often incinerated due to health hazards, but this increases the environmental impacts (e.g. volume of waste for incineration). Alternatives to incineration may need to be considered.
- Reducing the use of materials (including packaging materials) during processing. Some may consider reusable container systems as alternatives, but they also have separate sustainability considerations.
- Restricting the use of paper for tracking and documentation, by replacing paper with electronic systems.
- The prudent use of chemicals (e.g. detergents, chemical disinfectants), including not using chemicals that are considered persistent or damaging to the environment (this has become a legal requirement in certain regions).
- The minimal use of water, including the reuse of purified or critical water sources for other uses.
- Use of equipment that requires minimal water or energy, or providing water/energy recycling (when appropriate).
- Limiting energy use for equipment, including air handling (e.g. when not in use, running under conserved energy conditions).
- Use of event-related shelf-life of sterile, processed items rather than artificial time-bound lifetimes or labeling.

Index

A_0 242, 244, 420
AAMI *see* Association for the Advancement of Medical Instrumentation
Acanthameoba castellanii 118
accidental spillages and leakages 386–7
accountability 446
acids
    chemistry and chemicals 135, 137–8, 145–6
    cleaning procedures 179, 217
    disinfection 240–1
acquired immunodeficiency syndrome *see* HIV/AIDS
activated carbon filters 435, 437
acupuncture 55
additive manufacturing (AM) 71
adenosine triphosphate (ATP) 262, 419, 421–2
adeno-tonsillectomy 58
adhesive labels 413
aeration 326, 329–30, 334–5, 340, 353
AGVs *see* automated guided vehicles
AIDC *see* automatic identification and data capture
air-handling systems 60, 62, 63, 127, 192, 258
air removal 300–2, 308–9
alcohol-based cleaners 149–53
alcohol-based disinfectants 230–1
aldehyde-based disinfectants 232, 247–8
alkalis
    chemistry and chemicals 145–6
    cleaning procedures 217
    disinfection 254
    see also bases
aluminum 70
aluminum foil tests 423–4
AM *see* additive manufacturing
American National Standards Institute (ANSI) 14
    cleaning procedures 210–11
    disinfection 243
    inspection, assembly, and packaging 271, 283–4
    sterilization 321, 323, 333, 345, 349
    storage and distribution 364
aminoglycosides 114
amniocentesis 55
amoeba 117

amputation 58
analytes 169
anatomy and physiology 18–49
    cardiovascular system 18, 22–31
    digestive system 18, 24, 31–2
    endocrine system 25, 32–5
    human body structures 18–20
    integumentary system 25, 35–6
    lymphatic system 25, 36–8
    muscular system 26, 38
    nervous system 18, 26, 38–40
    reproductive system 27, 40–1
    respiratory system 18, 28, 41–2
    skeletal system 28, 42–6
    terminology 20–2
    urinary system 29, 46
anesthesia 54, 62, 67
angled micro scissors 78
ANSI *see* American National Standards Institute
antibiotics 5, 113–14, 124
antifungal drugs 117
antimicrobial activity 1–3, 6–9, 13, 442
    anatomy and physiology 37
    chemistry and chemicals 130, 133, 135, 138, 141, 146–55
    cleaning procedures 177, 179
    disinfection 218, 221–2, 227–47, 252
    microbiology 114, 125, 127
    sterilization 289–94, 299–302, 323–5, 328, 333, 337, 339, 345–6, 349–51
    water quality 432, 438
antisepsis 149–50, 242
antiseptics 252
AORN *see* Association of periOperative Registered Nurses
Apergillus fumigatus 116
apheresis 55
appendectomy 58
archaea 114
Aristotle 2, 4
arthroplasty 58
arthroscopy 60
artificial test soil (ATS) 213
AS/NZS *see* Standards Australia/Standards New Zealand

Ascaris lumbricoides 120
aseptic techniques 4–5, 62–6
aspiration instruments 84–5
Association for the Advancement of Medical Instrumentation (AAMI) 14
    cleaning procedures 210–11
    disinfection 243
    inspection, assembly, and packaging 259, 271, 283
    sterilization 321, 323, 333, 338, 345, 349
    storage and distribution 364
Association of periOperative Registered Nurses (AORN) 283
ASTM 283
atherectomy 55
ATP *see* adenosine triphosphate
ATS *see* artificial test soil
audit procedures 369, 418
Australia Regulations 13, 242
autoclaves *see* steam sterilizers
automated guided vehicles (AGVs) 97
automated systems 11
    cleaning procedures 144, 170, 178–9, 184–97, 204–5, 422–3
    disinfection 223, 225–6, 423
    point-of-use treatment 166–7
automatic identification and data capture (AIDC) 412–13

Bacillus anthracis 5
Bacillus atrophaeus 108–9, 291, 295, 323, 326
Bacillus atrophaeus-containing BIs 428–30
Bacon, Francis 3
bacterial infections
    chemistry and chemicals 147–50, 152
    disinfection 218–19, 220, 226, 229, 239
    historical development 5
    management and quality 427
    microbiology 102–3, 107–14
    safety issues 367
    sterilization 289–92, 300, 322, 326, 333, 339, 351
    water quality 434
bactericide 236
Balantidium coli 118

Decontamination and Device Processing in Healthcare, Second Edition. Gerald McDonnell and Georgia Alevizopoulou.
© 2025 John Wiley & Sons Ltd. Published 2025 by John Wiley & Sons Ltd.

Balfour retractors 86
barcodes 411–13
Basel Convention 386
bases
    chemistry and chemicals 135, 137–8
    cleaning procedures 179
    disinfection 240–1
    see also alkalis
bedside procedures 203
β-lactams 113–14
BI see biological indicators
biguanides 241
biochemical tests 261–2, 419, 421
biocides 135, 146–55, 221, 229–41
biofilms 108–10, 113, 213
biohazards 164, 166
biological indicators (BI) 295–6, 306, 311, 315–18, 351, 427–30
biopsies 55, 96, 97
Black Death 3
bladder 46
blood
    anatomy and physiology 22, 23
    cleaning procedures 207, 213
    infections 122
    inspection, assembly, and packaging 262
    instrumentation 81
    management and quality 421
    point-of-use treatment 158–9
    surgical and medical procedures 62
    transfusions 55
blood pressure (BP) monitors 99
bone cutters 77
bone gouges 79
bone holder forceps 79
bone marrow aspiration 55
bone screws and plates 88
Borgognoni, Theodoric 3
bovine spongiform encephalopathy (BSE) 104, 451
Bowie–Dick tests 296, 297, 307, 309, 321, 430
box joints 74–5
Boyle's Law 133
BP monitors see blood pressure monitors
brain 38–9
Brazil Regulations 242
Brearley, Harry 67
bronchoscopy 60
BSE see bovine spongiform encephalopathy

calipers 87
Canada Regulations 13, 242
Candida albicans 110, 116–17
capsules 108, 113
carbohydrates 19–20
carbon 169
cardboard packaging 359
cardiac catheterization 54
cardiovascular system 18, 22–3
cart washers 167, 196–7
CAs see corrective actions
CAT see computerized axial tomography

cavitation energy tests 422
cavities 20–1
CCD see charge-coupled device
CDC see Center for Disease Control
cell structure 19, 104–5, 107
Center for Disease Control (CDC) 243
central services department (CSD) 156
central sterile services departments (CSSD) 9, 156
cephalosporins 114
cesarean section 58
change management 403
charge-coupled device (CCD) 96
Charles' Law 133
checklists 269–70
chelating agents 135, 147
chemical indicators (CI) 426
    biological indicators 427–30
    disinfection 245–6
    in-pack internal chemical indicators 427
    management and quality 424–8
    process indicators 426–7
    sterilization 298, 306–7, 311, 315–18, 343, 351–2
    storage and distribution 364–5
chemical tests 261–2
chemical waste 377, 382
chemistry and chemicals 130–55
    antimicrobial activity 130, 133, 135, 138, 141, 146–55
    cleaning procedures 135, 138, 143–6, 170, 176–9, 181, 184–9, 191, 204–8, 213–17
    disinfection 131, 135, 138, 151–3, 221–2, 229–41, 247–51, 254–6
    elements 130–2
    light, radiation and electromagnetic spectrum 140–1
    measurement and physical properties 134–40
    mixtures, formulations and solutions 134
    pH scale 137–8
    phases of matter 131–4
    point-of-use treatment 158
    product selection and application 142–3
    safety issues 141–2, 366, 368–71
    sterilization 131, 133, 138, 154–5, 290–1, 319, 326–54
chemotherapy 55
childbirth 83
chisels 77
chlorhexidine 150–1, 160, 241
chlorine-based disinfectants 233–4
chlorine dioxide-based disinfectants 237–8, 247, 351
chloroxylenol 239–40
cholecystectomy 58, 97
CI see chemical indicators
ciliates 118
circulating nurse 54
civil laws 404–5
CJD see Creutzfeldt-Jakob disease
clamping instruments 75, 81

cleaning, definition, 169
    see also cleaning procedures
cleaning, monitoring 419–23
cleaning indicators 422
cleaning procedures 1–2, 169–217
    automated cleaning 184–207
    basic principles 176–80
    chemistry and chemicals 135, 138, 143–6, 170, 176–9, 182, 184–9, 191, 204–8, 213–17
    decontamination areas 9–11
    decontamination cycle 7
    disassembly and preparation 174–6, 182–3, 213
    endoscopy 174, 180, 191, 192, 196, 202–6, 438–43
    guidelines, standards and testing 184, 188, 198, 209–13
    infections 125–9
    inspection, assembly, and packaging 258–9
    management and quality 419–23
    manual cleaning 180–4, 204–5
    point-of-use treatment 159–62
    receiving and sorting 170–4
    regulations 15
    single-use devices 443–5
    Spaulding classification 6–7, 173
    special considerations 200–9
    sterilization 31, 305, 319
    troubleshooting problems 213–17
Clostridium spp. 108, 111–12
coagulated blood 213
coding and marking methods 413
cold forging 72
collagen 55
colonoscopy 60
communication 401–3
compatibility 142–3
complex instruments 173–4
computed tomography (CT) 54
computerized axial tomography (CAT) 55
conditioning stage 294, 300, 326, 334, 339
conductivity 139, 312, 435
conflict management 403–4
connective tissue 18
container/containment systems 164–7, 277, 279, 287, 359
contaminated waste materials 2
continuous process washers 193–4
controlled environments 257
conversion factors 136–7
copper 241
coronary angiograms 55
coronary artery by-pass 58
corrective actions (CAs) 418
corrosion inhibitors 135
corrosion-resistant steel (CRES) 70
cosmetic/plastic surgery 57, 58
COVID-19 pandemic 4, 105, 106
COVID-19 vaccines 37
CRES see corrosion-resistant steel
Creutzfeldt-Jakob disease (CJD) 104, 206, 451
criminal laws 404–5

critical devices 7
  chemistry and chemicals 153
  cleaning procedures 173, 196, 438–43
  disinfection 218–19, 222
  inspection, assembly, and packaging 237
  storage and distribution 355
crushing clamps 81
Cryptosporidium parvum 117–18
CSD *see* central services department
CSSD *see* central sterile services departments
CT *see* computed tomography
curettes 77, 79
customer needs, understanding 407
customer requirements 390–1
cutting instruments 75–7, 90
cysticide 236
cystoscopy 60
cytotoxic chemicals 158
cytotoxic waste 377

D-values 292, 346
DAI *see* device associated infections
data matrices 411–13
decontamination areas 9–12
decontamination cycle 7–9
dedicated lifts 361–2
deionization 437
delegation 401–2
dental caries 56
dental instruments 89, 173, 196
dental surgeries 51
dental system 44–6
deoxyribonucleic acid (DNA) 19–20, 104, 106, 109
Department of Health and Social Care, England 283
depth gauges 87–8
detection kits 212–14
device associated infections (DAI) 127–8
diagnostic procedures 50
dialysis 55
diathermy forceps 78
digestive system 18, 24, 31–2
digital calipers 88
dilators 73–4, 76, 87
dioxins 321, 386
disaster planning and management 388
disinfection 1, 218–56
  basic principles 221–3
  chemical disinfection 131, 135, 138, 151–3, 229–41, 247–51, 254–6
  classification 220–1
  cleaning procedures 177, 180, 184–9, 191–7, 205, 207–9, 215
  context 218–23
  decontamination areas 9
  decontamination cycle 7–9
  endoscopy 438–43
  guidelines and standards 223, 241–9, 251
  historical development 3–4, 6
  infections 125–8
  inspection, assembly, and packaging 259

management and quality 420, 423–4
monitoring 423–4
physical disinfection 222–9
point-of-use treatment 158–9, 166–7
prions 254–5, 452
regulations 13
resistance to inactivation 219–21
safety issues 369, 371
single-use devices 443–5
Spaulding classification 6–7, 152–3, 219
special considerations 246–55
storage and distribution 355
troubleshooting problems 255–6
water quality 432, 437
dispersion 147
disposable devices *see* single-use devices
disposal 2
dissecting instruments 75–7
dissecting SuperCut scissors 78
distillation 437
distribution *see* storage and distribution; transportation
documentation
  cleaning procedures 183, 201
  disinfection 222, 251–2
  inspection, assembly, and packaging 259, 270
  management and quality 426
  safety issues 368–70, 387
double-action bone cutter 78
double-sink set-up 181
downward displacement of air 302–3
Doyen retractors 86
drinking water quality 1–2
drug resistance 5–6, 113–14
dry heat disinfection 226
dry heat sterilization 318–25
drying procedures 192, 206, 208
  disinfection 250–1
  endoscopy 442–3
  laundry items 450
  sterilization 300
  storage and distribution 356
dryness test/fraction 315

E-beam radiation 324
ears 49
ebony finish 72
echocardiography 56
echo-endoscopy 97
ECM *see* electrochemical marking
Edinburgh test soil 213
efficacy
  chemistry and chemicals 143, 150
  disinfection 222, 236, 237, 246–8
  sterilization 290–1
EKG *see* electrocardiograms
EL *see* excursion limits
electrical equipment 201, 268
electrical hazards 372
electrical risks 387
electro-polishing 72
electro-thermal deactivation (ETD) 321–2

electrocardiograms (EKG) 55
electrochemical marking (ECM) 413
electromagnetic spectrum 140–1
elevators 361–2
emotional health 366, 373–4
employee engagement 400–1
emulsification 147
EN Standards 242
endocrine system 25, 32–5
endoscopes 89–97
endoscopic retrograde cholangiopancreatography (ERCP) 60
endoscopic ultrasound (EUS) 97
endoscopy *see* flexible endoscopy; rigid endoscopy
endotoxins 112–13, 324, 434–5
endotracheal intubation 56
Enterobius vermicularis 120
enveloped viruses 104–5, 147, 152
environmental disinfection 253–4
environmental factors 6
  safety issues 141–2, 369, 371, 372, 384–6
  sterilization 323
Environmental Protection Agency (EPA) 13, 241
enzyme-based cleaners 144–5, 160–1, 206
enzymes 135
EPA *see* Environmental Protection Agency
epithelial tissue 18
equipment requirements 393–4
equipment risks 366, 371–2
ERCP *see* endoscopic retrograde cholangiopancreatography
ergonomics 366, 373
ETD *see* electro-thermal deactivation
ethics 404–5
ethylene oxide (EO)
  basic sterilization principles 326–30
  chemistry and chemicals 154–5
  guidelines and standards 333
  properties and characteristics 326, 352–3
  sterilization 290, 326–32
  sterilizer design and components 331–2
European Union Devices Directives 405
European Union Directives 12, 242
EUS *see* endoscopic ultrasound
event related sterility 358
excursion limits (EL) 328
exotoxins 112–13
exposing instruments 76, 81–2
extended steam sterilization 308–11
external transportation 164–6, 362
eyes 47–9

facemasks 128, 171–2, 176, 182
fatal familial insomnia (FFI) 451
FDA *see* Food and Drug Administration
FFI *see* fatal familial insomnia
fiberscopy 96
filamentous fungi 116
filtration
  disinfection 227–9, 250–1
  sterilization 325
  water quality 435–7

fine-needle aspiration (FNA) 97
fire hazards 387
flagellates 118
flash sterilization 301, 307–8, 355
    see also immediate use steam sterilization
Fleming, Sir Alexander 5
flexible endoscopy 438
    anatomy and physiology 32
    cleaning procedures 174, 180, 191, 192, 196, 202–6, 438–43
    disinfection 234, 247–51, 255–6
    inspection, assembly, and packaging 266–7
    inspection of 441–2
    instrumentation 91, 93–7
    procedures and techniques 59
    storage and distribution 356–7
fluid-resistant caps 440
FNA see fine-needle aspiration
Food and Drug Administration (FDA) 13, 241
forceps 72–4, 77–83, 90, 91, 93, 264
formaldehyde 231
    basic sterilization principles 333–5
    chemistry and chemicals 154–5
    disinfection 233
    guidelines and standards 337–8
    properties and characteristics 332–4, 352–3
    sterilization 290, 332–9
    sterilizer design and components 335–7
formulations 134
Fracastorius, Hieronymus 3
friction 177, 182
functionality testing 262–3
fungal infections
    chemistry and chemicals 147–50, 152
    disinfection 220, 226, 231, 239
    microbiology 102–3, 114–17
    sterilization 290
fungicide 236
furans 386

Galen 3
gamma-radiation 324
gas laws 133
gas sensors 329, 336
gases 131–4
gastrointestinal (GI) tract 31–2
gastroscopy 60
genotoxic waste 377
Geobacillus stearothermophilus 108–9, 291, 333, 339, 352, 428
Geobacillus stearothermophilus spore-containing BIs 428
Gerstmann–Sträussler–Scheinker syndrome (GSS) 451
GI tract see gastrointestinal tract
Giardia lamblia 117–18
glucoprotamine 240
glutaraldehyde 231–2, 247, 249
glycopeptides 114
Gram positive/negative classification 107–8, 111, 114, 148, 149
grasping instruments 75, 77–81, 90

greenhouse gas emissions 386
GSS see Gerstmann–Sträussler–Scheinker syndrome
guidelines
    cleaning procedures 184, 188, 198, 209–13
    disinfection 223, 241–9, 251
    inspection 258–60
    management and quality 405, 406, 424
    packaging 271, 283–4
    sterilization 291, 296–7, 324, 326, 333, 337, 344, 349
    storage and distribution 364–5
    water quality 436

HAIs see healthcare-acquired infections
halogen-based disinfectants 233–5
hand and skin hygiene 1
    chemistry and chemicals 150–1
    historical development 3–5
    infections 123–6, 128
    safety issues 367
    surgical and medical procedures 61, 65
hand transport 360
handling 11, 15
    air-handling systems 60, 62, 63, 127, 192, 258
    management and quality 420
hard water 180, 184, 216, 313, 432–3, 436–7
hazard analysis and risk assessment 376
hazard labels see safety warning symbols
health and safety see safety issues
healthcare-acquired infections (HAIs) 5, 102, 127
heart 23
heat-sealing 278, 282
heavy duty gloves 175–6, 180
heavy metal-rich waste 382
helminthic infections
    chemistry and chemicals 146
    disinfection 219
    microbiology 102–3, 119–21
hematology see blood
hemorrhoidectomy 58
hemostatic forceps 264
HEPA filters see high efficiency particulate air filters
hepatitis viruses 106, 367–8
high efficiency particulate air (HEPA) filters 228, 356, 443
    disinfection 228–9
    inspection, assembly, and packaging 258
    microbiology 127
    sterilization 324, 337, 344
    storage and distribution 356
    surgical and medical procedures 62–3
high temperature formaldehyde/alcohol 333–6
highly infectious waste 382
hinge joints 74, 75
Hippocrates 2, 67
historical development 2–6, 67
HIV/AIDS 37, 105, 112, 367–8
holding instruments 75, 77–81, 90
hooks 85, 265
hormones 33

hot forging 72
HPV see human papillomavirus
HRC see Rockwell Hardness
Hugo™ RAS system 98
human immunodeficiency virus see HIV/AIDS
human papillomavirus (HPV) 105
hydrogen peroxide
    basic sterilization principles 339–43
    chemistry and chemicals 154–5
    disinfection 235–6, 247
    guidelines and standards 344
    properties and characteristics 337–9, 352–3
    sterilization 290, 337–46
    sterilizer design and components 343–4
hydrolysis 144–6
hysterectomy 58
hysteroscopy 60

ICN see infection control nurses
ICP-MS see inductively coupled plasma mass spectrometry
ICP-OES analysis see inductively coupled plasma–optical emission spectroscopy analysis
IDLH see immediately dangerous to life or health
IFU see instructions for use
immediate use steam sterilization (IUSS) 355
immediate use sterilization 301, 307–8, 355
immediately dangerous to life or health (IDLH) 352
immersion baths
    cleaning procedures 178, 188–91, 204, 214
    disinfection 226, 248, 254
    endoscopy 440
immunity 37
immunization see vaccination
implants 445–8
in-pack chemical indicators 428
in-pack internal chemical indicators 427
incineration 173, 318, 386
inductively coupled plasma mass spectrometry (ICP-MS) 140
inductively coupled plasma–optical emission spectroscopy (ICP-OES) analysis 436
infection control nurses (ICN) 5, 124
infection prevention and control (IPC) 102, 121
infections
    bacteria 102–3, 107–14
    cleaning procedures 176
    device processing 127–9
    fungi 102–3, 114–17
    helminths 102–3, 119–21
    historical development 2–3, 5
    human pathogens 110–14, 116
    management and quality 427–30
    microbiology 102–29
    microorganism types 102–21
    point-of-use treatment 156
    policy and practice 129
    prevention and control 102, 121–9, 367–8
    prions 103–4
    protozoa 102–3, 117–19

resistance to inactivation 219–21
safety issues 366–8
sources of contamination 122–3
sterilization 289–90
surgical procedures 51–2
viruses 102–7
water quality 434–5
see also disinfection
infectious waste 381–2
influenza viruses 105–6
infrared (IR) disinfection 227
inguinal hernia repair 58
inspection 259–60
    area design consideration 257–9
    cleaning procedures 182
    decontamination areas 9–11
    decontamination cycle 8
    disinfection 208–9, 212
    guidelines and standards 258–60
    laundry items 448–50
    maintenance, repairs and replacements 267–8
installation qualification (IQ) 426
instructions for use (IFU) 69
instrument trays *see* trays
instrumentation 1, 67–101
    aseptic technique 62–6
    basic, everyday instruments 73–5
    chemistry and chemicals 143–4, 153
    clamping and occluding 75, 81
    classification 75–6
    cleaning procedures 169–217, 438–45
    cutting and dissecting 75–7, 90
    decontamination cycle 7–9
    dental surgery 89
    device and tray assembling 268–74
    dilating 73–4, 76, 87
    disassembly and preparation for cleaning 174–6, 182–3, 213
    disinfection 218–56, 438–45
    endoscopy 97
    exposing and retracting 73, 76, 81–2
    grasping and holding 75, 77–81, 90
    historical development 5–6, 67
    infections 122, 124–5, 127–9
    inspection, assembly, and packaging 257–88
    instrument marking 72–3
    limited-use 68–9
    loan devices and sets 200–1, 445–8
    maintenance, repairs and replacements 267–8
    manufacturers and suppliers 71–3
    materials and manufacture 67, 69–72
    measuring and positioning 76, 87
    microsurgery 88, 90
    miscellaneous 76, 88–101
    point-of-use treatment 156–68
    powered tools 76, 87–9
    procedures and techniques 52, 62–6
    quality standards 71–4
    re-usable 68–9, 90, 157–8, 162, 172, 355
    safety issues 366, 371–2
    single-use 68–9, 90, 157–8, 162, 176, 443–5
    Spaulding classification 6–7, 50, 152–3

sterilization 289–354, 438–45
storage and distribution 355–65
suction irrigation/aspiration 74, 76, 84–5
suturing or stapling 76, 86
tattooing 90, 99
types and descriptions 73–99
viewing 76, 84–5
water quality 432
integumentary system 25, 35–6
internal chemical indicators 427
International Organization for Standardization (ISO) 14–16, 259, 280
    cleaning procedures 184, 189, 198, 209–10
    disinfection 223, 241–2, 245–6, 251
    inspection, assembly, and packaging 259, 283–4
    instrumentation 71, 74
    management and quality 406, 422–3, 430
    sterilization 291, 296–7, 320–1, 323, 333, 345, 349
International Regulations 242
intra-operative care 54, 65
inventory control 360, 409–10
inventory management 409–10
iodine-based cleaners 150–2, 160
iodine-based disinfectants 233
IPC *see* infection prevention and control
IQ *see* installation qualification
IR disinfection *see* infrared disinfection
irrigation systems 204–5
ISO *see* International Organization for Standardization
IUSS *see* immediate use steam sterilization

just-in-time (JIT) system 410

Keen, William V. 4–5
kidneys 46
Koch, Robert 5
Korea Regulations 242

label identification 283–5
labeling standards 141–2
labor requirements 392–3
landfill 384, 386
laparoscopy 60
large-chamber washers 197, 199
large intestine 32
laryngoscopy 60, 92–3
laser cutters 72
laser etching/annealing 413
laser surgery 57
LASIK eye surgery 51, 88
latex gloves 125–6
laundry items 2
    cleaning procedures 206–9, 449–50
    disinfection 252, 449–50
    point-of-use treatment 158
    post-procedure handling 448–50
leadership 401–2
leadership routines 408
leak testers 203–4

leak-testing procedure 440
leakages 386–7
lean principles 408
legal responsibilities 404–5
Legionella pneumophila 110
Legionella spp. 234, 241, 434
legislation 12, 376, 404–5
    see also guidelines; regulations; standards
leprosy 3
lifts 361–2
LigaClips 83
limited-use devices 68–9
linen *see* laundry items
lipids 19–20
lipopolysaccharide (LPS) 112–13
liquid chemical sterilization processes *see* immediate use steam sterilization
liquids 131–4
Lister, Joseph 4
liver 31–2
loading trays *see* trays
loan devices and sets 200–1, 445–8
low temperature steam formaldehyde (LTSF) 334–6
LPS *see* lipopolysaccharide
lumbar puncture (LP) 56
lymphatic system 25, 36–8

MAC *see* maximum allowable concentrations
Machinery Directive 12
magnetic resonance imaging (MRI) 53, 56
malleable retractors 85
mallets 88
management and quality 389–431
    change management 403
    cleaning procedures 419–23
    communication 401–3
    conflict management 403–4
    context 389–90
    customer requirements 390–1
    disinfection 420, 423–4
    effectiveness and goals 404, 408–9
    equipment requirements 393–4
    ethics and legal responsibilities 404–5
    handling 420
    inventory control 409–10
    labor requirements 392–3
    leadership and delegation 401–2
    materials management 409–14
    materials requirements 394–5
    packaging 420
    personnel management 393, 396–8
    point of use monitoring 420
    process management 405–9
    quality management 417–31
    recall situations 409
    resource requirements 391–2
    safety issues 374–6, 388
    space requirements 395–6
    standard work instructions 396
    sterilization 420, 424–31
    storage and distribution 420

management and quality (cont'd)
  teamwork 401–4
  tracking and traceability 410–11
  workflow 396
manual processes
  cleaning 180–4, 204–5, 422
  disinfection 222, 249, 423
  point-of-use treatment 166–7
mastectomy 58
material safety data sheets (MSDS) 386–7
materials management 409–14
  coding and marking methods 413
  inventory management 409–10
  scanning/identification 413–14
  tracking and traceability 410–11
  unique identification codes 411–13
materials requirements 394–5
maximum allowable concentrations (MAC) 335
Mayo curved scissors 78
Mayo straight scissors 78
measles-mumps-rubella (MMR) vaccine 37, 106
measurements 414
  outcome measurements 414–15
  process measurements 415–16
  waste measurements 416–17
measuring instruments 76, 87
MEC *see* minimum effective concentration
mechanical hazards 372
Medical Device Directive 12
medical equipment 52–3
medical instruments *see* instrumentation
medical procedures *see* surgical and medical procedures
medical teams 52
methicillin-resistant *Staphylococcus aureus* (MRSA) 110, 114
microbiocides 146
microbiological filters 228
microbiological tests 419
microbiology
  bacteria 102–3, 107–14
  fungi 102–3
  helminths 102–3, 119–21
  human pathogens 110–14, 116
  infection prevention and control 102, 121–9, 367–8
  microorganism types 102–21
  policy and practice 129
  prions 103–4
  protozoa 102–3, 117–19
  reprocessing 127–9
  resistance to inactivation 219–21
  safety issues 366–8
  sources of contamination 122–3
  sterilization 289–90
  viruses 102–7
  see also disinfection; infections
microsurgery 57
  cleaning procedures 198–200
  inspection, assembly, and packaging 265
  instrumentation 88, 90

microwave disinfection 227
minimal-risk devices 173
minimally invasive surgery (MIS) 51, 57
minimum effective concentration (MEC) 247
minimum recommended concentration (MRC) 247
mirror finish 72
MIS *see* minimally invasive surgery
mixtures 134
MMR vaccine *see* measles-mumps-rubella vaccine
moderate-risk devices 173
moist heat disinfection 223–6
moist heat sterilization *see* steam sterilization
moisture detection 353
molds 115–16
monitoring equipment 329, 343, 353
monolithic ceilings 357
most-resistant organisms (MRO) 291, 333, 339
MRC *see* minimum recommended concentration
MRI *see* magnetic resonance imaging
MRSA *see* methicillin-resistant *Staphylococcus aureus*
MSDS *see* material safety data sheets
multi-chamber washers 195–6
multidisciplinary teams 402
multi-drug resistance 114
muscular system 26, 38
muscular tissue 18
mycobacteria
  chemistry and chemicals 148–50, 152
  disinfection 220
  microbiology 114–15
  sterilization 290
mycobactericides 220
Mycobacterium species 110
Mycobacterium tuberculosis 5, 37
mycotoxins 117

natural orifice transluminal endoscopic surgery (NOTES) 59, 97
NCG *see* non-condensable gases
needles and needle holders 74–5, 82–3, 84, 86, 90, 158, 264–5
nervous system 18, 26, 38–40
nervous tissue 18
non-condensable gases (NCG) 314–15
non-critical devices 7
  chemistry and chemicals 153
  cleaning procedures 173, 196
  disinfection 219–20, 222
  inspection, assembly, and packaging 237
  storage and distribution 355
non-enveloped viruses 104–5, 147–8, 152
non-enzyme-based cleaners 145–6, 160–1
non-woven textile wraps 277–8
NOTES *see* natural orifice transluminal endoscopic surgery
nucleic acids 19–20, 104, 106
nursing staff 54

occluding instruments 76, 81
one (1) D barcodes 411
OPA *see* ortho-phthalaldehyde
open surgery 57
operational qualification (OQ) 426
ophthalmological devices 198–200
opportunistic pathogens 112
optical aids 260
OQ *see* operational qualification
oral cavity 31
organization 398
orthopedic instruments 176, 200–1, 447–8
ortho-phthalaldehyde (OPA) 221, 231, 232
oseltamivir 106
osteotomes 77
outcome measurements 414–15
ozone 154–5, 238–9, 252, 290, 350–3

PAA *see* peracetic acid
pacemakers 56
packaging 274–83
  area design consideration 257–9
  cleaning procedures 201
  decontamination areas 9–11
  decontamination cycle 8
  device and tray assembling 268–74
  guidelines and standards 271, 283–4
  label identification 283–5
  loading and unloading sterilizers 283–6
  management and quality 420
  material selection 276
  regulations 15
  storage and distribution 356–60, 362
  surgical and medical procedures 64
  types 276–9
pap smears 56
paper packaging 277–9
parametric monitoring 425–6
parametric release/monitoring 295, 306, 351–2, 422, 424–5
parasitic worms *see* helminthic infections
Paré, Ambroïse 3
partial colectomy 58
parvoviruses 105
PAs *see* preventative actions
Pasteur, Louis 4
pathological waste 377
patient safety 141, 369, 371, 434
patient soil 143, 160, 207–9, 214
PCD *see* process challenge devices
PCI *see* percutaneous coronary intervention
peel-open pouches 277–9
PEL *see* permissible exposure limits
penicillin 5, 113
people, managing 399–400
peptidoglycan 108
peracetic acid (PAA)
  basic sterilization principles 346–8
  chemistry and chemicals 154–5
  disinfection 235, 238, 247, 252
  guidelines and standards 349

Index

properties and characteristics 344–6
sterilization 290, 344–9, 351
sterilizer design and components 346–9
percutaneous coronary intervention (PCI) 56
percutaneous transluminal coronary angioplasty (PTCA) 56
performance measurements 414
performance qualification (PQ) 426
periodic table of elements 132
periosteal elevators 77
permissible exposure limits (PEL) 328, 352–3
persistent organic pollutants (POP) 386
personal protective equipment (PPE) 11–12, 141
   chemistry and chemicals 141–2
   cleaning procedures 175–6, 180–1, 189, 190, 208
   disinfection 232, 236, 251
   infections 106, 122, 125–9
   inspection, assembly, and packaging 258, 285–7
   laundry items 449–50
   point-of-use treatment 166
   safety issues 367–9, 371, 376
   sterilization 308, 348
personal safety 141–2, 369
personnel management 393, 396–8
   employee engagement 400–1
   managing people 399–400
   organization 398
   skills and knowledge requirements 398–9
   staff performance 400
PET *see* polyethylene terephthalate; positron emission tomography
PFD *see* process flow diagram
pH scale 137–8, 312–13, 435
pharmaceutical waste 377, 382
phases of matter 131–4
phenol-based disinfectants 151–3, 239–40
physical disinfection 222–9
physical health hazards 366, 373–4
physical sterilization 289, 299–325
physiology *see* anatomy and physiology
pin-hole leaks 441
plasma 131, 133–4, 340–2, 351
Plasmodium falciparum 117–18
plastic wastes 386
plastics 70–1
point of use cleaning 159–62
point of use guidance 362–5
point of use monitoring 420
point-of-use treatment 156–68
   chemistry and chemicals 144
   context 156
   point of use cleaning 159–62
   sorting 157–9
   tracking and traceability 168
   transportation 156
   transportation post procedure 162–7
polio 4
polyethylene terephthalate (PET) 71

polytetrafluoroethylene (PTFE) 71
POP *see* persistent organic pollutants
positioning instruments 87
positron emission tomography (PET) 54
post-operative care 54, 65–6
post-procedure handling
   decontamination cycle 8
   laundry items 448–50
   transportation 8
Potts vascular scissors 78
pouches 272–3, 277–9
powered tools 76, 87–9, 177
PPE *see* personal protective equipment
PQ *see* performance qualification
pre-cleaning 167
pre-cleaning, cleaning, and disinfection 406
pre-operative care 54, 64–5
pre-washing 177
preservatives 151–3
pressure pulsing air removal 301, 303
pressurized containers 381
preventative actions (PAs) 418
primary care 50
prions 450–3
   chemistry and chemicals 147, 152, 452
   cleaning procedures 206–7, 452
   disinfection 254–5, 452
   microbiology 103–4
   sterilization 311–12, 452–3
process challenge devices (PCD) 296, 298, 307, 315, 318, 321, 351–3, 430
process flow diagram (PFD) 396
process indicators 280–1, 426–7
process management 405–9
   leadership routines 408
   pre-cleaning, cleaning, and disinfection 406
   preparation and packaging 407
   process improvement 408
   recall situations 409
   sterilization and sterile storage 407
   understanding customer needs 407
process measurements 415–16
process monitoring 295–7, 306, 311, 315–18, 351–3
prostatectomy 58
proteins 19–20, 169, 212–13, 421
   see also prions
protozoal infections
   chemistry and chemicals 147, 152
   disinfection 219–20
   microbiology 102–3, 117, 119
pseudomonads 108
Pseudomonas aeruginosa 109, 434
PTCA *see* percutaneous transluminal coronary angioplasty
PTFE *see* polytetrafluoroethylene

QACs *see* quaternary ammonium compounds
QMS *see* quality management system
quality assurance (QA) 418
quality control (QC) 305–7, 351, 418

quality management 417
   chemical indicators 426–30
   cleaning, monitoring 419–23
   disinfection, monitoring 423–4
   parametric monitoring 425–6
   sterilization, monitoring 424–5, 430–1
quality management system (QMS) 71, 417–31, 453
quaternary ammonium compounds (QACs) 147, 153, 240
quinolones 114

racks 188, 287–8
radiation
   chemistry and chemicals 140–1
   disinfection 226–7
   sterilization 324–5
radio-frequency identification devices (RFID) 73, 411–14
radioactive chemicals 131, 158
radioactive waste 377, 382
RAS *see* robotic-assisted surgery
re-usable devices 90
   cleaning procedures 172
   point-of-use treatment 162
REACH Regulation 13
recall situations 409
receiving contaminated materials 170–4
reconstructive surgery 57
recycling 386
reels 278–9
reflex hammers 99–100
regulations 12–17, 222, 405
   see also guidelines; standards
reporting mechanisms 368
reproductive system 27, 40–1
resource requirements 391–2
respiratory system 18, 28, 41–2
restoration of dental caries 58
retractors 74, 76, 81–2, 91, 265
reusable devices 68–9, 257
   point-of-use treatment 157–8
   storage and distribution 355
reverse osmosis (RO) filtration 229, 437
RFID *see* radio-frequency identification devices
Rhizopus stolonifer 115
ribonucleic acid (RNA) 20, 104, 106
rigid containers *see* container/containment systems
rigid endoscopy
   cleaning procedures 174, 180, 192, 196, 438–43
   inspection, assembly, and packaging 265–6
   instrumentation 92–3
rinsing 177, 180, 205–6, 249, 432, 442
risk analysis 374–6, 405
RNA *see* ribonucleic acid
RO filtration *see* reverse osmosis filtration
robotic-assisted surgery (RAS) 57, 59, 67, 97–9, 201–2
Rockwell Hardness (HRC) 72

rubber gloves 5, 125–6
rusting
    disinfection 183, 213–17
    inspection, assembly, and packaging 268
    sterilization 310, 314
    water quality 432, 433

Saccharomyces cerevisiae 115
safe release 294
safety data sheets (SDSs) 141, 369
safety glasses 128, 141, 175
safety issues 366–88
    accidental spillages and leakages 386–7
    chemical hazards 366, 368–71
    chemistry and chemicals 141–2
    context 366
    device and equipment hazards 366, 371–2
    disaster planning and management 388
    disinfection 222
    fire hazards 387–8
    inspection, assembly, and packaging 259
    microbiological hazards 366–8
    physical and emotional health hazards 366, 373–4
    risk reduction and risk analysis 374–6
    sterilization 290
    waste management 376–7
    workplace hazard types 366
safety warning symbols 141–2, 330, 371, 372, 382, 384, 388
SAL *see* sterility assurance levels
sampling procedures 139
SARS-CoV-2 37, 103, 105, 106, 147
saturated steam 314
scaling 182, 187
scalpels 76–7
scanning/identification 413–14
SCBI *see* self-contained biological indicators
Schistosoma mansoni 120
scissors 73, 76–7, 90, 262–3
screw joints 75
scrub area 61
scrub nurse 54, 62, 64, 65
SDSs *see* safety data sheets
sealing and scalants 279–81
secondary care 50
self-contained biological indicators (SCBI) 295
self-retaining retractors 86, 265
semi-critical devices 7, 153
    cleaning procedures 173, 438–43
    disinfection 219–20, 222
    inspection, assembly, and packaging 237
    storage and distribution 355
semi-reusable medical device 69
Semmelweis, Ignaz 3
sensory nervous system 47–9
serrated instruments 75
severe acute respiratory syndrome coronavirus 2 (SARS-CoV-2) *see* COVID-19 pandemic
sexually transmitted diseases 112
sharpness testing 263

sharps
    point-of-use treatment 159, 160
    safety issues 371, 377, 382, 385
    storage and distribution 359
shelf-life
    chemistry and chemicals 151
    disinfection 231, 247
    inspection, assembly, and packaging 274, 284
    management and quality 431
    sterilization 319, 346
    storage and distribution 358, 360, 364
SI units 136
sigmoidoscopy 60
silver 241
single-chamber washers 196–7, 207–8
single-use devices (SUD) 68–9, 90, 454
    cleaning procedures 172
    point-of-use treatment 157–8, 162
    reprocessing 443–5
skeletal system 28, 42–6
skills and knowledge requirements 398–9
skin *see* hand and skin hygiene; integumentary system
skin grafting 58
small intestine 32
soaking caps 203, 440
sodium hypochlorite 254
soil tests 212, 422–3
solids 131–4
solubility 145
solutions 134
solvents 135
sonication baths *see* ultrasonic baths
sorting contaminated materials 157–9, 170–4
space requirements 395–6
spatulas 265
Spaulding, Dr Earl 5–7
Spaulding classification 6–7, 50, 152–3, 173, 219
speculums 84–5
spillages 386–7
splenectomy 97
sponges 182, 204
sporicides 236
sporozoans 118
sporulation
    chemistry and chemicals 152
    management and quality 427–30
    microbiology 108–9, 116
    sterilization 289–92, 300, 323, 326, 333, 339, 351
SSI *see* surgical site infections
staff performance 400
staff training
    cleaning procedures 180
    disinfection 223
    inspection, assembly, and packaging 262
    management and quality 398, 399
    safety issues 371–2, 373
    sterilization 290, 308
    storage and distribution 356
stainless steel 67, 69–72, 183, 213–17

standard work instructions 396
standards 14–16
    chemistry and chemicals 141–2
    cleaning procedures 188–9, 190, 209–13
    disinfection 223, 241–6, 251
    inspection, assembly, and packaging 271, 281–2
    instrumentation 71–4
    management and quality 405, 406, 422–3, 430
    sterilization 291, 296–7, 320–1, 324, 333, 337, 344, 349
    storage and distribution 364
Standards Australia/Standards New Zealand (AS/NZS) 283
Staphylococcus aureus 109
Staphylococcus epidermidis 109–10
Staphylococcus spp. 109–12, 114
stapling instruments 76, 82
steam purity 310, 312, 432, 435
steam quality 310, 312–20
steam sterilization 285, 287, 290, 299–318
    air removal 300–2, 308
    basic principles 299–301
    guidelines and standards 318, 320
    maintenance and quality control 305–7
    prions 311–12, 452–3
    process failures 315–18
    safety issues 386
    special considerations 307–15
    sterilizer design and components 304–5
    troubleshooting problems 315–18
    water and steam quality 310, 312–20
stereotactic surgery 88
sterility assurance levels (SAL) 290–2
sterilization 1–2, 8, 218, 289–354
    basic principles 290–301, 318–24, 326–30, 333–5, 339–43, 346–8
    chemical sterilization 131, 133, 138, 154–5, 290–1, 319, 326–54
    cleaning procedures 215
    context 289–90
    decontamination areas 9
    decontamination cycle 8
    disinfection procedures 220, 223, 226, 238–9
    endoscopy 438–43
    guidelines and standards 291, 296, 318, 320, 324, 333, 337, 344, 349
    infections 128–9
    inspection, assembly, and packaging 257–9, 267–8, 276–8, 280–8
    inspection and packaging 300, 321
    loading and unloading sterilizers 283–6
    management and quality 420, 424–31
    monitoring 424–5, 430–1
    physical sterilization 285–6, 290, 299–325
    prions 311–12, 452–3
    process failures 315–18, 353–4
    process monitoring 295–7, 306, 311, 315–18, 351–3
    regulations 15
    safety issues 369, 387

single-use devices 443–5
special considerations 307–15
and sterile storage 407
sterilizer design and components 304–5, 324, 330–2, 335–7, 343–4, 346–9
storage and distribution 355–62
surgical and medical procedures 62–6
troubleshooting problems 315–18, 353–4
water quality 432
STERIS SYSTEM 1® 348
STERIZONE® systems 350
STERRAD® systems 341–3
stethoscopes 100–1
stock rotation 360, 420
Stockholm Convention 387
stomach 31
storage and distribution 355–65
cleaning procedures 209
decontamination areas 9
decontamination cycle 9
environment and layout 356–60
guidance at point of use 362–5
guidelines and standards 365
handling of non-packaged or non-sterilized devices 355–6
inspection, assembly, and packaging 274–6
inventory control 360
management and quality 420
regulations 15
safety issues 382–4
sterile storage environment and layout 356–60
transport of sterile, packaged items 360–2
Streptococcus spp. 110
suction irrigation instruments 74, 76, 84–5, 91, 265
SUD *see* single-use devices
super-oxidized water 234–5, 247
superheat test 300, 301, 314, 315, 317
surfactants 135
surgical and medical procedures 50–66
aseptic technique 62–6
diagnostic procedures 50
disciplines and common procedures 56–7
endoscopy and endoscopic procedures 59
facilities 50–2, 59–62
medical equipment 52–3
procedures and techniques 52
see also instrumentation
surgical endoscopy 58
surgical scissors 73, 78
surgical site infections (SSI) 51–2, 127–8
surgical stainless steel 70
surgical teams 54
surrogate test devices 245
surveillance and monitoring 124
Sushruta 67
sustainability 453–4
suturing instruments 76, 82
syringes 91
SYSTEM 1 E™ 348

Taenia saginata 120
Tamiflu® 106
tapes 280–1
TASS *see* toxic anterior segment syndrome
tattooing 51, 57, 58, 90, 99
TDS *see* total dissolved solids
teamwork 401–4
telescope 93
temperature distribution testing 242
terminal waste disposal and the environment 384–6
tertiary care 50
test soils 212, 422–3
textiles *see* laundry items
TGA *see* Therapeutic Goods Administration
theatre sterile services units (TSSU) 9
THERABAND 263–4
Therapeutic Goods Administration (TGA) 13, 242
thermal disinfection 223–6, 252, 254–6
thermometers 100
3D printing 71
time weighted averages (TWA) 328, 352
titanium 70–1
titration 139
TOC *see* total organic carbon
tonsil snares 77, 79
total dissolved solids (TDS) 139, 435
total organic carbon (TOC) 139–40, 313, 435
toxic anterior segment syndrome (TASS) 198
tracheotomy (tracheostomy) 58
tracking and traceability 168, 270, 410–11
transmissible spongiform encephalopathies (TSE) 104, 206, 450–1
transplant surgery 57
transportation
chemistry and chemicals 144
cleaning procedures 209
inspection, assembly, and packaging 274, 276
point-of-use treatment 156, 162–7
post-procedure handling 8
safety issues 382–4
storage and distribution 355–6, 360–2
trays 188, 192–3, 214, 268–74, 287–8
triclosan 150, 239–40
trolleys 163–7, 197, 360–1
troubleshooting problems
cleaning procedures 213–17
disinfection 255–6
sterilization 315–18, 353–4
Trypanosoma brucei 117–18
TSE *see* transmissible spongiform encephalopathies
TSSU *see* theatre sterile services units
tungsten carbide 70, 72
tunnel washers 193–4, 207–8
TWA *see* time weighted averages
two-component blood test soil 213
2D barcodes 411
Tyvek® 273

UHMWPE *see* ultra-high molecular weight polyethylene
UIC *see* unique identification codes
ultra-high molecular weight polyethylene (UHMWPE) 71
ultrafiltration 229
ultrasonic baths 178, 188–91, 204–5, 214, 422–3
ultrasonography 56
ultraviolet (UV) disinfection 227, 437
unique identification codes (UIC) 72, 411–13
United States of America Regulations 13, 243
upward displacement of air 301
urinary system 29, 46
UV disinfection *see* ultraviolet disinfection

vaccination 1
historical development 4
microbiology 106, 121
safety issues 368
vacuum-assisted air removal 303
vacuum pulsing air removal 303
vaginal natural orifice transluminal endoscopic surgery (vNOTES) 97
validation 16
cleaning procedures 206, 209, 211
disinfection 251
inspection, assembly, and packaging 276, 283–5
management and quality 424
sterilization 311, 320, 323, 325, 333, 339, 345, 349
value stream map (VSM) 396
van Leeuwenhoek, Antonie 3
variant CJD 104, 206
variant Creutzfeldt-Jakob disease (vCJD) 451
ventilation 10–11
videoscopy 96
viewing instruments 76, 84–5
viral infections
chemistry and chemicals 147–50, 152
disinfection 220, 221, 231, 239
microbiology 102–7
safety issues 367
sterilization 290
virucide 236
virulence factors 112–14
visual cleanliness 260
visual inspection 183, 209, 212, 260–1
vNOTES *see* vaginal natural orifice transluminal endoscopic surgery
Volkmann bone curette 77, 79
VSM *see* value stream map

washer indicators 213
washing 177
waste management 376–7
context 376–7
segregation and types 377–82
terminal disposal and environmental safety 384–6
transport and storage 382–4

waste measurements 416–17
waste segregation and types of waste 377–82
waste transport and storage 382–4
water and water quality 432–8
   chemistry and chemicals 131–3, 134
   cleaning procedures 179–80, 197, 213–17
   disinfection 222–3, 246, 256
   sterilization 310, 312–20

wet heat disinfection 223–6
wet heat sterilization *see* steam sterilization
wetting 144
WHO *see* World Health Organization
workflow 396
workplace hazards *see* safety issues
World Health Organization (WHO) 206, 243, 283, 311, 377, 451
wound debridement 58
wound infections 2–3

woven textile wraps 277–8
wraps 272, 277–81
Wrigley's forceps 79, 83
Wuchereria bancrofti 120

X-ray radiation 324

yeasts 102–3, 115–16

Z-values 292, 300